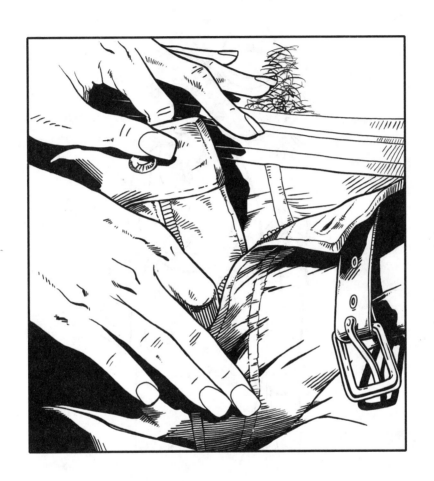

Welcome!

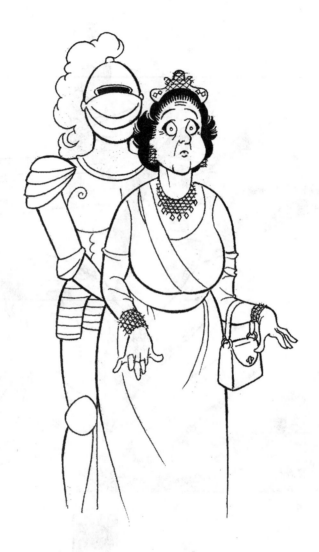

My favorite website?
www.GuideToGettingItOn.com

The eBook that changed the course of history?

The eBook version of the 'Guide To Getting It On'!
Less than ten of your US dollars. Bloody wonderful!

Guide To Getting It On

A book about the wonders of sex

author & publisher
Paul Joannides, Psy.D.

illustrator
Dærick Gröss Sr.

editor
Toni Johnson

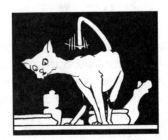

Goofy Foot Press
Oregon, U.S.A.

Guide To Getting It On!
Eighth Edition

V. 8.1 (8th edition, 3rd printing)

Publisher's Cataloging-In-Publication
Joannides, Paul N.
Guide to getting it on! / Paul Joannides, author;
Daerick Gross, illustrator.-- 8th ed.
p. cm.
Includes bibliographical references and index.
ISBN: 978-1-885535-45-0
1. Sex instruction. 2. Sex. 3. Man-woman
relationships. 1. Joannides, Paul. 11. Title.

HQ31.J63 2015   613.9'6

Goofy Foot Press
Oregon, U.S.A.
www.GuideToGettingItOn.com

printed in
Saline, Michigan
McNaughton & Gunn
Made in the U.S.A to bring smiles everywhere.

Fair Use

Bed of
CONTENTS

The Beginning

How To & Then Some

(more How To & Then Some)

Porn

Sex in the Real World

Your First Time

Beyond Vanilla

Below the Belt

Birth Control, Pregnancy & Parenting

Sex in History & Popular Culture

Orientation & Gender

Sex & the Human Condition

The End

Warning & Disclaimer

Hard as we tried, this Guide isn't perfect nor was it intended as a final authority on sex. There will be times when it is better to consult your beautician, bartender, or best friend. You might also speak to a physician or licensed sex therapist. Ultimately, it is your body and your sexuality—venture beyond the bounds of common sense at your own peril.

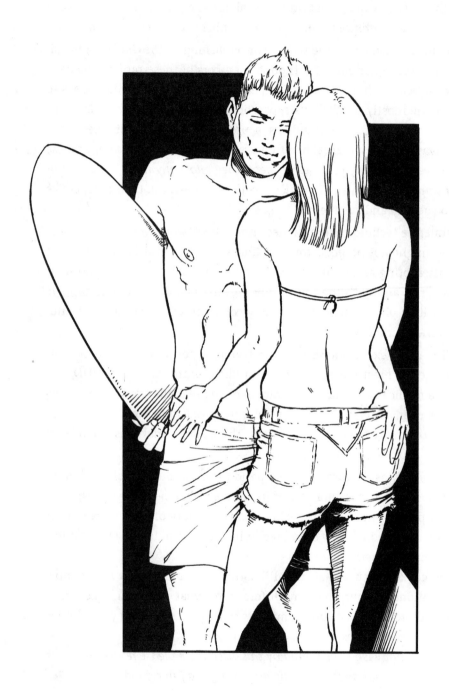

Changes — Then and Now

The founders of Facebook were nine years old. Dial-up was the way you got online. There was no texting, Twitter, Grindr or Tinder. Google? Amazon? YouTube? iTunes? They didn't exist. Porn was mostly in magazines you hid under your bed or it was on VHS cassettes you had to rent at a store.

When I started writing the *Guide To Getting It On,* scientists still clung to the notion that men wanted sex more than women and that women wanted to be in long-term relationships so they could have more children. I suppose we should be thankful that I began writing *The Guide* while sitting on the warm sands of a beach in Southern California. You couldn't help but look at the women on that beach and know that science had it all wrong.

The first edition of the *Guide To Getting It On* was 369 pages long. This edition is 1,152 pages. Many things have changed since the first edition went to press. Yet humans still have the same genitals and a lot of us still want sex to be special. Hopefully, you'll have as much fun with this new edition as readers did with the first.

The Guide Goes to College

I never expected *The Guide* would be used in more than 50 college sex education courses. Then students started telling me the book was the best sex-magnet ever. They would leave it out for others to see, and sex would often happen. (Why it's used in medical schools I'll never know. Medical students don't have time for sex.)

The first college to assign *The Guide* to students was Santa Barbara City College. I used to drive up to Santa Barbara to hand deliver the books. Santa Barbara City College will be one of the first colleges to receive this new edition. Now, however, students order the book online and there's even an eBook version with the illustrations in color.

Teens — The Missing Link?

Over the years, people have asked me "why don't you write a version of *The Guide* for teenagers?" As far as I could tell, this would have meant writing a watered-down version of *The Guide* with little purpose other than to make parents think their teens didn't need the real thing. I suppose I could have called it "the training wheels version" or the *Guide To Getting To First Base*. The idea of a teenage version of *The Guide* seems even more ludicrous now that boys are stroking it to porn from the time they are preteens, and girls in middle school are shaving their pubic hair.

To me, this version—the big people's version of *The Guide*—has always been as much for teenagers as for adults, but it's only recently that parents have been able to handle my saying so, and only in some parts of the country. (Given what kids see on their phones today, no one can accuse the illustrations in this book of being too explicit for teenage eyes.)

Not only do today's teenagers need accurate information about sex and making love, they also need help in understanding the roles that sex can play in people's lives. This isn't something they're getting from porn, which has become THE sex educator for our young.

A Million vs. Two Billion

The Guide is now in its 8th edition, and more than a million copies have been printed. The best way I know to thank those of you who have been so helpful over the years is to assure you that this new edition hasn't shed an ounce of attitude or taken a single short cut.

The Guide continues to provide a beam of hope during a time when more than two billion dollars have been spent on abstinence-based "sex education"—which is misinformation about sex and a thinly veiled attempt to make women feel shame about their bodies and shame for wanting to have sex. And now I'm hearing that way too many young women feel "it's nasty" for women to masturbate, and that only guys should do it. Seems like we still have a long way to go.

Ignorance remains this book's archenemy; the desire to know more about sex, its friend.

Paul Joannides, Psy.D.

Technology

Page Layout Software : Adobe InDesign CC
Hardware: Mac OS X on a 13" MacBook Pro
Cover Graphic Consultant : Rose Reed/Newport Lazerquick
Prepress/Press : McNaughton & Gunn
Copy Editing : Susanne Schunter & David Hoffert
eBook Conversion Guru : Ron Bilodeau

Occasional Typographical Issues

We are one of America's smallest presses producing one of the world's biggest and best books on sex. Every resource we have is spent on keeping this book as up-to-date as possible and helping it to evolve as technology and culture evolve. Unfortunately, this creates an environment where there can be typos. Hard as we try to catch them, some get by. For this we apologize.

If you find a typo and would like to tell us about it, please use the contact form at www.GuideToGettingItOn.com, which is the website for this book. Be sure to include the page number. People who do this are often surprised when they hear from the author. It's our way of saying thanks.

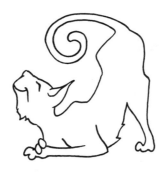

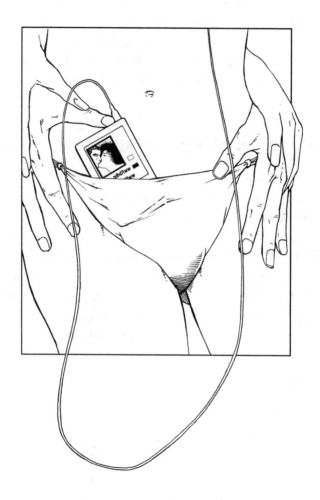

for Toni Johnson

1

The Alpha Chapter

Each of the lovers you have in life will want something different from you. Some will want you to touch them between their legs, others will want you to touch their soul. This book tries to help you with both. It encourages you to explore dimensions of sexuality that people usually aren't told about—from the emotional part of getting naked together to why a guy who takes his penis too seriously might have trouble pleasing his sweetheart. It covers subjects like hand jobs and heart throbs, kisses above and below the waist, friendship, and sex in different kinds of relationships.

Whether you have lots of experience or have yet to be with your first lover, a good place to start is with our Goofy Foot Philosophy:

It doesn't matter what you've got in your pants if there is nothing in your brain to connect it to.

Do With It What You Want

Since this is a book about sex, it makes sense to begin with a definition of what sex is. But trying to define sex is like trying to insert a diaphragm: just when you think you've got it in, the thing turns ninja on you. Here are a few things to consider if you are trying to define *sex:*

People think of intercourse as the ultimate sex act, the real thing—*ipsum fuctum*. But if intercourse is the ultimate act, then why can making out or holding hands be sweeter and more meaningful at times?

Almost all sex acts can be painful, obnoxious, or boring if you aren't doing them with someone who turns you on. Does this mean that the mental part of sex is more important than the physical part?

Why does one couple find a particular sex act to be highly erotic while another couple finds the same act to be disgusting?

💡A person has sex and an orgasm with a partner of many years, but the sex doesn't feel particularly exciting. The next afternoon he or she nearly bursts with excitement after catching the brief but intense gaze of a sexy stranger. How can a glance from a stranger take your breath away more than sex with a long-term lover?

💡You are getting a physical exam. You are naked and your genitals are being touched. Neither you nor the examiner is aware of any sexual excitement. However, if you were naked and being touched in this way after a romantic night out, it might be incredibly sexual. How much do we rely on the context of a situation to tell us what's sexual and what isn't?

💡How can a song, car, or piece of clothing be sexy?

Needless to say, we have given up on trying to pin a tail of definition on the big donkey of sex. It seems that any definition of sex needs to fit who you are as an individual as well as your particular situation. Instead of pretending to know what that might be, consider this:

> Learning about sex and intimacy is a lifelong adventure. Even with years of experience, we still blow it on occasion. The best we can do in the pages that follow is to tell you what we wish we had known about sex many years ago. Do with it what you want.

Morality & What's in Your Pants

In much of America we still try to equate morality with whether you keep your pants on. We also associate morality with religion. But the truth is, there are Christians, atheists, Jews, and Muslims who are moral people and there are Christians, atheists, Jews, and Muslims who are immoral people. The same is true for people who are sexually active and for those who aren't. Morality, from this Guide's perspective, is about respecting and caring for your fellow human beings. It has little to do with how you enjoy your sexuality, unless what you do breaks a special trust or is not mutually consensual.

Hmmm. A Book on Sex

Consider the books on sex that were written between 1830 and today. Some of these books gave a girl a psychiatric diagnosis if she masturbated or wanted to be on top, while the theories about male sexuality could be contradictory and bizarre. Today's sex books make all sorts of claims as well. Yet the writers of these books consider themselves to be paragons of reason and truth. So, please keep two things in mind: that books on sex don't often pass the test of time and this is a book on sex.

While there are plenty of sexual traditions, there are no *Ten Commandments of Sex*. Sex books are merely a reflection of the time and culture that spawn them. Sexual fashion will change many times between now and when you are a resident of the old folks' home.

Birth Control and Beyond

This book talks about everything from scruffy sex rodents to things you can do to make a condom feel right. Hopefully, this will help you avoid things like unwanted pregnancies and an early funeral. In the meantime, it might be helpful to remember that just about anything in this world that's worth doing will kill you if you're stupid about it. Having sex can be far less risky than driving on the freeway or even driving across town. It just depends on how smart you are about sex and how badly you drive.

How It Fits In

When your mom was in school, she couldn't sneak a phone between her legs during a lecture, snap a picture of her pre-mom crotch, and send it to one of your potential fathers with CU2NITE, Wet4U or IWSN.

Although today's technology is more interesting than ever before, the reasons why people have sex are pretty much the same. Love and infatuation still top the list, but feeling horny and having fun are frequent motivators. People also have sex to make babies, to feel more grounded, to make money, to help them feel more desirable and less lonely, and the list goes on.

Sex with the same person can mean different things at different times. Early in a relationship, it might excite you and rev you up; later it might be a source of comfort and calm. In most relationships, there will be times when the sex is boring or when it makes you feel more distant than close.

For those of you who are younger, people sometimes refer to matters of the heart as puppy love and treat them with disrespect. That's silly. The most powerful feelings in life are often puppy love. Cherish them. As for having sex with your puppy love, far be it from this Guide to say yes or no. It might be wonderful but, then again, it might not. Just be aware that there's usually more to a good carnal experience than the hydraulics of sticking hard into wet. For some people, what separates good sex from bad are intangibles like fun, friendship, love, and caring.

As you get older, your expectations about sex may change. If you just turned 17, getting laid in and of itself can be a huge thing. But by the time you turn 34, you'll have more experience under your belt. By then you might want your sex life to take you some place different than when you were younger. Perhaps you will be searching for different qualities in a partner as well. Hopefully, you will want sex to be special no matter what your age.

A Red Flag—Matters of the Heart

Some sexual relationships are mostly physical. Others are emotional. Keeping it just physical is not an ability that everyone has or wants. Sometimes it depends on your situation and where you are in life, other times it's a matter of chemistry.

The emotions that accompany sexual relationships can be magical, enchanting, and wonderful. Then again, they can be awful. A cherished relationship can fizzle and go flat, leaving you empty or in agony. It can cause you so much heartache that you might wish you were dead. The tears can pour from a place so deep that you'll wonder if they will ever stop.

Fortunately, lovemaking can also be a way of working through fears and uncertainty, as well as a place for growth, forgiveness, fun, and friendship. If you make it a priority and keep working at it, sex can help you be more present, honest, and alive with yourself and your partner.

No Assumptions Here

Most of us make assumptions about the sex lives and relationships of other people. Consider Tim, a quiet, college-aged computer geek, and Jake, a well-liked 27-year-old shortstop on his company's baseball team. Tim is bicep-challenged while Jake looks like he just leapt from the pages of *Men's Health*. Yet Tim-the-geek has a creative and fulfilling sex life with his girl-friend, while Jake-the-hunk lives in fear that someone will discover his sex life consists of watching porn with his hand between his legs.

This book is just as much for Tim and his girlfriend as it is for Jake. It makes no assumptions other than you are curious about sex and might want to enjoy it even more.

Charts, Graphs and Sex Surveys

There are no charts or graphs in this book. If you are the type who insists on having such things, consider this: how do you graph the value of a loving glance or a heartfelt hug? Yet try to enjoy sex in a relationship without them. Rather than assuming which graph is best for you, this Guide tries to accommodate a full range of sexual tastes and beliefs, be they conservative, eclectic or kinky. Are any of us just one or another?

This book also avoids the latest in popular surveys, such as one recently done by a large news organization. This study found that the top seven traits women find most important in a male partner are humor, intelligence, honesty, kindness, values, communication skills, and dependability. That sounds fine, until you realize things like "loves me," "shares my interests," "exciting sex partner," and "acceptable to parents and friends" were not on the list of characteristics that women could check. And while the attractiveness of a partner's teeth came in 16th, you can bet that "attractive teeth" would have ranked much higher if the study had been funded by a company that makes toothpaste.

Final Beginning Note

Most people would probably agree that sex is best when it's honest, caring, and fun. The same should be true for books on sex. Hopefully, you will find *The Guide's* attempt at explaining love and sex to be honest and true.

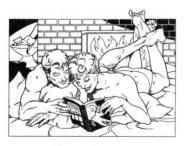

Dear Paul,

In my intro psych class, they wanted us to take a detailed survey about sex. My boyfriend and I really like sex, but I didn't feel comfortable doing the survey and left most of it blank. Does this mean I'm weird?

Athena from Mt. Holyoke

Dear Athena,

My own suspicion about sex surveys was born two days before I took my first intro-to-anything class in college. Perhaps some background will help.

I had spent my first 18 years in a small town that didn't have a lot of stop lights or two-story buildings. It did, however, have as many bars as churches, and a number of girls who feared a life of loneliness if they didn't get knocked-up by the end of high school.

So I had spent the totality of my life in the nape of America's red neck. Then, I suddenly found myself as a freshman at UC Berkeley, where there were Krishnas instead of cows, and "weed" was no longer the hallmark of poor pasture management.

Back then, I had no idea that the nice, neanderthal-looking guy who lived upstairs in my dorm would become a co-founder of Apple, or that I would someday write a book on sex that people like yourself would have on their shelves.

What I did know is that I had to show up at the student health center to take a physical exam. That's when I became one of hundreds of guys in their boxers or briefs, waiting in a mile-long line to pee on command. First, however, we got to stand in front of a row of doctors who pulled our briefs down and reported what they saw to the young nursing students who were sitting next to them with charts in their laps. Not being ones to take it on faith, the nursing students looked up and checked as well.

Then, when I got back to the dorm, there was a thick survey sitting on my desk. It wanted to know about my personal sexual habits. Being barely a man and just two days in the big city, I wasn't ready to confess "how many times I masturbated during the past week." But I did know that no matter how far from home you are and no matter how fast of a lane you have fallen into, what's personal is personal, and nobody has a right to take that away from you. So, like you, I left the survey blank.

As I think back over the sex survey from my first few days in college, I am reminded of how complex and personal sex is for some of us, as it seems to be for you. At the same time, I appreciate that your roommate might be uploading videos of herself having sex on Spankwire. And what about all of the people who post intimate details of their private lives on social media?

Are you "weird?" Perhaps. But I suspect that's true for many of us.

CHAPTER

2
Romance

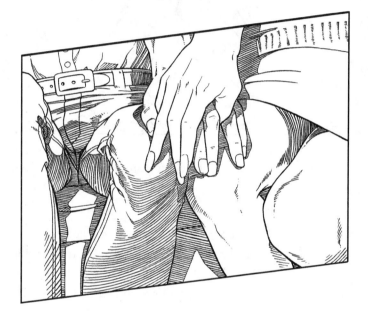

Romance is something thoughtful you do for someone you love. It's the Gorilla Glue that holds relationships together. It's lube for above the belt instead of below.

Romance can be as simple as leaving a note on the refrigerator that says "I love you" or giving an unexpected hug. It can include heroic gestures like helping your partner do his taxes or scouring the tile in her skanky-looking shower or taking a whole day to organize a lover's *Nightmare-on-Elm-Street* closet.

Contrary to what the ads and commercials tell you, romance does not need to cost a thing. There's not a single thing about being romantic that should require an increase in your credit limit. You are deluding yourself if

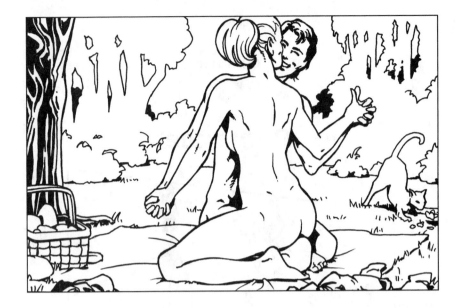

you think the only way you can be wildly romantic is by single-handedly jump-starting the economy.

Romance vs. Sex

Try not to assume that romance will result in sex. Romance resides in a special universe somewhere between Platonic love and carnal lust. Romance can evolve into sex, and the sex can be incredibly romantic, but it's just as possible to have a romantic evening and end up in bed alone. When that happens, you do what the rest of us have done since the beginning of time: you romance your penis or clitoris yourself.

Romance When You Are Dating as Opposed to When You Are Married

Getting the oil on your partner's car changed and having it washed can be a romantic thing if you are dating. However, if you are married, it's probably one of those things that's migrated from the romance column to being just another job on your to-do list. Hopefully it's something your partner appreciates, but it's unlikely to get you a night of oral sex because "you're so darned wonderful."

On the other hand, when you were dating, going to a movie might not have been particularly romantic, given how you would do it at the drop of a hat. But once you have kids, going to a movie involves hiring a babysitter and

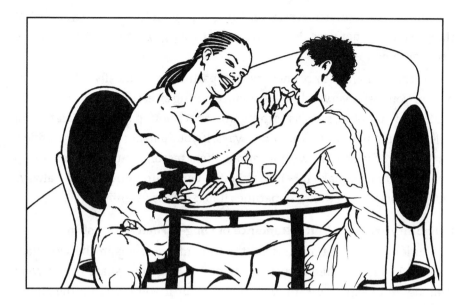

maybe picking her up, getting dinner made for your children, and finding some way to defy the laws of parenting and get to the theater on time. By virtue of the wedding ring and your most excellent breeding skills, going out to see a movie goes from routine to romantic.

Likewise, your partner may have loved receiving stuffed animals before marriage, but after having children, the population of stuffed animals in your household will have reached critical mass. She's thinking, "How do I sneak this bag of stuffed animals to Goodwill without little Sophia having a meltdown?"

Married or not, getting a lover her favorite chocolate is almost always romantic regardless of the number of notches on the side of her uterus. Chocolate works on the same part of the brain as cocaine and heroin.

Getting Your Romance Meters in Sync

When it comes to being romantic, people can have very different styles. If the person you are lusting over feels like a keeper, try to figure out what is romantic to him or her. This might be different from what's romantic to you.

While things that make a big splash could be what catches your romantic eye, your partner might prefer the understated. Just because his or her romantic style is different from yours doesn't mean you can't be wonderfully romantic in each other's eyes. Over time, you should make a mental list of things your partner goes "Wow!" over. That way you won't panic when the need for romance arises.

It can be harder to connect with a partner romantically when one or both of you feels overwhelmed. Romance during stressful times can require a different approach, such as turning into a rock your partner can lean on or quietly taking up the slack in other ways. If your partner has a huge project coming up or is dealing with a serious life stressor, plan ahead for things you can do to help make it better, although being supportive doesn't always require "doing" something. Sometimes it just means listening.

Reliability vs. Excitability: Romance in Long-Term Relationships

In long-term relationships, all the romantic gestures in the world are meaningless if you aren't trustworthy or don't do your share of the work. Sending an unexpected card won't get you far if you didn't do the chores your partner was counting on you to do. For romance to work in a long-term relationship, it helps if both of you are reliable. Then, the kind and thoughtful gestures have a footing to stand on.

On the other hand, when you hear people in long-term relationships say the sparkle has gone in their relationship, it's possible they have worked so hard on being reliable that they have forgotten about the gestures that help make a relationship hot.

Consider some of the sexually exciting moments during the first few months of your relationship. Maybe you were more playful or more daring. Maybe you were so excited that you ripped at your partner's clothes in a way that made her feel incredibly attractive and exciting. Now, you wait until each other has watched their favorite TV show, brushed their teeth, and checked their phone for the umpteenth time. How do you make each other feel sexy and exciting when things have become so predictable?

There's a balancing act in any long-term relationship, given how "reliability" means going to work and keeping your commitments, while "erotic" is more about dropping everything and surrendering to the moment.

The Thrill Is Gone

Some neurobiologists believe when a relationship is new, during the first six months to a year, we process our lovers in the wild'n'crazy part of the brain. Our good judgment is mostly shot to hell and even a lover's most annoying habits seem endearing. We pine over them, obsess about them, and want to have lots of sex with them.

Then, after a year or so, we start to process our long-term partners with the "long-term relationship" parts of the brain. Reality rears its sometimes ugly head, and the warts in your relationship start to show. It can also be a time when partners begin to take each other for granted, and sometimes stop trying as hard to be romantic. To protect your sex life from being lost in the kids-and-a-mortgage part of your brain, it helps to add novelty. Novelty is a way of lobbing your relationship back into the sexually-exciting part of the brain.

So if you find yourself thinking more about getting new matching recliners for in front of your 900-inch TV than about doing something fun with your partner, it might be time to think outside the grandma/grandpa part of your cranium. Maybe you can visit new and different places, or perhaps the two of you can try snuggling in one of the recliners and make out during the movie.

When the Pool Boy Looks Way Better Than Your Spouse

This header is misleading. That's because a lot of people fantasize about someone other than their partner. It's perfectly normal and doesn't mean there's a problem with the sexual excitement in your relationship if you are thinking about someone else when you are making love or masturbating.

On the other hand, let's say your partner of fifteen years is the most trust-worthy and hard-working man on the face of the earth. He's a great father to your kids, and you love him dearly, but the romance in your relationship is kaput. And let's say you have been noticing the pool man a lot more than you did before. By the time he leaves each week you are wetter than the pool deck. How do you get that kind of passion back with your husband?

It's quite possible that in your husband's mind his way of being roman-tic is by working his tail off for you and the kids. Worse things have hap-pened. Be sure that at least a couple of times a week you tell him how much you appreciate how hard he works. Do this from now until the end of time. Then, think back over the past fifteen years and come up with things the two of you have enjoyed doing together—without the kids. Maybe it's river rafting, maybe it's shopping for antiques or going to a carnival. Maybe it's working in the garden together. If it's possible, find ways for the two of you to start doing some of these things together again, or find new things you've talked about trying but have never gotten around to.

This kind of approach is a traditional one that doesn't reach too far into the world of sexual novelty. Someone who is less traditional might suggest you broach the subject of trying a threesome with your husband and the pool boy. But swinging is more apt to work if the primary couple has a solid and satisfying sexual relationship to begin with. Unless your husband is secretly lusting after the pool boy as well.

This is a complex subject that requires way more consideration than the few pages it receives here! There are plenty of books on the subject that can help, or seeing a couples' therapist or sex therapist could be an important next step in getting your relationship back on track.

What Readers Have to Say about Romance

"Romance is being kind, gentle, and thoughtful. Sometimes intense as when making love, sometimes only on pilot light, but never off."
male age 70

"Romance is being naked in the sun." *male age 42*

"Romance is when she and I can absolutely forget that the rest of the world exists. Just today we both had a million things to do to prepare for the coming work week, but I turned on the CD player and played a great Spanish song about a bull that falls in love with the moon. Soon we had dropped our work and were spinning each other around the living room like two people who had no idea how to dance flamenco." *male age 25*

"What is romance? Stroking my hair, holding my hand, helping me with the housework, cooking, talking, sharing the day with me."
female age 43

"Romance is waking up in my partner's arms and being told that he loves me." *female age 27*

"Romance is when we go Rollerblading at the beach." *male age 32*

"Romance is sitting on a hammock together reading our books."
female age 26

"For romance, I enjoy a great bubble bath together with candles and wine, lots of great smelling scents whether it's perfume, incense, or just the smell of my man." *female age 36*

"It's bringing home a single rose or a little something to say I was thinking of you today." *female age 34*

"Doing things that show he values me as a life partner and not just a bed partner." *female age 45*

"If he brings you flowers or jewelry and he's not there in any other way, it's not romance." *female age 45*

A Highly Evolved Thanks to anthropologist Helen Fisher from Rutgers.

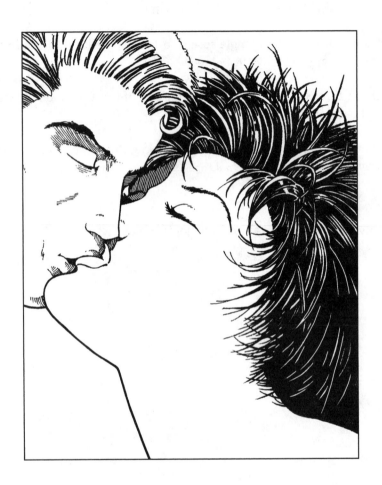

3
Kissing

This chapter is about kissing on the lips as opposed to kissing on the genitals, although one often leads to the other. Sometimes kissing is the start of sex. Other times, kissing is the main course. Either way, it's hard to find a better way to pass an hour when you're hanging out together.

Kissing can be awkward at times, especially at the start. It's also one of the rare things that doesn't cost you a dime but you can remember for the rest of your life. It's what causes panties to become drenched and precum to flow.

It's funny how guys will worry about the size of their penises when they should be worrying about how well they kiss. Kissing usually says more about you and is more likely to be a deal breaker.

Talking in Tongues

Kissing a partner on the lips makes more of an emotional statement than kissing him or her on the genitals, even if the latter often feels better. One of this book's advisors, who makes her living by having sex with different men, won't let anyone but her husband kiss her on the lips. And when a relationship starts to go sour, couples usually stop kissing on the lips long before they stop having intercourse.

There are reasons why kissing can be more intimate than getting into a partner's pants. From the moment we are born, most of us are kissed by moms, dads, aunts, uncles, grandparents, and anyone else whose approaching lips we can't successfully dodge. Being kissed symbolizes a profound love that we hopefully come into the world experiencing.

Another reason for the added power of kissing is so many of the major senses—vision, smell, hearing, and taste—have their outlets on the human face. Not to mention the lips and skin are exquisitely sensitive to touch. There are so many sensory centers located on or near the human face that we have terms such as "You're in my face" or "Get out of my face" to express annoyance or social discomfort.

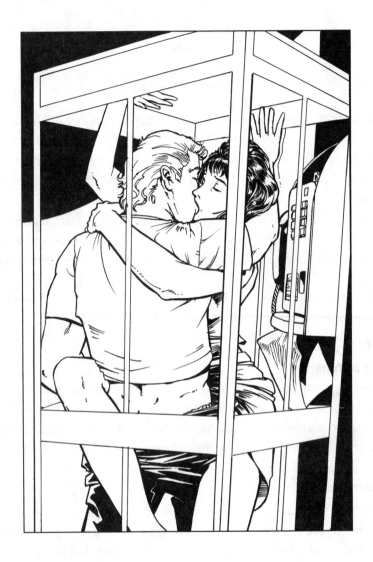

1960

Same Couple

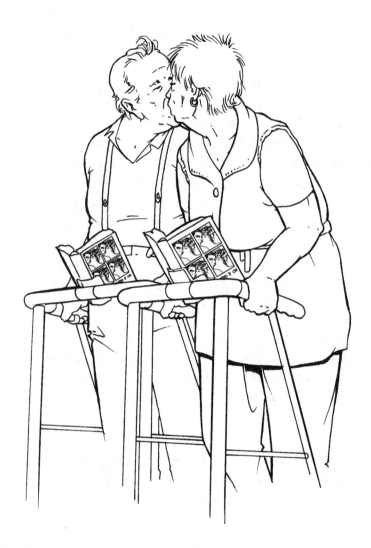

Today

Same Kiss?

Look at the importance of lips in style and fashion. You can buy a zillion different colors of lip gloss and lipstick, with some that sparkle and others that make your lips look wet. (Be sure to see the section "Kissing and Lip Gloss.")

When Kissing Is the Main Course

Kissing is often a prelude to other things, but there are plenty of times when kissing is all you get. Like when you are fifteen and necking all night long. Or when you are older but want to feel like you are fifteen. Or when a woman has started her period and she hasn't yet read *The Guide's* most excellent chapter on period sex, Chapter 50: *Surfing the Crimson Wave.*

Don't for a moment think that monster make-out sessions are kids' stuff. Some people experience these as hotter than much of the intercourse they've had.

If all you plan on doing is making out, be sure to put your gum in a safe place where you can find it afterward. It will help take the edge off until you can go home and masturbate.

Great Kissing Advice

"The best thing you can do during a good kissing session is to ask your partner to kiss you the way he or she likes to be kissed. It really works. Just sit back and let him or her take over; you'll learn all kinds of things." *male age 26*

Kissing can be so powerful, yet we seldom take the time to ask a partner how he or she likes to be kissed. Maybe delicate butterfly kisses are what get your partner going rather than the dramatic lip-lock action you saw in a movie. You'll never know unless you ask.

Movie Kiss Remake

Maybe you are too shy to ask a lover how she or he wants to be kissed. Here's a playful way to achieve the same result.

In her how-to book on kissing, Violet Blue lists some of the best movie kisses, from *Bull Durham* and *Sixteen Candles* to *Gone With The Wind* and *The Matrix Reloaded.* Why not do a search for "best movie kisses" and make a list of cinematic spectaculars to download?

You and your partner can try to imitate each of the kissing scenes. (Actors often do several reshoots before they get a scene right. The same should be true for the two of you!) If your partner gives you an Academy Award for best kissing performance, that was probably how he or she wants to be kissed. Hopefully, your partner's favorite kissing scene isn't from *Lady and the Tramp*.

Readers' Smooch Advice: The Basics

"Please don't eat my mouth. A good kiss can make me wet with desire, with only the softest touch." *female age 23*

"Start really light. Barely brush your lips against hers. Be very aware of her response. Increase the pressure ever so slightly when she begins to meet your lips. Eventually, touch the tip of your tongue to her lips. If she opens her mouth, you can let your tongue enter just the smallest bit, but try not to force her mouth open." *male age 25*

"Kissing is not just a preliminary to fucking. Gently explore with your tongue, lightly suck on her lips and tongue. If she is into it as much as you, kiss with good suction, not lazily." *female age 45*

"When you're kissing, be gentle; don't swallow a woman's entire face or dig your teeth into her cheeks." *female age 36*

Breathe or Die, and Don't Forget to Swallow

People who are new to kissing sometimes ask if they should kiss with their eyes open or closed. We don't know.

Another question is what to do with your nose. When you are kissing, your mouth is often busy, while your nose is mostly in the way. Breathing through your nose gives it a purpose and keeps your partner from feeling like you are attempting mouth-to-mouth resuscitation. Tilting your head to the side can help avoid a collision of oncoming beaks.

You might find it helpful to take an occasional pause in the make-out action. Maybe you need to catch your breath; if you're a guy, maybe you need to adjust your erection if it's pointing in an uncomfortable direction. You can keep the momentum going during these intermissions by gently stroking the side of your partner's face with the back of your fingers, or you can tell them how much they turn you on or how lucky you are to be with them.

As for the wisdom in swallowing often, take these comments to heart:

"Try not to slobber!" *female age 25*

"Turn off the water works! There is nothing worse than a big slobbery wet kiss." *female age 27*

"An overly wet mouth is a turn-off." *female age 32*

"Girls love slobber. At least that's what they tell me. Maybe that's 'cause I slobber. Hey, wait a second!" *male age 22*

French Kissing

French kissing is spelunking with your tongues. The reason it is called "French kissing" is that French women found it to be an effective way to make French men stop talking.

French kissing is not a tongue-to-tonsils regatta. Try swallowing first, and go gently. Pretend your tongue is Baryshnikov instead of Vin Diesel, and you will do just fine. There is always time for tonsil-sucking later.

Mouths enjoy variety. Don't occupy your partner's mouth like it's a parking space in New York or Chicago. Bring your tongue out for air. Try changing the pace by kissing your partner's neck before re-probing the deep.

Some people think their tongues should act like a penis when they are French kissing. A penis gets hard and likes to thrust in and out of anything that will have it. It can't help itself. But a tongue shouldn't thrust in and out like a penis and you shouldn't try to deep throat a partner with it.

"Take it slow and easy, but not too easy." *female age 26*

"Don't jam your tongue down someone's throat until she invites you in." *female age 38*

"Getting deep throated for fifteen minutes at a whack is no fun." *fem, 48*

First Time French Kissing Advice

You don't want to put your tongue in a partner's mouth if it's not welcome. But how do you know?

Fortunately, you don't need to leap from closed-lip kissing to tonsil hockey in one fell swoop. If your partner is into kissing you and you've been at it for awhile, you might try opening your mouth a bit so there's a space between your lips. You can then gently run the tip of your tongue around the edge of your partner's lips. That way, you're not invading their open-mouth space, but you're not being a weenie either. See how your partner responds.

If they want your tongue, they'll let you know. They might even put their tongue in your mouth. Or maybe it will feel nice to gently suck on an upper or lower lip without anyone's tongue leaving its bullpen.

Once your tongue gets the green light, you might want to explore a partner's mouth with your tongue, including the sensitive corners of their lips, the ridges on the roof of their mouth, and their gums and teeth. But how do you do this without them feeling like they are at the dentist? Your best bet is to forge ahead in small steps, seeing how your partner responds before exploring further.

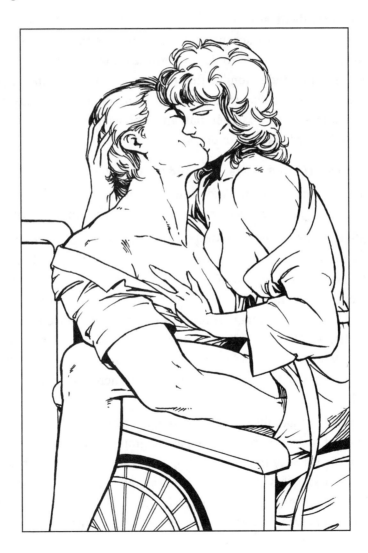

Tongue Sucking

There's not much to say about sucking on each other's tongues except that you might find it to be enjoyable. Tongue sucking can be wildly sensual and suggestive. Some lovers get very turned on by doing it as well as by having it done to them. Others will pass.

When sucking tongue, you are basically doing the same thing to your partner's tongue that you would to a lollipop. Sometimes you can suck your partner's tongue into your mouth, which can be kind of cool. Be gentle and brief your first few times as a tongue sucker to see if your partner likes it.

Tongue Tips While Kissing

Books on kissing list dozens of different kisses and tongue tricks. More power to you if you're able to do an entire gymnastics routine with your tongue. As for this guide's tongue tips, there is only one. The tip of a pointed tongue is hard, and a flat tongue is soft. Experiment with making your tongue hard when you kiss, then flat, and whatever feels good in between. (This might be good practice for oral sex!)

Hands on a Partner's Breasts, Butt and In Their Hair

What you do with your hands when you are kissing can put a kiss into hyper drive or it can mess everything up. Here are some things to consider:

Hair: Once you've been kissing for several minutes and the situation is warming up, a partner might enjoy it if you run your fingers through their hair while you are kissing. But if a woman has a head full of hair extensions or has done serious moussing, she might grab your hand and pull it away. Respect this. Run your fingers through a partner's hair once and see what their reaction is. Also, hair follicles contain nerves. Some partners will want you to run your fingers gently through their hair to barely tickle their hair follicles; for others, a firm and confident grip on their hair makes their scalp feel good.

Breasts: Just because a woman might have her tongue down your throat doesn't mean you have a free pass to grope her breasts. A guy should never assume it's okay to put a hand on a partner's breasts just because he and she are locking lips. If a woman wants a man's hands on her breasts, she should grab them and put them there. Unfortunately, not all women realize that if they want something they need to speak up and ask for it.

So if it seems like a woman's breasts are calling to you for attention but she won't put your hand there, you might try sensuously running your hand up and down her side. Go slowly and stay away from her breasts. Don't move your hands closer until you get a loud and clear signal to do so. Otherwise, you risk killing the moment and making a mockery of mutual consent.

Backs and Butts: It can feel really good when a partner gently runs a hand up and down your back while you are kissing. The same is true with a hand on the butt. However, fondling a partner's butt crack and the area under the butt cheeks is best left for couples who have made out before and both enjoy it.

Body Contact When Kissing vs. Dry Humping

It's pretty hard to ignore that your chests and crotches are speaking to each other when you are making out. You don't want to stop the conversation, nor do you want your partner to feel like they're being dry humped if all they want is to be kissed.

There will be times when making out turns into dry humping, but kissing passionately and dry humping are not the same. The safest and smartest route is to let it be a mutual decision, with plenty of mutual feedback.

Flossing, Brushing and Death Breath

It is raunchy to kiss with pieces of food stuck in your teeth.

Flossing and brushing can make you far more attractive than wearing cologne or sucking on breath mints. If you are concerned about bad breath, check with your dentist. Dentists know all about bad breath, as many of them have it themselves. Ask if you should scrape the surface of your tongue with the edge of a spoon. The white gooey stuff that the spoon picks up is said by some to cause certain kinds of bad breath. But it's only a temporary fix and won't take the place of brushing.

If you are eating food with garlic or onions, make sure the person you plan to smooch with shares some big bites. Flossing and brushing won't put a dent in breath that is laced with garlic. Your only defense is to share the offense.

Kissing when You Are Wearing Lip Gloss

Some partners will refuse to kiss a woman who is wearing lipstick or lip gloss. They prefer lips to be natural. Others like it when a woman is wearing a particular flavor. You usually can't go wrong with a natural hydrating beeswax gloss like Burt's Bees, but the greasy glosses can feel gross.

Plenty of women will pull out a tissue and do a quick lipstick wipeoff when they're about to start kissing. This can be a wise maneuver if you are kissing someone for the first time. Once you get to know them better, ask what they prefer. You might try out your favorite flavors and see if they bite. As for glitter gloss, be sure to ask.

Out Darn Gum!

Even if you just popped in a new piece of gum and it's still bursting with flavor, do not try to hide it in the back of your mouth when you are making out. There are couples who have no problem passing gum back and forth, but until you and your partner are that kind of couple, take the gum out.

If You Are Wearing Braces

For people who have braces with rubber bands, consider taking the rubber bands out ahead of time. One reader barely escaped mid-smooch tragedy when a rubber band on his sweetheart's braces came unhooked and nearly shot him in the uvula. A direct hit would have triggered the same reflex that causes vomiting.

Also, an incoming tongue might get scratched or caught on metal edges that don't pose a problem for the wearer of the braces. For a practical but sexy come on, tell a new partner it might be better if he or she explored the inside of your mouth with their tongue to make sure everything is okay.

Putting the "Neck" in Necking

In hundreds of sex surveys, both male and female readers of *The Guide* have said that they wished their partner would spend more time kissing them on the neck. Lots more time.

So don't forget the neck. Few people wanted vampire action, but something this side of raising a hickey might help create a welcome reception in parts of the body that are between the neck and knees.

What about Hickeys?

Hickeys are what happen when a lover sucks on your neck or other body parts with enough force to cause internal bleeding. The hickey is the resulting bruise. Some people love the feel of getting hickeys. Some are proud of their hickeys and display them the way bikers do tattoos. Other people are mortified and even wear turtlenecks in the middle of summer to cover their hickeys up.

To prevent hickey mortification, point to the area between your legs and tell your lover to suck there. Unless your name is Sookie.

How to Hide a Hickey

Hickeys go through stages, so you will need to change your cover-up makeup as the hickey goes from three-alarm to one-alarm.

- If the hickey is blue-black-purple, use a yellow-based concealer. If it's reddish, try a green concealer.

- If the hickey is greenish-yellow, use a pink-based concealer. Be sure to blend out the edges.

- If your hickey is blue-black-purple at the epicenter and reddish around the perimeter, dab on yellow in the center and green over the reddish part.

After the concealer is on, dab on your normal foundation. Do not rub. Then use your normal powder. If not being found out is of the utmost importance, try a translucent powder on top of the whole mess to help set it.

If you don't have green, use an oil-based concealer that is lighter than your natural skin color. That's because the hickey color will cause the lighter concealer to look darker. But focus the lighter concealer only on the hickey area and not on the skin beyond it. Otherwise, the unbruised skin around the hickey perimeter will look like a big smudge, and everyone will know.

The Real Estate between Your Ears & Knees

Lovers who enjoy each other will often explore kissing a partner from head to toe, discovering and rediscovering where he or she likes to be kissed. Here are a few areas to consider:

Skin Folds The places on the body where the skin folds or creases tend to be sensitive and love to be kissed. These include the backs of knees, the fronts of elbows, the nape of the neck, under breasts, on eyelids, armpits, crotches, between fingers and toes, and behind ears.

Lower Back & Buns The lower back and rear end can be exquisite places to kiss and kiss again.

Bellies & Navels Think of the navel as a little vulva rather than a collecting point for lint. Some people love to have their navels licked and caressed. This will seriously annoy others.

Long Licks Don't hesitate to get your tongue really wet and take a long lick up your partner's body, from tailbone to neck or hip to armpit (known as "Australian" in some circles.)

Human Serving Tray Fruits, dessert foods, and certain liquors can be served on various parts of the body with pleasing results.

Love Bites Teeth on skin can feel really nice or really ugly. Lube your lover's skin with oil or saliva so your teeth glide along the surface. Then raise your lips up and run your teeth back and forth. You might try a little biting action on large muscle groups such as the shoulders or buns. Be sure to get lots of feedback from the bitee and try not to violate your local cannibalism statutes.

Eskimo Pies & Eskimo Kisses: Kissing in Other Cultures

You may have heard that Eskimos don't kiss like we do. Instead of kissing on the lips they allegedly rub noses. What's closer to the truth is that Eskimos put their noses in close proximity to inhale the breath of a loved one. Perhaps they do this to keep their lips from freezing together.

Eskimos find that inhaling the breath of a lover is erotic; those of us from more temperate climates prefer exchanging wads of saliva. People raised in different cultures may define what's sexy in different ways.

Kissing on the Edge of Town

In nearly every community where people have lips, there are certain places where the locals go to make out.

In the town where your author grew up, there were two favorite places where people went to kiss and grope—well, three if you counted the drive-in theater, but that was more like an extra bedroom. One of those places was at the river, which was in the mountains east of town. Another was in the orange groves.

Perhaps there were places where you grew up that lovers went to for making out. Maybe there is still a place where you and your sweetheart go.

Passion Pits & the Phone Booth—Symbols of the Past

Not long ago, there were more than 4,000 drive-in theaters or *passion pits* in America where younger couples kissed, groped, and petted themselves into a frenzy. While the population is nearly double today what it was then, there are now fewer than 500 drive-in theaters in America.

It never hurts to have a "Drive-In Night" in your living room where all you do is grope and make out in front of a big-screen TV, or in your back yard if you have a projector. Don't forget the condoms and popcorn.

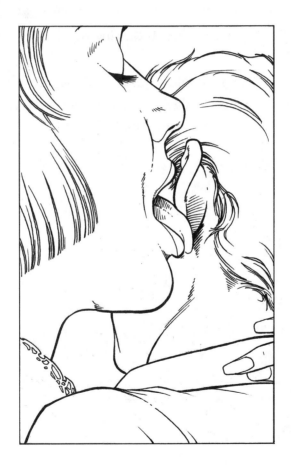

Be sure to see our video on kissing at www.GuideToGettingItOn.com.

For the latest info about sex
and our how-to videos, get naked at

www.GuideToGettingItOn.com

The Guide is also available in
a spectacular color eBook version for
your iPad, Kindle or Nook.

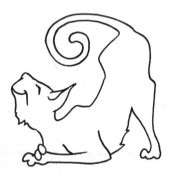

4
The Importance of Getting Naked

In relationships, there are different kinds of nakedness. Sometimes, we just get physically naked. Other times when we take our clothes off, we get emotionally naked. Whatever your situation, this chapter suggests a kind of nakedness that has emotional as well as physical grit. It also talks about different ways of getting naked, and the more delicate things we cover ourselves with that can be as inviting as wearing nothing at all.

Getting Naked — An Overview

For some people, getting naked in front of a lover is easy and natural. Some sext naked pictures of themselves. For others, getting naked can cause distress or embarrassment. They might engineer situations where they can get it on without taking their clothes off in front of a partner. Perhaps this gives you an idea of how powerful getting naked can be, and how vulnerable we can feel about our bodies.

As a culture, we are so uptight about nakedness that we don't have street-corner fountains with marble cherubs peeing into pools of water or public paintings of naked Botticelli babes. A bare crotch on network television is about as common as a snowstorm in Siam. Even the suggestion of body parts beneath a person's blue jeans on the public airwaves can result in a massive fine from the FCC. No wonder why a free-for-all of nakedness has evolved over the Internet in the form of porn.

Don't Sell Near-Nakedness Short

Porn aside, many of us are more aroused by near-naked images than by actual nakedness. Perhaps that's because near-nakedness allows more space for our fantasies to imagine what's under the skimpy thongs, bikinis, and whatever else is used to cover prime breast and genital real estate. With the suggestion of impending nakedness, the illustrations in this chapter may have more intrigue than if the couples in them were buck naked.

The Naked-Nipple Rule

In North America, we believe that a woman isn't really naked unless her nipples are showing. In Europe, they still don't understand the big fuss over naked breasts.

On mainstream television, we have the naked-nipple rule. Show a naked nipple on network television, and thousands of dollars in fines will soon follow. We also have the naked-nipple rule on most beaches in North America. Hopefully, you are able to violate the naked-nipple rule with a partner as often as you like.

Getting Naked — Hidden Possibilities

Porn gives a distorted idea of nakedness, yet it's how we sometimes think nakedness with a partner should be.

If you and your sweetheart are in the process of becoming more physical, you might consider some of the hidden possibilities that getting naked can offer. A lot of honesty and trust can be generated when you are naked together, something that rarely develops if the sole purpose of taking your clothes off is to have sex. It's how you can learn to relate physically with more than just your crotches. It's how a guy can learn to have his penis resting on a woman's soft, warm skin without feeling like he has to perform with it, and how her vulva and breasts can be pushing against him while she dozes off.

Naked Logistics

If it feels like your relationship is ready, you might consider planning a time and place where you can work on getting naked. Some couples enjoy undressing each other, while others make a game out of taking their clothes off, from playing strip poker to lighthearted wrestling. There are occasions where one partner blindfolds the other before undressing him or her.

Getting naked happens naturally if you shower together or go skinny-dipping. Sometimes it happens when you are hot-tubbing, and some couples enjoy undressing each other while dancing. If you try this, be sure to have birth control handy in case you end up doing the polka.

It can sometimes be helpful for partners to tell each other some of the things they do and don't like about their bodies. It used to be that women would worry about their butts being too big or their breasts being too small or mismatched. But since porn became our main source of sex education,

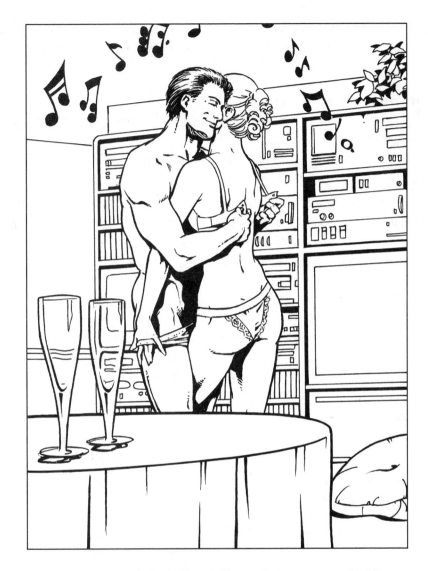

some women are worried about their labia not being porn perfect. Some guys worry they aren't hung well enough, or they might be hung too well, or that their penis might bend the wrong way when it gets hard. Getting your fears out in the open with a partner will usually help you feel more comfortable.

For couples who are particularly self-conscious, writer Jay Wiseman suggests getting naked in total darkness. Each partner then takes a turn examining the body of the other with a small flashlight. This can be a fun game that taps into your fantasies and helps decrease the anxiety of being seen naked all at once. Another way for the shy to share their nakedness is by getting a fun top or T-shirt to wear with nothing on underneath. Or maybe you'd like to try a pair of silk boxers.

Guys Worry: Wood Good, Wood Bad?

When it comes to getting naked, men sometimes worry whether they should or shouldn't have a hard-on. It doesn't matter. It's fine either way. The point is learning to associate nakedness with something other than just sex or bathing.

Some people don't have the slightest hesitation to get naked for sex, but if it's getting naked just to talk or hold each other, good luck. They may become fidgety and fire off a rapidly dismissive, "Sure, we'll have to try that sometime...." Perhaps that kind of nakedness feels too intimate.

Naked & Getting Off

While getting naked together doesn't need to include orgasms, some couples find it uplifting to have one or two somewhere along the way. So plan your naked time to include lots of holding and touching, try an orgasm or two, and then even more holding and touching afterward. (One reader comments, "Good luck on this one. I've spent a lot of lonely time while my partner sleeps immediately after orgasm.")

Coming is usually the last thing that couples do when they are having sex. Yet it might be nice to spend extra time holding and touching each other after you have orgasms. Coming clears the senses in a way that allows many of us to share a special kind of warmth and tenderness.

Sex Tips with a Cranky Marxist Edge

We now have a multimillion-dollar lingerie business, which has made a handsome profit selling flimsy wisps of underwear to women in the name of lingerie. Manufacturers are starting to gouge men with similar intent, charging $10 to $20 for a pair of men's briefs that could otherwise be bought at Walmart or Costco for $3.00.

Counterpoint: "I have read portions of *The Guide* out loud to my girlfriend, and we are enjoying it very much. I have but one complaint: stop the lingerie bashing. It is perhaps the only good thing about American consumerism."

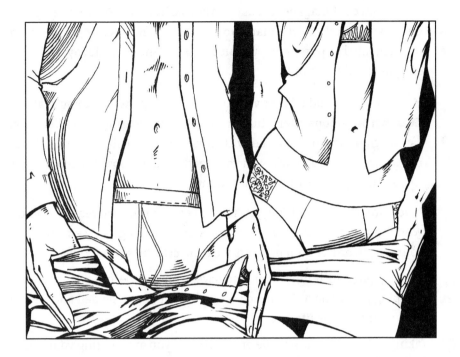

If you find underwear to be erotic, here are a couple of possibilities:

 Women who wear nylons and garters might consider putting their panties on over the garter belt instead of under, so their panties can come off while leaving the stockings and garters intact.

 A common garter *faux pas* is wearing the rear garter all the way back instead of to the side. On the right leg, the front garter should be worn at dead center (12:00), and the rear garter should attach to the nylon at 3:30 to 4:00 as opposed to 6:00. On the left leg the front garter attaches at 12:00 and the rear garter at 7:30 or 8:00. This helps keep the seams straight.

 If you wear a push-up bra, put it on, and then reach across your chest with your right hand. Grab your left breast from under your armpit, lifting it up and dropping it into the bra cup. Do the same thing with your left hand and right breast. Another bra misdemeanor: incorrectly adjusting the straps so the bra rides up too high or droops down too low.

Here's a piece of shagadelic seduction advice from the 1960s: When going out, a woman might let a man know that she is not wearing underwear, or reach into her purse and pull out a pair of panties while saying, "Oops, I forgot to put these on!"

 Here's a way to add a bit of variety and challenge when doing oral sex: Go down on your partner while she or he is still wearing underwear. You can reach under the material with your tongue, push it to one side for proper access, or pull it off with your teeth. You'll probably need a fingertip assist, but the gesture is what counts!

 If you are having a quickie, you might keep your underwear on and try working around it. Also, some couples enjoy having oral sex and intercourse with one or both partners wearing crotchless underwear.

 Dry humping with only your underwear on can be fun. Plenty of dry humping gets done at the beach when it's not very crowded and people are wearing swimsuits.

 Taking a shower or bath while one or both of you are wearing your underwear can be fun.

 Women shouldn't hesitate to take their lovers with them when shopping for lingerie. Shopping for a new bra or other intimate apparel might seem mundane to a woman, but it could be a fun treat for a man. It will help give him ideas for when he wants to get you a special gift. If it's possible, ask him to accompany you into the dressing room. A drawback is that a man's presence might cause other women to feel self-conscious.

 For men, the next time you are in a department store with your lover, nudge her into the men's underwear department and ask her what style and colors she thinks might look best on you.

Men's Underwear

Although men have a choice of wearing briefs, boxers, boxer-briefs, thongs, nothing, or even women's underwear, most of us end up wearing whatever our mothers bought for us as kids. Each provides a different kind of feeling that a man gets used to, thus casting him for life as either a briefs guy or a boxer guy. Some men find that boxer-briefs offer the best of both worlds.

While a briefs man might experiment with boxers for a couple of months or even years, there is a tendency to go back to what he started with. Same with a boxer man. A woman shouldn't push the issue one way or the other, unless the man doesn't care. What she should encourage is that his underwear be clean and not full of holes.

Cramped Penis Alert

A guy's penis usually hangs downward when it's soft, but as it stiffens it needs extra head room to accommodate the expansion. If a man is wearing jeans, the expanding penis often gets trapped in a downward position (ouch!) or gets stuck in a horizontal pickle. So if you are fooling around with your clothes on, the penis will often need a quick adjustment to point in the right direction. While it might be presumptuous for a woman to lend a helping hand if you are making out on a first date, this can be a nice gesture once you are on groping terms. When the bulge starts to grow, reach inside his pants and pull the penis up so its head is pointing toward the man's chest, unless it naturally bends down.

Jocks

Some women get turned on by seeing a lover in an athletic supporter, as long as it isn't wringing wet from playing hours of basketball or soccer. The athletic supporter emphasizes a man's rear end by keeping it naked while highlighting his genitals by keeping them covered.

Learning from Lady Lawyers

During the second half of the 1900s, lady lawyers suddenly began to penetrate the traditional male lair. Being confused about how to be taken seriously, most of these women started wearing boring wool suits with blouses that had floppy bows (the "lady lawyer" uniform). The intent was to look as nonsexual and unalluring as humanly possible, as femininity was considered to be a liability when arguing matters of law. Short of wearing a body bag to court, most of the women succeeded handily. Some of these lady lawyers made it a point to wear steamy lingerie under their boring suits. It was a way of saying to themselves, "At least some part of me is still feminine."

In our society, wearing lingerie has been an important way for women to feel feminine. Some women feel sexier wearing lingerie than they do being naked. And some women feel better masturbating while wearing lingerie or panties. Some will masturbate with their fingers over their underwear, while others will masturbate with their fingers inside their underwear. What often feels best of all is when a lover pulls off the underwear you are wearing.

Girls UnderGear

Here's a brief list of what women are wearing under it all:

Thong—A narrow piece of material that passes between the legs and up through the butt where it attaches to a waistband. Thongs were traditionally the underwear of strippers. Then, women in Brazil started wearing them, and it was only a matter of time before they worked their way under North American dresses and jeans. There are different types of thongs, including G-strings or T-backs, which are the underwear equivalent of dental floss; the Tanga, which has more material in the seat; and the Rio, which has straps on the sides. *Sorry, but our gyno-experts say thongs can cause the lips of women's genitals to chafe. Also, the butt-floss part of the thong provides a zipline for bacteria from the anus to move into the vagina and cause an infection.*

Hipsters or *Boy Shorts*—The comfort favorite of many girls, hipsters and boy shorts are like low-rise briefs that offer full coverage without looking like granny panties. Materials can range from cotton to lace. *Hipsters* stop higher on the thigh while *boy shorts* have the start of a leg.

Bikini—The modern bikini was born in 1946. It was named after the island Bikini Atoll, which is part of the Marshall Islands in the Pacific Ocean where nuclear weapons were tested. It was so revealing that the only model who would originally wear it was a nude dancer. It did not become popular in the US until the early 1960s when Brian Hyland's song *Itsy Bitsy Teenie Weenie Yellow Polka Dot Bikini* hit the charts. Then, American women suddenly started gearing up—or down. (The *Itsy Bitsy Bikini* song sold nearly a million copies in its first two months, which was an obscene amount of records in those days.) No one then would ever have dreamed that bikini panties would become commonplace. And today's G-strings and thongs would have been unthinkable.

String Bikinis—String bikinis are called string bikinis because they have strings on the sides that connect the front and back panels.

Granny Panties—These occupy the women's underwear niche that's between bikinis and Depends.

Visible Panty Line—VPL or *Visible Panty Line* is a female fashion felony. The biggest cause is panties that are too tight. Some types of thongs and boy-shorts can help prevent VPL, but not if what you are wearing is extremely tight or transparent.

Stripping

Getting naked for an audience is called stripping. Until the advent of Chippendales in the 1980s, stripping was something that only girls did, and it usually fell into one of two categories. The first was the playful, private stripping that a woman does for her significant other. Even evangelical marriage manuals nod and wink when a good Christian wife puts on a show to get her man's baby-making gears going. The other kind of stripping is for pay in front of strangers. Society frowns on women who do this. If you doubt that, try telling your mom you are dating a girl who strips at the Kitty-Kat Lounge.

Contrary to what you might think, it's the women at the male strip shows who go wild and get aggressive, while the male audience members at girlie strip shows are expected to be more subdued.

US News and World Report says that Americans spend more money at strip clubs than at the opera, ballet, Broadway and Off-Broadway theater, and classical music performances combined.

If the thought of stripping for your partner turns you on, a great book to consult is *The Stripper's Guide to Looking Great Naked* by Jennifer Axen and Leigh Phillips, Chronicle Books. The authors interviewed strippers from all over the country for suggestions that could be helpful to women who want to make an impression in front of their partners.

According to *The Stripper's Guide*, a cornerstone of a stripper's appeal is how each stripper needs to adopt her own unique look. It does a woman no good to try looking like someone else. It's all about attitude and having your own style rather than sporting the perfect body. Forget buying expensive products, going on strange diets, and spending hours at the gym.

The Stripper's Guide offers a number of tips based on general body types. For instance, when it comes to trimming your pubic hair, women with a voluptuous or well-endowed body might try a landing strip. The vertical line balances the curves and draws the eyes downward. A woman with an I-shaped body might go for a more natural-looking pubic bush, which helps make her hips look more round and curvy.

Playing Strip Poker

A time-honored and frequently fun way of getting naked together is by playing strip poker. While you don't need a book to tell you how to play strip poker, *The Stripper's Guide* offers hilarious advice for a woman who unexpectedly finds herself in a game of strip poker but hasn't trimmed her pubic hair in a month and is wearing a granny bra. The authors suggest that she head for the bathroom for her three minutes of ABT "allowable bathroom time." She should stuff the granny bra into her purse or into a drawer (better to be totally topless than shirtless with an ugly bra). She should run her fingers under cold water and tweak her nipples. And if the cards aren't running her way and she loses her pants, she should make a show of taking them off, but sit with her legs crossed.

Technology Gives Nakedness a New Dimension

Years ago, when the first edition of this book was being written, this chapter stopped right here. That's because there was no such a thing as sexting or women who got naked on webcams.

Now, an entire book could be written on webcam communities alone. The expansion of nakedness beyond what was once the almost exclusive domain of strip clubs and Peeping Toms has been phenomenal.

The first and most famous cam girl was Jenni Ringley. Jenni's willingness to broadcast every aspect of her private life on the new invention of the webcam was unprecedented in the history of nakedness or technology.

Cam Girls — Nakedness Makes Online History Through Lifecasting

Until the invention of the webcam in the late 1990s, if you wanted to see a stripper strip, you went to a club that featured strippers. But then came JenniCam, featuring the World Wide Web's first cam girl.

JenniCam was broadcast live from 19-year-old Jennifer's Ringley's dorm room in Dickinson College in 1996. This was when there was only dialup. So for the first year or two, JenniCam would only refresh once every three to five minutes.

Unlike today's webcams, which stream in real time and are more of an x-rated peep show, the first webcams would broadcast live 24/7. Early cam girls like Jennifer were referred to as "lifecasters." The early webcams were the forerunners of reality TV shows like *Big Brother*.

The webcam was on in Jenni's dorm room 24/7. Much of the time, viewers would see nothing but an empty room. Other times, they would see Jenni eating or reading. Sometimes they would see her naked, masturbating, or performing a striptease. Jennicam viewership skyrocketed when her webcam started showing Jenni having sex with her boyfriend.

It wasn't long before 3 to 4 million people a day were watching Jenni do the same things they would see you doing if there were a webcam in your bedroom or living room 24/7.

Even then, there were far more graphic pornographic images available on the Internet, which viewers didn't have to sit in front of their computer screens like peeping Toms to see. But that was the magic of the early cam shows. Viewers could be the ultimate voyeurs.

A key part of the early cam girl experience was the blog or website where the cam girl would keep her diary or post her daily journal, answer viewer questions, and provide an archive of images. The early cam girl blogs were the forerunners of Facebook pages. But only a handful of cam girls would ever experience the level of celebrity and early social networking fame that Jenni Ringley did.

JenniCam was live for seven years. It was the perfect intersection of technology, exhibitionism, and voyeurism.

The early cam girls don't exist anymore online. They've been replaced by thousands of women who have joined cam sites that cater to customers who want to see women masturbate and act out special fantasies. The women set up cams in their homes or dorms where they perform several hours a day. These are the new sex workers. They are the strippers of the electronic age.

As for Jenni Ringley, she is almost entirely absent from the Internet today, and says she prefers it that way.

Sexting

Modern technology has thrown nakedness another twist in the form of sexting, where a person takes pictures of their naked body (or parts of it) and sends them to someone else. So the cameras on phones have taken what would have formerly been a slice of the pornographic pie and personalized it.

Sexting has had so much media play and will continue to do so that it's hard to even know where to begin discussing it. For now, the best advice for people who are of a legal age and want to sext is to make an attempt to find creative and seductive ways of sexting rather than simply being porn-actor wannabes. There are now books and articles on how to sext creatively and how to show less flesh and more allure when you sext. Why not research the subject and try to use the amazing capacity of your phone to create your own unique style?

As for guys sending dick pics, gay guys might be fine with it, but think twice before sending a dick pic to a woman. Few women are as impressed with dick pics as the men who send them.

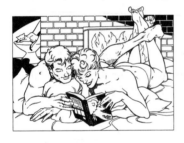

Dear Paul,

I get seriously turned on when my girl-friend is wearing pantyhose. There's some-thing about the feel of them on her legs that makes Mr. Winky pop straight in the air. Any advice about this?

Seamless in Seattle

Dear Seamless,

Given how most of our mothers wore nylons or pantyhose, and considering how often our toddler selves stood next to them with arms wrapped around their legs, it's a wonder more guys aren't stirred into action by the feel of a woman in pantyhose.

Assuming your girlfriend is understanding and willing, ask her to cut out the cotton crotch on a pair of pantyhose. Thanks to the new ventilation system, you'll be able to go down on her as well as have intercourse while she is wearing her customized pantyhose. Make sure she cuts out the crotch on the inside of the seam so they don't unravel. Also, consider helping her to arrive orally before slipping your penis in, because it isn't likely that you will be lasting for long if nylons are your thing. If she isn't handy with scissors, she can purchase crotchless pantyhose in some stores, but probably not at places like Walmart or Target.

For those of you who are wondering about the difference between a guy with a healthy appreciation of girls in pantyhose versus one with a fetish or paraphilia, see Chapter 46: *Kinky Corner.*

Thanks to the writings of Barbara Keesling, Linda Levine, Lonnie Barbach, Cynthia Heimel, and Jay Wiseman for naked inspiration. Ditto to the folks at Los Angeles' Trashy Lingerie, and to Katherine Liepe-Levinson, author of *Strip Show.* Thanks also to Leslie Davisson who was involved in the original launch of *The Guide.*

CHAPTER

5
On the Penis

This chapter was written for women readers, although the men who have seen it claim to be amused. The topic is boys and their toys. Hopefully the following pages provide some insight into the love, and sometimes hate, relationship between a man and his weenie.

Toys, Pain & Pleasure

As a woman, the first thing you will find out about penises and testicles is that most guys take them way too seriously. There are reasons for this:

💡The penis is the only childhood toy that a guy gets to keep and play with throughout his entire life. It is the only toy he will ever own that feels good when he tugs on it, that constantly changes size and shape, and is activated by the realm of the senses. Try to find that at Toys'R'Us.

💡One of the first things a man does when he wakes up in the morning and the last thing he does at night is to touch his penis and testicles. It's a male ritual of self-affirmation that has little to do with sexual stimulation. A daytime extension of this is known as pocket pool.

💡The average male pees between five and seven times a day. Each time he pees he has a specific ritual, from the way he pulls his penis out to how he wags it when he's done. When he is peeing alone a guy will often invent imaginary targets in the toilet to gun for. An especially fine time is had when a cigarette butt has been left behind. Gunning for floating cigarette butts is the male urinary equivalent of playing *Halo* or *World of Warcraft*. While this may be a difficult concept for a woman to fully grasp, it does make for a certain amount of familiarity, friendship, and even self-bonding between a man and his penis.

🔅Another bathroom-related matter has to do with visual reinforcement. How many women look down when they are peeing to see what's coming out of their bodies? Guys look down often. As a result, we males get visual reinforcement for the feelings we have in our genitals when we pee. While women experience a hand-eye-genital experience when they use tampons, it's usually not all that visual, and it doesn't start until after puberty. Between erections, pocket pool, package adjustments and peeing, guys have far more sensory experience with the penis than most women have with their vaginas. This must be why women sometimes call us "Dicks!"

🔅You wouldn't believe how often the human male experiences a jolt of pain in his testicles. It is a discomfort that gives a guy the kind of extra-personal relationship with his reproductive equipment that menstruating women have with theirs. The source of agony can be anything from an elbow during a game of basketball to simply bending over and having your pants crimp the very life force out of you. One of the great culprits in male testicular angst is the horizontal bar on the bicycle frame. Why is it that girls' bicycle frames are V-shaped when it is guys who need the V? Not only did this confusion among bicycle makers result in our younger selves not getting to look up girls' dresses when they were mounting their bikes, but many of us still have the word Schwinn engraved on the underside of our testicles from each time a foot slipped off the pedal.

🔅This may be difficult to fully appreciate, but there is the matter of the unwanted hard-on. The unwanted hard-on usually strikes with predictable ferociousness first thing in the morning. Not only does it interfere with the ability to relieve a full bladder, but it provides logistical problems for a guy who has to traverse shared hallways to get to the bathroom. The unwanted hard-on can be excruciating and even painful for its most frequent victim, the adolescent male. The unwanted hard-on is much less of a problem after a man turns thirty, and by the time he's forty it is an event accompanied by a sigh of relief and a moment of thanks.

🔅Our society teaches us that sexual pleasure between a man and a woman depends on the man's ability to get hard and stay hard. What a demented view of sex. This puts a lot of pressure on guys to be consummate cocksmen. It makes us more dick-centered than necessary, at the expense of everyone.

💡When life is full of despair, the one thing that a guy can usually count on for a good feeling is his penis, unless matters are totally out of hand, in which case he needs to consider something stronger like tequila or prayer.

These items aside, the most important thing for a woman to know about a penis is how it figures into a man's concept of his own manliness. Ridiculous, but important.

Weirdness in the Locker Room

You might think that a man's primary concern about penis size has to do with what a sexual partner likes. But how he stacks up among his buds is just as important, if not more. When we asked men if they feel comfortable about being naked in the locker room, the majority answered the question as if we'd asked about penis size, even if the words "penis" and "size" were never part of the question. These are the exact answers men gave when asked:

"How do you feel about being naked in the locker room?"

"I used to feel uncomfortable back in my freshman year of high school. Then I realized that I was really a little bigger than average."

male age 21

"I used to think that my penis was really small, and so I was shy about it. As it turns out, I'm on the high end of average when erect: I'm just not a hanger." *male age 32*

"I have an inferiority complex about the size of my penis. I don't care how many studies tell me that I am right in the middle of the curve, I will always feel small." *male age 25*

"I was raised in a fairly strict and religious environment, so nudity of any kind was a no-no. My equipment is pretty small, and I was a late bloomer. All this adds up to being very shy about my own appearance. In junior high and high school, when 'naked locker time' was mandatory, I would arrive as early as possible and change quickly so that others wouldn't see me. If others were around me without clothes on, I gave myself tunnel vision or imaginary blinders so I wouldn't see other guys' equipment. I didn't want to be perceived as gay, and glancing around was a good way to get yourself taunted at least, beat up at worst." *male age 41 (And this guy was straight!)*

The men who said they were comfortable in the locker room often made reference to their penis size as well, indicating they were well hung. You can almost predict how a man feels about being naked in the locker room by asking how he feels about the size of his penis. Hopefully, the following from a Marine who has been in combat helps provide perspective:

"The tradition of group showers is still strong in the Marine Corps. It makes us more comfortable with each other, and if you are trusting a guy to save your life, do you really think penis size is that big a deal? Before the military though, I worried I didn't 'measure up.'" *male 27*

As for guys checking out other guys, you would think this curiosity would decrease as they get to be adults. Not so, according to a study by a group of Ph.D. students. These students hung out in rest rooms at a San Diego Padres game and secretly studied a hundred different men who were peeing. They claim that many of the men made an attempt to check out the equipment of whomever was peeing next to them. Furthermore, men who were well-endowed went out of their way to show their bigger units to the other men who were peeing. These tendencies might be more true of Padres fans than, say, Phillies fans, who are usually too busy weeping in the men's room to check out the size of the other boys' bats. So if you are a man who has ever glanced down at another man's penis when you are peeing, take comfort in knowing that you are probably normal.

Size, Shape, Plumbing & The Goofy Dick Game

Ads like those below have flooded the backs of newspapers and magazines since the 1800s. We now have TV infomercials and e-mails promoting products for "natural male enhancement." The products don't work—they never have—but the scams still do.

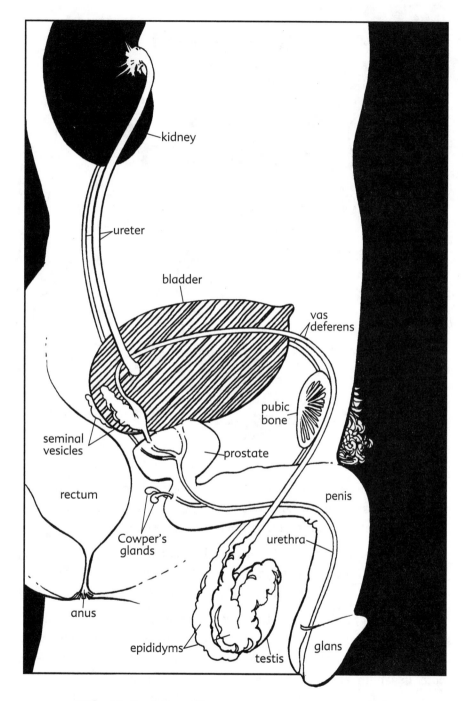

kidney

ureter

bladder

vas deferens

pubic bone

seminal vesicles

prostate

rectum

penis

Cowper's glands

urethra

anus

epididyms

testis

glans

What's Inside a Guy

The Bone Yard

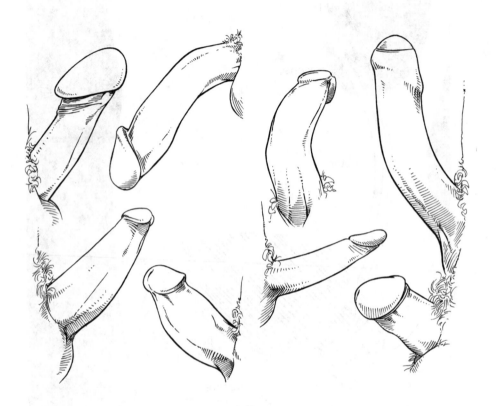

Shape From these drawings of real-life erections, you can see that terms like "6 inches" or "normal" are somewhat meaningless. All of these erect penises are normal, yet very different from each other. One points down.

Size. In a review of studies that included 15,521 penises, the average length of an erect penis was about 5.25 to 5.5 inches. The average circumference was about 4.5 inches. The length of a penis when not erect was about 3.5 inches.

A penis that is 7 inches long when erect is in the upper 97th percentile of all penises. It's reasonable to assume that guys who are in porn or who upload videos of themselves to porn sites have the largest 1% to 5% of all penises both in length and circumference. Also, when men measure their own penises, the length ends up being way longer than when researchers do it.

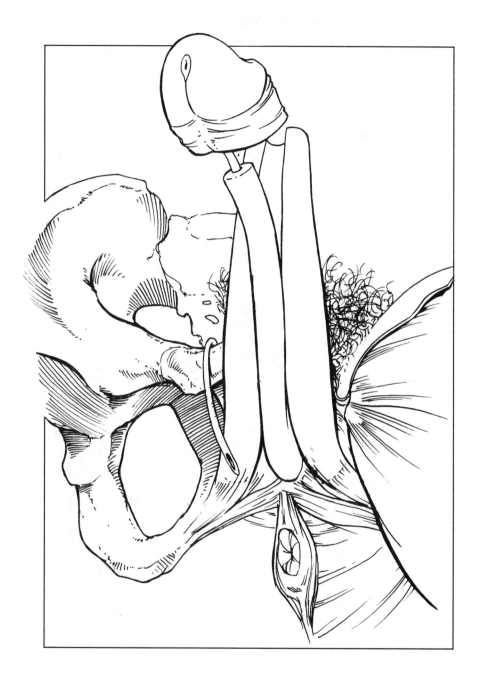

The Wrecking Yard

THE GOOFY DICK GAME
Real Penises of Real Guys

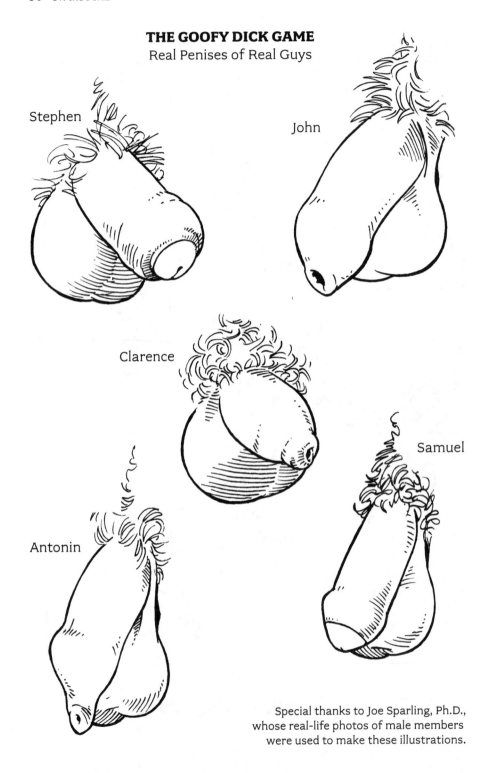

Stephen

John

Clarence

Samuel

Antonin

Special thanks to Joe Sparling, Ph.D.,
whose real-life photos of male members
were used to make these illustrations.

You Be the Judge!
Match Each Soft Penis On
The Other Page With Its Erection
On This Page

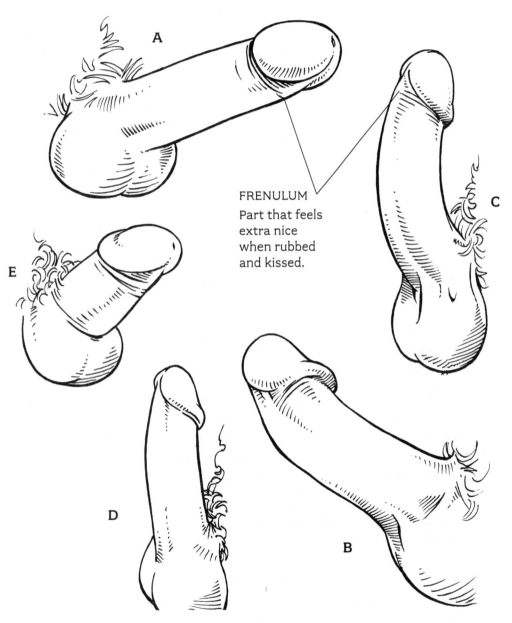

A

C

FRENULUM
Part that feels
extra nice
when rubbed
and kissed.

E

D

B

Stephen–A Antonin–C Clarence–E Samuel–D John–B

Manliness — What Is It?

In our culture, being manly means you don't act gay. It also means if you have girly parts to your character, you keep them hidden. But this is defining masculinity by saying what it isn't.

What is being masculine? Is it a physical way of being? Is it a state of mind? Is it having the right politics? Is it what your dick gets hard over? Can you still be manly if you sound like a prissy snap-queen? This Guide's definition of masculinity keeps evolving. Here it is in its current state:

> Masculinity is mostly an invention of modern culture. It doesn't have a huge foundation in science or nature, yet it remains a powerful force in the way we view ourselves and each other.

> To be manly or masculine in American culture, a guy should be a fairly responsible person who can be independent when the occasion demands. As often as not, he should be caring, comforting, and kind. He should be able to give and receive physical and emotional tenderness without being too controlling. He should have values and a good work ethic, and he shouldn't need to prove his masculinity by trying to scare or intimidate others.

> He doesn't need to have a pussy-seeking sensor at the end of his penis, and his physical appearance can range from Bill Gates geek to movie star perfect. Showering to prevent smelly balls and pits should be a priority.

There are plenty of males who have none of these qualities, but appear to be total studs nonetheless. These are guys who usually take their penises way too seriously. That is because the only way they can convince themselves they are real men is by performing manly activities or drinking lots of beer or doing drugs, and then having a vagina nearby they can stick themselves into. They tend to be more show than substance.

Penis As Camouflage: Why It's Difficult to Be Satisfied By a Guy Who Takes His Penis Too Seriously

A hard penis is sometimes used to camouflage what's missing inside a man, as well as what's missing in a relationship between a man and a woman. If a guy is all hung up about his penis being a symbol of his manliness or demands that it have a disproportionate amount of attention, then it gets in the way of his being at one with a lover. The same is true for a male who needs to always play a manly role. He sometimes feels more warmth for his car or computer than for his partner.

Unfortunately, a lot of women grew up thinking that a distant, self-involved, dick-centered type of guy is what manhood is all about. As a result, they end up being attracted to males with whom they can never really get close, and spend the rest of their lives bellyaching about what duds men are.

Narcisso 'Gasms

Biologically, most women can have a couple of orgasms to the average man's one. This is fine with most men, since most of us would like to see our partners have as much pleasure as their hearts desire. But for a man who takes his penis too seriously, orgasm giving can become too important. A partner's orgasms become reassurance that he is a total guy. We all do this to some extent, but for some it's a matter of narcissistic life and death.

If your man is like this, you may discover that your main function in life is to look good and have lots of loud orgasms. Or maybe it's just to look good. Consider yourself an offering to the great Dick God.

The Penile-Pumping Regatta

Some men lose emotional connection once intercourse begins. The woman starts to feel like she's become a masturbation machine. Sex becomes a pumping regatta in order to prove dick-worthiness. This can be really boring for both partners.

To give you an idea of how much insecurity is involved in all this, consider the words of a 29-year-old man who is starting to question why he takes his penis so seriously:

> "It's like, I attack sex. I'm afraid of slowing it down. If I'm gonna be fucking, I'll fuck like crazy, gotta have a huge dick and fuck like crazy to avoid dealing with whatever's making me anxious. Women have always said to me, 'God, you can't get enough.' But I think the reason I can't get enough is that if I slow down, the fears start to crowd in on me. Does this woman really want to be with me? Is she going to leave? Is my cock good enough? It's hard for me not to use sex as a seal of approval."
> —From Harry Maurer's *Sex: An Oral History,* Viking Press

Of course, there are plenty of women who have their own insecurities. Is getting breast implants or wearing a padded bra all that different from this guy's need to have a perfect penis?

Note: Porn merely reinforces paranoia about dick worthiness. The fact that most porn actors consume nearly fatal amounts of boner drugs to stay hard is lost on most men and women.

The Diagnosis & Cure

How do you distinguish a man who takes his penis too seriously from one who doesn't?

The man who doesn't take his penis too seriously doesn't flake out when it comes to doing the dishes. He may have various passions in life, often sports, music, gaming, work, or trying to fix things (sometimes successfully), but these usually help to center rather than isolate him. Sex with him is a natural extension of your friendship. It makes all the sense in the world.

As for "curing" the kind of man who takes his penis too seriously, you can't. Hard as you might try, no human being has ever changed just because someone else wanted him or her to. It's something that has to come from within. Friends and lovers can sometimes help if they are willing to call the guy on his nonsense, but they can't make the changes for him.

Sexual Awareness: Hood Ornaments vs. Wet Triangles

When it comes to sexual awareness, the penis is positioned like the hood ornament on a car. It's difficult to ignore what your hood ornament is telling you when it's making a tent in the front of your pants. Sometimes we guys aren't even aware we are sexually aroused until we feel ourselves starting to get hard.

Women are not conditioned from early childhood to associate sexual arousal with specific body cues in the way that men are. While their genitals often swell and lubricate, no flags get waved. Most of the changes happen on the inside and can be chalked-up to a nice tingly sensation between their legs. Besides, "good" girls are often taught to ignore their body's sexual cues.

While the penis can be a reliable indicator of sexual excitement, it does have its share of false positives and occasional negatives.

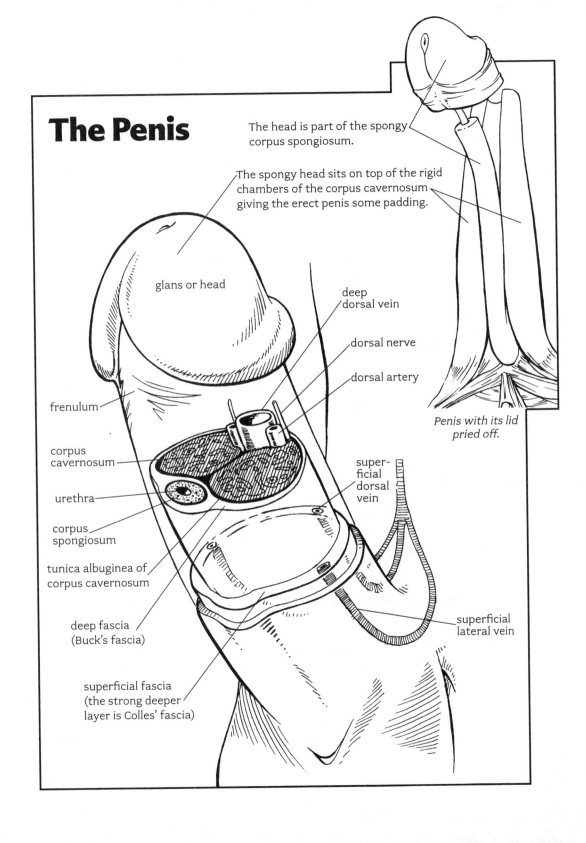

The Penis

The head is part of the spongy corpus spongiosum.

The spongy head sits on top of the rigid chambers of the corpus cavernosum giving the erect penis some padding.

glans or head

frenulum

corpus cavernosum

urethra

corpus spongiosum

tunica albuginea of corpus cavernosum

deep fascia (Buck's fascia)

superficial fascia (the strong deeper layer is Colles' fascia)

deep dorsal vein

dorsal nerve

dorsal artery

super-ficial dorsal vein

superficial lateral vein

Penis with its lid pried off.

How a Penis Gets Hard

The penis has three chambers inside that run the length of it. Two of the chambers are responsible for making it hard or rigid. They are called the corpus cavernosa. They run parallel to each other up the shaft of the penis. Think of a double-barrel shotgun, and that's how they sit next to each other. These two chambers or cylinders are made of spongy material that are covered by a thin but extremely tough exterior. To get an erection, they fill up with blood. As a result, the blood pressure in an erect penis is way higher than the blood pressure in the rest of a man's body.

The third chamber is made of a similar spongy tissue and it encircles the urethra, or the tube that a man pees and ejaculates through. While this third tube expands during erection, it doesn't get hard or rigid like the other two tubes. If it did, it would crimp shut the urethra and there's no way a guy could ejaculate through it.

This third chamber, which is called the corpus spongiosum, also forms the head of the penis. While the head of the penis expands or mushrooms during erection, it stays relatively soft.

Unwanted Wood

"For some reason, out of nowhere, your penis starts to get hard, and it is extremely difficult to stop." *male age 25*

"It's totally embarrassing. You just want to get up and go, but you can't. So you start pulling on your shirt or sweater to try to cover up the bulge. You become very self-conscious; you think everyone is looking at your crotch." *male age 43*

"It's like being in an elevator with an umbrella that will not go down." *male age 42*

"It can physically hurt when your penis is trapped in your jeans pointing downward and it suddenly gets hard for no reason whatsoever." *male age 26*

"Most of my memories of unwanted erections were at school, generally during class, and I was terrified that someone would notice." *male age 24*

"I travel a lot for business and sometimes wake up erect after a flight. It's terribly embarrassing. If I can't think the damn thing down, then I have to go through the tricky maneuver of flipping it up, trapping it under my waistband without being noticed, and then keeping my briefcase in front of me when I stand." *male age 25*

Women usually assume that the presence of a hard-on means that a man is sexually aroused, and that no rise in his pants means he isn't. If only it were that simple. Consider the occurrence of the unwanted hard-on. The average teenage male is capable of getting a totally unwanted hard-on in the middle of an algebra test for absolutely no reason, unless he is a member of that rare breed who finds polynomial equations sexually arousing. When you are a young man, hard-ons just happen; nobody is more befuddled than the possessor of the penis. To say that all hard-ons are a sign of sexual arousal badly overstates the case. One reader took a bad grade in an early-morning high school class because he couldn't go to the chalkboard due to his unwanted erections. His only thoughts were of embarrassment, not sex.

In addition to getting unwanted hard-ons, there are times when a man can feel highly aroused, yet either fail to get hard or have it go limp when he needs it the most (floppus erectus).

Hiding an Unwanted Erection

A large portion of unwanted erections have little to do with being sexually aroused, and guys usually have no more control over them than women do over getting their periods. So thinking about awful things like french-kissing your grandmother isn't going to bring a raging hard-on down because it's probably not about sex to begin with. Pinching yourself until you bleed won't help, and jerking off more often than you already do won't change anything. Since you can't prevent unwanted erections, it helps to have ways to hide them.

If unwanted erections are a problem, avoid wearing sweat pants in public places. Wear pants that are have more rigid material like denim, because the sweat pant material is more likely to drape around your erection and show it off. You might avoid skinny jeans as well.

Baggy untucked Ts or sweat shirts have been saving young men from boner embarrassment since the beginning of time. The same is true for a briefcase, backpack or laptop bag with long straps that you can casually shift in front of your crotch. If your erection feels comfortable in the up direction, put your hands in your pockets and nudge it under the waistband of your briefs or boxers. Men call this maneuver the 'waistband tuck'.

False Negatives: When Gravity Dings the Dong

Confucius says

If limp dick is worst thing that happens to your relationship,
you live charmed life.

Hopefully, your lovemaking isn't solely dependent on the man's ability to get hard. If it is, your sexual relationship might be somewhat limited. It's also disconcerting to think that your entire sex life might be centered on the whims of the average penis, hard or soft.

Regarding the biology of erections, it is perfectly normal for a hard penis to partly deflate every fifteen minutes or so. Regarding the psychology of erections, hard-ons have been known to fly south for varying periods of time, from a single day to who knows how long.

The most unhelpful thing a woman can do when a guy can't get it up is to become defensive. Women often assume that erection failures mean the man doesn't find them attractive or that he might be gay. These are possibilities. But there are a billion other reasons for not being able to get an erection, from fearing you won't be good in bed to what just happened on Wall Street. Physical problems like diabetes can also be a factor.

Given the stress of living in the modern world, it's a wonder we men are able to get it up as often as we do. And given the lack of tenderness or excitement in some relationships, an unerect penis might be a signal that the man and woman need to get closer emotionally.

While most of us have been raised to think of a limp penis as a sign of failure, perhaps it might be more productive to view it as an opportunity to bring a man and woman together. (For a more complete discussion of male hydraulic failure, see Chapter 55: *When Your System Crashes*.)

Betty on Dick

The following passage is from Betty Dodson's classic *Sex for One* from Harmony Books. In addressing the issue of misbehaving penises, Ms. Dodson speaks with welcome concern:

> "Although I ran only a dozen men's groups, the experience helped me to let go of my old conviction that men got a better deal when it came to sex.... I thought they could always have easy orgasms even with casual sex, and I envied their never having to worry about the biological realities of periods or pregnancies. But the truth is that not all men are able to be assertive studs who make out all the time.... The most consistent sex problem for many men in the workshops was owning a penis that seemed to have a will of its own. An unpredictable sex organ that got hard when no one was around and then refused to become erect when a man was holding the woman of his dreams in his arms...."

If this situation sounds familiar, tell your man that there probably isn't a woman alive who wouldn't be happy to receive a long, lingering back rub and oral sex in the place of intercourse. Or what about a go at an extended orgasm from Chapter 15: *The Zen of Finger Fucking?* If his woody won't work, let him know in no uncertain terms that there are plenty of other ways to please you sexually.

This Guide's philosophy:

Never, ever let a recalcitrant penis ruin sex for either of you!

When Young Men Use Boner Drugs Recreationally

Ordinarily, a discussion of using erection drugs should be in the chapter on erection problems. But there is an increasing number of young men who don't have erection problems but take erection drugs for recreational purposes. This might be due to unreal expectations that their penis needs to be like that of porn stars, who are taking erection drugs themselves.

The problem is that once young men who don't need erection drugs start taking them, they become less confident in their own erections. They expect erections that are harder than normal and quicker on the rebound. So they give themselves a false expectation of what an erection is supposed to be, and they start to lose confidence in themselves to get it up without taking boner drugs.

One of the disappointments older men with erection problems can have with erection drugs is they aren't able to recreate the rock-hard erections

men had when they were young. But for 20 year olds without erection problems, drugs like Viagra and Cialis don't have the difficult job of raising the
dead. So the drug is more able to create a porn-like erection.

Nature didn't create erections to be like baseball bats. Normal is not
porn perfect. And no matter what your age, if you don't need erection pills,
don't take them. The latest research is showing that when men who don't
need erection drugs start using them, they can end up giving themselves a
needless dependency on the pills, when the money would be better spent on
flowers and romance. The following personal account from a reader echoes
this very concern:

> "I was dealing with a pretty complicated personal life, along with
> stress and mild depression. So my erections weren't as consistent
> as I would have liked. My doc prescribed Viagra, at my request. I
> was able to take it and get a good effect from very small doses,
> which means it was probably just working as a mental crutch.
>
> Later I found myself with an interesting feeling of psychological
> dependence on the Viagra pills. They made me lazy. I didn't have to
> worry about relaxing, clearing my head, being present, the pills did
> all the work. Plus, I would psych myself into problems, by worrying
> about not taking the Viagra, then worry myself into having prob-
> lems, and then feeling shitty if I had problems and hadn't taken it.
> It was a very interesting dog-chasing-its tail syndrome.
>
> So when they describe folks as addicted to Viagra, I get it. Even for
> young men, it can serve as a psychological crutch, taking off a lot
> of the very significant pressure we feel to get hard at a moment's
> notice. Even now, after not taking them for months, if I have the
> slightest twinge of low response, I can start to panic, and this can
> create a cascade effect where I keep thinking about how that little
> pill would solve everything..."

In case you are concerned about your erections not being perfect, take
solace in knowing that after receiving 5,000 sex surveys from women over
the past ten years, it's difficult to remember complaints about a lover's ability
to get an erection.

Also keep in mind that as soon as a guy thinks more about what he can
do for a woman with his penis than what he can do for her with his fingers,

lips and imagination, then you can pretty well assume his lover will be finding herself increasingly bored with what happens in bed. When it comes to good sex, a perfect penis is the most expendable part.

Penis Perceptions Driven By Porn

Dr. Stephanie Buehler, a therapist with years of experience, reported the following to the author of *The Guide* about the increasing number of normal young men who are scheduling appointments with her because:

> "They believe they should be studs who are able to perform any time, anywhere, with anyone at a moment's notice."

These normal young men think there is something wrong with them because they can't perform like the guys in porn. This is particularly sad because one of the things women want most in a potential partner is a good personality. However, men in porn aren't defined by their personalities. All that counts is their penises, which better be erect and better be able to come on command. Porn is also helping drive unreal expectations in some women about the sexual abilities of men!

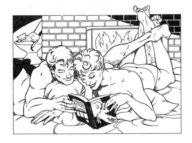

Dear Paul,

My boyfriend always wakes up in the morning with an erection. But when we start having intercourse, it goes down. He doesn't have this problem any other time. What's up?

Gretta in Marietta

Dear Gretta,

Contrary to how it seems, the kind of erection your boyfriend has when he first wakes up is little more than a limp penis trapped inside of a raging hard-on. It happens because he wakes up while in the middle of a dream.

Men usually have three or four erections during a normal night of sleep. These erections are caused by the changes in the body that happen during REM or dream sleep. They are triggered by a different part of the brain than normal erections. So rather than being caused by a dream about sex, sleep erections are automatic. Men get them whether they're dreaming about being chased by wolves, or kissing the love of their life. So your BF is basically waking up with a leftover sleep erection.

Although his penis looks hard and feels hard, it's not the kind of erection your guy gets when he's been thinking about you all day. So even if it seems like your man is ready for action, treat his penis like it's a floppy one that needs to be aroused. Try kissing or playing with it before jumping his bone(s). This will help turn it into a waking-state erection that's sex worthy.

Since his erection was not born from sexual desire, don't assume that your boyfriend feels like having sex. He might feel better if he could pee and brush his teeth. Or he may be just fine boning the babe of his dreams with a full bladder and dragon breath. For some guys, waking up next to a lover is enough to make them feel sexually excited. Others always wake up feeling horny. *Do a search for "morning wood" at www.GuideToGettingItOn.com to see how men from our sex survey describe morning wood versus the erections they get when they are fully awake and sexually aroused.*

A Wet Warning—Ain't Love Grand!

Every once in a while a girlfriend will ask a guy if she can stand behind him and hold his penis while he pees. This is a completely normal request born of completely normal curiosity. But be forewarned that you are sometimes giggling so hard that the entire bathroom becomes a target. On the other hand, women sometimes do a better job of aiming the thing than we men. As for penile calligraphy skills, one female friend of this Guide loves grabbing her husband's penis and writing their names in the snow with its amber stream.

First Ejaculation

Before puberty, a young dude can stroke his pecker until it almost falls off, but his orgasms will mostly be dry except for a few drops of clear, slick, slightly viscous fluid which is probably precum. This changes during puberty. Puberty kicks the prostate gland, seminal vesicles and testicles into semen-making mode. This creates a real ejaculation which is white and thick.

The process of going from a few drops to a full wad can be wonderful if you know what to expect and know it's normal. It can be disturbing if a guy hasn't been told about ejaculation and he masturbates for the first time after entering puberty. Here's how a lot of boys used to react to their first ejaculation before porn was so easy for preteens to access:

"I didn't really know what I was doing. I was eleven and discovered this new feeling when I rubbed this silky part of my blanket over my penis, so I kept doing it. Eventually, I got this intense feeling in my groin and then there was this goop everywhere. I was completely freaked and grossed out. I thought that I broke myself, but was too afraid to tell my parents." *male age 34*

"I was sure anything that felt THAT good had to be sinful and that my ejaculate was evidence that I was damaging my insides. Each time I'd masturbate (almost daily) I would feel horrible guilt afterward and swear to God that I would never do it again." *male age 44*

"I had heard about masturbation while sitting in the back of the school bus. When I tried it just the way the kids told me, it was almost like pain. For weeks I would stop short of actual orgasm for fear that I would do some sort of internal damage to myself. Finally, one day I kept rubbing through my fear and found that I enjoyed the hurting tremendously." *male age 35*

Now, most boys have watched porn before puberty and they know it's normal for men to produce a wad of semen. Instead of feeling fear that they've broken something by playing with themselves, they can feel relief and hopefully pride that their body has reached a manly milestone.

The Couch-Potato Penis

As things get older, they start to petrify or harden. This is true for logs, fossils and the human brain. Unfortunately, it is not true for the human penis. As a penis approaches its fifth decade, it tends to petrify less fully than it did earlier in life. It also squirts less fluid during ejaculation. Some women will cling to this information like a ray of hope, while others will be disappointed. Whatever your situation, it shouldn't make much difference. As the bearer of the penis gets older, he becomes wiser in the ways of love. By then, he can compensate with wit and wisdom for what he loses in hardness and volume.

Older men don't always make an effort to stay in good shape. It's being out of shape, rather than increasing age, that often causes the couch-potato penis and decline in libido. However, age alone is responsible for changes in ejaculation, with the middle-aged man sometimes feeling nostalgic for his teenage genitals, which could sometimes propel ejaculate two feet or more.

Bebop & Squirt — Men & Multiples

Most males experience orgasm as an overlapping two-part process—sensation and ejaculation. Some guys have learned to separate the two events, experiencing a series of orgasmic sensations before they finally ejaculate. According to Dr. Marian Dunn, who interviewed a number of men with this ability, the one common thread was that their partner remained in a state of high sexual excitement after the man's first feeling of orgasm. This seemed to provide an essential path of feedback that the man could feel in his penis as it remained inside her vagina.

Some of the men had small ejaculations with each orgasm, while others didn't ejaculate until the end. Some of these men had been able to do this all of their lives; others had learned it recently. The men who had always been able to do it assumed that all men could and were surprised when a sexual partner pointed out the difference.

This should not be confused with delayed ejaculation, a situation where the man wants to have an orgasm but is unable to (see Chapter 54).

Hormone Advisory: The Impact of Testosterone

The bulk of men's testosterone is produced by the testicles. What do we know about the impact of testosterone (T) on men's behavior? It seems that a male with higher testosterone is more likely to be on the football or rugby team than a man with lower levels of testosterone. He's more likely to be aggressive, want to show off more to women, want to pump iron, and he'll probably want to have sex more often than a guy with lower testosterone.

Men with high levels of testosterone are also more likely to be in prison and they are more likely to be unemployed.

Men with lower or more moderate levels of testosterone tend to be more agreeable and less reactive than men with high testosterone. So a general or a diplomat whose effectiveness depends on consensus building rather than impulsivity is more likely to have a lower level of testosterone than a soldier who loves the rush of battle. Along these lines, a prosecuting attorney is more likely to have a higher level of testosterone than a patent attorney.

A male with lower testosterone is more likely to be introverted, is less likely to perform extreme skateboard tricks and is less likely to do dangerous, risky and otherwise stupid things. However, there is no association with testosterone level and courage or bravery. So the terms "he's got balls" or "grow a pair" really aren't accurate. Nor does having low testosterone have anything to do with cowardly behavior or with being a sissy.

More important than the absolute levels of hormones is how a man has been socialized to behave. There are also situations when our hormones increase as a response to the sexual feelings we are having, rather than it being the hormones that are causing the feelings.

Men and Estrogen

Contrary to what you might think, testosterone in men is also converted into estrogen. The estrogen is very important for how a man feels. So if a healthy twenty-year-old male were to suddenly lose his testicles and not produce testosterone, he would suffer negative effects from having no estrogen in addition to having no testosterone. He'd essentially go through menopause. He would have hot flashes and his bones would become brittle. These are things that estrogen protects men from experiencing—in addition to feeling depressed and having little sex drive which would result from his having so little testosterone.

The Great Testosterone Sham

Drug companies are making millions of dollars selling testosterone to men who may not need it. They have created ads that make men over the age of forty think they'll get their twenty-year old selves back by taking testosterone. This is dumb and probably dangerous, but good luck talking sense to a middle-aged man who is being promised a pharmaceutical miracle.

Guys & Horniness

It is sometimes assumed that the average male wants to have sex every hour of the day as long as the opportunity presents itself. There are plenty of men for whom this axiom does not apply. It could be the man has a nervous system that's sensitive enough to be impacted by some of the really disturbing things that happen in the world. Or maybe he is tired and needs a good night's sleep. Whatever the case, it is sometimes difficult to drop everything and have sex. There are plenty of times when it's just as nice to cuddle up close to a sweetheart and enjoy falling asleep in each other's arms.

How Often Do Men Think about Sex?

Two of the more common urban myths about sexuality are that men think about sex every minute or two, and that men think about sex way more than women do.

Researchers have found that the college-aged males they studied think about sex once an hour on average, and the women they studied think about sex once every two hours. This can vary greatly from person to person and from hour to hour.

To help put it into perspective: *College students think about sleep and food as often, if not more often, than they think about sex!* Also, not all sexual thoughts are created equal. Sexual thoughts can range from a brief and fleeting stirring that lasts a millisecond, to an elaborate sexual fantasy that can cause a tent in your pants or a flood between your legs. Researchers need to explore whether there's a difference in the kind of sexual thoughts men and women have, and which types of sexual thoughts we have more of.

Something that can influence a woman's sexual thoughts more than men's is if she feels discomfort about her sexuality or if she worries that others will think badly of her for being interested in sex. If that's the case, she'll be less likely to have sexual thoughts, or less likely to admit to others that she has sexual thoughts.

Mercy Sex Basics — Making a Man Come Sooner

Let's say you are getting your man off as an act of kindness and aren't particularly into it, or you really need a good night's sleep but won't be able to get one until your guy's glands have sneezed. Here are a few suggestions that might be helpful in making a man come sooner. The latter suggestions, which deal with increasing his level of mental excitement, will likely be more effective, but they might be more taxing on you if you are not particularly into it.

Tighten the Foreskin Pulling the foreskin taut around the base of the penis can cause a man to feel more sensation when his penis is stimulated.

Focus on the Frenulum The frenulum is the most sensitive part of the penis. It's just below the head of the penis, on the side where the seam runs up the shaft. During oral sex, you might focus on this area. If doing him by hand, make sure that your fingers run over this part of the penis with a fair amount of pressure during each stroke. Pumping too quickly may numb out the penis and be counterproductive. Also, using a well-lubricated hand rather than masturbating him dry might help to speed up his ejaculation.

Adding a Squeeze or Twist Try giving a well-lubricated hand job where your entire hand wraps around the penis and twists up and down it as though it were following the red stripe on a barber's pole. Try a similar twisting motion with your head during oral sex. Just a slight turn of the neck is all that's needed, nothing to give you whiplash. At the same time, work the area between his testicles with one of your hands.

Visuals If the man is turned on by your naked body, crank up the lights and park the parts he enjoys most in full view. If there's a particular bra or panties that gets him going, wear them.

Play with Yourself Never hesitate to play with your nipples or vulva. Some men will be so turned on by watching you play with yourself that they will begin to masturbate and finish themselves off with their own hand.

Pleasure Toggles Some men have a spot along the part of the penis that is buried beneath their testicles or all the way back to the rim of their anus which deepens the degree of sensation when pressed upon. Knowing your man's sexual anatomy and keeping a finger on this spot may help move up launch time. Women who give superb blow jobs often work these areas with one hand while tending to the end of the penis with their tongue and lips.

Nipples Some guys' nipples are quite sensitive; others aren't. If your man's are, tweaking them with your fingertips or caressing them with your lips and tongue can speed up arrival time.

On or Up His Rear It doesn't matter if it's your bum or his, the human anus is probably the second-most sensitive part of the body. A wet finger on it, swirling around it, or pushed into it can speed some men up considerably.

Extras If he gets turned on by you talking dirty to him, do it if you are in the mood. If he likes porn, put his laptop or iPad where he can see it. If you are having intercourse, try slowing down the thrusting rather than speeding up, or change his pace. If he is thrusting shallow, have him thrust deep. If you usually do it in the bedroom, switch to the kitchen or living room if you can. A change in routine can help increase the level of excitement and speed of launch time.

If His Weenie Goes Pop

A penis should never make a cracking sound or go "POP." Although rare, the pop might be from a fracture of the penis, which has nothing to do with what most of us consider a fracture to be. Unlike an arm or a leg, there is no bone in the penis to break. A "fracture" of the penis can only happen when a penis is erect, and when one of the chambers or cylinders in the penis tears. Think of what happens if you put a knife through a balloon or jab it into the side of a can of soda. While a knife is not involved in a penis fracture, that's what happens when the side of one of the erectile chambers tears. The way they fix a penis fracture is by sewing up the tear in the side of the chamber.

A penis fracture can also be related to a snapping of the ligament in the penis that acts like the suspension cables on the Golden Gate Bridge. If it breaks, internal bleeding might permanently damage the penis.

A fractured penis will often make a cracking sound, followed by rapid loss of erection, pain, swelling, and hemorrhage. The outcome is excellent if the penis is surgically repaired within a couple of hours. If you wait longer, the damage could be permanent, including a penis that's shaped like a deflated circus balloon, or an Allen wrench.

Warning The intercourse position that can cause the most potential damage to the penis is when the woman is on top. Be sure the vagina is plenty wet and understand that bad things can happen if the penis pulls out too far and then gets sat on it when the head is not inside the vaginal opening (or anus, if that's your sport). Any kind of genital pain that lasts more than ten minutes needs to be tended to by a physician. Serious long-term damage can often be averted if you get medical help right away.

Two Strange Causes of Penis Fractures

While fractures of the penis only seem to happen during sex, they are fortunately quite rare. But in a recent study of sixteen men who had fractured their penis, half were having extra marital affairs when the injury occurred, and none of the fractures were caused by an angry wife. Only three of the men were having sex with their own spouse in their own bedroom. As a result, the sex was often rushed, aggressive, awkward, and it tended to happen in unusual places like cars, elevators, offices and public rest rooms, where the men were unable to protect their penis from the sudden downward thrust of their partner.

Another cause of penile fracture can be a seriously aggressive form of masturbation. There is an area in Iran where this kind of penis bravado is practiced and it results in several fractured penises each year. Hopefully, no one will make a YouTube video of it. It would be an awful thing for men in other cultures to start imitating!

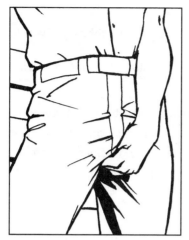

Dear Paul,

Why are guys always touching and grabbing at their genitals?"

Eva from Evanston

Dear Eva,

When the skin on the balls sticks to the thighs, or the skin on the penis sticks to the skin on the balls, you get a claustrophobic feeling. It's like if you had to keep your arms pressed against your sides all the time. Try it for just five minutes without lifting them. When this happens with a guy's penis and scrotum, he's gotta dig to lift and separate or it starts to feel like he's going to go nuts. Body powder can sometimes help. Underwear that doesn't fit right can make matters worse.

Dear Paul,

When guys are peeing, why can't they aim it right? Would it kill them to get all of it in the bowl?

Nancy in Niagara Falls

Dear Nancy,

The problem is not with the aim, but with the unpredictable nature of the stream. It breaks up about as often as the signal on a cell phone.

Sometimes a rebel tributary appears and shoots off to the side, sometimes a healthy stream will suddenly turn into a spray, and sometimes it goes exactly where you aim it, but the toilet water splashes up and makes a mess on the rim.

This is no reason why a guy shouldn't grab a wad of toilet paper and clean up after himself (bowl, floor, walls, shoes, ceiling). This is something that parents should teach their sons. Also, I don't know if you are aware of the first law of fluid dynamics, but a man never pees on his pants leg unless it is one minute before an important meeting, first date, or job interview.

I'm told that women can be wickedly messy when they pee, especially in public rest rooms. But that's a different story for a different chapter.

Dear Paul,

The skin on the shaft of my husband's penis is a lot darker than the skin on the rest of his body. Is this normal?

Amber from Brownsville

Dear Amber,

It's perfectly normal. Penises vary as much in skin tone as they do in size and shape. One man's penis might be darker than his normal skin color, another's might be lighter, and a third might even have freckles or blotches. You can't predict the tone of the bone until the pants are down.

_____

Dear Paul,

When my husband's penis is erect, it almost points down instead of up. Is this normal?

Diane in Bend

Dear Diane,

Penises often point up, at approximately a 30-degree angle from the stomach, assuming the guy doesn't have a big beer belly. But plenty of erect penises stick straight out, and others point down. You might try an intercourse position where you are on top but facing his feet. From this position, his funky rooster may be able to tickle parts of you that a man with an "uppie" would miss. Most important is that you and he experiment with positions that feel good for both of you.

_____

Dear Paul,

My penis has a curve in it, but it only shows when I'm hard. Did I cause the curve by the way I masturbate?

Curly in Canton

Dear Curly,

It's perfectly normal for guys to have a curve in their penis which only shows up when they have an erection. Contrary to the urban myth that curves are caused by the way men masturbate, most curves happen before boys are born—when they are still fetuses in their mother's wombs and their penises are still forming.

In a very small minority of men, the curve can be so extreme that intercourse is not possible. But for most men with curves, this is not a problem. A curve can be a strength if there are special spots in a lover's vagina that can benefit from the focused attention that a curve can offer.

––––––––––––––––

Dear Paul,

When it comes to pleasing guys, why are they so focused on their penises? There's so much of the body that feels good when it's kissed and touched, yet they seem to want everything to focus on the penis.

Flabbergasted in Frankfurt

Dear Flabby,

Let me start by asking you a few questions. Let's say you've just cooked your lover a romantic, candlelit dinner. You've gone to the gym, feel really good about your body, and you are wearing a killer dress with your sexiest lingerie underneath. You want him to want you more than he wants his car, a new phone or Monday Night Football.

But when the lights finally go down, much to your surprise, there's no party in his pants. No matter what you try, he's not able to have an erection. So tell me, what's going through your mind? Are you thinking that he's not interested? Are you worried that he doesn't find you attractive? Let's say you call it a wash and go for it another time. If he still has no erection, are you thinking maybe he's a wimp? Gay? If you are married, do you start to wonder if he's having an affair?

The truth is, you are probably just as focused on his penis as he is, as the ultimate indicator that you are attractive and that he is excited about you. So once a penis gets hard, a guy figures he'd better start doing something with it ASAP. If the thing suddenly goes down, especially if it deflates while your legs are wrapped tight around his waist and you've just cried out, "Fuck me harder," heaven help the poor boy. He'll be a big disappointment to you and an even bigger disappointment to himself.

Also, whether it's due to our biology or simply the things we teach ourselves about sex, a man sometimes feels a strong need to ejaculate once he becomes aroused. This need is much more pronounced in the teens or twenties than later in life. It makes us focus on having to do something with the penis rather than being able to enjoy what's going on around us.

In Praise of Geeks!

What better way to end a chapter like this than with the following sentiment from a female reader:

"I don't know about other women, but I have discovered that the *geek* crowd which doesn't often get laid in high school has a great deal of time to contemplate what they'd do if they ever got their hands on a woman. They are far better lovers because they've taken the time to contemplate something other than *scoring*. As a friend of mine used to say, 'Nine-tenths of sex happens in your mind; the rest is all in your head.' Geeks think, while jocks avoid it at all costs because in high school, thinking is not cool. Besides, geeks know how to be passionate rather than just *stoked*. Give me a geek any time."

Special Thanks to Richard Wassersug, University of British Columbia, Terri Fisher, The Ohio State University at Mansfield, Marian Dunn, SUNY Downstate Medical Center, Dr. Stephanie Buehler, Newport Beach, California, and Dr. David Ley, Albuquerque, New Mexico.

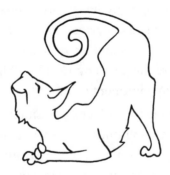

CHAPTER

6

Semen Confidential

Awoman from Utah asked, "Why does male ejaculate smell vaguely of cleaning products?" It's funny how one question can lead to an entire chapter—about semen, not cleaning products. In addition to the bleach-like smell, this chapter looks at semen stains, semen allergies, upset stomachs after swallowing semen, why semen gets clumpy in water and sticks to hair on the shower drain cover, and it answers the mother of all semen questions: "Why does my boyfriend's jizz burn when it gets in my eyes?"

Lock and Load

Semen doesn't pour out of a penis fully homogenized like milk from a carton, even if a guy has been bouncing on a trampoline. The first squirt has secretions from the Cowper (bulbourethral) and Littre glands. The prostate gland manufactures the next wave of man chowder, which is 15% to 30% of the total volume of each ejaculation. This is followed by the relatively small but potent contribution of sperm from the testicles. The seminal vesicles hold up the rear of each ejaculation with a blast that produces 65% to 80% of the entire wad. The total volume of an average ejaculation is between a half and a full teaspoon.

Why Semen Smells Like Clorox

When Ms. Utah asked why male ejaculate smells "vaguely of cleaning products," we assume she is referring to a bleach-like smell, unless the semen of men in Utah smells like Windex, 409, or Janitor in a Drum.

The lion's share of semen comes from two sources: the seminal vesicles and the prostate gland. The testicles make less than 5% of semen. So which of these sources cause semen to have a bleach-like smell?

Urologists know that when you cut open a testicle, there is no odor. So we can rule out testicles and the sperm they produce as being the source of the bleach-like smell. The seminal vesicles aren't the culprit, either. That leaves the prostate gland, which produces a chemical called spermine. This is what gives semen its characteristic cleaning-product smell. Spermine is a member of the polyamine family of chemicals. (Semen also smells like fresh bean sprouts, which makes perfectly good sense because bean sprouts contain the chemical spermine.)

Changes in the pH of semen and variations in how the body buffers it explain why some men's ejaculate smells more bleachy than others, or why one guy's semen might smell more like Clorox one day and less so the next. That's because pH impacts how spermine behaves.

For science and history buffs, spermine phosphate crystals were first found in semen in 1678 by Anton von Leeuwenhoek, father of the modern microscope and the first microbiologist. Semen was one of the first things Leeuwenhoek looked at under his new microscope. Two hundred years later, German chemists gave spermine its name, although women have known about the cleaning-product smell of semen since the time of Aristotle.

As a man is about to ejaculate, the components that make up semen collect in the part of the urethra that runs through the prostate gland. To create an ejaculation, the muscle fibers surrounding this part of the urethra squeeze it like you might the bulb of a turkey baster. At some point during this process, the phosphate in the spermine-phosphate molecules gets pried off. This allows the free base of spermine to be released which creates the bleach-like smell. Semen stops smelling like bleach after it's been in the air for a while because the free bases in spermine start linking together to form an odorless compound.

When a Penis Spits in Your Eye

A few years ago, a reader asked why her boyfriend's ejaculate burns when it gets in her eye. We had given up on ever knowing why after receiving a curt and nasty response from an optometry professor at a leading university. He apparently thought our inquiry was from trolls. Fortunately, an answer has finally emerged and it, too, points to spermine.

While the concentration of spermine in semen isn't nearly as high as when you order it from a chemical supply house, pure spermine carries harsh warnings. The material safety data sheet for commercially produced spermine says:

Danger! Corrosive. Causes eye and skin burns. May cause severe respiratory-tract irritation with possible burns. May cause severe digestive-tract irritation with possible burns. May cause central-nervous-system effects. May cause cardiac disturbances. **Causes eye burns.** May cause chemical conjunctivitis and corneal damage. Causes skin burns.

While there might be other chemicals in semen that cause your eyes to burn, the number one culprit is spermine. Also, semen can be a bit alkaline, which could possibly cause eyeball irritation.

Why an Upset Stomach?

Some women report getting a stomach ache after swallowing their lover's splooge. This is usually blamed on the prostaglandins that are in semen, which might make it similar to the kind of stomach upset that some people get after taking aspirin. However, after reading spermine's material safety data sheet, you can't help but wonder if spermine is also involved.

What Makes Boy Batter Taste Like It Does

A thorough explanation of why male ejaculate tastes the way it does is beyond the scope of this book. However, in looking at the chemicals in semen, the amount of citrate ions stick out as possible culprits. These ions help semen to be a strong buffering agent; they also make for a lot of calcium citrate, which tastes both salty and sour.

Semen has a number of other ions, namely magnesium, potassium, sodium, and zinc. As for how zinc tastes, there's a fairly well-known taste test that's used to determine if people have low levels of zinc. You are given a solution of zinc to drink, and if you can't taste anything, it's because your body has a zinc deficiency. However, if you've got an acceptable level of zinc, the zinc solution tastes "strong and unpleasant." This means that semen may taste better to people who have a zinc deficiency, although it's probably not wise to phone your healthcare provider and say, "My boyfriend's cum tastes really yummy to me. Does this mean I'm zinc-deficient?" Let's just say there's a fair amount of zinc in spunk, and zinc doesn't taste very good unless you have a zinc deficiency or the semen is low in zinc. Ditto for magnesium. And we all know what sodium tastes like.

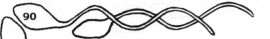

On the bright side, semen does contain fructose and glucose. However, in their "Review of the Physical and Chemical Properties of Human Semen," Owen and Katz discovered that the amount of fructose and glucose can vary as much as four-fold from man to man.

Semen is home to low concentrations of other polyamines by the names of putrescine and cadaverine. These compounds are essential for cells to live. They also announce themselves when cells die. Both putrescine and cadaverine are well-named and are responsible for the rotting flesh smell after things die. This familiar smell is an important indicator of spoilage in food.

Most cheeses that are really smelly and sharp-tasting are high in putrescine, but so is fermented soy sauce, shrimp, and certain citrus fruits. Putrescine and cadaverine are what bring us the fishy smell when women have bacterial infections in their vaginas. One reason why semen doesn't ordinarily smell fishy is because it has a very low concentration of cellular matter, so there are fewer dying cells to produce a fishy odor.

When Semen Smells Bad Rather than Just Bleachy

After being with a couple of men, most women have a baseline sense of what semen usually smells like. However, semen can occasionally have a pungent odor that our andrology-urology consultant says can be the result of a hidden prostate infection. He's referring to a combined bleach-like and fishy odor. The fishy part comes from the polyamines that are released from decaying white blood cells that end up in the semen as a result of the infection in the prostate.

Semen normally contains some white blood cells, but at a very low level. When a man has a prostate infection, the white blood cell count in his semen increases, which results in more of the smelly polyamines like putrescine being liberated:

> "Since I do a lot of semen analysis in my office, I can tell the semen that has lots of white blood cells when we open the container. It has a really strong, bad odor—to the point that my research assistant is able to suspect that men have an infection just from the odor of semen when we are preparing slides to be examined."

Men who have prostatitis might notice yellowish, jellylike globs in their semen. Suspicions also rise when semen has a honey-like sweet smell. This

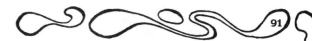

can be the result of a staph infection. Healthy man-jam tends to be mostly white and has the smell of clean, fresh bleach.

Out, Damn Spot

Ever notice that some boys' semen stains are worse than others? Semen contains a lot of protein, much of which is albumin. This is the same kind of protein that is in egg whites, although we don't recommend making omelettes with semen.

As protein dries it changes optical qualities and color. The yellowish staining quality of semen is related to the concentration of protein in it. The concentration of sperm can also have an impact. The higher the sperm count, the more opaque or yellowish semen will be. These factors determine why one guy's semen may have a greater tendency to leave yellowish stains in underwear, sheets and socks he might have used for clean up when jerking off than another guy's semen.

How Thick Is Splooge?

Viscosity is a measure of how fast or slow a liquid flows from a container. The viscosity of male ejaculate fresh from the penis can vary from 1.3 cP to 23.3 cP at room temperature. For reference, the viscosity of water is around 1.0 cP. Given such a range, this means some men's wads are almost as thin as water while others nearly need a grease gun to squirt it out. (Some women cite the texture of semen as being the reason they don't like to swallow when giving blow jobs.)

The viscosity of semen starts to change as soon as it is ejaculated. That's because during ejaculation, a protein made by the prostate gland called prostate-specific antigen (PSA) mixes with the rest of the semen. This starts a reaction that makes semen become more watery so sperm can swim in it. Due to the liquefying power of PSA, semen becomes almost like water within 5 to 30 minutes. If you doubt this, have a guy ejaculate in a glass and watch it for the next 30 minutes. This liquefaction happens even faster when semen is in the vagina. It's why semen drips out of a woman's vagina when she stands up after intercourse.

Volume and Why You'll Probably Never Shoot Like a Porn Star

Semen researchers masturbate a lot. This is why so many studies have been done on the volume of human ejaculation.

These studies show the average volume of a wad is between 2.3 ml and 4.99 ml. For reference, a teaspoon is a pubic hair shy of 5.0 ml. So it's safe to say that the average man shoots between half a teaspoon and a full teaspoon each time he ejaculates. (The average bull weighs between 1,000 and 2,000 lbs. He ejaculates between 4 ml and 8 ml, or not much more than the average human male.)

Semen Allergies

A semen allergy is caused by an allergic reaction to a particular protein in semen that's made by the prostate gland. The onset can vary. A woman could have been just fine with a partner's semen for a couple of years, and then suddenly start having an allergic reaction to it for no good reason. Or she may have had a semen allergy from her very first contact with semen. Symptoms can include pain, redness, burning, swelling, and itching.

Semen allergy is very uncommon. Up to 40,000 women in the United States are thought to have it. One way to decide if the problems are due to semen or chronic vaginitis is to use a condom during intercourse. (It's best to use a polyurethane condom, given how the symptoms might also be from a latex allergy.) If the symptoms stop when you are using a condom but begin again when you don't use a condom, it's time to consider a semen allergy.

Aside from a complete gynecologic exam, a woman will need to get intradermal testing to see if she has an allergy to semen. This is where a small amount of semen is injected under the skin. If this were done on the Syfy Channel, an alien child would start incubating at the injection site. But in real life, it simply determines if there's an allergic reaction.

Fortunately, there is a desensitization treatment for semen allergy that is safe and effective. You need to do it under the supervision of an allergist or immunologist. It is called a "graded challenge" where diluted solutions of semen are placed in the vagina every twenty minutes until the woman is able to tolerate undiluted semen. The "downside" is that the couple has to have intercourse at least two to three times a week from that day forward to maintain the desensitization.

Another thing about semen allergy is a woman doesn't get a bad reaction to the semen of just one guy. If she did, switching partners would be a treatment option, although not always a practical one. If she gets a semen

allergy, it's to all semen from all men. Also, once she develops a semen allergy, it's not just to semen in her vagina. The burning and itching can occur any place where semen touches her skin, including in her mouth or up her bum. As with food allergies, a semen allergy might go away as fast as it arrived.

Why Semen Gets Clumpy in the Shower or Bath

You may have noticed that semen gets clumpy, stringy and sticky when it's in water—like when a guy masturbates in the bath and the semen clumps up and sticks to his skin and body hair, or when he masturbates in the shower and the semen sticks to any hair that's collected on the drain cover.

When semen first comes out of the penis, it's hydrophobic which means it hates water. Even though it's a liquid, when fresh semen makes contact with water, it will form clumps, like the bubbles in Lava lamps. These clumps are semen's way of protecting as much of itself as possible from water. You can see this occur if a guy will ejaculate into a glass of water. His friends will be amazed.

These sticky semen clumps will stick to your skin or shower floor or the hair that's on the shower drain. This is why if a man has roommates and shares a shower, it's only right for him to clean up the shower drain after he's masturbated and his clumpy semen has collected there. (Dorm shower drain covers—YUCK!)

Semen will only clump up if it makes contact with water as a guy is in the process of ejaculating. Otherwise, semen will liquefy or get watery in ten to fifteen minutes. This is why you should tie off the end of a condom, to keep the liquefying semen from dripping out.

Spying on Sperm

It can be very cool to look at your own or your partner's semen under a microscope. What you thought was a gob of sticky goo is actually a metropolis of biological activity. It's like looking down at New York during rush hour, only with sperm instead of Taxi cabs. Here's how you do it:

Materials: You'll need access to a microscope that has 100x and 400x magnifications, a microscope slide and coverslips, and a human male with a hard-on. Make sure the microscope has a good light and that you can focus on the edge of a coverslip that's on a glass slide.

Producing the Sample: This is the funnest part! If you don't know how to produce semen, there are chapters in this book that can help. If you need lube, only use saliva. Most commercial lubricants do evil to sperm.

Timing: You'll want to have the semen under the microscope within 60 to 90 minutes after it is produced.

The Container: As you might recall from the start of this chapter, semen doesn't squirt out pre-mixed. So you'll need to collect the entire ejaculation in the same container. If you don't, you might not be collecting the squirts that have sperm. Be sure to use a container large enough to fit the head of the penis into while it splooges. Do not collect the specimen in a condom unless it's a condom made from polyurethane and has no lube inside. The materials in most condoms are not sperm friendly.

The Semen: While it tends to come out thick, your semen will liquefy within 15 to 20 minutes—so much that it will become almost as thin as water. After it has liquefied, give it a close look with your naked eyes. According to our sperm consultant:

> "If it is clear (transparent), the sperm count is probably low. If it is cloudy but you can see through it (translucent), it is a medium sperm count. If it is creamy white or yellowish and you cannot see through it, it is probably a fairly high sperm count. This is not a measure of fertility, just something interesting. Besides, it only takes one sperm for paternity, and the number of sperm depends on many things, including how often you ejaculate, if you've been in hot tubs or hot baths, what medications you are taking, etc."

The Temperature: Keep your specimen between body temperature and room temperature. Any colder or hotter, and sperm start dropping like flies. If you're taking the semen from your dorm to the biology lab, keep it warm and safe.

Slide Prep: Lightly swirl the semen in the container to mix it. Put a drop or two on the slide, and then place a cover slip over it.

Look-See: Put the slide on the microscope's platform and observe it with the 10x objective (at hopefully a 100x magnification). The sperm are going to be very small and difficult to see. Once you spy sperm, change to the 40x objective, but don't make any significant changes in focus or you risk breaking

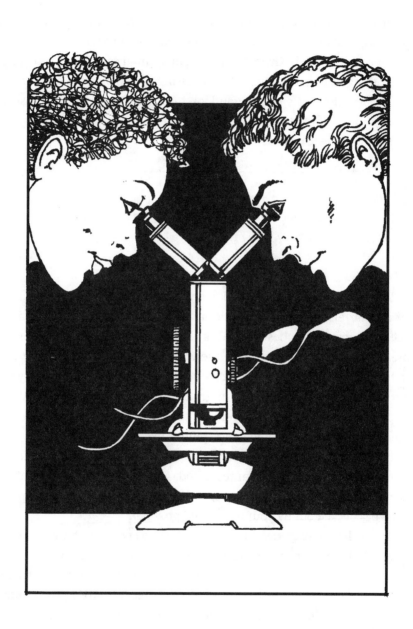

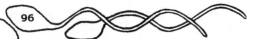

the slide with the lens. If you need to make changes in the focus, go back to the 10x objective and do it that way.

Other Gunk in Your Junk: Semen has more than 300 constituents, including proteins, fats, immature sperm cells, dead parts of old sperm, and occasionally blood cells. Given the less-than optimal conditions you are probably working under, it wouldn't be surprising if 50% or more of your sperm were dead as doornails before you look through the microscope. Also, only about 15% of sperm are the beautiful type with flowing tails, the rest are not like you see in the textbooks.

Dear Paul,

When I have an erection, it starts dripping like I've come before I actually come. Is something wrong with my penis?

Marty from Manitoba

Dear Marty,

It sounds like precum, which is one of nature's finer sex lubes. Unlike your regular ejaculate, precum is clear and oozes out gradually instead of shooting across your chest. It makes the head of your penis slippery and more disposed to slide kindly into the vagina of the love of your life. It may also help make the urethra less acidic so your ejaculate is more likely to get a girl pregnant. You can tell precum from urine by touching it with your fingertip and then pulling your finger away. Precum will stay connected to your finger, making a clear, cool-looking spindle, like bubble gum when you pull part of it out of your mouth. Precum can also drip out with a morning erection or when you've got unwanted wood. Any other fluids of an unknown origin that drip out of your penis, especially if they are a bit green or pus-like, should be checked out by your healthcare provider.

As for the popular idea that precum has no sperm in it, that is not true. Up to 40% of men's precum has low amounts of sperm in it. This could potentially get a woman pregnant, and is why you should not rely on withdrawal or coitus interruptus for birth control. You can also get HIV from an infected person's precum. So make sure a condom goes on early if you are concerned about getting an STI from a male partner.

Be sure to see our video "Pregnant from Precum?" at GuideToGettingItOn.com.

Readers' Comments

*What did you think
the first time you saw a guy ejaculate?*

"I was a little shocked. I was young, 15, and I don't think I understood exactly what was going on. It's also when I realized that tissues weren't just for noses anymore." *female age 27*

"I did it right! Good job! I was proud of me. Then I thought, 'Geez, I hope my mom doesn't come home early.'" *female age 22*

"I remember being disgusted and oddly fascinated at the same time, and I couldn't believe how far that stuff could shoot out!" *female 32*

"It just kind of oozed out. For some reason I thought there was supposed to be more of a stream." *female age 37*

"I was jealous he could actually project it from his body and I couldn't."
female age 23

"I was kinda grossed out by the whole thing." *female age 45*

"I was proud that I made him ejaculate, but I couldn't believe that people actually would let that go in their mouths. I was a senior in high school."
female age 25

"I wondered what it felt like. I wondered what it tasted like. Also, I wondered what it would feel like to have that happen inside of me."
female age 25

"I vaguely remember thinking, it's amazing how their bodily process is. Also, there is what is needed to help form a human being." *female age 36*

A Very Special Thanks: to Steven "Dr. Sperm" Schrader, Ph.D., Darius A. Paduch, MD., PhD, Urology & Reproductive Medicine, Weill Cornell Medical College, and Jennifer Collins, MD, Albert Einstein School of Medicine.

For the latest on what's inside a girl, visit:

www.GuideToGettingItOn.com

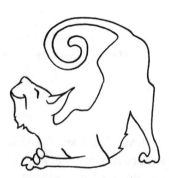

7
What's Inside a Girl?

What follows is an experience the author of this book had with women's genitals when he was 11-years-old. He had been in the big city for a week visiting relatives and it was time to catch the Greyhound bus to return home.

Busses didn't always have bathrooms, so it was good to go before you boarded. The men's bathroom in the Greyhound bus depot was a palace of porcelain fixtures and horrible smells. At the end of a long row of sinks sat three vending machines.

One of the machines had men's colognes; you could spritz yourself with Old Spice or Brut for a dime. The next machine had a strange looking product from France that claimed to tickle women. And the third machine said *Instant Pussy—2 Quarters.*

To put this into perspective, candy bars weren't much more than a nickel, and two quarters amounted to a near fortune. Then again, the front of the third machine promised a facsimile so exact that you couldn't tell the instant pussy from the real thing.

For the next fifteen minutes, the boy pondered the ultimate existential question: ten candy bars or instant pussy, ten candy bars or instant pussy, ten candy bars or instant pussy.

It was different for boys back then. There was no Wikipedia, and porn consisted of hard-to-find nudist magazines with women who had so much pubic hair that Pomeranian dogs might as well have been sitting on their laps. Women at the beach were of no help either—bikinis as we know them today were a dream of the future, and the bottoms of two-piece bathing suits looked like a cross between granny panties and ill-fitting Spanx. Whatever information you could find about women's genitals came from reading the encyclopedia or from the instructions in your sister's tampon box.

So you can understand why a boy might have left the men's bathroom with two fewer quarters and a sense of hope that a box of Instant Pussy would reveal at least something about one of life's greatest mysteries.

The rest of the day was spent in quiet anticipation, with thoughts of instant pussy overwhelming whatever sights and sounds the long trip home had to offer. After hours on the bus, the boy arrived home and anxiously opened the small box. The instructions said, "Place capsule in a large glass of warm water." He took out a thermometer and tried to make the water a perfect 98.6. Then came the big moment. He crossed himself and revved up his courage. His trembling fingers dropped the capsule into the glass. Then he waited for the hidden mystery to unfold. And he waited. And he waited.

Forty minutes went by before the gelatin capsule melted and revealed a thin piece of sponge in the shape of a cat.

A grown man would have known to go for the candy bars. But the boy was still clinging to the hope that there were answers to questions that felt so much bigger than he.

Porn vs. Reality

Times have changed when it comes to seeing what's between women's legs. Porn has become the gateway for all things having to do with sex. In porn, a woman's vagina is ready to accept any penis at any time. There is no discussion, preparation, or need for permission. There's no sense of how complex women's genitals can be, especially the parts you can't see.

Although men's and women's genitals are made from many of the same cells, if a man approaches a woman's genitals in the same way he does his own—or the way he sees it done in porn—he and his partner might be missing out on a lot of fun.

Women's Sexual Anatomy — The Nerve of It All

In the late 1950s, a scientist named Kermit Krantz dissected the genital regions of eight dead women. He explored how women's genitals are wired. It is difficult to find a single research report on the topic of women's sexuality that is of more value than the one produced by Kermit Krantz.

He found a great deal of variation in the way the nerve endings are distributed throughout the different women's genitals. While there tended to be a higher concentration of nerve endings in the clitoris, the amount varied significantly among the different women. Some had more nerve endings in the labia minora (inner lips) than in the clitoris, and some women's nerve endings were highly concentrated in one area while other women had nerve endings that were spread out over a larger area. To quote Dr. Krantz:

"The extent of innervation in different females varies greatly."

What this suggests is that no two women get off sexually in the exact same way. Each woman needs to explore her own unique sexual universe, from where to touch to the kinds of fantasies that get her off. One woman might love oral sex and only be so-so about intercourse, while the next craves a penis between her legs. Another woman might prefer oral sex with Trevor, but intercourse with Isiah.

A man won't know exactly what a woman likes in bed until she tells him. It's not the sort of awareness he is going to assimilate during a one-night stand or from watching a lifetime of porn. He needs to feel comfortable asking questions and taking direction.

Unfortunately, porn has given a lot of women the idea that a man should magically know how to please a woman in bed. Nothing could be further from the truth.

Show & Tell

"While women speak to each other in graphic terms about things like menstruation, blow jobs, and the ratio of penis size to male ego, we usually don't talk to each other about what our crotches look like; not that we'd necessarily want to." *female age 34*

Most guys know what their penises look like. That's because male genitals stick out. You can't help but notice. But women don't usually look at their own genitals, and even when they do, much of the sexually reactive parts are inside their pelvis where they can't be seen without an ultrasound machine.

Before the easy availability of porn, there were politically correct beaver books published by feminists to show women how much variation there is in different women's genitals. This was helpful, because there is way more variation in women's genitals than we see in today's porn.

But the muff shots in the politically-correct beaver books had a sterile edge that was not particularly inviting. The new-age beaver books were missing a woman's perspective that said, "What we have between our legs is a good thing. It's cool, it's nice, we like it." There is something reassuring about a woman who finds her genitals to be sexy. Perhaps it's why some men nearly ejaculate on the spot if a partner enjoys masturbating and lets him hold her or watch while she's doing it. Maybe it explains some of the allure of lingerie. It's in knowing that a woman finds her genitals sexy enough to cover them in a sensual or erotic way.

Busy Little Beavers

People refer to everything between a woman's legs as her vagina or "down there." Yet this is far from true. What sits between a naked woman's legs is her vulva.

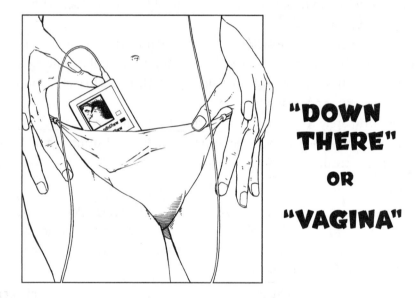

"DOWN THERE" OR "VAGINA"

You might ask, "What difference does it make if you call it a vulva, vagina or 'down there'?" One female educator answered this question with a question of her own: "What if parents taught their children that they had no eyes, ears, nose or mouth, but instead gave them one word for their entire face and called it 'tongue'?" This would be confusing. And it might suggest that parents are afraid of faces and all the wonderful things they can do.

Some men see no need to learn about the different structures that are between a woman's legs. They figure, "My penis goes in there just fine. She likes it, I like it, what's more to learn?" And some women are more concerned with how to wax their genitals than in knowing more about them. Hopefully, you'll want to know what's inside a girl's genitals. It can made a big difference in the pleasure you are able to give and receive.

The Vulva

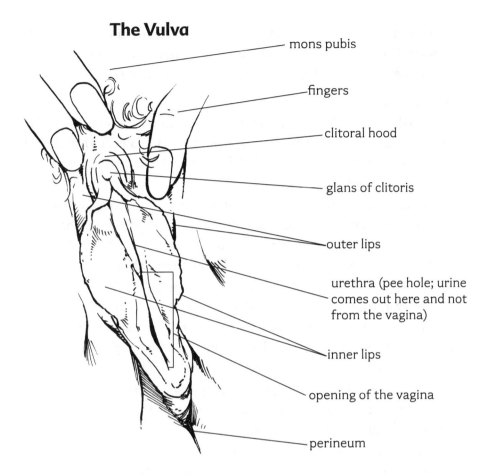

mons pubis

fingers

clitoral hood

glans of clitoris

outer lips

urethra (pee hole; urine comes out here and not from the vagina)

inner lips

opening of the vagina

perineum

The Mons: Love-Making Ally

The mons pubis is a fleshy mound of tissue that sits on top of the pubic bone. It is made up of fat and is usually covered by pubic hair, unless a woman shaves.

The tissue inside the mons is sensitive to estrogen. So when a woman goes through puberty, the added estrogen turns the mons into a mound. The mons pushes the upper part of the larger labia out and forms the pudendal cleft, which is the top part of what some people call "the camel toe." Some mons are very prominent, others not so much.

The suspensory ligament of the clitoris has its base in the mons pubis, and the neck of the clitoris runs through part of the mons. This is why some women will push, pull, or make a circular motion with their fingers on their mons when they masturbate. A woman might enjoy it if a partner pushes his fingers against the mons and rubs it in a circular motion or pulls it upward. This might also apply pressure to the deeper parts of the clitoris. Some women like the feeling when a partner tugs on their pubic hair.

Lips, Lips, Lips

Even the ancient Romans got it wrong. They named the outer lips "labia majora" (big lips) and the inner lips "labia minora" (small lips). They should have called them "inner" and "outer," given how the inner lips are often more major than the outer lips.

The outer lips are made from the same embryological tissue as the scrotum. This is why their skin is so similar to that of the scrotum. Both have the same sweat glands, nerve endings and hair follicles, and both produce the same nice sensations when they are kissed and caressed by a lover.

If a baby is going to be a boy, nature fuses the outer labia to make the sack that eventually covers the testicles. The seam down the middle of the scrotum is where the outer labia fused together. If the baby is going to be female, the opening between the labia remains and two lips fill with fatty tissue. The labia majora can vary greatly in size, shape and color.

The labia minora or inner lips often give vulvas their unique personalities. They start just beneath the clitoris and can run all the way to the bottom of the vagina. They fan out in different ways and shapes, and when a woman is aroused, they perk up and deepen in color.

The inner labia are made of the same tissue as the head of the penis, only they are thinner. They are sexually reactive, which means the tissue becomes engorged and can double or triple in thickness when a woman is sexually aroused. The skin on the inner labia has no hair, and the edges of the labia minora are packed with nerves. As a result, touching and caressing the inner labia can signal the brain to make woman's genitals ready for sexual intercourse.

Since the inner labia attach at the bottom of the glans of the clitoris, some women find it feels really nice when a partner gently tugs on them or massages them. This is an indirect way of stimulating the most sensitive part of the clitoris.

The inner lips can be from three-quarters of an inch long to four inches long, and they can be from one-quarter of an inch to two inches wide. They

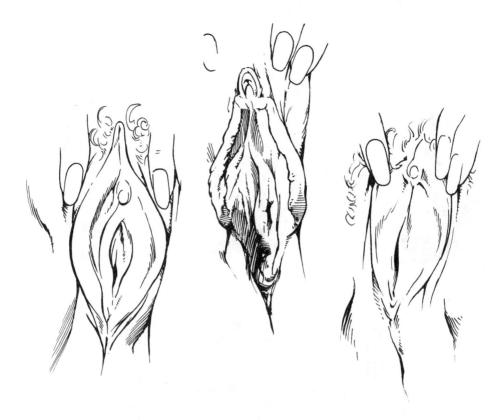

can stretch a bit when tugged. Just like breasts, they can be asymmetrical and it's normal for one to be double the width of the other. In some parts of Africa the labia minora can be as large as eight inches because the women intentionally stretch them. Here in the States, women worry their inner labia are too big and some even consider having them surgically downsized with an operation called labiaplasty.

The inner lips attach to the glans of the clitoris. Some women play with them or stroke them when they are masturbating. Caressing the inner lips or gently tugging on them can provide a neat way of stimulating the clitoris.

During intercourse, the inner lips are pushed and pulled with each stroke of the penis, which can tug and stimulate the glans of the clitoris.

The Perfect Puss?—Porn Is No Friend of the Inner Labia

Porn loves small inner labia. Some porn actresses have inner labia that are naturally petite, while others had theirs trimmed through a surgical process known as labiaplasy. As for perspective on what labia or real women

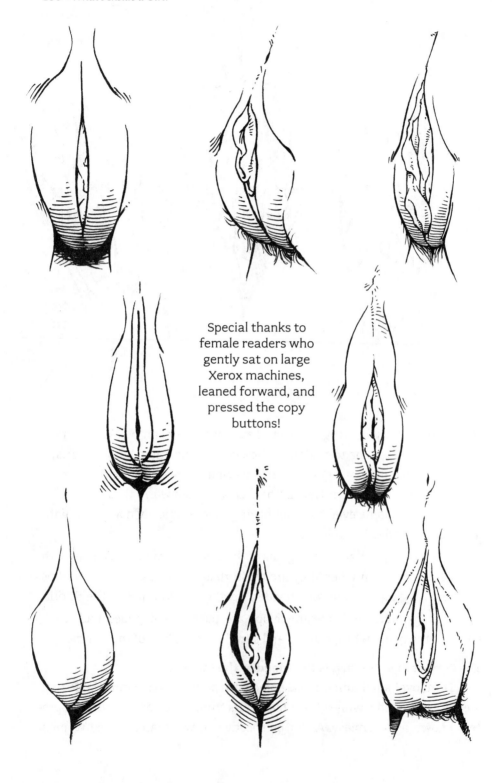

Special thanks to female readers who gently sat on large Xerox machines, leaned forward, and pressed the copy buttons!

really look like, one of the best people on the planet to ask would be a lesbian photographer and pornographer:

> "Lesbians are at an advantage in the vaginal knowledge department because we see our lovers' pussies all the time. We get up close and personal with real cunts in all of their real imperfection. But most straight women don't have the kind of access to vaginas that you get from licking box all the time. Many of my straight female friends have told me that the majority of up-close-and-personal views they've had of various vulvas have come from porn. And worse than that, some women feel insecure about their own coochies when they don't look like the ones in *Playboy*.

> "Well, let me just set the record straight: Cunts don't really look like that. Trust me. I'm a pornographer."

> –From Diana Cage's *Box Lunch: The Layperson's Guide To Cunnilingus*

Perfection is no more common between a woman's legs than it is between a man's. A lack of symmetry is one of the wonderful things about being human.

Clitoris: Point Guard for Women's Genitals

Most people think a clitoris is the little knob you see when a woman spreads her legs. But as you can see in the illustrations on the following pages, there's much more to the clitoris than that.

The glans or tip is a small but potent part of the clitoris. The hood-like structure that drapes over the glans is just that—the hood. It's like the foreskin on a penis. When women masturbate, they often press a fingertip against the hood and rub it in a small circle or back and forth.

The hood of the clitoris can usually glide over the glans without it feeling abrasive. However, some hoods are bonded to the clitoris. This is perfectly okay and the sexual sensation usually feels fine. Surgery to separate the hood from the glans is seldom necessary or wise.

Some women find their clitoris changes sensitivity with the time of the month, in others it keeps an even keel.

As a woman approaches orgasm, it can seem like the tip of her clitoris disappears or retracts. This can be confusing for the man who is trying to stimulate the clitoris by hand or mouth. Should he play Hercule Poirot and give chase, or wait until the clitoris returns?

The Clitoris and Surrounding Structures

All you see of the clitoris when looking between a woman's legs is the tip or glans. There's much more of the clitoris inside a woman's pelvis.

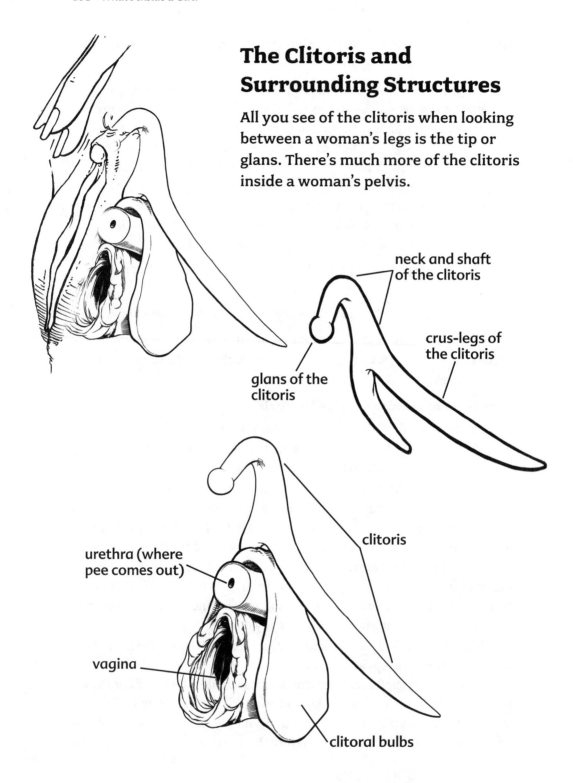

neck and shaft of the clitoris

crus-legs of the clitoris

glans of the clitoris

clitoris

urethra (where pee comes out)

vagina

clitoral bulbs

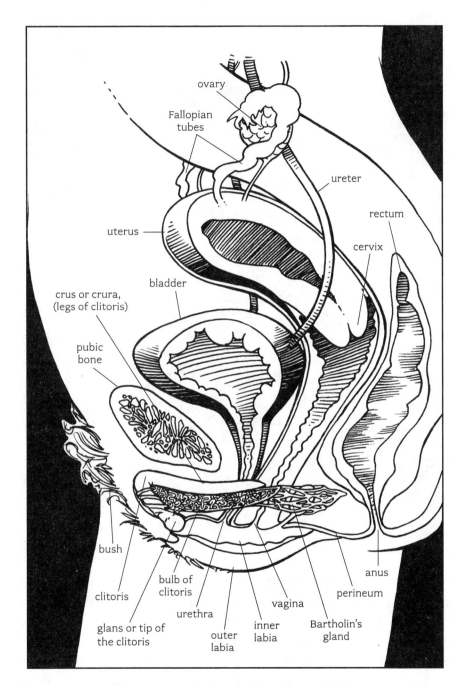

ovary

Fallopian
tubes

ureter

rectum

uterus

cervix

crus or crura,
(legs of clitoris)

bladder

pubic
bone

bush

clitoris

anus

perineum

bulb of
clitoris

vagina

Bartholin's
gland

urethra

glans or tip of
the clitoris

inner
labia

outer
labia

What's Inside a Girl

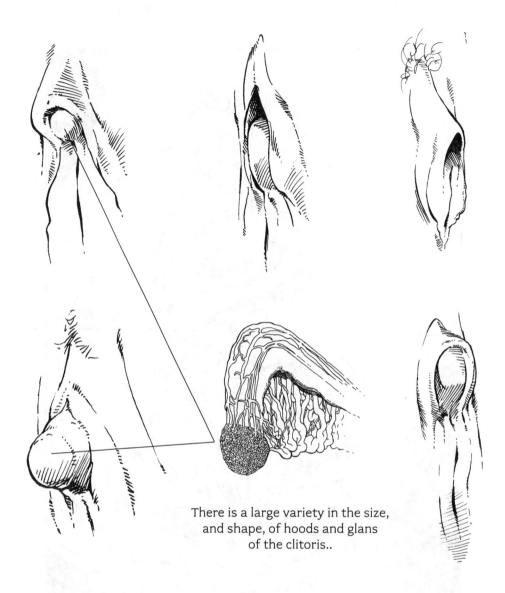

There is a large variety in the size,
and shape, of hoods and glans
of the clitoris..

No one quite knows why the clitoris seems to sometimes disappear at the height of sexual arousal. The mystery could be due to pelvic muscle contractions that cause the shaft and glans to straighten out. If you are stimulating the clitoris with your finger or tongue, it might feel like it suddenly starts to hide or retract. If whatever you were doing managed to get it to throb or spasm, don't change now unless the woman indicates otherwise. Let the clitoris play its game of cat and mouse.

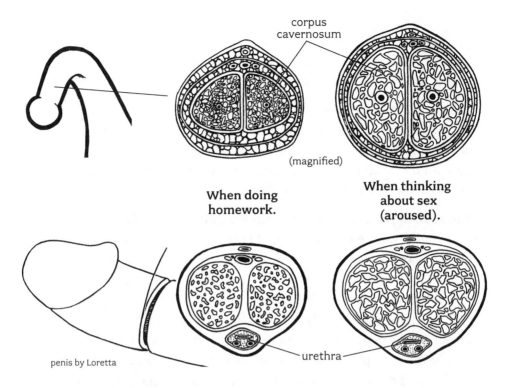

corpus
cavernosum

(magnified)

**When doing
homework.**

**When thinking
about sex
(aroused).**

penis by Loretta

urethra

X-Section of the Shaft of the Clitoris and a Penis

The Size of the Clitoris

Guys aren't the only ones who worry about genital size. Some women worry that the tip or glans of their clitoris is too big, others wish theirs was more easy to find.

The size of the tip or glans of the clitoris can vary greatly. In some women, it nearly pops out to shake your hand; in others it can hardly be seen. It is usually a little smaller than a pencil eraser, but it can range from being barely noticeable to being the size of a toe or a small penis. The clitoris also becomes from 50% to 300% larger when a woman is sexually aroused.

It's unfortunate anyone worries about the size of a clitoris, because there's no relationship between its size and the sensations it is capable of producing. So there is no limit to the enjoyment a woman can have with her clitoris regardless of how big or small it is. Also, there is no relationship between a woman's height or weight and the size of her clitoris, although childbirth probably makes it larger.

The size of the clitoris is impacted by hormones which rev up during puberty. As a result, by the time a women is in her early thirties, the tip of her clitoris will be up to four times larger than it was when she began puberty.

The Crura of the Clitoris

The clitoris proper has three different parts: the glans or tip, the shaft, and the crura or legs. The crura look like the legs of a wishbone. They run beneath the labia. The shaft and crura contain bodies of erectile tissue that are called the corpus cavernosum, just like the cylinders that are in the penis.

The Bulbs of the Clitoris aka "Vestibular Bulbs"—Clitoris Adjacent

Mother Nature planted a pair of bulbs inside her favorite garden. They are called the bulbs of the clitoris, and they swell and blossom each time a woman is sexually aroused. They are close to the clitoris and communicate with it through blood vessels, but they are made of slightly different tissue.

The bulbs of the clitoris are more elastic than the clitoris. They expand proportionally more than the clitoris or penis when a woman is aroused and they have larger spaces that blood can rush into than the clitoris or penis.

There is debate about whether the bulbs are actually part of the clitoris and if they should be called the bulbs of the clitoris or simply the vestibular bulbs. Whatever the case, they appear to be sexually reactive.

The Axis of Arousal—Clitoris, Clitoral Bulbs & Labia Minora

When a woman becomes sexually aroused, her clitoris, clitoral bulbs and inner lips become engorged with blood. These structures seem to communicate with each other when a woman is becoming sexually excited. It's not like they text each other, but all three are highly involved when sexual excitement is in the air. (Researcher Helen O'Connell might suggest we include the urethral sponge, making the axis of arousal a quartet. And changes the tissues surrounding the vagina are also part of women's arousal.)

Suggestion: Take a moment and look at the diagrams of the clitoris in this chapter. See the placement of the crura and the bulbs? Some women enjoy it when a partner does a deep fingertip massage of the tissue that's beneath their labia. It might seem like it would be painful, but you may be stimulating rich vascular beds. With plenty of feedback and a willingness to explore, you'll learn what feels good and what doesn't. (For more, see Chapter 15: *The Zen of Finger Fucking*.)

The Clitoris during Intercourse

"I rub the heck out of my clitoris during intercourse. I do it to reach an orgasm when my partner is almost there." *female age 25*

"I almost always rub on my clit during intercourse. I usually make small circular motions, which is not how I move my finger when I masturbate. I love when he does it too, although sometimes I have to move his hand into the correct spot." *female age 24*

"I have tried rubbing my clit once or twice, but prefer to focus my attention on his dick inside of me." *female age 20*

The glans of the clitoris is seldom positioned to rub noses with an incoming penis. Many women enjoy the added stimulation of a finger or vibrator during intercourse, or they push the clitoris against the shaft of a sweetheart's thrusting penis or grind it against his pubic bone.

More than 85% of the women who have taken our sex survey and who have orgasms during intercourse do not have orgasms by thrusting alone. Either they or their partner stimulate their clitoris with fingers while the penis is thrusting, or they grind their clitoris into his pubic bone. Other women do just fine with thrusting alone. Research is beginning to suggest that a woman may be more likely to have orgasms from intercourse if the glans of her clitoris is located closer to the opening of her vagina, possibly allowing it to get more stimulation from the penis.

Be sure to see our videos on The Clitoris at GuideToGettingItOn.com.

A Final Note on the Clitoris — How Do You Pronounce It?

Years ago, the author of this book had to address a classroom of students and he needed to say "clitoris." There he was, with more than a decade of college under his belt, not knowing how to pronounce the word "clitoris." To prepare, he wrote "clitoris" on one card and "penis" on another. He showed the card to friends of both sexes and asked them to say the words out loud.

No one hesitated in pronouncing penis, but almost everyone approached clitoris with a perplexed look and said, "Well, here's how I have always pronounced it." Some said cli-TOR-is, others said CLIT-or-is. Either pronunciation is correct, although many people call the clitoris "it."

Urinary Meatus — Might Be More Fun Than It Sounds

In the area between the inner lips, which is called the 'vestibule,' there is a small circle of firm tissue around the end of the urethra (where pee comes out.) Vertically, it is between the tip of the clitoris and the mouth of the vagina. It is sensitive enough that some women rub it when they are masturbating. It is called the "urethral meatus," which is Greek for "pee through it and play with it if you like."

The Vagina

The human body is made up of many different tubes. The favorite tube of many straight males and lesbians is the vagina, a hollow canal with walls that contain four layers of tissue, nerves and blood vessels. When not aroused, the walls of the vagina lie flat against each other like a firehose without water. When aroused, the vagina straightens out. The first third of her vagina becomes narrower, while the back part may balloon a bit.

Some women particularly enjoy stimulation at the opening of their vagina. That's because the opening of the vagina has touch receptors.

> "The main request I ask of my partner is to tease me with his cock. That's because most of the sensitivity in my vagina is at the opening."
>
> *female age 25*

While the first third of the vagina is often sensitive to touch, the back two-thirds are more sensitive to pressure. This is why having a thicker object such as a penis or dildo in the back of the vagina can feel extra good when a woman is masturbating or when her clitoris is being stimulated.

Vaginal Ruggae

During the years between puberty and menopause, the surface of the vagina has tiny folds or ridges that make it seem corrugated. These are called the vaginal ruggae. They help the vagina to expand during intercourse and childbirth. But before puberty and after menopause, the surface of the vagina is mostly smooth.

Vaginal Tenting

As a woman becomes more aroused, the back of her vagina will often expand or balloon open, and her cervix will raise up. This is called vaginal

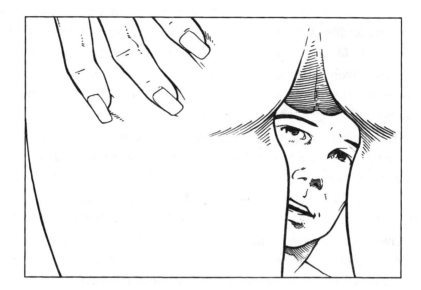

tenting. You can feel it with your fingers if you have them extended into the back part of a woman's vagina when she's highly aroused. This might cause a woman to long for something inside her vagina which the rear walls can grasp.

Vaginal Farts

"My boyfriend was performing oral sex on me and fingering my vagina. When I sat up, all of the air in my vagina came rushing out and made a huge fartlike noise. I was totally embarrassed; it was completely unexpected. I looked at my boyfriend with shock on my face, and then we both started laughing." *female age 25*

Air can get trapped inside a vagina and make a fartlike noise when it comes out. This happens frequently. It's normal room air that is seeping out. Unlike real farts, it doesn't smell and won't peel the paint off the walls.

Vaginal farts are more likely to happen after you have had an orgasm and the rear part of your vagina ballooned open. The noise can happen when your vagina is returning to its resting state and the collected air rushes out. The Scottish utilized this principle to create the bagpipe. Vagina farts can also happen when you are not having sex, like in a yoga class.

A Tipped Uterus

The uterus is an upside-down pear-shaped organ that is located between a woman's bladder and her rectum. It is where human infants spend their first 40 weeks. Many people consider it to be the strongest muscle in the body.

In most women, the uterus tips toward the front of her body. But up to 30% of women have a uterus that is tipped, retroverted or tilted, meaning that the uterus points up or more toward the back.

This might be why some women with a tipped uterus experience period pain more as a back ache than a pain in their abdomen, and why they tend to have more back pain and diarrhea when they are menstruating. Some women with a tipped uterus know when their period is coming because they start having loose stools that might be caused by a release of prostaglandins.

Given how the vagina and uterus are positioned, a reversal in the direction of the uterus can make certain intercourse positions painful for a woman with a tipped uterus that are not painful for a woman whose uterus is pointing forward.

If you have a tipped uterus and experience pain during rear entry intercourse, it might be due to the penis banging into your uterus or your ovaries. The pain might also come from extra air that can accumulate during intercourse in the vagina of a woman with a tipped uterus. So your lover needs to realize that while his former partner might have been the Reverse Cowgirl Queen, this position could cause you a lot of pain. On the other hand, you might excel at intercourse in the missionary position.

Here's what three women who took our sex survey say, but what works for you may be very different than this.

"My uterus is tilted. It makes doggy-style intercourse painful. I prefer to be on top of my boyfriend."

"I have a very tipped uterus. Unless I'm pregnant they can't pick it up on a regular ultrasound because it leans so far backwards. Intercourse feels best with me on top or missionary. I've found that doggie style isn't very comfortable for me, nor is me being on top while facing his feet. As long as we are close to each other, belly touching belly, deep thrusting is fine. If we are separate, like if I'm laying down and he is in an upright position, deep thrusting can

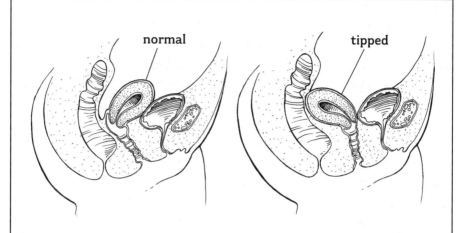

Uterus Alignment

*A tipped or tilted uterus points toward the back instead of the front
or it can be aligned at any point in between.*

be uncomfortable. Where I'm at in my cycle also plays a role in how comfortable or uncomfortable things are."

"I have a tipped uterus, and this may be why it hurts when my partner thrusts too deep. It may also be why I don't like to be penetrated from the rear. Being on top is the most comfortable position for me and the one that provides the highest likelihood of orgasm."

There is a popular myth that women with tipped uteruses can't conceive as easily as other women. Don't believe it. Many women with a tipped uterus go their entire lives without even knowing it's tipped. Poorly fitted bras will cause far more inconvenience in life for most women than a tipped uterus.

Some women with a tipped or tilted uterus refer to it as an "inverted uterus." However, an inverted uterus is a rare event that happens when your uterus turns inside out right after you've given birth.

Also, the uterus can sometimes become tipped due to a problem such as endometriosis, so if you start having discomfort with intercourse, be sure to tell your doctor. As with all questions regarding matters of health, the information in a book can never take the place of an exam from a gynecologist.

The Cervix and Fornix

The cervix is a small, fleshy dome in the rear of the vagina. It acts as a gatekeeper that joins the uterus and the vagina. The cervix can be as small as a cherry in a woman who has not delivered a baby through her vagina, or it can be much bigger. It has a dimple in the center that menstrual fluids flow down and male ejaculate flows up. Science doesn't yet understand the role of the cervix in sexual response.

The cervix sometimes feels softer during ovulation, when mucus passes through it to help bathe the vagina. This keeps the environment clean and more acidic, which are conditions that encourage conception. At mid-cycle, when conception is most likely to occur, the mucus becomes clear and slippery, like raw egg-whites.

The cervix has a space around it called the fornix. This is a delightful area to explore with a finger. When women are approaching orgasm, this part of the vagina will often balloon open. (See "Vaginal Tenting" on pages 114-115.) Some women find stimulation of the space around the fornix to be pleasing. It is also a good space to know about when a woman's vagina isn't particularly deep or her lover has a long penis. Couples in this situation might experiment with intercourse positions that encourage the penis to slide under the cervix and into the fornix.

From a sex therapist: Women often report feeling pain during sex that is deep in their vagina. What they may be feeling is the pain of their partner's penis hitting the cervix. Women are often surprised about this and don't realize what they are feeling is their cervix! In many cases it happens because they are not aroused so their vagina is not fully tilted. They should slow down and get aroused or change position.

There are at least two ways to see a cervix. The first is by using a speculum. This is a metal or plastic device that physicians insert into a woman's vagina to help push the walls apart. It allows the physician to see parts of a woman that few women or their sexual partners ever do. If you have a healthy curiosity, get a speculum from your physician or medical-supply store. Lube it with KY jelly, gently insert it into the vagina and add the beam of your favorite flashlight or phone. For the woman to see her own cervix, she will need to incorporate a hand-held mirror or the camera from a phone into the process. (For more on pelvic exams and using a speculum, please see Chapter 47: *Vulva Care: Keeping Your Kitty Happy.*)

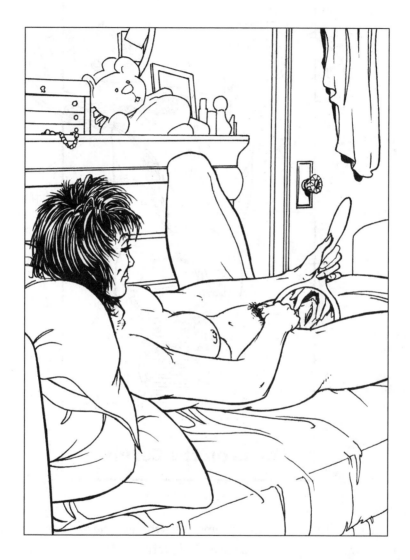

You might try using the camera on your phone instead of a mirror. Even without a speculum, it's always good for a woman to check out her genitals. They shouldn't be a part of her body that only a lover gets to see and enjoy.

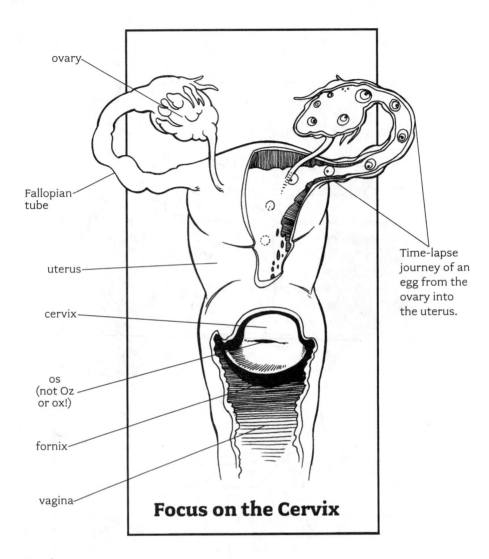

ovary

Fallopian
tube

uterus

cervix

os
(not Oz
or ox!)

fornix

vagina

Time-lapse
journey of an
egg from the
ovary into
the uterus.

Focus on the Cervix

Ovaries

A man's testicles announce themselves wherever he goes. Not so with a woman's ovaries. It's possible to have a long-term relationship with a woman and not even know her ovaries are there, except indirectly through events like periods and pregnancy.

The best time to feel a woman's ovaries is when she is lying on her back and is in an "It's okay if you feel my ovaries" mood. Rest one hand on her lower abdomen below her belly button. Place a lubricated finger or two from your other hand deep into her vagina. When you encounter the rear wall of her vagina, veer to the left or right and push up gently while push-ing down with the hand that's on her abdomen. You will need to rely on her instructions. If a woman doesn't know where her ovaries are, she might ask her gynecologist to show her.

Sponges Around the Urethra

There is a spongy area above the walls of the vagina called the urethral sponge. The urethral sponge is tissue that surrounds the entire length of the urethra, which is the tube that takes urine from the bladder to the toilet. It runs along the roof of the vagina. If a woman his sexually aroused and you put your finger in a vagina and make a "come here" motion, you are pushing into the urethral sponge. Some women find this feels good. Others find it to be annoying.

The tissue of the urethral sponge contains tiny periurethral glands that have an embryological and histological similarity to the prostate. However, there is no prostate gland in the female pelvis.

G-Spot Area

Over the past ten years, the G-spot has become a major industry, com-plete with G-spot books, G-spot vibrators, G-spot toys, and G-spot videos.

While researchers don't question the orgasms that some women have with G-spot stimulation, there isn't any special wiring or trigger-tissue in the G-spot area that would make its stimulation universally wonderful for all women. So what is it about stimulating this area that makes it feel really good for some women but not others?

One of the problems is that until recently, we've mainly been limited to doing research on cadavers. And while some of these dead women might still be orgasming in the afterlife, researchers can't see how different parts of a person's sexual anatomy interact when they're dead.

With newer technology, we'll find more answers regarding the G-spot area. However, the debate will continue for a while longer.

One explanation of the G-spot has been proposed by one of our gyne-cology consultants. She says, "I always felt that the G-spot was actually a stimulation of the area that corresponded to the trigone of the bladder and that was why many women felt even greater sensations when their bladders were slightly full during sex. I have some patients who intentionally drink fluids to fill their bladder prior to sexual play because it 'feels better'. When they do this, I think the trigone presses down more on the anterior vaginal wall and is more easily stimulated." This corresponds with the experience of many women who find that G-spot area stimulation causes a feeling of bladder fullness:

> "When my partner is going down on me and inserts his finger, placing pressure upwards on the top wall of my vaginal canal, it feels really really good if I ignore that it also feels like I need to pee."
>
> *female age 24*

One of the top sex researchers in the world was kind enough to weigh in the G-spot controversy for readers of *The Guide*. His take on the G-spot area is that when you are stimulating the anterior wall of the vagina you are stimulating parts of the urethra, the urethrovaginal 'space,' the clitoris via the ligaments connecting to it, the vaginal wall, and possibly Kobelt's plexus. He believes that all of these participate in arousing the brain. But he also says that where and how you fit the G-spot into an 'anterior vaginal wall complex' is a challenge.

The G-Spot Bottom Line

With all of the media hype and sex-store attention about G-spot stimulation, some readers will be thinking, "Why spend so much time with a woman's clitoris when I could be stimulating her G-spot?" The answer should depend totally on what your partner wants rather than on what someone else tells you.

Mercifully, Claire Yang, M.D., a neurophysiologist and researcher in the Department of Urology at the University of Washington, has the following to say:

> "I think that because the sexual response is so closely linked to emotions, the experience of pleasure, and in particular sexual pleasure, it is not going to be tied directly to anatomical structure, even during sexual arousal. For instance, why do women not feel sexual stimulation when those same areas that you describe are being examined during a gyn exam? The bottom line is: the entire genital area has nerves (as does the entire body), and in the context of

sexual arousal, the processing of the messages is what makes the experience, not just the manual stimulation. I think the processing of sexual stimulation by the female brain is extremely variable, and to pin down a particular area (or situation) that is universally arousing is not possible at this time. That is why the concept of the G-spot has not gained universal acceptance. That is why the pursuit of a female sexual-arousal drug has been elusive. That is why the female sexual response will remain a mystery for a little while longer."

The writers at the major women's magazines routinely call the author of *The Guide* to ask about this spot or that spot, and the latest position that's supposed to be mother of all intercourse positions. It's seldom enough if he says, "This might feel good for some women, but not for others. A woman should explore for herself and find what does and doesn't work for her."

For more on the mechanics of G-spot area exploration, please see Chapter 15: *The Zen of Finger Fucking.*

Variations in Wetness

When sexually aroused, some women's vaginas get so wet that the woman needs to wring out her underwear. Other women can be every bit as aroused, but their vaginas remain dry. Wetness also varies during certain phases of a woman's menstrual cycle. Contrary to what you might think, some women need to add lube for period sex. That's because a woman's estrogen levels are at their lowest point during her period, and this can result in a decrease in natural lubrication.

Men shouldn't be so silly as to gauge a woman's level of sexual arousal on vaginal wetness alone. It's possible for a woman to be very aroused, but not very wet. On the other hand, there's been a lot of ridiculousness regarding women's sexual wetness thanks to porn. In porn, a woman's vagina is always ready for anything a guy (or guys) want to ram up it.

We used to say that most women require at least twenty minutes of making out and fooling around before a partner should even reach between her legs. But people assume sex in real life is supposed to happen like sex in porn. Maybe this is one of the reasons why so many women in their teens and twenties are experiencing pain during intercourse.

Female Sexual Arousal

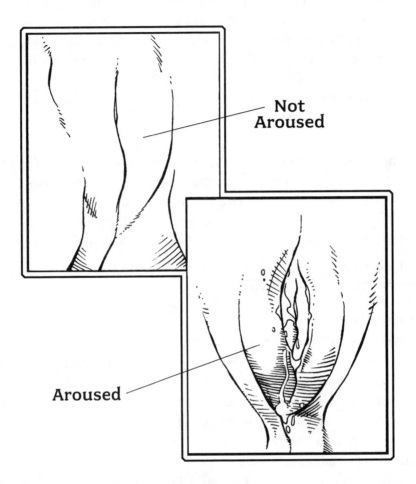

**Not
Aroused**

Aroused

Not all vulvas show this degree of change with sexual arousal, but the changes inside a woman's pelvis during arousal can be extensive.

While some women are quickly aroused and are ready for fingering, oral sex or intercourse as soon as the women in porn, most women require actual effort on the part of a partner in the form of kissing, caressing, and fun before they are ready to have sex. This doesn't mean women like sex any less than men. It's probably because sexual arousal occurs differently in women's brains than in men's, but no one knows for sure.

As for extra wetness during or just before orgasms, some women have a little, others have a lot. The combined sex fluids of both partners have been known as the wet spot on the mattress. Its diameter can vary from couple to couple.

If you happen to be a gusher or a bed-drencher, please don't think that any man in his right mind is going to have a problem with it. Why not have fun shopping together for sets of towels that are just for sex? And if you are worried about the mattress, take solace in knowing that they now make waterproof mattress-pad covers that feel and sound like normal mattress-pad covers. They are wonderful!

Female Ejaculation, Squirting or Gushing

Some women expel extra fluid at the time of orgasm. The biggest problem with this is that women who do it sometimes feel embarrassed and try to prevent it. As a result, they keep themselves from fully relaxing, and this can inhibit orgasms and pleasure.

The second problem is what porn has done with it. A few years ago, a porn actress wrote a book on "female ejaculation." She began giving workshops where she claimed that "female ejaculation" was nothing short of amazing, and that any woman could become a female ejaculator with the right training. Rather than just a few milliliters of "female ejaculate," women were being encouraged to ejaculate a cup or more of fluid.

Now, a decade later, we know that the paraurethral glands can only produce 2 to 4 mls of fluid. This is similar to what the male prostate gland produces during ejaculation. Much more than that, and it's urine from the bladder that's being released. Some experts in female sexual health are starting to be concerned that women who have been forcing themselves to squirt during sex might be causing their bladders to prolapse. However, this has done nothing to put a dent into the "gusher," "female squirting" and "female ejaculation" categories of porn.

As for what we currently do and don't know about female ejaculation, some women release up to a teaspoon of fluid from their urethra at the time of orgasm. This is not urine. It is most likely produced by the paraurethral glands and it may often go into the bladder instead of squirting out of the body, so the woman is not aware of it. (More studies need to be done. For now, the best we can say is this is what seems to happen.)

We also know that when women release more than a teaspoon or two of fluid, it seems to be a dilute form of urine that comes from the woman's bladder.

For women who don't squirt or release fluid during orgasm, please do not attempt to train yourself or force yourself to do this. Forcing yourself to ejaculate might not be good for your bladder over time.

For women who do release fluid during orgasm, there is absolutely nothing wrong about it and hopefully you will not feel embarrassed by it. It could be a result of how your body is wired, combined with becoming extremely relaxed during sex and the way your partner is stimulating you. What's not to like about that?

If you release fluid during orgasm, why not put towels on the bed before making love? Also, they now make waterproof mattress pads and covers that don't crinkle or feel weird, but the manufacturer doesn't mention anything about squirting on the package.

FEMALE EJACULATION SUMMARY: There is nothing wrong with squirting and nothing wrong with not squirting. Squirting is not a sign of better sex. Not squirting is not a sign of inferior sex.

Being Wet When You Are Not Aroused

Our gyno consultant says that too many women think there's something wrong with their vaginas because they are moist during the day when they are not thinking about sex. She says this is perfectly normal, assuming a woman is in good gynecological health.

Also, a woman shouldn't feel there's something wrong with her if she gets really wet from thinking about sex when she's alone, but needs to add lube when she's with a partner or before intercourse—assuming she and her partner have spent enough time on the arousal part of sex before trying to have intercourse.

Menopause

Menopause is what naturally happens to a woman's body when she is over 40 and stops having her monthly periods and no longer has to worry about getting pregnant. People have always believed that a woman's sex drive

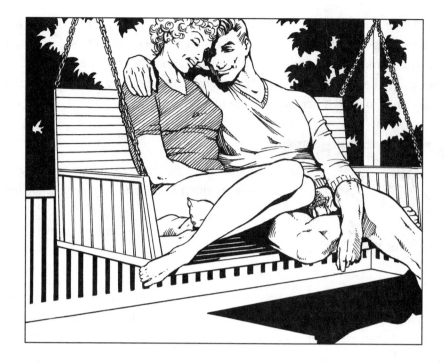

goes down as she enters menopause. Yet researchers have discovered that when a menopausal woman gets into a new relationship, she can be as horny as many 20-somethings. It could be the excitement she is feeling toward her partner, rather than the level of her hormones, that determines how much she wants sex. Then again, it can be difficult for any person, male or female, to feel sexual excitement if their hormones are below a certain threshold.

As for vaginal lubrication, some menopausal women become less wet when they are sexually aroused. The skin in their vagina may begin to feel less elastic or more sensitive during menopause. While there are hormonal creams that can help, the women from Touch of a Woman strongly recommend that a woman or her partner massage her vulva and the opening of her vagina every day with a moisturizer to help keep it more elastic. If you are approaching menopause, please give this totally free, drug free program a look. And keep in mind that the woman who has written this protocol is an MD and is extremely knowledgable about women's sexual health. The title is "Still Juicy: Maintaining Sexual Health Through and Beyond Menopause." Go to www.sexualityresources.com and enter "still juicy" in the search box.

There are also life stressors that a menopausal woman will commonly face, such as if her own mom and dad or her partner's parents are in declining health and she has to deal with their situation. On the plus side, her children might be starting to live on their own, which can be good for a relationship, or not so good if her children are high maintenance.

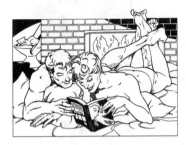

Dear Paul,

My girlfriend thinks her genitals are ugly. Is there anything I can do to help her change her mind?

Bobby in Beaver Falls

Dear Bobby,

It's the strangest thing how women can harbor negative feelings about the way their crotches look. A lot of girls don't even look at their own genitals until they are older, and even then, they refer to them as "down there." Men end up knowing more about women's genitals and how they look than a number of women do.

Then again, our society has never wanted girls to be curious about their genitals. While it is natural for a child to fall asleep with a hand between her legs, parents often assume this kind of self-comforting will turn an innocent girl into a slut-in-the-making. Heaven help a girl who is caught bringing her fingers to her mouth or nose after touching herself "down there."

A number of young women won't use OB tampons or the NuvaRing because they find it disgusting to put their fingers inside their own vagina. What are we doing when we raise intelligent young women to think it's "icky" to stick their fingers inside their vaginas? And now we've got young women who think "it's nasty" for women to masturbate.

I recently received a video about a sex educator's workshops where women check out each other's genitals. One of the women here at the Goofy Foot Press, who prides herself on her independence and liberation, felt uncomfortable when she first saw the tape. Then she remembered that she is just fine with porn where men's penises are wagging all over the place, so she made an effort to relax and watch the video. She had never realized her own discomfort with women's genitals.

How can you help your girlfriend be more positive about her genitals? First, begin by realizing this is part of a cultural disease. Then, perhaps with patient and creative encouragement on your part, maybe her own eyes will start to reflect the delight that's in yours when you look between her legs.

Reader Comments

What does it feel like in your genitals when you are sexually aroused?

"Tingling starts in my clitoris and spreads to my labia. My whole vulva starts to throb, literally. The throbbing is extremely pleasurable. Then my vulva gets swollen and almost hot. Once it is swollen, every slight touch sends lightning bolts of pleasure all around my whole body." *female age 23*

"Sometimes it's an ache not unlike having a full bladder. Other times, a sensation of heat and congestion in my labia, clitoris and vagina. If I'm highly aroused, or if my clothing is tight, I'll be able to feel my pulse between my legs. Sometimes I'll feel my tendons and muscles twitching as well." *female age 36*

"My labia feel swollen and tight; my clitoris becomes hard. Sometimes my clitoris feels like it's huge, and it sort of throbs. If I am extremely aroused, my whole vulva feels as though it's pounding, with my clitoris as the center." *female age 26*

"You know the feeling you get right before your leg or arm falls asleep? I mean, before it's annoying or hurts. It's a really intense tingling feeling. It makes my whole body feel warm and excited. There are moments, however, right before my partner enters me, when my vagina actually aches." *female age 27*

When did you first make the connection between being sexually aroused and being wet?

"When I was around 10 or 11, while watching a sex scene in a film. My panties got wet, and I realized that was why. If I'm really turned on, I'll drip down to my ankles." *female age 25*

"I first connected being wet with sexual arousal when I was 13. I was watching a silent, vintage erotic film with a friend. When I went to the bathroom, I was soaked!" *female age 26*

"The first time I connected wetness with sex was when I was 9 or so and got all wet and throbby when I was watching a couple kissing at the beach. But I don't always get wet when I feel aroused; it isn't an indicator for me." *female age 38*

"When I first masturbated, I only touched myself on my clitoris, so I was very surprised when I eventually felt my vagina and it was dripping fluid." *female age 23*

About being wet...

"Being wet is hard to explain. I don't know if I can offer insight because it just happens. The most annoying thing is that if you don't wear panties and get wet, it tends to be very messy, but arousing!" *female age 36*

"For me, the degree of my wetness varies greatly from time to time and seems to be largely affected by how mentally 'into' having sex I am at that given time." *female age 34*

"If my boyfriend just starts kissing me and wants to have sex, I am not automatically wet. I need to be turned on. This could be my way of slowing down and paying attention to my body, or it could be by talking sexy, reading, looking at, or listening to erotica."

female age 26

"It does not work when my partner concentrates solely on doing mechanical things to get me wet. Yet a simple, very tender kiss can do it." *female age 48*

"I enjoy sex a great deal, but seldom get wet." *female age 32*

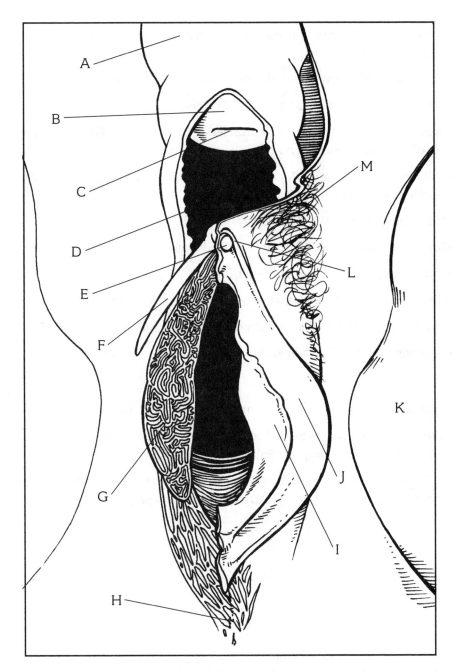

Female-Anatomy-as-Modern-Art Quiz

A—uterus; B—cervix; C—os; D—vagina; E—glans or tip of clitoris;
F. crus or leg of clitoris; G—bulb of clitoris; H—perineum;
I—inner lip or labia minora; J—outer lip or labia majora;
K—inner thigh; L—hood of clitoris ;   M—pubic hair

A Very Special Thanks to these highly regarded experts for their generous help and advice:

•Claire Yang, MD, Department of Urology, University of Washington

•Alessandra Rellini, Ph.D., University of Vermont

•Marca Sipski, MD, Director of Neuroscience Rehabilitation Research, University of Alabama at Birmingham

•William W. Young, MD, Department of Obstetrics and Gynecology, Dartmouth Medical School

•Maureen Whelihan, MD, Gynecology

•Roy Levin, University of Sheffield, Sheffield England

•Carol Tavris, Ph.D. and Leonore Tiefer, Ph.D.

•Ellen Barnard, MSSW, A Woman's Touch, Madison, Wisconsin

•Myrtle Wilhite, MD, A Woman's Touch, Madison Wisconsin

•Christine Vacarro, DO, Madigan Army Medical Center, Tacoma, WA

Some of the illustrations in this chapter were strongly influenced by:

Atlas of Human Sex Anatomy, Second Edition, Robert Latou Dickinson, The Williams & Wilkins Company, Baltimore, Maryland, 1949

A New View of a Woman's Body by the Federation of Feminist Women's Health Centers, Illustrations by Suzann Gage: www.progressivehealth.org

CHAPTER

8

The Hymen

The hymen is a collar of tissue around the opening of the vagina. It is the source of myth and legend, and it remains a mystery to much of modern medicine. Not many primary care physicians can even accurately locate the hymen. When we recently polled a group of gynecologists and women's sexual health experts, few could say what happens to the hymen of a sexually-active woman over time.

Some of the better studies on the hymen have only been done in the last couple of years, and some of these contradict each other. Most of the research on hymens concerns sexual abuse, so it's not particularly helpful if you are trying to understand the hymen in a context of healthy sexual activity.

This chapters presents what is currently known about the sexually-happy hymen. If there are holes in our knowledge, it goes with the territory.

How Your Hymen Came to Be

The hymen is located just inside the opening of the vagina. Unfortunately, people often refer to everything between a woman's legs as her vagina. So for clarification, you won't see her hymen if a woman simply spreads her legs. To locate the hymen, you would need to pull apart her labia and look inside the opening of her actual vagina. The opening of the vagina is called the introitus.

To understand how the hymen came to be and why it is where it is, it is important to know about the difference between the vulva and vagina. That's because each had a hand in the development of the hymen while the woman was still a fetus in her mother's womb.

VULVA: This is the part of a woman's genitals that are on the outside—the part you actually see when you are looking at an adult magazine centerfold. It includes the mons pubis, the tip of the clitoris, and the lips or labia.

VAGINA: To find the opening of the vagina, separate the lips or labia. The vagina is an elastic tube-like structure that a tampon or penis slides into. The average vagina is a bit less than 4 inches long or deep when not aroused and perhaps 5 to 6 inches or more when a woman is sexually turned on.

The Hymen—Where East Meets West

The vulva and vagina are not made from the same kind of embryonic tissue. This is where the hymen comes in. It is the ridge of tissue that is formed where the tissue from the vulva meets the tissue from the vagina, or where the vulva stops and the vagina starts.

Think of when two different land masses collide and a mountain range is created at that spot. That's somewhat how the hymen was created. Because the tissue on the inner side of the hymen comes from the vagina, it is estrogen-sensitive like the rest of a woman's vagina. The tissue on the vulva side of the hymen is sensitive to testosterone, as is the rest of the vulva.

When a girl begins to go through puberty and her estrogen levels rise, the hymen changes considerably. It becomes more elastic and no longer covers the opening of her vagina.

It's Puberty and Not the Penis That Causes the Hymen to Change

As the body changes during puberty, so does the hymen. Before puberty, a girl's hymen is often crescent-shaped, although there can be significant variations. The hymen is stretched across the opening of the vagina and it is almost translucent. You can see some of the capillaries in it and it covers much of the opening of the vagina.

By the end of puberty, the hymen no longer drapes across the opening of the vagina, but becomes more like an O-ring or collar, allowing a penis to have entry. This change is due to the impact of estrogen on the hymen tissue, which has estrogen receptors in it just like the walls of the vagina. Since the estrogen makes the hymen more elastic, our modern notion that the hymen "pops" like a cherry during the first intercourse is silly.

The estrogen that comes with the start of puberty causes the hymen to become shorter and thicker, more like a hedge or collar than the former drape or a wall that it was during childhood. With this thickening comes elasticity.

So it is puberty that changes the hymen, not the first intercourse. It's as if nature is changing the girl's hymen to make it ready for intercourse.

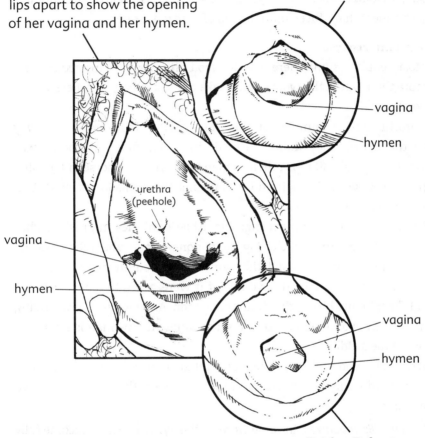

Adulthood

This woman is stretching her lips apart to show the opening of her vagina and her hymen.

Before Puberty The hymen is almost translucent and is often crescent shaped. The opening of the vagina is often hidden behind the hymen.

vagina

hymen

urethra (peehole)

vagina

hymen

vagina

hymen

During Puberty

The increase in estrogen causes the walls of the hymen to become thicker, shorter and more elastic.

The Changing HYMEN

Far from making hymens that pop, nature made the hymen ready for intercourse by changing its shape and making it more elastic during puberty.

From Saran Wrap into Spandex

Researchers often have trouble distinguishing between the hymens of teenage girls who are sexually active and hymens of teenage girls who are still virgins. That wouldn't be the case if hymens were like "Cherries that pop."

Still, it's hard to dispel the myth that the hymen is a seal of virginity, like the plastic sheet that's fused onto the top of a frozen dinner.

Your First Intercourse

Most people assume there will be blood after the first intercourse. Yet way more than half of the women who take our sex survey say there wasn't any blood.

Unfortunately, a number of the women who answered our survey believe the reason they didn't bleed during their first intercourse was because they had already torn their hymen while riding a horse or by doing the splits, or while their boyfriend was feeling them up. So the myth that hymens pop is alive and well

Researchers who were investigating athletic injuries in girls' crotches where bleeding occurred, including splits-gone-wrong and inline-skating related trauma, found it wasn't the hymen that bled. In cases where the hymen most certainly should have torn if it were going to tear, it was the vagina that split and bled rather than the hymen. And why horseback riding would wear away a hymen makes no sense unless the woman is sitting on the horn of the saddle.

While a hymen will most likely be stretched during a first intercourse, it shouldn't ordinarily tear. If it does, or if there is pain, there are at least two possible causes:

Not Fully Estrogenized: In some women, the hymen doesn't become fully estrogenized or elasticized during puberty. One healthcare provider who does premarital exams says she sometimes prescribes estrogen cream for soon-to-be married women whose hymens haven't become very elasticized. So if you haven't had intercourse and are concerned, it would be a good to ask a gynecologist if your hymen appears to have been adequately estrogenized for intercourse. (No one knows if the estrogen in hormonal birth control helps the hymen become more elasticized. No research has been done.)

Clumsy or Not Aroused Enough: Another reason for why a first inter-course can be painful is when the male partner is inexperienced, rough, has poor aim, is really big, or the woman is not sufficiently aroused and there's not enough lubrication. As a result, the hymen might tear or bruise, in the same way your gum might when you accidentally chomp on it.

There is an entire chapter on your first intercourse later in the book, Chapter 40: *Bye Bye V-Card—Losing Your Virginity.* Hopefully, it can help prevent a painful first time.

Another thing researchers have discovered is how fast the hymen heals. Medical examiners have been surprised at how normal the hymen can look in girls who they know have been sexually molested. The latest research has found that tears in a hymen usually heal quickly, often within 24 to 48 hours.

Tag

A hymen can start bleeding for the first time years after a woman has been having intercourse. This might be due to a tear in a "hymenal tag," which is a remnant of the hymen. These tags are like any of the other folds of skin inside the vagina, except they might look like pointy bits where there would otherwise be smoothness. Hymen tags are fairly common, but most women never detect them because they don't feel any different from other parts of the vagina.

What Happens to the Hymen Over Time

One gynecologist we consulted believes the hymen wears away with intercourse. The larger the penis, the more it wears. She believes she can accurately guess the size of a partner's penis based on how worn the hymen appears to be. Another gynecologist disagrees, saying you can't predict anything about the number of sexual partners or their girth by the appearance of the hymen.

Needless to say, a bit of research would be helpful, but one would need to examine the hymens of women who are virgins and then a few years later. You would also need to know the dimensions of their partners' penises, approximately how many thrusts per average intercourse, and how often they've had intercourse. It is unlikely Congress will be approving funding for such a study any time soon.

The experts did agree it's not unusual to see fronds of the hymen protruding from the vagina. These might have been tags from the hymen that became stretched. Also, childbirth might be a hymen's worst nightmare, causing a fair amount of stress on the hymen.

Warranty Repair or Revirginization

"Revirginization surgery," is when a surgeon takes the tattered edges of a hymen and purse-strings them together. None of our consultants were excited about it. The explicatives they used in describing the wisdom of "revirginization surgery" are not appropriate for a family book like this. However, if the alternative is being stoned in the village square...

Hymen Issues

If you have trouble removing tampons, intercourse is uncomfortable and your gynecologist says you have a septate hymen, a bit of local anesthetic and a small snip can often do wonders. A septate hymen is one that hangs vertically through the center of the vagina and looks a bit like the uvula at the back of your throat except it usually attached at both the top and the bottom. The ridge around the head of the penis can catch on this kind of hymen during the out strokes of intercourse.

An "imperforate hymen" is more rare than a septate hymen. It is where the hymen completely covers the opening of the vagina. If you really do have an imperforate hymen, having it taken care of surgically is essential.

If you are having discomfort during sexplay, don't assume the problem is your hymen. One thing to discuss with a gynecologist is whether the pain is at the opening or the back of your vagina. Before blaming your hymen, you might want to rule out things like vaginismus, vulvar vestibulitis syndrome, chronic constipation, certain infections, adhesions under the clitoral hood, or when the woman is not adequately aroused or there's not enough lubrication.

Vaginsimus is when the ring of muscles around the opening of the vagina automatically clamps shut. Vulvar vestibulitis is where the vestibule and the hymen are very tender when touched lightly with even a cotton swab, not to mention an incoming penis. See Chapter 56: *Damn That Hurts! When Sex Is Painful.*

No matter what your symptoms are, if a hymenectomy is suggested, get a second opinion. This is not only wise but important.

9

Orgasms

Define orgasm? It's somewhere between a hand grenade and a sunset."

—Mr. Billy Rumpanos, lifetime surfer and
early friend of Goofy Foot Press

One of the many nice things about sharing sex is having orgasms, also known as coming. But orgasms are not without their mystery. Perhaps it might be helpful to consider a few comments about orgasm from Dr. Frieda Tingle, the world's leading expert on sex:

Q. Dr. Tingle, what do you think of sex in America?
A. I think it would be a good idea.

Q. Do you think Americans are too concerned about orgasms?
A. Whose? Their own or their neighbor's?

Q. In general.
A. Orgasm is very important for many Americans because it tells them when the sexual encounter is over. Most of these people enjoy competitive sports, where some official is forever blowing a whistle or waving a little flag to let them know the event has ended. Without orgasm, they would be fumbling around, never knowing when it was time to suggest a game of Scrabble or a corned-beef sandwich.

Q. What kind of things affect a person's ability to have an orgasm?
A. One important factor is diet. Many times I have been told that it is impossible to have an orgasm after eating an entire pizza. I assume this has something to do with the Italian religious taboo against sexual abandon. Another factor is the weather. Many patients have told me that if the window is open and they are being rained on, it is particularly difficult to have the orgasmic experience....

(Dr. Frieda Tingle is the alter ego of Carol Tavris and Leonore Tiefer.)

Orgasm Defined

The best way to define orgasm is to put your hand in your pants and give yourself one. But this assumes you are able to give yourself orgasms and that you don't have six different kinds when you do. Perhaps you will find the following definition to be helpful:

💡 Orgasms are extra-special sensations that people sometimes experience while being sexual, either alone or with a partner. They occur after a certain threshold of excitement has been crossed and can last from seconds to minutes or longer. A sense of well-being or relief often follows. This might be due to a release of pain inhibitors following orgasm. For instance, studies have shown that people with arthritis sometimes get pain relief for three to four hours after having an orgasm.

💡 Orgasms often feel as if they are being broadcast from the genitals or pelvic floor, although there is no reason why they can't come from other parts of the body.

💡 Some people experience orgasm as a single, tidal-wavelike surge of sensation with a couple of brief aftershocks; others experience it as a series of waves, genital sneezes, or bursts of light, color, warmth, and energy. Some describe orgasm as creeping up on them and slowly flooding their senses. Some of us experience it as an explosion while others call it a whisper.

💡 Some orgasms make you feel great; others can be wimpy and disappointing. Some orgasms are strictly physical; others are physical and emotional. Some reach into the body; others reach into the soul. Some are intense and obvious; others are diffuse and subtle.

💡 The way an orgasm feels can vary with different types of sexual activity; for instance, oral sex orgasms might feel different from intercourse orgasms. Masturbation orgasms are often the most intense, but not necessarily the most satisfying.

💡 Orgasms with the same partner are likely to run the gamut from totally spectacular to downright disappointing. It depends on the particular day, and whether your worlds are colliding or are in sync.

💡 Some people have orgasms when a lover kisses them on the back of the neck; others need a stick or two of dynamite between their legs. The amount of stimulation needed to generate an orgasm has nothing to do with how much you enjoy sex.

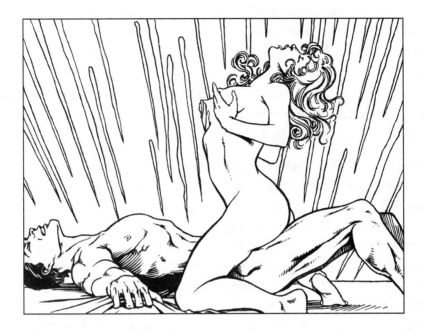

When shared with someone you love, the feelings that follow orgasm can make it possible to experience a special kind of intimacy.

Some people feel pleasantly amped or energized following orgasm, while others feel mellow and might want to sleep. For some people, one orgasm begs for another. For others, it calls for hugging and tenderness.

Genitals can become extremely sensitive after having an orgasm. Stimulation that may have felt wonderful moments before orgasm often feels painful or abrasive immediately after. It never hurts to ask your partner about this, since it's true for some but not all.

Some people are easily derailed on the road to orgasm. For others, the phone can ring, the earth can shake, and a dam can break—they come no matter what.

A philosopher named Sartre noticed that as he was having an orgasm he entered his own private orbit which caused him to lose awareness of his partner. Some couples make up for this temporary separation by feeling extra-close immediately following orgasm.

It is not necessary or even desirable for partners to come at the same time. It can be wonderful to feel or watch your partner have an orgasm, which is difficult to do if you are coming simultaneously. And it can be nice to occasionally blast off together. Just be aware that not many couples are able to pull this off.

Some people have orgasms with their legs squeezed together, while others come with their legs wide apart (innies vs. outies). People who prefer coming one way sometimes find it difficult to come the other way.

Does Orgasm Alter Your Consciousness?

When people are coming, they often experience a change in consciousness. Some of the latest brain research suggests why.

Doing high-tech scans on orgasming brains is very new and fraught with technical difficulties. They are highly suspect for technical reasons that are not the fault of the researchers. That said, PET scans of the brains of orgasming people show that parts of the conscious brain are shut down or turned off when a person is having an orgasm, while other parts are quite energized. From the scans, it appears that people enter into a deep, emotionless state while coming—with women going into an even deeper state than men.

Past editions of this book described some women's orgasms as transporting them into another dimension such as an orbit or two around the moons of Jupiter. The new brain-scan data suggests this might result from a combination of what's being shut down in the orgasming person's mind in addition to what's being lit up.

Your Partner's Orgasms

We often assume that a partner who has an orgasm is fully satisfied, while one who doesn't is disappointed. But while most of us can give ourselves really intense orgasms when we masturbate, not many of us can get feelings of closeness and intimacy when we do ourselves solo. For some people, these latter feelings are the most important part of lovemaking. So try to be sensitive, but not too paranoid, about your partner's orgasms.

Increasing Your Chances

If wanting orgasms were the sole reason for doing a particular sex act, not many women would bother with intercourse.

Things that increase your chances of having an orgasm: being seriously into your partner, exercise and a healthy diet, reading romance novels,seeing erotic images, and anything else that turns you on or increases your level of excitement. (Going to college increases the chance of a woman orgasming from masturbation; guys have never needed a degree to figure that one out.)

Things that decrease the chance of orgasm: being annoyed or angry with your partner, smoking (chemicals in tobacco constrict blood flow to the genitals and may lower the level of testosterone in both men and women), stress (notice how you tend to have more sex while on vacation), not sleeping enough and taking certain drugs. Antihistamines will dry up more than just your nose, and there's a huge list of drugs that will dent your libido or seriously delay your orgasm, especially SSRI anti-depressants such as Prozac, Zoloft and Paxil. Hormonal methods of birth control can have sexual side effects in some women, as is reported in Chapter 59: *The Pill & Your Sex Drive.*

Almost twice as many Protestant women as Catholic women report they orgasm during sex. Perhaps one problem for Catholic women is the Catholic church's strident prohibition against touching yourself or masturbating, which is how a lot of women learn to have orgasms. Information on how Catholic boys learn to have orgasms is still under litigation in many dioceses throughout the land.

Expressions, Decibels & The Way People Come in the Movies

Some people worry about how they behave when they are having orgasms. Some are self-conscious because they lose control, others because they don't. There is no correct way to come. Sexuality is an altered state of mind; what you do with it is a matter of personal choice.

Some people worry they will look weird if they allow themselves to be overwhelmed by an orgasm. They fear their partner will laugh or find them ugly. Quite to the contrary. It is far more likely that a partner will think:

> "Wow! Her face got all twisted and contorted. She looked like she was tripping big time. She must have had a major orgasm. Maybe I'm not so bad in bed after all...."

There are also plenty of people who have sensational orgasms but hardly show it. Their orgasms are an internal phenomenon that remains hidden from the outside world.

Many of us assume that women are supposed to make noise when they are coming, even though there is no correlation between decibels and delight. Some women sound like freight trains when they orgasm; others become completely quiet except for an occasional twitch and sigh. The same is true for men. If your partner comes in a quiet way and you would like to know more about it, why not ask?

Many of us learned to come quietly at a very young age. That's because there might not have been much privacy where we masturbated. Letting out a loud bellow would have informed the entire household. This was particularly true if you shared a room with siblings, and even worse if you had the top mattress in a bunk bed. The same difficulties are faced by people living in dorms, sororities, fraternities, and military barracks, where roommates often sleep only a few feet away. So we pretend to be asleep when masturbating—a funny notion when you consider our roommates are probably pretending they are sleeping as well.

The great sex-noise dilemma is also faced by parents while making love (or trying to make love) when there's a household full of kids. Depending on the ages of the children, their response to hearing mom and dad can range from "Mommy sounds upset" to "That's SO gross, where's my earbuds?"

Is It Possible to Have Too Many Orgasms?

Some Tantric types nearly hemorrhage at the notion of a man ejaculating. They think the male body is depleted when it ejaculates. As a result, they hoard the white sticky stuff like generals do weapons-grade plutonium. Some even teach themselves to have dry orgasms.

Is there much reality to this seed-spilling fear? The Nazis apparently pondered this same question. So they forced a prisoner of war to masturbate every three hours, day and night, for the duration of World War II. Thanks to the Allied invasion, the prisoner finally got to stop jerking off. He went on to father several children and lived to a ripe old age, certainly as old as most seed-retaining monks if they didn't fib about being 128 when they are really only 64. As for other living examples, one friend of Goofy Foot Press is now in his early 70s, but his mind is incredibly sharp, and he doesn't look a day over 50. He currently has at least five ejaculations per week, down from the ten or so he had been having since he was a teenager. According to semen-retention theories, he should be among *The Walking Dead*.

Regarding women and orgasm: nobody in his or her right mind has ever worried about a woman having too many orgasms, except for the people who live next door or in the apartment below.

Please see our "No Fap" video at www.GuideToGettingItOn.com, where we explain how bogus science from the 1800s is rearing its head yet again, .

Where Does Coming Come From?

The following quote is from a woman who had a spontaneous orgasm while riding public transit — a rather scary thought if you have ever taken the bus in places like Los Angeles or Detroit:

> "I've perfected this wonderful ability to orgasm without touching myself. It started one day on the commuter train when I was ovulating, and I felt myself throbbing. I started running a fantasy in my mind and discovered I could bring myself to orgasm. The only trouble with a public place is you have to control your breathing...." [Words of a former high school homecoming queen from the Midwest, as found in Julia Hutton's *Good Sex*, Cleis Press.]

One sex therapist tells about a time in college when he and his friends were talking about different ways of masturbating. One guy said he could ejaculate without touching his penis. Bets were quickly made. The room became quiet, and Mr. Spontaneous whipped out his penis. After his eyes were closed for a while, his penis became erect. The student began breathing faster, and eventually had an ejaculation without ever touching his penis.

Not only is it possible for some people to have an orgasm without genital stimulation, but it can even happen without sexual thoughts. Some women have spontaneous orgasms during highly charged debates or intellectual discussions that have nothing to do with sex. One female reader had her first orgasm as a teenager while her hair was being brushed, and as a 40-year-old she still has orgasms when her hair is brushed. Some women have spontaneous orgasms when working out, especially when doing crunches or exercises that involve the abs.

While not many of us are able to have orgasms without genital stimulation, the existence of hands-free orgasms does suggest that there is more to orgasm than genital contact. People who have suffered nerve injuries and can no longer feel sensation in their genitals can learn to have orgasm feelings in other parts of their bodies, such as their faces, arms, necks, lips, chests, and backs. That's because the power to experience orgasm resides in our brains and not simply in our groins.

One woman whose clitoris and vagina were removed due to cancer was able to experience the same kind of intense multiple orgasms after the surgery as before.

People who have lost one of their senses do not suddenly grow new ones to compensate. They are forced to better use the senses that remain. This suggests that many of us could achieve greater sexual pleasure from other parts of our bodies if we learned to allow it. One way of doing this is mentioned later in this Guide, where the woman stimulates her partner's penis with one hand while using her other hand or lips to caress another part of his body not normally associated with sexual feelings.

Orgasm-Chapter Letdown

One of the failings of this book is that it doesn't define "orgasm" more broadly. For instance, in talking about male orgasm, it is assumed that this happens when a penis is squeezed, stroked, fucked or sucked. But what if a man has an intense full-body orgasm when his partner kisses his neck for hours? In assuming that an orgasm needs to squirt out of our genitals, we keep ourselves from exploring other possibilities. But to include the full range of possibilities would add another hundred pages to this book, and if that doesn't make you cry out in horror, nothing will.

Pain Next to Pleasure

Receptors for pain and pleasure are located next to each other throughout our bodies. These receptors often fire at the same time. It is our brain's job to decide whether the overall experience feels good or bad. To make such a decision, our brain will sort through its database of everything from whether we are ticklish to how we feel about people with brown hair and green eyes who are trying to get us off. As a result, our brains each make their own decisions about what is pleasurable and what is painful.

While one person might enjoy masturbating to the fantasy of seeing Johnny or Amber naked, the mere hint of Johnny or Amber's presence might make another person feel sick to his or her stomach. Or one person might find spanking to be painful and a turn-off, while another might find spanking to be painful and erotic. The stimulus is the same, but how we feel about it depends on how our brain interprets it.

The way we interpret pain is also impacted by our level of sexual arousal. People who enjoy an occasional slap on the rear during sex usually don't like the pain unless it's done when they are sexually aroused. Being aroused can cause the brain to throw routine caution to the wind, converting sensations that are otherwise painful into sensations of pleasure.

Possible Assist for Women's & Men's Orgasms

When women are about to come they often pull in or tighten their pelvic muscles. Yet trying to totally relax or perhaps pushing out just a little might make their orgasms more intense. Some women will hesitate to do this from fear that it might cause them to pass gas or pee, but you'll both live if she does. And if you consider the gas-passing habits of most couples, chances are she owes him a few.

Whether you are male or female, you might occasionally experiment with relaxing the muscle tone in your pelvis when you come. Some men find they can prolong the feelings of orgasm if they relax their crotch and anus as orgasm is about to come.

What Was It Like?

Lovers sometimes ask each other if they came, but not what coming feels like. Sexual experiences can be hard to put into words, since they often exist on the cusp between physical and emotional sensation. But asking a partner to describe what an orgasm feels like might lead to some interesting insights and discussions.

Guys Faking Orgasm?

When the first edition of *The Guide* was published, it was assumed that women are the ones who do the faking. Yet up to 30% of young adult males have faked orgasms at one time or another.

Researcher Karen Yescavage found that guys fake orgasm for reasons like: "I was tired," "I faked it so she wouldn't see me go limp," "So she would think she was doing a good job," or "I wanted to get it over with." The reasons women gave for faking tended to fall into the "I-was-tired-bored-or-it-was-hurting" category.

A number of people who faked orgasms felt it helped increase the intimacy in sex. For them, the intimacy was more important than whether they really came or not. Others feel that deceiving a partner is wrong no matter what the justification. They can't see how you can lie and feel more intimate at the same time.

The people who admitted to faking orgasms didn't fake them very often. Lesbians fake orgasms as often as straight white women, while straight white women faked orgasms twice as often as Hispanic women. One possible explanation is that lesbians and white males may expect their partners to have more orgasms than Hispanic males do, and so the white females and lesbians felt more compelled to fake orgasms.

If Your Partner Fakes Orgasms

One of the worst things you can do when a partner fakes an orgasm is to go on a mission to help him or her have real orgasms. This usually makes matters worse.

When it comes to orgasms, there is sometimes a fine line between helpful concern and obnoxious fretting, especially if the reason you need your partner to have an orgasm is for your own reassurance that you are a good lover.

Rather than trying to help your partner have an orgasm, why not try to discover the things that give him or her pleasure and comfort? Contrary to what you think, this might simply be holding each other for an extended time or not grabbing for your lover's crotch the minute you feel horny. If your partner has suggestions about technique, all the better, but this might not be where the issue lies.

Far more relationships crumble from a lack of emotional pleasure than from a lack of orgasms. As long as you are able to give each other emotional pleasure, there are plenty of ways to achieve orgasm. This book lists several hundred of them.

Orgasm Dementia

Sometimes it's fun to count orgasms and go for it like pigs to mud. But for some people, orgasm production and/or procurement has a suspicious edge. Here are a few reasons why:

Some people get a sense of smug superiority by claiming how many orgasms they either had or "gave" a partner. They confuse sex with pinball or Halo.

Some people use pleasure-giving as a way of controlling a partner. They might hardly come while making sure a partner comes several times. This might not sound like such a bad problem, but partners who won't surrender the reins sexually are sometimes controlling in other aspects of life, as well.

There are people who expect their partners to supply them with constant sex and orgasms. This can breed resentment over time, as the other partner starts to feel used.

Some people need to have sex or masturbate several times a day to help numb a chronic sense of anxiety or ease feelings of deadness. A constant stream of orgasms can be their way of keeping an emotional funk at arm's length. Do not confuse this with sexual pleasure, even if they might.

Reinventing the Sexual Wheel — Marketing & Orgasm

During the last couple of years we were supposed to buy books and DVDs on G-spot orgasms, female ejaculation, extended orgasms, one-hour orgasms, Tantric-sex orgasms and extraordinary orgasms for boring people. Now, TV infomercials have been hawking better orgasms through pills and herbal enhancement, which we suggest you stay far, far away from.

While learning more about your body and sexuality is almost always a good thing, it's also important to use your judgement and common sense. You will usually know what works better for you sexually than the so-called experts.

Readers' Comments

For men: What does an orgasm feel like?

"My knees get weak and I tingle everywhere. It feels like I am numb all over." *male age 21*

"Like an energy emanating in the soles of my feet, up the back of my legs, in and through my rear end, to my belly button, and out through my balls and penis. Awesome, warm, exhausting." *male age 26*

"When I'm getting close, it feels like every ounce of fluid in my body has been forced into my penis. My whole body is in anticipation of the moment when my penis can no longer take the incredible pressure and bursts. Flames envelope the entire thing and the shock reverberates throughout my entire body." *male age 25*

"Orgasm makes me feel very connected to my lover, like I'm becoming a part of her." *male age 39*

"It feels like all your vital matter collects in your penis and then shoots out of you!" *male age 22*

For women: What does an orgasm feel like?

"Every orgasm I have is different! Sometimes I feel like I'm just melting, floating away. Sometimes I feel like I'm running or pushing into the orgasm. Sometimes an orgasm will sneak up on me; other times I will be able to control its arrival and duration." *female age 45*

"All my orgasms seem to be the same beast, but with varying levels of intensity from 'Gosh, was that it?' to an ache so sharp it's almost hard to bear. My most intense orgasms tend to come from using a vibrator but, oddly enough, they're not always the most satisfying."

female age 36

"Orgasms range for me from a simple response in my genitals, without much sensation and even some numbness, to a mind-blowing, explosive force of nature that permeates my whole body, mind, and emotions, encircles my partner and fills the room around us. Sometimes it's the physical sensations that are the most intense part of orgasm; other times it's the emotional quality and being with my partner that take top billing. Even when the physical sensation isn't very intense, I generally feel much more whole and integrated after an orgasm."

female age 47

Your first orgasm?

"With a vibrator at age 38. Finally!!!" *female age 49*

"It didn't happen until seven months after my first sexual experience. I had no idea what was happening. We were through having sex. When I began to put my clothes back on, I started to tingle and fluids started flowing out. It felt great, but I was actually kind of scared and embarrassed." *female age 21*

"I had an electric shaver that had an attachment which was a massager. After about an hour of moving it around on my clit (and praying that the pillow between my legs was muffling the sounds so my parents didn't hear) I had an orgasm. I'd already had sex many times with my boyfriend, but I felt like I was really sinning now!" *female age 25*

"I didn't really know what I was doing. I was about 10 or 11 and discovered this new feeling when I rubbed this silky part of my blanket over my penis, so I kept doing it. Eventually I got this intense feeling in my groin and then there was this goop everywhere. I was completely freaked and grossed out. I thought that I broke myself, but was too afraid to tell my parents." *male age 24*

"My first orgasm took place at age 18, when my fiancé introduced me, despite my initial revulsion and disbelief, to the delights of cunnilingus. I thought he was depraved. I was sure I was going straight to hell. I couldn't wait for it to happen again!" *female age 55*

"I had my first orgasm during one of my first menstrual periods. The feeling of a clean pad against my genitals made me feel a warmth I had never experienced before. I rubbed against it to see if I could prolong the sensation, although I had no idea what the sensation was. I just knew it felt good!" *female age 45*

"I didn't know what was going on. My body felt like it was convulsing. I tried not to let the guy know this was happening. I didn't know at the time I was supposed to let myself go and enjoy it." *female age 26*

"The first one I had was clitoral—it tickled (I was probably 10). The second type of orgasm I had was when I was 20. I felt it more in my vagina. It was overwhelmingly emotional and I came in a flood, and I do mean flood. I thought I had peed all over my partner. Now I have both kinds of orgasms. I get to pick, let's see, lobster or steak?"

female age 26

"My first orgasm was when I was making out in the back seat of a car. I was on top of my boyfriend and there was a lot of bumping and grinding going on, and I just climaxed, with my clothes on." *female age 49*

"I was surprised by how sensitive my clit was, but I wasn't sure the actual orgasm was an orgasm because it didn't seem nearly as explosive as what happened in the bodice-rippers I'd been reading. I couldn't believe I'd gone through all this work for that. Happily, many years of practice improved the results!" *female age 36*

"Age 20. One morning before arising I was idly rubbing my clit and fantasizing, and from out of nowhere excitement began building more intensely than it ever had before. I rubbed myself quite vigorously and for a very long time, until suddenly there was a mind-blowing explosion. I was certain that everyone in the house figured out what I was doing. I was very embarrassed. However, I repeated the experience every night—it took over an hour of heavy-duty stimulation at first."
female age 51

"My first orgasm was by a male friend (not a lover). I told him that sex was not that great. He used his fingers to teach me what it could feel like. I remember thinking 'Oh God, this is an orgasm!'" *female age 48*

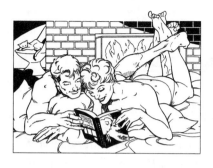

Dear Paul,

My girlfriend doesn't like me to play with her breasts, and the only way she can have an orgasm is when I give her oral sex. My former girlfriend didn't like me to give her oral sex, but sometimes had an orgasm from breast stimulation alone. Both women enjoy sex, but seem so different. How come?

Confused in Kalamazoo

Dear Confused,

For some people, you play with their breasts, and BOOM! their genitals are on fire. For others, you are better off reading them their constitutional rights.

As for why the different responses, I'd like to share with you an idea that was proposed by Herbert Otto, author of *Liberated Orgasm*. He feels that the kind of orgasms we experience are in part determined by what our culture teaches us to expect.

For instance, in the 1950s, a lot of teenagers enjoyed extended kissing and petting sessions, but intercourse before marriage was seriously frowned upon. So a woman who was a teenager in the 1950s might have learned to have orgasms from necking and nipple-play sessions in the front seat of a car—without a single touch or lick below the belt. This same woman's great granddaughter pays no social price for messing around with her pants off. She has read *Cosmo* since she was 12 and saw her first porn even earlier. As far as she's concerned, nothing short of a partner's mouth welded to her clitoris is going to give her an orgasm. And so her body responds differently than her great grandmother's.

I've focused on some of the less obvious factors that might play a role. A simpler explanation is that your current girlfriend's breasts aren't as sensitive as your former girlfriend's, or it hurts when you touch them. And perhaps your former girlfriend felt there was something uninviting about her genitals, so she wasn't comfortable with your face being between her legs.

Do you think it's possible your girlfriend is wondering why you like something one way while her former lover liked it another way?

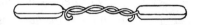

Hi Dr. Paul,

I'm a writer from a major women's magazine. I'd love to interview you for a story to ask if there's any evidence pointing to how many orgasms a woman is able to have, whether there's a "limit," and how women can achieve orgasm after orgasm after orgasm. Are you interested?

Echo

Hi Echo,

Thanks for thinking of me for your article.

Here's the problem—I deal with real people who have real sex lives. You deal with editors who want sensational articles in order to sell magazines.

The idea of "orgasm after orgasm after orgasm" sounds bizarre to me. It's just one more burden we are placing on women to act like porn stars.

The thing that matters is if the sex is satisfying for a woman and her partner—not the number of orgasms. Whether it's one orgasm, two orgasms or none, what's important is the quality of the sex and if it's achieving what a woman wants for herself and for her relationship, if she's in a relationship.

So I'm thinking I'm not the person who's going to make your article shine, or put a smile on your editors' faces!

This was a real inquiry from a real writer
for a real women's magazine made shortly before
this edition of The Guide went to press.

10
The Orgasm Talk

There are a lot of talks about a lot of things. But the one talk couples almost never have is the orgasm talk which is an honest discussion about orgasms rather than just "Did you come?"

The lack of conversation makes perfectly good sense. We live in a culture that's so at war with its sexuality that it spends almost as much money on abstinence-based sex education as it does on porn—neither of which is going to teach you much about pleasing a partner. The love we make is sometimes a frantic attempt to get into each other's pants while avoiding deeper meanings and possibilities.

It doesn't have to be that way. Sex can be even more fun after you have the orgasm talk.

Why Women's Orgasms, Rather than Men's, Are a Lovemaking Trophy

The male orgasm is usually a given during intercourse, and women will sometimes freak out if a man doesn't come from a blow job, even though they know that men don't always orgasm from oral sex. You'd think they would be jumping for joy at getting to avoid the "Do I have to swallow?" dilemma. Instead they worry something is wrong.

Women's orgasms aren't as predictable as men's. Women who are masturbating will usually have orgasms in the same amount of time as men do, but things can be different when you throw a partner into the mix.

Also, men's orgasms announce themselves with a fluid and sticky fanfare. Not so for women's orgasms. Men are often at the mercy of women to inform them if they did or didn't have an orgasm. Otherwise, men would never need to ask, "Was it good for you?"

These are some of the differences that make the occurrence of men's orgasms seem pedestrian, while women's are a topic of conversation.

Is the Lack of Orgasm a Deal Breaker for Women?

If the only reason a woman wants sex is for an orgasm, she'd be ahead of the curve if she sent her partner off to play video games with his friends and took matters into her own hands. It's the elusive nature of women's orgasms during partner sex that elevates the female orgasm to the realm of the love-making holy grail. Adding further to the mystery for men is how women do not always associate satisfaction during sex with having an orgasm. The mere idea of sex being satisfying without an orgasm is a foreign concept for most men.

In our sex survey, we ask women what they would prefer if they had to choose between receiving really good oral sex and intercourse. The vast majority say they'd rather have intercourse, even if they might orgasm more frequently from oral sex. Many prefer the intimacy and full body contact of intercourse. Plus, some women say they are more present during intercourse, while oral sex will often transport them into a different dimension of time and space. At the same time, women fiercely complain when a partner is not concerned about their orgasms.

Hopefully you are starting to see how helpful it can be for women to discuss orgasms with their partners and what they do and don't consider to be a satisfying sexual experience.

Men Often View Orgasms One Way, Women Another

When a man fails to have an orgasm during sex, he will probably feel that sex was a failure or it didn't qualify as sex. He will often assume that women feel the same way if they don't have an orgasm.

Women may have a different view of orgasms. Researchers are finding that women split the orgasm issue into separate male and female roles. They view the male's role as needing to provide them with enough physical stimulation to cause an orgasm. However, they think it's their responsibility to be in the right mental space to enable themselves to have an orgasm. If a woman can't get in the right mental place, she will often assume it's her own fault and not his. But is it really this simple?

Instead of assuming men know how to provide the right kind of physical stimulation, it would be helpful if women knew just how different any two women can be. Porn gives the idea that men magically know how to please women, when in real life, men need and often want guidance from a partner. This means that a woman's ability to show her partner how to stimulate her physically is often the key to his being able to provide her with the kind of physical stimulation she needs.

As for being in the right mental space, it is unlikely a woman will magically forget everything that has or hasn't gone on between her and her partner during the past week just because they are about to have sex. It's unlikely that feelings of anger, frustration or disappointment will evaporate the second he pulls out his penis. Helping to create the right mental space is just as much his job as it is hers.

Women's Orgasms: A Bonus or The Goal?

Is a woman's orgasm the goal of making love, or are other things more important?

It could be that a lover's ability to make a woman feel sexy and desired is more important. Maybe it's his ability to be playful and to make sex fun. Or what about acting out fantasy scenarios or being a little kinky if that's what turns her on? Perhaps a woman wants her partner to be more "take charge" in bed. Some of these qualities might rate higher than having an orgasm. And when these qualities are in place, the chances are greater that a woman will have an orgasm or will at least feel sexually satisfied.

Orgasms Before Intercourse? Orgasms After?

Some women prefer to have an orgasm before intercourse begins. There can be a couple of reasons for this. By the time a woman has been able to have an orgasm, it's very likely that the tissue around her vagina has become engorged in the best possible way. Orgasms also release compounds into the blood stream that can decrease pain and create more relaxation and feelings of closeness. These factors can help intercourse feel better.

Also, having an orgasm prior to intercourse can help take the pressure off of a woman. It might allow her to enjoy the closeness and intimacy of intercourse, especially if she thinks her partner will feel like a failure if she hasn't had an orgasm at some point during their lovemaking. Or maybe a woman will feel more comfortable having an orgasm after intercourse. She might enjoy it if a partner holds her while she gets herself off with her fingers or a vibrator.

Talking about how and when a woman prefers to have an orgasm can be an important part of the orgasm talk.

Orgasms during Intercourse

A common assumption is that the penis directly stimulates the clitoris during intercourse. Yet if you look at where the tip of a woman's clitoris ends and where her vaginal opening begins, you might start to wonder what nature was thinking. The tip of the clitoris is an inch or more above the opening of the vagina.

Perhaps that's why so many women who take our sex survey say they need external clitoral stimulation during intercourse in order to have an orgasm. They either need a finger or vibrator on their clit while a partner is thrusting, or they need to grind their clitoris into his pelvic bone.

So if either of you is assuming all women should have orgasms from thrusting alone without a clitoral-stimulation assist, this would be a good time to dispel such a notion.

Fingers Okay, But Not a Vibrator?

Men tell researchers it's perfectly okay with them if they or their partners stimulate the clitoris with their fingers during intercourse. However, they aren't nearly as enthusiastic about a partner using a vibrator during intercourse. It seems they interpret the vibrator as a rival or as indicating a failure on their part.

But what does it matter if a woman is using a vibrator or her fingers during intercourse? Intercourse should be about pleasure. Any guy whose partner enjoys using a vibrator during intercourse should consider himself a lucky man. That's because she'll be having some intense orgasms, and she'll associate them with him and the feel of his penis inside of her. (If a woman likes vibrations, another thing to experiment with is a vibrating cock ring.)

It's different with anal sex. Guys usually don't mind if a woman uses a vibrator on her clitoris if they are having anal sex. Perhaps one of the allures of anal sex is that it's more "anything goes" than vaginal intercourse. Or maybe it makes more sense to a man that a woman would use a vibrator on her clitoris when his penis is in her rear.

The Final Approach But No Landing

Women will often get close to having an orgasm, but something happens or changes in the last minute and they suddenly career away from it. So when you have the orgasm talk, be sure to ask what a woman needs as she approaches orgasm. Is it for you to be verbal? Quiet? Gentle? Firm? Rough?

Does she want your penis involved, or your fingers or lips, or does she just need you to hold her while she gets there by herself? Does she need a vibrator or anal stimulation? Does she want you to kiss her neck or touch her breasts or butt?

One of the worst things a partner can do when a woman is approaching orgasm is to start going faster or harder, or to change the rhythm. It's as easy to push a woman off a trajectory toward orgasm with too much stimulation as with too little. This is why it's so important to talk about what works best for her in the minutes before orgasm—when she's close to having one but isn't there yet.

You'll also want to find out what's best once she starts to have an orgasm. Should you keep doing exactly what you were doing before she started to come, or something else?

And what about the minutes immediately after? How should you be then? Some women might want you to put steady pressure on their vulva after they orgasm. Others will want you to keep doing what you were doing but at a greatly reduced intensity. For others, hands off is the only sensible approach.

Orgasm Obsessed

There is no more certain way to have a terrible time in bed than to become obsessed about orgasms. If you are obsessed about sharing pleasure, no problem. But being obsessed about a woman's orgasms is a recipe for lovemaking disaster. She'll feel pressured, and you will feel like a failure.

A very special thanks to Claire Salisbury at Western University in Ontario, Canada, to Tristan Taormino, and to Nina Hartley, who, in her excellent book *Nina Hartley's Guide to Total Sex*, suggested having a talk with a woman about what she wants her partner to do just before she starts having an orgasm as well as during and after.

Massage your senses with regular visits to

www.GuideToGettingItOn.com

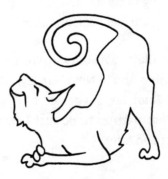

11
Body Massage
The Ultimate Tenderness

In doing research for this book, almost every way that humans give each other sexual pleasure was considered. Attempts were made to view sex through the eyes of mate swappers, Tantric-sex masters, gays, lesbians, born-again Christians, bondage enthusiasts, and those whose sex lives are really boring. Having left no sexual stone unturned, one and only one universal truth about human sexuality emerged:

No matter what your sexual beliefs, fantasies, kink, or persuasion, nothing beats a good back rub.

Nobody, absolutely nobody, had a single bad thing to say about a good back rub. Ditto for foot massage.

Hard vs. Soft? Male vs. Female?

Just about every book ever written on sex loves to state that men touch women too hard, and that women touch men too soft. Baloney, says a straw poll taken by the Goofy Foot Press. There are two types of touch that both men and women like a great deal:

Feather-Light to Light This is where the fingertips lightly dance across the surface of the skin, resulting in a delightful tingling sensation that may or may not raise goose bumps. It can also be done with the flat of the hand doing light, long, gentle strokes.

Deep & Hard This is when muscles are kneaded with a strength and authority that chases away stress and tension. The men commented that they often fear they are doing this too hard, but their female partners almost always say it's just right or to do it harder.

Fortunately, numerous books on touch and massage have been published in the last twenty years. There are also several nicely done videos on the subject. An hour spent reading one of these books or watching a video will do a great deal for your relationship. Pay special attention to the chapters on foot rubs, hand rubs, and scalp and facial massages. These body parts are often ignored because they aren't considered blue-chip erogenous zones.

Spectators vs. Participants

Some people struggle to get fully into their bodies. Some have trouble relaxing enough to enjoy what is being shared with them sexually. They need to be hypervigilant about what is going on around them. The same thing happens when a person always needs to perform and has difficulty becoming passive enough to allow sexual things to happen to his or her body.

Learning to massage and be massaged is one way that might help you to relax your body's armor. This might be anxiety-producing at the start, so go slowly and try to enjoy the gains you are able to make.

Combining Sex & Massage

One reader comments: "My husband often massages my shoulders while I'm giving him head. It feels wonderful and serves to relax me so I can become more easily aroused." Another reader ties her naked partner's hands together above his head, lets him watch as she slowly removes her satin panties and then caresses his entire body with them. A third reader drags her hair across her lover's naked body and eventually wraps it around his genitals. One man reports that the best way to drive his partner into total ecstasy is by brushing her hair or massaging her scalp with his fingertips. Another couple takes long, candlelit showers together, shampooing each other's hair and soaping each other's body.

Perhaps you have your own favorite ways of combining massage with sex play. Whatever your inclination, if there is only one thing you take from this book, it will hopefully be the resolve to make massage an integral part of your sexual relationships. Touch and massage might be the most important aspects of human sexuality, outside of the occasional need to replenish the species.

12

Sex Lubes —A New Look

We can place a webcam on a comet that's 300 million miles away and less than 3 miles in diameter, yet we have almost no medical research on something as important as sex lubes. We now know more about that comet–67P/Churyumov-Gerasimenko–than we know about the safety and effectiveness of the chemicals that millions of women put in their vaginas to help them have better sex.

You would think that something which impacts so many people would have been a top priority for research. But since it has to do with sexual pleasure and not disease, and since the lube-making companies have worked overtime to keep lube classified as a cosmetic and not something the FDA could get its mitts on, there has been no oversight. This is changing, but a number of the former lubes on the market have been grandfathered in as cosmetics with little or no oversight. Some lubes remain on the market that could increase your chances of getting an STI like herpes.

Fortunately, some research is being done on sex lubes as antimicrobials to help prevent the spread of HIV. But that research is mostly asking "Will women actually use this gunk in their junk?" So please read this chapter with the knowledge that some or all of it may be wrong. If you have any concerns, please consult with a gynecologist, not that gynecologists know a lot about sex lubes, but they can tell you if your vagina is healthy. *To learn about the ecosystem that keeps a woman's vagina healthy and why it would be helpful to know how sex lubes effect it, see Chapter 49: Inside Amber's Vagina.*

Who Uses Lube and Why?

It's surprising how many young couples are using lube—couples who you'd think would be dripping wet without store-bought lube. Perhaps their lack of natural lube is a side effect of using hormonal birth control or condoms. Or maybe they are not taking enough time for the woman to become adequately aroused before having intercourse. Or they may be taking plenty of time, but the woman's vagina doesn't get as slick as they would like.

Some couples need lube for marathon lovemaking sessions—especially when they are in distance relationships and are making up for lost time. Lubes can be helpful when size discrepancies make for a tight fit. Couples sometimes need lube for menopause-related dryness. Lube helps some women avoid UTIs, causes other women to get vaginal infections, and is often a must for sex if you are receiving chemo for cancer.

People use lube when they are giving each other hand-jobs, finger fucking, masturbating and for anal sex. Some couples like to incorporate lube into oral sex. It also helps with certain sex toys and it can work wonders for sex in a hot tub.

While this may be counter intuitive, the lack of estrogen during a woman's period may cause her vagina to produce less natural lubrication than normal. So some couples need lube for period sex.

Marketing Hype

Companies that make sex lubes are spending millions of dollars on slick marketing campaigns. They want you to believe that couples who coat their crotches with expensive lubes will experience dimensions of bliss that the poor idiots who rely on nature's own lube are missing out on. But what about things like communication, fun, romance and respect? Does squirting chemicals up your crotch make up for a lack of that?

Don't Spit on Spit!

Given that people need lubrication for sex, we contacted a professor of gynecology at a medical school and asked, "What about the old standby of saliva? It seems to have gotten a bum rap these days. Is that because stores can't sell it or has science discovered something really bad about it?" This professor checked in with one of the world's leading experts in vulvar pain, and both shared the same opinion about saliva—*it can be an excellent sex lube as long as you don't need something that's very slippery.*

If you wonder why these experts might recommend saliva over the pricey stuff, let's look at the ingredients in a well-respected lube that is water-based, hypo-allergenic and fragrance free. While that sounds good, here's a list of the chemicals in the lube that will end up inside your body:

Propylene Glycol, Isopropyl Palmitate, Dimethicone, Cellulose Polymer, Polysorbate 60, Sorbitan Stearate, Stearyl Alcohol, Glyceryl

Stearate NSD. B.N.P.D, Di Sodium EDTA, Phenoxy Ethanol, Methyl Paraben, Butyl Paraben, Propyl Paraben, BHT

Fortunately, only a couple of these ingredients are listed in the *Hazardous Chemicals Desk Reference*. And why do they call it hypoallergenic when paraben and glycol are known allergens for some women? A staff member of the FDA couldn't find any criteria for what a hypoallergenic lube is or how the FDA defines "hypoallergenic."

Until very recently, sex lubes have been classified as cosmetics. As cosmetics, there was no need to evaluate them for use in mucus membranes such as the vagina, rectum or urethra—where absorption of chemicals into the bloodstream can be quite high.

Also, no agency checks to make sure that what's in the bottles of sex lube is what's listed on the label. A few years ago, researcher Bruce Voeller found toxic chemicals in one of the brands of lube that he tested. Bruce suggested only buying sex lube from companies that manufacture pharmaceuticals, because of increased FDA oversight. But one of the largest sex lube manufacturers in the world has been the pharmaceutical giant Johnson & Johnson. Johnson & Johnson has now paid $2.2 billion in healthcare fraud violations and has had enough recalls to fill half this book. This icon of health care products has finally started to remove known carcinogens from its baby care line of products due to extreme pressure from consumer advocate groups..

Another large pharmaceutical company was selling vaginal moisturizer for humans whose active ingredient was too dangerous for use in cow vaginas. Does this mean you shouldn't use store-bought lubes or vaginal moisturizers? No. But it does speak well for spending a few extra minutes kissing and caressing before automatically grabbing for the sex lube.

Lube Basics #1

People confuse sex lubes with automobile lubes. With auto lubes, you want to eliminate as much friction as possible. But if you eliminated all of the friction when having sex, no one would ever have an orgasm. Sex needs friction in order to feel good. With too much friction, sex hurts. With too little friction, there's not enough sensation. So the best sex lube for you is not necessarily the lube that's the most slick.

Lube Basics #2

Different lubes allow different amounts of sensation. So the brand of lube to use may depend on the kind of sex you are having and the kind of feeling you and your partner enjoy. Some lubes are thin, which allow you to feel more sensation, others are more cushioning. Rub the lube between your fingers and see if you can still feel the ridges. If so, it's a thinner lube that will act more as an assist to a woman's natural lube. If you can't feel the ridges, it's probably a more cushioning lube that might be better for weekend-warrior sex or anal sex.

Silicone Lubes

Consultants to *The Guide* say that some of the best sex lubes currently available for general sexplay for most couples are silicone-based lubes. But considering how little research there is, this could change with changes in the scientific literature. Also, you may have specific needs that require something else.

Some people love the feel of silicone lubes, others don't. You might say, "I've heard that silicone is unsafe in breast implants. Why would I want to stick it in private places?" If you have ever been on the receiving end of a penis that's wearing a pre-lubricated condom, you've had silicone inside of you. Silicone molecules are supposedly too large to be absorbed into the body. The problem with leaky boob implants is the silicone gets trapped inside a woman's chest with no way to get out.

You can use most silicone-based lubes with latex condoms—but check the package to make sure. Unlike water based lubes which tend to dry out quickly, the silicone keeps the lube slicker for longer. A lot of people prefer it for anal sex as well as for vaginal sex and handjobs. The downside is it doesn't come off very easily, which is one of its upsides for use during sex.

Silicone lube can be incredibly helpful if you are having sex in water. Water washes away natural lubrication, making intercourse in hot tubs and pools difficult. Silicone-based lubes are slow to wash off and will help keep a penis pumping longer for intercourse in hot tubs, bathtubs, lakes, rivers and oceans. The trick is to slop it on your genitals while they are still dry.

A problem with silicone lubes is their effect on silicone sex toys. It's not pretty. Put a condom on silicone sex toys before using silicone lube. Silicone lubes can also stain your sheets. You might try treating the stains with Dawn dish detergent or a fabric-safe degreaser, but the prognosis is not good. (Do not use lube-stained sheets on the bed when your mom is visiting.)

If you are into electric sex—the serious kind with probes and electrodes—never use silicone-based lubes. The silicone acts as an insulator.

Slipping Danger: Silicone lubes become a slipping hazard if they drip on the floor, especially if you use them in the shower. We're talking ice-rink slick. So apply it to your genitals before you get in the shower or tub.

Natural Products as Sex Lube — Coconut Oil vs. Olive Oil

If you want a natural oil for sex lube, and don't care that there's no scientific research to say if it's safe, the current choice seems to be coconut oil. Coconut oil absorbs nicely into the walls of the vagina. However, it's not very slippery. As for olive oil, it can collect around the cervix, resulting in a rancid-smelling crotch. A recent study that evaluated the use of olive oil for skin massage found it significantly damages the skin barrier. While olive oil can be great on vegetables and salads, do not use it for sex.

Some types of coconut oil are marketed as "virgin coconut oil." This does not mean you can only use it if it's your first time. Although if there's one time a woman should consider using lube, her first time would be it.

While the words "saliva" and "coconut oil" sound better for a vagina than propylene glycol, hydroxymethylcellulose, sorbitol and polysorbate 60, there's no science to guide us one way or the other.

Glycerin in Lubes

Lubes that are glycerin-based tend to be slicker than other lubes, which means if you rub them between your fingers you won't feel the ridges as much as with lubes like *Liquid Silk*. People who prefer lubes with glycerin say they feel "really fast." One problem some women have with glycerin is that it's similar to glucose. Glucose is one of the things that yeast feeds on inside a woman's vagina. Too much of it can encourage a robust yeast colony where you don't want one. So if you are prone to yeast infections, are immunosuppressed, or have diabetes, consider a sex lube without glycerin.

Friction Burns from Sex Lube?

Believe it or not, women can get friction burns in the vagina when a lube is too gloppy or gets thick from drying out. So avoid gloppy lubes if you are experiencing discomfort. If you are having sex and your lube is getting gummy or is drying out, try adding a few drops of water or saliva to rehydrate it instead of adding more lube.

Other Sources of Lube Woe

The propylene glycol in some lubes can be an irritant for some women. So can lubes with a high pH, such as Astroglide. For more on pH and a woman's vagina, please see Chater 49: *Inside Amber's Vagina*. As for petroleum jelly, what limited research there is indicates that it's not a good choice.

When a Woman Feels Too Wet

Some women lubricate so much that they can't really feel the penis going in and out. If you are having this problem, have your partner pull out every now and then and dry the both of you off with a towel. Some people suggest trying an over-the-counter antihistamine to help dry up your natural lube if it's a problem, but check with your healthcare provider first. The opposite problem can occur if you are taking an antihistamine for sinus issues and it is drying up your natural sex lube.

Lubes for Anal Play

Historically, the lube of choice for all things anal was a famous brand of vegetable shortening. Then came the '80s and the plague, and since then the sex-lube wars with sex lube manufacturers fighting for market share. (You might not think of your anus as a profit center, but companies that make toilet paper and sex lube certainly do.)

Nowadays, just about everyone who is into anal sex has a "slippery top ten." Good luck finding a consensus on which is best.

Vegetable shortening remains the standard that anal-sex lubes are trying to copy, but without its downsides. Vegetable shortening has no antibacterial properties, so dipping back into the can might contaminate it. While fine for your fries, vegetable shortening melts latex condoms, which are thought to be safer for anal intercourse than polyurethane condoms. Vegetable oil tends to leave rancid-smelling sheets with wicked stains. Also, there might be problems with vegetable-shortening-fecal-ooze dripping from a woman's anus into her vagina if she is in an ass-over-tea kettle position when having anal sex.

There are no warnings on the side of vegetable shortening containers that say, "Use only in your oven and not up your bum." But there are no scientific studies on the safety of vegetable oil for anal sex. So while there are plenty of opinions, no one really knows what's best. As for the lubes for anal sex which say they use "FDA-approved ingredients," this means absolutely nothing, as the FDA does not have a list of approved ingredients for anal intercourse.

Silicone-based lubes are the current front runner for anal sex. They should do the job for anal sex without your butt dripping grease like the grill at McDonald's. Ask around, do a browser search, and check the reviews on Amazon.

Be careful with lubes that contain pain-killers. They tend to have names like *Anal-Eze*, and *Tushy Tamer*. Using lube with numbing agents is like disabling the smoke alarms in your home. Pain during anal sex is an important indicator that you are being too rough, aren't relaxed enough, aren't turned on enough, that your partner is too big, or that anal sex is not for you. Also, if something numbs your anus, it will numb your partner's penis, setting the stage for an unwise marathon in your rectum.

Gnarly Anal Warning: Sorbitol and glycerin are used in a number of sex lubes. They are also an active ingredient in laxatives and suppositories. Think about it before grabbing just any lube for anal sex.

Anal Fisting

The fisting world is divided into camps of traditional vegetable-shortening fisters and camps of postmodern oil-based fisters who prefer *Elbow Grease, Boy Butter, ID Cream* and *Men's Cream*. There are also reformed fisters who use thick water-based and silicone-based lubes like *Astroglide Gel, Probe Thick and Rich, Eros Silicone Gel* or *Eros Cream*. Anal fisting is beyond the scope of this book and can be dangerous, so please research it carefully beforehand.

Lubes for Hand-Jobs and Masturbation

Avoid hand creams for hand jobs and masturbation. Most hand creams and moisturizers are designed to be absorbed by the skin so people won't feel like greased pigs after they use them. The macro-molecules in moisturizers are designed to go flat fast. As a result, most hand moisturizers are poor performers for sex or massage.

Whether it is for giving your partner a handjob or just for jerking off, you'll want a lube that stays wet and slippery. A popular and nearly legendary jerk-off lubricant is a facial cleanser called *Albolene*. Newer products include *Men's Cream, Boy Butter, Gun Oil Stroke 29, Swiss Navy Masturbation Cream, Hardware Wank Wax, ID Cream, and ManUp.* A jerk-off standard since 1979 has been *Elbow Grease.* For those of you who like roasting your nuts, there's *Elbow Grease Hot* with menthol.

Men who are not circumcised are less likely to use lube for masturbation. Their factory-equipped foreskins usually do the job.

J-Lube Precaution: *J-Lube* is a powdered veterinary lube that is water activated. It is also used for jerking off. Beware that a tiny amount of *J-Lube* in the peritoneal cavity (gut) of a horse or cow will quickly kill the animal. We're talking a few moos and all four hooves are sticking straight in the air.

Women's Genitals (On the Outside)

Women have used saliva for masturbating since the beginning of time. Coconut oil might work well for masturbation or vulva massage. Scented lubes and anything containing nonoxynol-9 should be avoided because they can cause irritation. If you like lube with oral sex, why not try food-grade coconut oil, unless you are following up with latex-condom intercourse.

Vaginal Moisturizers and "Arousal Creams"

Vaginal moisturizers are for situations like vaginal atrophy or post menopausal issues as opposed to when you need a lube for sex. One popular vaginal moisturizer, *Replens,* might actually work like a chemical peel.

Estrogen creams are often prescribed for vaginal dryness. Do not use estrogen products or an *Estring* as lubes for intercourse! These are for vaginal atrophy, which is different from the dryness a 21-year-old might have.

We are also at the dawn of a new age in "arousal creams." It's strange what a huge disconnect there sometimes is between the claims of the companies that make the creams and the women who actually use them. While the creams claim to bring more blood flow into the crotch, some users say it feels like rubbing *Vicks VapoRub* on their clits.

Would five minutes more of kissing before intercourse have the same result as arousal creams, which sometimes smell like old bacon grease? Then again, if you like it and the product works for you, more power to it and you.

CHAPTER

13
Consent

For the past twenty years, almost every page of this book has been about consent. It's always been a proponent for asking, respecting and never pushing or pressuring a person to have sex. It doesn't matter if you are together an hour or a lifetime, if there isn't consent, then there shouldn't be sex.

Now, in more and more states, sex without mutual consent is not legal. It is incumbent upon men to know what this means, and to help prevent sex without mutual consent from happening.

Then vs. Now

For too long, too many males have defined consent in sex as whatever they could get away with. But the government has instructed colleges to implement new rules requiring mutual consent before and during sex. Laws with similar provisions are being enacted in states, where the excuse of "But she didn't say 'no'!" will no longer offer protection for a man who is charged with sexual assault or rape.

The new consent rules also address situations where there was coercion but the woman isn't sure if she was actually assaulted. While it is perfectly normal for a woman to wonder if the sex was worth the effort, the last thing she should be asking herself is "was it rape?"

"I'm Not a Rapist!"

No one wants to see himself as a rapist. But if you have pressured a woman to have sex when she didn't want to have sex, or you have had casual sex with a woman who was under the influence of alcohol, drugs, or was asleep, then you may have committed sexual assault or rape.

It may sound extreme to tell you that a man should no longer have casual sex with a woman who has had alcohol or drugs. But you can now be guilty of sexual assault if you "fondle or "grope" a woman who is under the influence. And you don't want to tell the court "But she only had one beer."

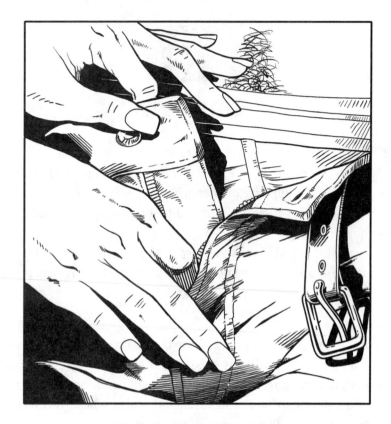

**Sex needs to be something you BOTH want,
without alcohol or being pressured.**

Even if a woman didn't say 'no' to sex, you can still be charged with sexual assault. The same is true if a woman said "yes," but suffers buyer's remorse and it becomes her word against yours.

With the new consent laws, if it's a "he-said she-said" situation, the chances are high the male will lose. So men need to start asking themselves if casual sex is worth the risk of being arrested for rape. We don't believe it is, and this would be one of the most liberal, pro-pleasure books on sex that's ever been written.

There's nothing in the new laws that say you have to buy a woman a wedding ring before asking for a handjob. But it's important that the decision be hers every bit as much as yours—without coercion, pressure, alcohol or drugs.

Rules for When To Keep Your Zipper Up
And When It's Okay to Pull It Down

An agreement to kiss is not an agreement to have intercourse. It never has been. Feeling each other up and discovering the woman's vagina is wet is not consent to put a penis in it. If a woman chooses to wear a short, sexy dress, it is not an invitation for you to reach underneath it or to take it off.

If a potential partner doesn't want sex as much as you do and isn't willing to say so, go home and masturbate. If the relationship is worth it, call or text the next day and talk things over.

If you need to convince someone to have sex with you, then it's wrong. If they need to convince you to have sex with them, then it's wrong.

Just because someone gave you permission before doesn't mean you have permission now. Always ask. Having had sex with a person in the past is not a rain check for sex in the future.

Not being sure how far you want to go is normal. If a woman wants to get physical with you but isn't sure how far she wants to go, you absolutely must talk it over with her to find what she is comfortable with. In the eyes of the law, hesitation is the same as the person saying "NO!" If you proceed, you can be charged with rape.

If a potential partner who you've not had sex with before has been drinking or doing drugs, wait until the next day when she is sober and can legally consent before pursuing sex. Otherwise, you can be charged, even if she was the one who asked you to have sex.

What Should You Do

Let's say you meet someone who you'd like to have casual sex with. Talk, flirt, ask for her contact info, then go home and masturbate. Get in touch with her the next day.

Text. Meet for coffee. Do something together besides grope and make out. If she wants to have casual sex with you, make sure she's known you for at least a day and has had time to think about it. This will hopefully reduce the chances she might have second thoughts afterward. And if she does, it will more likely be because you weren't satisfying in bed as opposed to her feeling she was pressured or coerced.

If you think "She was letting me feel her breasts, so I figured it was okay to fuck her," imagine the fun you'll have explaining that one to a female police officer or to a judge and jury.

You can't justify bad behavior by saying, "Women aren't always clear— 'no' just means you need to try harder!" It is now incumbent upon the man to make sure the woman wants to have sex without being pressured.

Why the Changes?

For too long, a woman who was assaulted and had the courage to file charges against the man who assaulted her was raped a second time by the legal system. She's the one who was put on trial. This is changing. The onus for consent is being placed more and more on the male.

This is fair. When it comes to being sexually assaulted, most males have had the ability to keep themselves out of harm's way by being sensible. That's a much better deal than women have had over the years.

No Longer Hiding in The Shadows

Until the last twenty years, people thought of sexual assault as something that was committed by a stranger who lurked in the shadows or pried a woman's bedroom window open. No one thought of it as something your date did after the two of you started making out. They did not think of it as something that happened when you were at a party. But as researchers interviewed more women, they started hearing accounts of men who would not stop, in spite of a woman's protests.

There are men who are adept at engaging women in kissing or petting, and then assaulting them in the same manner as "traditional" rapists who lurk in corners. Men like these can come from wealthy families who are on the social A-lists. They can be sports heroes, Boy Scouts, altar boys, and divinity students at a Bible college.

To help prevent this kind of sexual assault, the courts have pushed the limits of what consent is into a somewhat artificial and at times awkward place. The onus of stopping sexplay now rests on the male the moment a woman says, "Stop!" or "Maybe I should go" or "This doesn't feel right." A woman may have agreed to have intercourse, but if she changes her mind after 300 thrusts, a man needs to pull out immediately and not after thrust number 310.

In a decision for the State of California Supreme Court called *People v. John Z*, a woman agreed to have intercourse, but at some point during the intercourse, she indicated she might want to leave. She didn't say "Stop" or "I don't want to keep doing this." The court found that she was raped because the man did not stop the moment she indicated a change of heart.

Making sure a woman can legally consent to sex is now the job of the male, and it is very different from what you might think. Even if a woman bought the first two rounds of drinks or brought the pot and rolled the joints, she is not legally able to consent to sex if she has been drinking or doing drugs. This can be true even if she voluntarily went down on a man to help him get hard and put in the penis herself.

It doesn't matter if both of you were equally drunk or stoned. The mere fact that she was drinking can turn intercourse into sexual assault in some states, depending on the situation. Also, there are times when it is not legal to have sex with a woman if you are her boss, her teacher, her minister, her physician or her coach.

Don't assume a woman is playing a game when she hesitates or says "No." Anything less than an exuberant "Yes!" should be understood as a "NO!" Never, ever try to win a woman over by pressuring her to have sex. The courts have made it clear this will not be tolerated.

In the absence of a woman making it clear she wants sex, a man needs to assume that sex is neither desired nor legal. *Prison is no place you want to be, and it's become easier to find yourself there if you push sex on another person.*

What About Dick Pics?

Never send unsolicited pictures of your dick, or post pictures of you and another person having sex. These can result in your being arrested for sexual assault, stalking and multiple other crimes.

If You Know You Have a Communicable Disease

If you know you have a communicable disease and do not inform a new partner, you can be sued. Not only is it morally right to inform someone you are about to have sex with that you have a contagious condition such as herpes or HIV, warning them will help you cover your legal bases.

Yes Means Yes

There are a number of new programs on college campuses that are designed to teach mutual consent in sex.

"Yes Means Yes!" is one such program. It's where a young woman is supposed to suddenly feel comfortable proclaiming to a male "I want to have sex with you, and here's exactly what I want us to do!"

This program is well intended. But for a reality check, it is being promoted by the same government that has spent more than $2 billion to fund programs that teach young women to feel shame about their bodies and shame for wanting sex. The Department of Education now expects these same women to suddenly jump for joy and shout "YES!" to casual sex.

These are the same young women who were encouraged to take "purity pledges" in middle school and high school, and who men in Congress are still trying to tell what they can and can't do with their bodies. These are the same young women who were called "sluts" and "hoes" if they admitted to wanting sex as much as males in middle school and high school, and they can still face dire consequences in some cultures for having premarital sex.

For a much more realistic take on "Yes Means Yes," consider the following by social psychologist Carol Tavris: "How do you know what you want until you start doing something you think you want and then don't? Or do? People married for 40 years are often unable to say clearly what they want, or don't want, and we expect 18-year-olds to know what they want?"

Until society makes some radical changes, programs like "Yes Means Yes" could result in even more young women getting drunk before having casual sex, so they can feel less conflicted about rattling off the new mantra of "Yes, I want to have sex with you, and here's exactly what I want us to do!"

While "Yes means yes!" is something we'd like to see become a reality, we still have a long way to go with "No means no!" Too many men feel that being relentless in the pursuit of a woman is okay, and it's acceptable to try to wear a woman down. A woman should not have to repeatedly say no to a person's advances.

Bystander Intervention

There is a program based on "bystander intervention" that is one of the cornerstones of consent. Bystander intervention is when a bystander intervenes on behalf of a woman who, for whatever reasons, is not able to legally give consent to sex.

If you're a man and you hear a woman screaming in a burning house, you'd most likely try to find a way to save her. You wouldn't say to yourself "She was probably smoking a cigarette in bed, it's her own damn fault." But that's how we often feel about a woman who arrives at a party wearing next to nothing, or is blowing a .025. We figure whatever happens is her own fault.

Guys will sometimes say, "If I was *sure* she was in trouble, I would have intervened. But how do you really know?" The answer to that is easy. If you aren't sure, then you need to intervene. You need to see her and hear from her that she's okay. And if the numbers are seriously against you, call the police or MPs. Uncertainty should be a *guide to action*, not an excuse for inaction.

It's not hard to understand how a guy who wouldn't hesitate to run into a burning building to save someone else might hesitate or feel paralyzed when confronting the bad behavior of his friends. And he might feel justifiably afraid. When a woman is being sexually compromised, we have generations of herd behavior telling us to ignore the situation.

The best we can tell you is rather than ignoring it, take a moment and try to tap into some inner resource—perhaps connecting emotionally with someone who you admire or who you looked up to for his strength and courage. And then you need to find your inner bad ass and become certain about a situation you are uncertain of. Or at the very least, call the authorities who might be able to help.

This will take courage, and it will help define you as a person. It will also help the world become a better place for half the people in it.

Answers to Questions from Inquiring Minds

To Mark at the University of Georgia who feels he was misled: When it comes to sex, we've all been misled (or led on) at one time or another. Some of us have misled others. Even if it seemed like she wanted sex as much as you, the second she looked at her watch and said "Gotta go" you should have had your penis in your pants faster than a tachyon through a crack in the cosmic egg.

To LouAnne at Texas Women's University who can't understand why consent laws apply to women as well as men: The two of you had been slamming down shots of tequila in his bedroom and he was wearing blue jeans three sizes too small in all the right places. LouAnne, it wouldn't matter if he were buck naked and had a red tassel on the end of his penis, when a person says "No more" you need to respect his wishes. Even if a partner has their tongue halfway down your throat for the better part of an hour, if they suddenly pull it out and wag it in a way that says "This is all you're gonna get," then you'd better stop. The same is true if the two of you have been married for ten or twenty years. A ring or wedding vow is not consent to rape.

To Randy, formerly at Fairleigh Dickinson University and currently residing in the New Jersey State Prison system: The two of you had been flirting for weeks. She invited you to a party. Both of you had been drinking when she saw you from across the room. She threw her arms around you and said, "Let's go upstairs, find someplace private, and have the sex we've always dreamed about." The following Monday, you find yourself arrested for rape. How can this be? "Informed consent" implies your partner was sober enough to make a rational decision. It doesn't matter if the two of you had been flirting for weeks. If she was not sober when she put the moves on you, it is you who can be charged with a crime in some states. And even if the jury had found you innocent, it would still cost you thousands of dollars to defend yourself and the personal toll would be immense.

———————

Why Was this chapter addressed to straight males? While consent can certainly be an issue for gays and lesbians, the vast majority of consent violations involve sex that's between men and women. And while plenty of women have pressured men into having sex, when the subject is rape or coercion, we are usually talking about the behavior of straight males.

14

Handjobs
Different Strokes
For Different Blokes

Women often ask, "Why should I give him a handjob? I can't possibly compete with the hand that knows him SOOO well. Besides, there's nothing special about it. He can give himself a handjob any time he wants."

After reading hundreds of men's sex survey responses about masturbation vs. handjobs from a lover, the vast majority of men—more than 90%, would rather receive a handjob from a lover. A number of men said that technically speaking, masturbation often feels better, but they still enjoy the experience more when it's a partner who is doing the stroking.

Think about it: Who is he fantasizing about when he is jerking off? It's you! When it is your hand instead of his, you are there in person to flood his senses with what he can only fantasize about when he is alone. And that's just giving him a garden-variety handjob. There are extreme handjobs that can turn his entire body into a giant sex receptor.

What You Bring To It

Perhaps it might help to explain two different reasons why guys masturbate. There can be lots of other reasons—these are just two.

One reason is for fun time when he's alone. It's like playing his favorite video game—with the controller being in his pants and the display in his mind when he closes his eyes. Some women get upset when they discover their partner still jerks off; they don't understand what this kind of masturbation is about and they view it as rejection. That's unfortunate, because people usually masturbate throughout life, whether they are in a relationship or not.

There's another reason why a guy might masturbate. It has to do with longing for the presence and touch of a partner. He imagines a woman he loves is there and it helps him feel less alone. For a lot of us, this kind of jerking off helped us keep our sanity until someone like you came along. It was a form of sexual life support.

Depending on the mood and the situation, your handjob might be casual and fun—like the way he does himself when it's a form of sport—or it might be to supply comfort and intimacy. Either way, it's all good.

Although your hand may be doing the same thing that his hand has done thousands of times before, it's your presence that makes your handjob special and superior. That's why it's important for you look at it as being something special. Try putting more into it than just moving the muscles in your arm. Make it a fun and intimate act. Cuddle close to him. Take control. Give him tender kisses on the neck or nipples while you are doing him with your hand. Your handjobs can be more emotionally comforting than you might know.

A handjob can be an opportunity for intimacy and closeness that a lot of women underestimate. And you don't have to worry about STIs, getting pregnant or needing to swallow while giving a guy a handjob. What's not to like?

Getting a Grip—Learning Boy Basics

"I could never move my fist that fast for so long. He really manhandles that sucker, and it doesn't seem to hurt!" *female age 55*

A frequent complaint from men about the way women give handjobs is that they use too light of a touch.

One of the common slang terms for masturbation is "beat your meat." It's not "tickle your meat" or "caress your meat." It's BEAT your meat. Terms like "jerking off," "slap the monkey," "bash the bishop," and "whacking off" do not imply gentleness. The technique that men use most when they masturbate can be summarized as: Grab it and give it a good workout.

A mistake women commonly make is they don't ask their partner to tell them how firmly to grab. Does he want your hand tighter? Looser? Get the grip right, and you're halfway there.

Position, Position, Position

To find the optimal hand position, lie parallel to your partner and reach across his body as he does when he is masturbating. Ask him to form your fingers around his penis in the same way he does when he's alone and thinking about you.

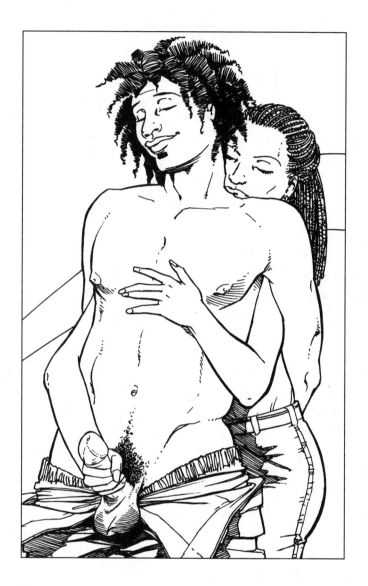

Her fingertips are on the side of his penis, rather than digging into the front. That way, her fingers glide smoothly over the sensitive frenulum area. Also, she's kissing his neck and caressing his chest with her other hand. All signs of excellent form.

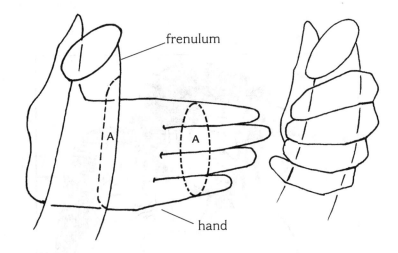

This is a rough approximation of where your hand should go when giving a hand job. Actual placement will depend on the size of your hand, the size of his equipment, the amount of foreskin (tight or loose circumcision or no circumcision) and the preferences of your partner.

Where he puts his hand on the shaft is more significant than you might think. Try to imitate the exact place where he grips himself. He probably positions his hand so it stimulates the most sensitive area of the penis called the frenulum. It's just below the head on the side that's away from the man's belly when he has an erection. It shows good form to rub your fingers—not your fingertips—over this spot with each stroke, especially if you plan on getting this over with before next Christmas.

Wrap your entire hand around the penis so your thumb and index finger would touch if there weren't a sausage in the way. Your hand should be in the same position as if it were holding a mug of coffee or a cup of tea. That's how we guys learn to masturbate, by drinking tea.

Make sure your fingertips are resting on the side or the back of the penis rather than in front. Otherwise, your fingertips would go over the frenulum, which can be uncomfortable. Guys usually position their hand so the crook of their finger rather than their fingertips rubs over the frenulum.

The Stroke

After your partner shows you where to place your hand on the shaft of his penis, have him show you how high and low to stroke. Different foreskins allow for different stroking distances. If your former boyfriend had a tight circumcision, his stroking distance might be a bit limited. If your current partner is not circumcised, he has more yardage to work with, and his stroking length is probably greater. That's why each guy needs to show you what he's used to.

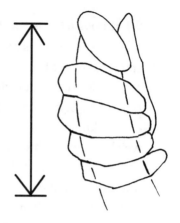

Some men will pull the foreskin all the way over the top of the head of their penis, others won't. Some will pull the foreskin all the way down to the scrotum, others won't. The main part of the sensation will come from rubbing your fingers over the frenulum.

Practice, Patience and Taking Control

Don't be surprised if it takes a few tutorials before you learn to give a handjob just right, especially if your hand is considerably smaller than his. If your own man is too uptight to teach you, any number of his friends will probably be willing to let you learn the basics on them, or maybe one of your BFFs can demonstrate on her boyfriend!

Once you learn the basics, all that's left is what you do with your lips and the fingers of your other hand, and then to feel comfortable taking control. Part of the fun of receiving a handjob is being able to kick back while your partner takes total control.

Dry or Lubed?

When you are circumcised, it can feel better to masturbate with lube. Masturbation or a handjob with lube can feel more like intercourse for a man who is circumcised and it lets him get more sensation from the head of his penis. However, masturbating dry is more practical. It is less of a production and there's less clean up.

An intact foreskin usually provides a really nice sensation without lube. This is one of the advantages to not being circumcised.

What Does a Penis Feel Like?

When a penis is soft it feels a little like human lips. The skin has a silky smooth, almost translucent texture that slides over the tissue beneath it. A soft penis is extremely flexible. It can be warm or cold to the touch and feels more like a squid than a hotdog. Some people describe it as being squishy.

To know what a hard penis feels like, find a fairly buff guy who lifts weights and ask him to flex his arms. A hard bicep feels similar to a hard penis, although a hard penis won't be nearly as big around. Poking a finger into a man's unflexed pecs will give you an approximate idea of what a semi-erect penis feels like. Here are some women's recollections about the first time they touched a penis:

> "It was sort of like 'Oh my God, what do you do with it?' I knew if you did something to it in the right way, that was good. I felt it very, very carefully, not sure what I was dealing with. It was like an alien creature that you were supposed to automatically know how to please. As I listen to myself describing it, I must have considered it as separate from the individual who it belonged to!" *female age 34*

> "It was not a pleasant experience then, but it sure is now."
> *female age 42*

> "I had intercourse a number of times but never touched it. I didn't get into that until much later." *female age 26*

> "I didn't like the way it felt when flaccid. A couple of years later I finally got around to making friends with it, and it became exciting."
> *female age 21*

> "It took me a while to figure out that you could really handle it, that it wasn't fragile." *female age 27*

Your Touch vs. His

Men sometimes view their body and their penis as two unrelated entities. They stroke the penis without caressing the other body parts that can help jerking off to feel more like a full-body experience. This is one of the ways that your giving a man a handjob can be so special—you will hopefully be adding your own special magic, perhaps by straddling some part of him and pushing your crotch into him, or by caressing him with your other hand, or by kissing him with your soft lips, or by whispering into his ear...

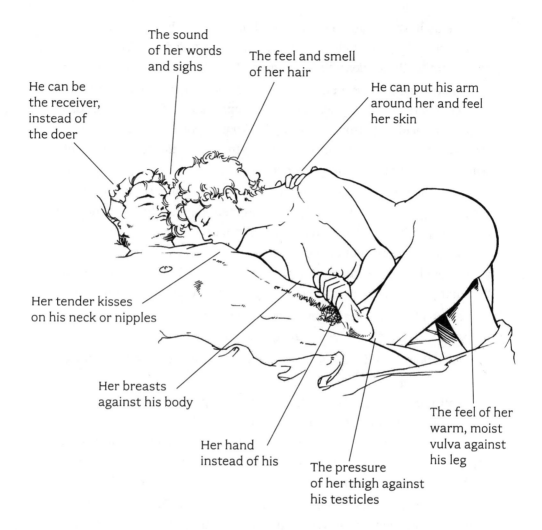

The sound of her words and sighs

The feel and smell of her hair

He can be the receiver, instead of the doer

He can put his arm around her and feel her skin

Her tender kisses on his neck or nipples

Her breasts against his body

Her hand instead of his

The pressure of her thigh against his testicles

The feel of her warm, moist vulva against his leg

Things a woman brings to a handjob.

Few women realize that they have the potential to control nearly every cell in a man's body with each stroke. Instead, they just jerk away until things get sticky.

Technical Points

Some women give handjobs that are jerky. After all, it's called "jerking off." And it might appear that when guys masturbate we use a single upstroke followed by a single downstroke, in rapid succession. But that's not how we do it. We usually have a more fluid motion. The hand doesn't stop or even slow down as it changes direction from up to down. The motion is smooth rather than jerky, which means the term "jerking off" is a misnomer.

Another issue is when a woman slows down or stops pumping as the man begins to ejaculate. Most guys will appreciate it if you keep stroking after they ejaculate ("stroking through") *although you need to ask him about making direct contact with the head of his penis, which can become incredibly sensitive as soon as a guy starts coming.*

Some men might want you to milk out each drop of semen. As part of the draining process, some guys push with their fingers into the hidden part of their penis that's between their balls, or into the perineum.

As his handjob motion becomes familiar, you might want to caress your lover's testicles with one hand as you are jerking him off with the other. Whether you kiss or stare into each other's eyes as he is coming is up to you.

Panty Play If he likes lingerie, take your panties off and drape them over his penis and testicles while you are giving him a handjob.

Variation Consider doing your man when he is standing or kneeling as opposed to lying on his back.

Ball Trick When masturbating, some guys push the little finger of the stroking hand against the lower part of the shaft near the scrotum. This causes the scrotum to jiggle or vibrate with each stroke, providing a secondary source of sensation. It's always best to seek a man's input when first trying to do this, since your pinky might inadvertently poke him in the balls.

Alternating Caresses and Stokes In his wonderful *Tricks to Please a Man* (Greenery Press) author Jay Wiseman lists several tips to make a traditional handjob more fun. He suggests caressing the penis and balls for ten seconds with your fingertips, followed by one quick up-and-down hand stroke. Then caress for ten more seconds, followed by two quick up-and-down hand strokes. After every ten-second period of caressing, increase the stroke total by one.

Thigh Sensation While facing him, have him straddle your thigh so it is touching or pushing up against his testicles as you are stroking his penis.

When a Man Helps a Partner Learn How to Please Him

A man can help both himself and his partner if he will turn the lights up, get naked, and let her learn about his genitals. The purpose is for her to tickle, squeeze, tug, and prod each part of your sexual anatomy so she can learn your comfort zones and become more confident in handling your penis and testicles. She should gently increase the pressure on each part until you say "Ouch!" Then back off just a bit. Here are a few specifics:

Penis Have her tug it, yank it, and squeeze it until she's able to distinguish your *Ouch!* zone from your *Ahh!* zone. Then help her learn how to grasp your penis to give you a handjob. Indicate how far up and down you like the strokes to go, as well as how fast to do them and how long you wish she would keep stroking after you come.

Testicles If the room is cold and your testicles have retracted almost to your armpits, turn up the heat and put something warm over your scrotum until you have coaxed your testicles back down. Once they are hanging freely, have her tickle, caress, and play with them, letting her know what feels good and what doesn't. Then have her slowly squeeze each testicle, helping her learn about your comfort zone. Also, have her put a finger or two in the space between your testicles and push in until she is massaging the buried part of your penis.

Extreme Hand-job Techniques For an Extremely Good Time

The next couple of pages talk about techniques for doing an extended handjob when your goal is to enhance sensation with each stroke as opposed to simply getting him off. Lubricating your hands and his genitals is essential. Any number of oils will work nicely, as long as you're thinking coconut or peanut oil instead of Penzoil.

Extreme Technique: Lube Him Up

The first thing to do is to get your partner completely naked. This is usually not a difficult task.

The most civilized way of lubricating a groin is to cup one hand over the man's genitals and drip massage oil over your hand. Gravity will pull the oil through your fingers and onto his genitals. Make sure his testicles and penis are thoroughly basted with oil. To catch the excess oil, put a thick towel under him with a sheet of plastic under that.

Different Strokes

When doing a man dry, it's best to be by his side so you can imitate his strokes. But when giving an extreme handjob, you will be using lube, so you can do a fine job from wherever you sit.

These strokes make it possible to give a man full-body sexual pleasure that he is not capable of giving himself. It is not necessary for him to have an erection for this to feel great. Some people think it feels best when the penis isn't erect, so please reassure your partner ahead of time that you don't expect him to stay hard, and it may feel better if he's only semi erect.

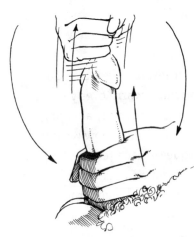

Fists Going Up Be sure all skin surfaces are well lubed. Wrap one hand around the base of the penis, squeeze lightly and pull it up along the shaft and into the air. As this hand is making its upward stroke, grab the base of the penis with your free hand, squeeze and do the same thing. Create a fluid motion with one hand constantly following the other. Slow the pace if the man shows signs of impending orgasm. Some folks suggest giving a little extra squeeze or snap on the upward stroke as your hand reaches the head of the penis.

Fists Going Down Same technique as above, only in the reverse direction with your hands going from the tip of the penis to the base. This usually requires an erection. Otherwise, his penis will just flop there in your hand. Also, don't grip as tightly as you might with fists going up. There's no point in shoving his penis into his body.

Thumbs Up While facing the man's crotch, clasp your fingers together as you might do while deep in prayer. The only difference here is that your hands are clasped around your man's penis. Use the pads of your thumbs to massage the front part of the penis that has the seam going up it. Spend extra time rubbing the area where the head attaches to the shaft. Just below this juncture is the sensitive frenulum. Some people compare the sensitivity of the frenulum to that of the clitoris, although they are overstating the case.

Open Palm Rubbing Head of Penis Some guys might like this; others won't. Hold the shaft of the penis in one hand. Open your other hand flat and rub it in a circular pattern over the head of the penis as though you were buffing it. Make sure the palm of your hand is well-lubed.

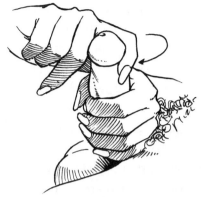

Twisting the Cap Off a Bottle of Beer Hold the shaft of a well-lubricated penis near the base. With your other hand, grasp the head of the penis as though it were the cap on a bottle of beer. Twist it as if you were opening a beer bottle, with your thumb and forefinger running along the groove under the ridge where the head attaches to the shaft.

Wringing a Towel Dry Grasp the lower part of a well-lubed penis with one hand and the upper part of the shaft with the other. There should be no gap between your hands unless nature endowed the man with exceptional proportions. Twist your hands back and forth in opposite directions.

Strokes to Try When The Foreskin Is Pulled Taut

The penis can usually be made more sensitive by pulling the foreskin down against the scrotum to make it tighter. Guys who masturbate with lubrication often use one hand to pull the foreskin taut while stroking the shaft with the other. This also helps keep the baggy skin on the scrotum from rising up onto the shaft of the penis.

To make the foreskin more taut, clamp your thumb and forefinger around the shaft of the penis nearly an inch above where it joins the testicles (scrotum). Pull the skin down so your other fingers and palm rest on the testicles. This will make the foreskin feel tighter.

If the man is uncircumcised, reach higher up on the shaft to pull the extra skin down. If a penis is circumcised, you won't have as much foreskin to pull taut. But these strokes can still feel good regardless of a man's circumcision status. *Only do genital massage on a penis when the foreskin is pulled taught if you are using lubrication.*

Penis-Belly Rub The penis should be lubricated and resting flat against the man's belly. Pull the skin taut at the base of the penis. Open your other hand and lay it flat on top of the penis; then drag it toward the man's chest, as if you were trying to push or pull the good feelings out of his penis and onto the skin of his belly. Repeat.

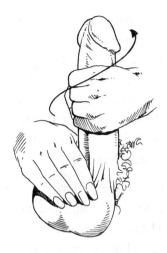

The Corkscrew or Following the Stripe on the Barber's Pole Pull the skin taut at the base of your partner's well-lubricated penis. Wrap your other hand around the base, squeeze lightly and twist it upward as though you were following a corkscrew or the stripe on a barber's pole. If his penis is hard enough, you can do a reverse downstroke. This should return your hand to the same position where it started, or just do a series of upward strokes. Whether you are simultaneously giving oral sex or just a lubricated handjob, don't hesitate to use a twisting motion up and down on the shaft of the penis, especially just beneath the head.

Thumbs Up — Thumbs Down There are two ways to grasp a penis that is lubricated. One is with your thumb upward, so your little finger is closest to the base of the penis. The other is with your hand facing down, so the thumb is around the base and your little finger is around the head end of the penis. It can be quite impressive when a woman alternates hand orientation with her stroking hand, so he never knows if the next stroke will be thumbs up or thumbs down.

Octopussy Fingers Pull the foreskin taut with one hand. Lay the palm of your other hand over the head of the penis and drop your fingers down along the sides of the shaft. (Your hand will look like an open parachute or an octopus.) Your fingers will stimulate the sides of the penis as you move your hand up and down. You can also twist your hand sideways, or do a corkscrew stroke that combines both motions.

Massaging Under the Testicles

If his scrotum is tight, heat the room and put a warm washcloth over the man's crotch. Let it warm up for a couple of minutes until the testicles hang freely. Press into the middle of the scrotum with the pads of your fingers. You will be touching the part of the penis that is covered by the testicles.. There is often a single spot on this part of the penis where a number of ligaments, muscle fibers, and nerve endings seem to converge. Putting fingertip pressure on this spot while massaging the "regular" part of the penis with your other

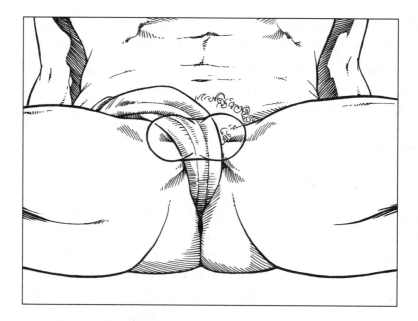

The Man with Invisible Balls

Women often assume the penis is somehow glued or stapled to the front of a man's pelvic bone. In reality, it runs beneath his testicles and anchors inside his pelvis. Some men enjoy having the "invisible" part of the penis massaged. Push into the space between the testicles with your fingertips and gently rub. Also massage the flat space behind his testicles (aka "taint").

hand can create a subtle, warm feeling that some men will find enjoyable. This nerve bundle might be on one side of the shaft rather than in the middle. You might also try massaging this area when giving a blowjob.

You might also try massaging the area behind the scrotum, that runs from the scrotum to the anus. This is called the perineum or "taint."

Additional Testicle Massage Techniques

Here are a few techniques to try on the testicles, as well as some strokes that include the testicles and penis. None of these strokes should cause any pain or discomfort. If they do, stop. There is more information about testicles and testicle massage in Chapter 17: *Balls, Balls, Balls.*

Simple Testicle Massage Explore with your fingertips the space between and around the testicles. Be gentle at first, and seek plenty of feedback. Once you find a form of massage that feels pleasing for your partner, do it often. For some men, the sensation feels like it's part back rub and part orgasm.

Ball Rub With the thumb and forefinger of one hand, make a ring around the part of your partner's scrotum where it attaches to his groin. Squeeze gently until his testicles are popping out a bit, but not enough to cause pain. Run the fingertips of your other hand up and down the sides of his scrotum with a light tickling touch.

Flat-Handed Doggy Dig Straddle your partner's chest while facing his feet. Lay his penis flat against his belly with the head pointing up toward his navel. Place one of your well-lubricated hands between his legs with your fingertips resting below his testicles. Pull the hand all the way up to his belly, dragging your fingers over his testicles and penis. Repeat with your other hand, rhythmically alternating strokes as a dog might when digging in the dirt. This same stroke is illustrated in Chapter 15: *The Zen of Finger Fucking.*

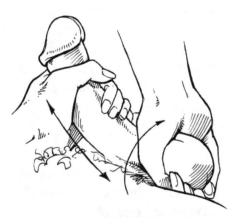

Penis Up, Balls Down Be sure your hands are well-lubricated. Grasp the lower part of the penis with one hand. Clamp the fingers of your other hand around the base of the scrotum where it attaches to the groin. This should cause the testicles to pop out a bit, and the skin covering them should become taut. Squeeze both hands lightly. Then do an upward stroke with the penis hand while the testicles hand pulls gently in the opposite direction. Find a tempo that works for both of you, and keep repeating these strokes.

The Point of No Return

When doing an extreme handjob, you might want to keep a man highly aroused for long periods of time without letting him ejaculate. It is possible!

Consider a scale of 0 to 10 where 0 means no sexual arousal and 10 is an orgasm. Let's say your partner starts to ejaculate when he reaches a 9 on this scale. Past that, there's no turning back. Try to keep him between 7 and 8 for as long as possible. When he finally does ejaculate, it might feel quite intense.

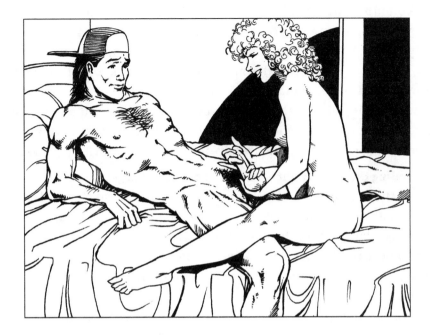

This position can be great for hand jobs with lube, but not so good for doing it dry. Worse yet, her form is poor (fingertips on the frenulum). But he doesn't care, what with his washboard abs and cool cap.

One way to keep a guy at such a high level of excitement is to learn his body language for when he is about to ejaculate. There are physical signs for this: the veins in his penis may start to bulge, or his penis might give a sudden throb, the color of the head might darken, his testicles may suck up into his groin, his muscles may suddenly tighten, his hips may thrust, and he might start to groan or invoke the names of the saints. To help delay his ejaculation, decrease the intensity when this starts to happen.

Some women find it very helpful if the man is able to report his levels of excitement. This will help you learn when to up the pace and when to back off. After a while you will become so familiar with his body language that you won't need him to tell you.

Ready, Set, Relax

It never hurts to begin genital massage by finding those parts of your partner's body where tension gathers. Who knows why, but the shoulders and back often become the body's collecting points for tension. There is no point in doing good work on a man's genitals when the weight of the world is parked between his shoulder blades. This is also true for women's bodies.

Some men believe that the only important part of sex is when a penis is being rubbed, sucked or fucked. They might not care about the tension in their shoulders. They will sometimes direct your hands straight to their crotch with the idea that an orgasm will help relax them. While this is true, think of how much more pleasure they could receive if they were relaxed to begin with.

Spreading the Excitement — Pavlov Between the Legs

Handjobs can be used to help a man link the sensations in his crotch with other parts of his body. For instance, you might gently stimulate the man's genitals with one hand while caressing other parts of his body with your other hand. It may help if he inhales deeply while you are doing this, as though he is sucking the warm glow from his genitals into the upper part of his body.

Or you might try kissing or caressing your partner's neck, shoulders, nipples, or chest while massaging his genitals. At various intervals, stop stroking your partner's genitals but continue to kiss or caress the other parts of his body. If he were a dog and his name was Pavlov, he might eventually learn to have genital sensations when you caress these other body parts without reaching between his legs. Likewise, he might learn to have pleasant sensations in other parts of his body when his penis is stimulated. The goal is to help a man experience sensation over his entire body.

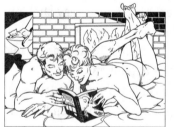

Dear Paul,
What if a guy is uncircumcised? Do you give him the same kind of handjob as a guy who is cut?

Helen from Troy

Dear Helen,
An uncut penis has plenty of foreskin that slides up and down with each stroke. The foreskin also keeps the head of the penis moist. As a result, it's even easier to give a guy a handjob who is not circumcised, and it doesn't require lube. (The skin on a circumcised penis is tighter and the head is dry. The foreskin doesn't glide up and down as smoothly.)

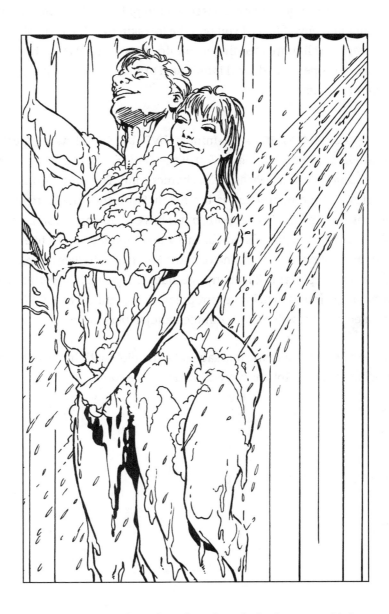

The shower is a fine place for a handjob. If you need lube,
try hair conditioner instead of soap. Soap can burn if it
gets into the urethra.

If your partner is not circumcised, you might try a few foreskin tricks—like asking him how if feels if you pull the foreskin over the head of his penis. Then insert a well-lubricated fingertip into the space between the foreskin and head of his penis, and swirl it around. For more tips, see Chapter 27: *Fun with Your Foreskin.*

HIGHLY RECOMMENDED: A 20-minute DVD by The Pleasure Mechanics titled *Guide to Handjobs, How to Touch the Penis for Prolonged Arousal and Powerful Orgasms* (www.PleasureMechanics.com). The tone in this video is wonderful and the instruction is top notch. Since they use a lifelike penis instead of a real penis, it is not porn, but it has everything a woman needs to know about giving a great handjob. This video should be given to every teenage girl and young woman in the country. Being able to give an exceptional handjob is an important skill at any age, but it's especially important if there is no condom around to help prevent pregnancy or the spread of STIs. Watching a video like this will help guarantee handjob perfection.

Also, there are several erotic massage (aka handjob with lube) videos at the New School of Erotic Touch: www.EroticMassage.com.

15
The Zen of Finger Fucking

" Rubbing lightly is what I do when I masturbate, so I like it even more when my boyfriend does it. I love it when he runs his fingers along my inner lips, up and down. I also love my genitals to be rubbed and tickled when I wear jeans or corduroy. I can come from that kind of stimulation." *female age 23*

Some men take the term "finger fucking" quite literally. They think a woman's idea of a good time is having a man cram his fingers up her vagina. Or they attack a woman's clitoris as if it were a doorbell button, believing that the harder they push it the closer she will come to having the big "O." The only "O" she is likely to experience is "OUCH!"

Finger fucking is not something a man does to a woman, but something he does with a woman. It's all of him — his smile, kiss, laughter, strength, and tenderness focused in the ends of his fingers.

Hopefully you will find this chapter to be helpful, especially if you are able to leave your jackhammer behind and are willing to try things with your fingers that you might not have tried before. But none of it will make a difference if your partner isn't already turned-on before you touch her clitoris. If she isn't already feeling at least somewhat aroused, that's what you need to focus on rather than sticking your hand between her legs. (Being highly aroused usually changes the way a woman experiences touch on her clitoris.) Feedback is also crucial. It won't help if she doesn't give you feedback.

Please forgive the term "finger fucking." It's just an expression. The last thing you'll want is for your fingers to be doing a bony imitation of a penis fucking a woman's vagina unless that's what she wants you to do. If your fingers were supposed to do the job of a penis, something white and gooey would squirt out of the tips when you rubbed your knuckles.

Backseat Groping

There are different kinds of finger fucking. One involves the hot-and-heavy groping that's an extension of making out. It's when a guy gets his hand between a woman's legs because she wants it there and because there's all kinds of passion and kissing and drooling going on. It's all about the moment. You don't need a chapter on that.

What follows is learning how to please a woman with your fingertips. It's nothing you do in the dark or while you are stoned or drunk. The first few times, it requires lights, looking, and lots of feedback. And if the stars are lined up just right, and you and she are truly into each other and your phones are turned off, you might just end up giving her incredible amounts of pleasure.

Altered Process, Altered Goals

The first thing to do is to banish the usual guy-goal of giving a girl an orgasm. She'll have one if she has one: maybe you'll be the medium, maybe not.

With the kind of finger fucking that's in this chapter, you'll try to help her walk along the edge of something intense and sweet for longer than she may have with guys before. It's something she might do when she's alone and masturbating, but it's not always easy to achieve when the fingers and game plan are not her own.

While an orgasm at the end of the rainbow is a worthy goal, sometimes goals can get in the way. You'll be way ahead if you stop trying to orchestrate an "Oh-my-God-I'm-Coming!" type of orgasm. The experience you are going for is different from the kind of fast blast you get when you are jerking off, which is great for a guy but doesn't always achieve full bandwidth for a girl.

Coaching, Patience & Practice

"I had to learn how to touch her clit... I can remember being clumsy about it early on. She'd have to stop me — I was going too fast, going too hard. I can remember her saying, 'You're in the wrong place.' 'Well, show me where. I mean physically, show me. Rub so I can see it. OK, now I understand.' Over time, I've learned where the places are. I can find them in the dark now. But early on I couldn't.... She would take my hand, or my finger, and she would put it right exactly where it was supposed to be, and she'd move it the way she wanted me to move it, and she would apply pressure to the back of my fingers, the amount of pressure she wanted, until I got the hang of it, and then she would take her hand away. If I got out of sync or something, she'd put her hand back and show me until I got it right. A few weeks later I might need some re-education, so she'd show me again." —From *Sex: An Oral History*, by Harry Maurer, Viking.

First, try to learn how to do your sweetheart in the same way she does herself, assuming she does herself. Start by making an agreement with her that she will provide lots of coaching and patience, and you will provide an eager willingness to learn.

Also take heart in knowing that hands that are used to throwing a baseball, digging with a shovel, abusing a game controller, or torquing down engine bolts can get frustrated when it comes to finessing a woman's genitals. Fingers that spend hours each day on a keyboard might fare better, but probably not. There's the matter of knowing when to speed up, slow down, push softer or harder, or stay your course. It requires patience and practice.

For some excellent videos on The Clitoris, visit the book's website
www.GuideToGettingItOn.com.

Penis vs. Clitoris — Course Correction Required!

"I've seen a couple of guys masturbate. I can't believe how rough they are with themselves!" *female age 26*

The reason this woman can't believe how "rough" we guys are with ourselves is because she would never dream of touching her genitals in that way. Think of how you squeeze or wag your penis when you are finished peeing. Approach a clitoris with that kind of careless abandon, and you are likely to be a dead man.

It's usually fine to handle a penis that's not aroused. A man doesn't feel pain when he does this, and he rarely minds it when a partner strokes or touches his penis when it is not aroused. But that isn't how it usually works with a clitoris. It's best if a woman is sexually aroused before you touch her clitoris. If she's aroused, the right kind of touch can feel wonderful. Otherwise, it can feel painful.

Ways That Women Stimulate Their Clitoris

Rub their entire hand up and down, stimulating the clitoris, inner labia, and outer labia.

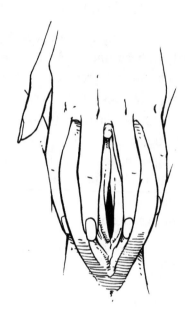

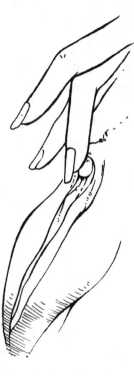

Softly stimulate the glans or tip of the clitoris.

Adapted with thanks from Sadie Allison's
**Tickle Your Fancy — A Woman's Guide
To Sexual Self-Pleasure**

Place three or four fingers between the outer labia and massage.

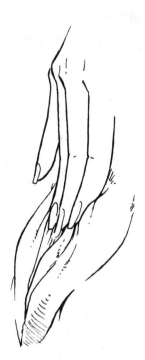

Separate the outer labia with their index and ring fingers while stimulating the clitoris with their middle finger.

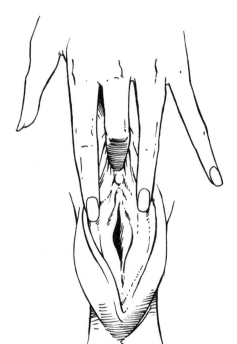

More Ways That Women Stimulate Their Clitoris

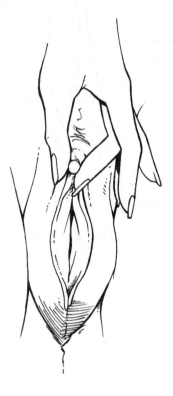

Roll, squeeze, tug, or lift.

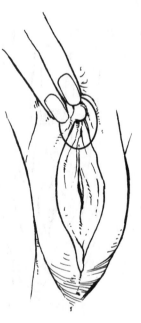

Rub along the side (up and down) or in circles.

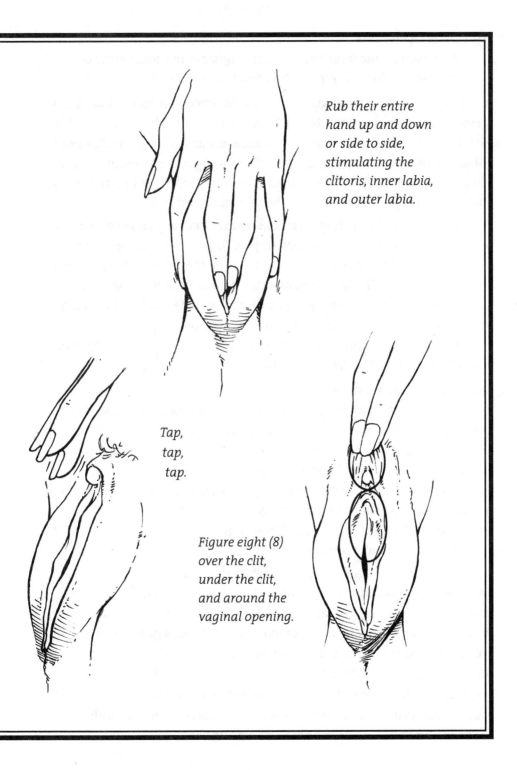

Rub their entire hand up and down or side to side, stimulating the clitoris, inner labia, and outer labia.

Tap, tap, tap.

Figure eight (8) over the clit, under the clit, and around the vaginal opening.

Try a Little Tenderness

"When women moan or gasp, it encourages me to press harder or faster on the clit. Always with poor results." *male age 41*

When it comes to touching a woman's clit, always err on the side of tenderness. Assume that softer is better. Push just hard enough to move the skin back and forth over the shaft of the clitoris, assuming you can find the shaft of the clitoris. And don't even get near the naked glans of the clitoris until you've paid your respects to a woman's inner thighs, larger lips and mons pubis. The tip or glans of the clitoris should be your last stop.

The tip of the clitoris is often more sensitive than any single part of the penis. You don't want the rough skin of your fingers to suddenly rub across it. This is why you should gently push and pull on the clitoral hood and labia (lips) as a way of indirectly simulating the clitoris until a woman lets you know it's ready for further engagement. Ultimately, it depends on the woman, how sensitive her clitoris is, and on how sexually aroused she is.

There are other kinds of genital massage where your lover may want you to be more vigorous. We'll get to that.

Showing Instead of Telling

Be aware that a woman's understanding of her own sexuality is sometimes on a body level and she may struggle when trying to put it into words. Getting all frustrated and yelling "Just tell me" does absolutely no good. She probably would if she could, but it's like asking someone to tell you the meaning of life. She may simply have to show you by putting her own hands over yours and guiding your fingers as they go. Or she might say, "Keep trying different ways—I'll let you know when it feels right" or "Maybe my clit wouldn't be so shy if you weren't pressing quite so hard..." or "Try it here."

Also, a woman might say "harder" when she means faster, or vice versa. And never make the mistake of thinking that if a little pressure feels good, a lot of pressure will send her through the ceiling. This may happen, but not in the way you intended. Guys also reason that if slow feels good, fast will feel even better. This distortion in thinking will get you nowhere. If faster is what she wants, work on establishing signals so she can let you know.

Mix-ups will happen. You can get really frustrated. But it's not like anybody is going to die or lose their job because you confused harder with faster. You have your hands between a woman's legs. Be happy.

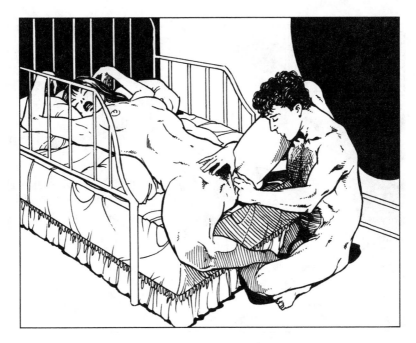

*The Prince is fingering a very happy Snow White
while the Dwarfs are away in the forest.*

Intrigue along the Inseam

In matters of love and sex, it never hurts for a man's fingers to have a sense of humor. Fingertips that tease and dance will find an especially warm welcome. Gently running your fingertips up and down a woman's inner thigh is a million times more enticing than shoving your middle finger up her crotch. If and when she's ready to have your fingers inside of her, she will let you know. Even then it's sometimes wise to tease and play some more.

Instruments of Pleasure or Weapons of Mass Destruction?

Make sure there are no rough edges on your fingernails. Keep your fingernails smooth and clean. Pry out any grease or dark gunk that's under them. And if your hands are rough, put hand lotion on them every day.

Learning Her Style

"It's not a dish of salted peanuts down there, don't just grab and hope for the best. It's very sensitive. Even the slightest movement can produce a reaction, good or bad." *female age 45*

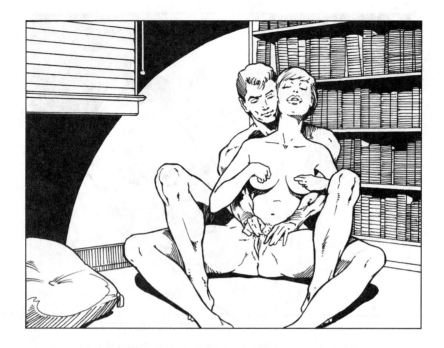

So you're going to learn how she masturbates,. Grab a boddice-ripper (romance) novel with one hand, and have a bowl of popcorn or chips close by. That's how some women do it. Read a few pages, rub a little clit, read a few pages, eat some chips... And if she doesn't masturbate, maybe you'll want to learn the fine art together.

When a woman masturbates, she often rests her wrist on her lower abdomen just above the pubic bone. Try to do the same, since it will influence the way your fingers feel on her vulva.

Lie next to her and reach your arm over her body until your fingers are between her legs. This allows your fingers to approach her vulva in the same way that her own fingers do. Or try sitting like the couple in the illustration above. Don't try to "masturbate" her while sitting between her legs and facing her vulva. This is a great position to use for the kind of genital massage, but it's not particularly effective if you are trying to imitate the way she touches herself.

Here are some observations and tips for learning how to do a woman the way she does herself.

☂ Dry fingers on a dry clitoris do not make for the best of times. Try to bring lubrication up from the bottom part of her vaginal opening, where the lips make a "U." This is where a woman's natural lube tends to initially pool. Drag the fluid up with your fingertips, or use saliva or lube. This assumes you have spent the time and effort to help her become aroused.

☂ Ask if your partner uses extra lubrication when she masturbates, such as saliva, baby oil, Vaseline, coconut oil, KY, or Liquid Silk. Never be shy about using extra lubrication, especially if you'll be at it for long periods of time.

☂ When men try to masturbate women, they often use all fingers and no wrist. When a woman does herself she will sometime incorporate her wrist into the motion, with only one finger touching her vulva. This can be a subtle but significant detail, and it requires practice. (If you think your tongue wants to fall off during oral sex, wait until you try doing the wrist-thing for 20 minutes. There are reasons why women use vibrators.)

☂ Find out if your partner 's a favorite side of her clitoris or labia that she likes to stimulate. Be su   v her lead.

☂ Some women v   ll back the hood of the clitoris to more directly stimu   will allow for much higher lev-els of stimulatio   fficiently aroused or if she's not someone wh   -fucking felony.

☂ An excellent   ut pleasing your partner is to rest your fingers over hers w   sturbating. Then do the reverse, with her placing her fingers on t   rs, acting as guides. A woman shouldn't hesitate to take a man's finger and put them exactly on those parts of her body where she likes to be touched. Most men will appreciate the assist, and after about the 500th time, most will remember how to do it just right.

☂ Another advantage of having your arm resting across your partner's body is it allows you to feel how her body is responding. This is important, because as a woman becomes more aroused she may need you to stimulate her in a different way. Or it might be a cue to keep stimulating her in exactly the same way. Being able to read her body's signals is essential.

☂ Some women direct the stimulation to just one spot. Others might stimulate themselves in a more global way when they are masturbating, tugging and pulling on the surface of the entire vulva.

🌂 Since the shaft of the clitoris runs though the mons pubis, some women push and pull on the mons or push into it and make a circular motion with it.

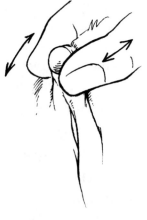

🌂 Some women move their finger side-to-side across the clitoris, or up and down like when plucking a guitar. She will assume it's all very simple and have no idea why you don't get it.

🌂 Novelty is not always good. Try to achieve a steady tempo and rhythm with your fingers. That way, if she says "faster" or "slower," you'll have a point of reference to work from.

Whether you should roll the shaft of the clitoris depends on how long it is and if she wants you to.

🌂 Some women may need an array of sensations because they habituate to the same finger motion and it loses its effect. However, they may be in the minority. Always discuss this first.

🌂 Ask if your partner puts something inside of her vagina when she masturbates. This can provide a feeling of fullness, which can help amplify the sensations. Other women prefer external stimulation only.

🌂 Some women like something in or on their anus. If you are trying to duplicate everything she does, it's not going to work if she forgets to tell you about the vibrating butt plug that she can't get off without.

It's Time for Genital Massage

Giving a woman the kind of genital massage that is described in the pages that follow differs from trying to "get her off by hand" in a number of ways. You will be working her into a high level of sensation and then trying to keep her there. By using specific finger movements on her clitoris, you might be able to help her stay near peak levels of pleasure for several minutes or more. But this will require finding the right spots around her clitoris to keep your fingertips on, and maintaining a consistent rhythm.

The Vulva: XBox for Grown-Ups?

Aside from the satisfaction of being able to truly delight your partner, doing genital massage might also allow you to see her genitals open up, puff up, brighten, contract and perhaps even pulse.

In addition to the visual feedback, you'll be receiving sensory feedback from the tip of your finger. Eventually, you might be able to tell from the feeling in your finger where it's best to be. Sometimes you can help her reach different levels of sensation as you change the length of your finger's stroke by just a hair, or by changing the speed, or pressure.

Getting Started with Genital Massage

The woman should be lying on her back. Her partner sits between her legs, facing her with her vulva in front of him, or he can sit to one side of her, with one of her open legs across his lap. The point is for him to have good access to her vulva with both hands, and to have a good view so he can see the changes that are occurring in her vulva as she becomes more aroused.

You might start by caressing her inner thighs to help her relax and to build excitement. This seems like a contradiction, but the more relaxed a woman feels, the more sexually excited her body can become.

This is a good time to start talking to each other, because you will need lots of feedback to learn where and how to touch. This simply won't work without a woman's input. Likewise, you will want to tell her what you are going to do before you do it.

No matter how wet your partner is or gets, use and reuse lots of lube that's good for massage, such as coconut oil or some of the masturbation lubes mentioned in Chapter 12: *Sex Lubes—A New Look.*

Put at least a tablespoon or two of lube on your fingers and start at her perineum. This is the area between her vulva and bum. Pull your fingers and the lube up from there, through her labia, all the way up into the pubic hair area on her mons pubis. It's fine to not directly touch her clit just yet. Avoiding it can be part of the build-up.

Make sure she tells you how the lube feels as you are applying it. She should especially tell you about anything you are doing that feels good.

CLIT MASSAGE: The clit-massaging aficionados from *The Welcomed Consensus* who are referenced at the end of the chapter still recommend using old-fashioned KY in the tube, and/or Vaseline on the clit itself. This may be too gooey, goopy or thick for intercourse and not the best for massaging her lips and the rest of her vulva, but they haven't found anything better for direct clit massage

Clit Clocks—Finding Her Mark

Imagine a clock—the old-fashioned type that has a big hand, a little hand, and perhaps even a cuckoo bird at the top. Mentally superimpose the clock over the tip of her clitoris. This will give you a map for how to find any special spots that you will want to focus on in the future.

Also, look at how the inner lips of her vulva are sitting, their color, and observe the opening of her vagina. The landscape of her vulva will be changing as you find the right spots to massage. Visual cues will be helpful and kind of amazing. People think nothing of a penis swelling when it is aroused, but we seldom think of a woman's vulva as changing. (If she's okay with it ,you might take before and after pictures so she can see the changes.)

Next, put a glob of lube on the tip of your index finger. Depending on your inclination and her anatomy, you might pull the hood on her clit back

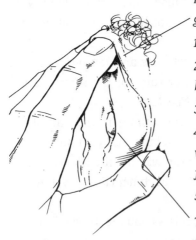

Reaching under the hood for the glans of her clitoris.

1. She needs to feel very aroused first.

2. Be sure there is a thick layer of lube between your finger and her clitoris.

3. Make very light, gentle movements.

4. Give each other lots of feedback, to find what spot feels best and how to move the finger tip over it.

5. Relube or add water to keep surface slick.

The opening of her vagina may become round if her vulva is engorged enough.

This is a form of stimulation that might work for some women. For others, it will be too much or too little.

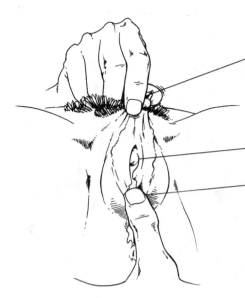

Clitoris stimulation by the hand above while the hand below puts pressure on the lower part of the vaginal opening and the perineum area.

The opening of her vagina.

Thumb pressure from below might help amplify the sensations, or you might try using your entire hand against her perineum area at the same time that you are massaging her clitoris.

with the fingers of your other hand or you might simply push into the space between the hood and the glans. Gently circle the glans of her clit with the lube. Ask her to tell you what it feels like. Ask if she wants you to push harder or more lightly. Make sure you notice what her clit feels like on your fingertip. How does it respond when you touch the spot? How does the rest of her vulva respond? Does it make her anus contract? Observe as much as you can.

What you are trying to do is to find spots that generate nice feelings when you stroke your fingertip across them. For instance, you might try a linear motion, as if you are flicking a tiny light switch on and off. If you find any spots that she says feel good, experiment with the pressure and the length of the "on-off" motion.

Fist or Thumb on the Lower Part of Her Vaginal Opening

To help create a sensation of groundedness in your lover's vulva, you might try pushing the thumb or palm of your other hand against the lower part of her vaginal opening or on her perineum (see illustration above). This helps some women to feel a sense of solidity or comfort.

Remember, you are providing comforting pressure to the outside of her genitals. This isn't the time to be putting your fingers inside of her vagina unless she specifically asks you to.

Sexually reactive structures that are inside a woman's pelvis where they can't be seen.

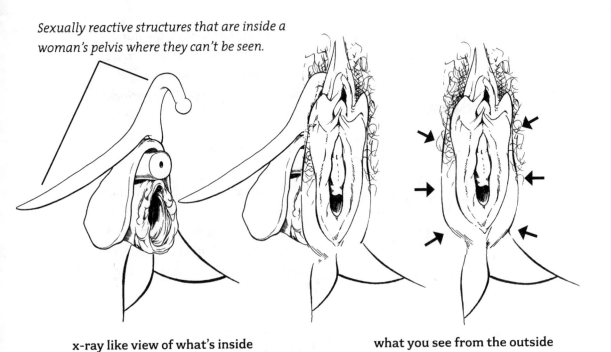

x-ray like view of what's inside   **what you see from the outside**

Finger pressure into the groin along the base of the labia majora (bigger lips) can feel very pleasing to some women. You are not only massaging the labia, but you might be stimulating parts of your partner's sexual anatomy that are buried far beneath her labia. (Push in with your fingertips; let her feedback be your guide.) Some women also enjoy it when you squeeze your fingertips together over the labia, massaging the tissue that way.

Anticipation vs. Dread

If it stops being fun for the two of you, or if it starts to feel uncomfortable or overwhelming, stop!

If you go beyond what feels good, her body will tense up the next time, and that's what you don't want to have happen. If this is something the two of you try again, she needs to look forward to it. Anticipation can work for you, and it can work against you.

While the next part of this chapter describes techniques for stimulating the inside of a woman's vagina, it does so only in the name of exploration, and because some women find it enjoyable. Others don't like it.

Don't expect sexual pleasure to have rules and to be universal, which is what porn, some of the women's magazines and the sex-toy business wants you to believe.

Fingers inside Her Vagina

A lot of guys think the goal of finger fucking is to get their finger all the way to the back of a woman's vagina. This would show a profound misunderstanding of how a woman's vagina is wired.

You never want to surprise a woman's vagina by suddenly shoving a finger into it. A more satisfying approach is to ease your finger in slowly and in stages, one joint at a time, and only after she has reached a level of arousal where she's spreading her legs and arching her hips in a good way.

Think of the vagina as a tube that's about four inches long. Once a woman is sexually aroused, start at the rim (opening) of the vagina. Put pressure on each part of the tissue around the opening as your finger eventually makes a complete circle. She needs to give you feedback about any spots that she might want you to revisit. Then move your fingertip a little deeper inside and do the same thing all over again. Keep repeating this until you have done her whole vagina.

It helps to be extra thorough about exploring the first third of the vagina, because that's a part that can be most sensitive to touch. Pay special attention to the upper half of her vagina between 9:00 and 3:00. A number of women report pleasurable responses in this part of the vagina.

Eventually, she might want you to do an in-out motion with your fingers, or maybe not. Don't assume she'll want your finger to thrust in and out like a penis. When it comes to sexual stimulation, fingers and penises are two very different tools and should be used differently.

A woman may want you to stimulate the roof of her vagina. Maybe she will want you to jiggle your hand or pull upward, so your finger makes an "L" or a hook, where the first part of your finger stays inside her vagina and your inner knuckle pulls up against her clitoris.

If you give each other lots of feedback, you will discover what does and doesn't work. Just don't assume that what worked for a former partner will be well-received by your current lover.

If you have been stimulating her clitoris with good results and her genitals are puffed up, you might want to keep pleasing her clitoris with one finger while placing a finger from your other hand in her vagina. Stimulation from your other hand may feel good for some women, but will be too much or distracting for another woman.

If Old-Fashioned Finger-Fucking Is What She Wants

In reviewing lesbian porn movies, author Jay Wiseman noticed that when lesbian performers put their fingers in a partner's vagina, they almost always use two fingers—not one or three. Wiseman asked a number of women about this, and most replied that two fingers simply feel better. This will also depend upon a woman's level of arousal, the size of her partner's hand, and sometimes upon her body's menstrual status.

You might consider wearing latex gloves when putting your fingers inside a woman's vagina. The smooth latex surface sometimes feels nice for

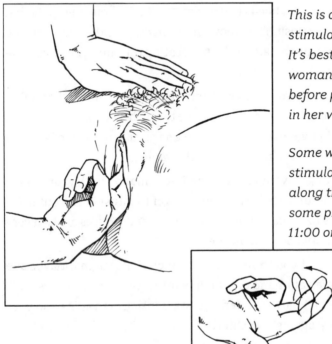

This is a common way to stimulate the G-spot area. It's best to wait until the woman is highly aroused before putting your fingers in her vagina.

Some women prefer you to stimulate the G-spot area along the roof of the vagina; some prefer a fingertip at 11:00 or 1:00.

Some women enjoy G-spot area massage, others find it to be unproductive or uncomfortable.

the woman and helps keep your fingers from stinging when they marinate in vaginal fluids, which are fairly acidic. Try putting a dab of water-based lube inside each fingertip of the glove. See if it makes any difference for you or her.

Isn't She Supposed To Scream with Delight?

Actually, no. Some women who are relaxed and receiving maximum sexual pleasure zone out and go into another world. While they might moan or smile, hip-bucking and screaming aren't usually part of it. With other women, you might need to give the neighbors ear plugs. There is no correlation between decibels and delight.

Other Things to Consider

When massaging different parts of a woman's genitals, apply just enough pressure to move the skin back and forth over the tissue that's under it. Press harder if she asks.

Finding a man's peehole is not a particularly taxing exercise; finding a woman's can take a bit of work. Why would you want to? Because there is a small dome of tissue that surrounds a woman's urinary opening. Some women might enjoy it if you stimulate this area.

Some women feel a certain dull but enjoyable sensitivity around the base or deepest part of the vagina, a full finger deep. This part of the vagina might be more sensitive to pressure than touch.

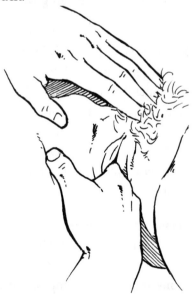

Place your free hand over the lower part of your lover's abdomen. Experiment by applying different kinds of pressure with your top hand while you are exploring inside her vagina with the fingers from your other hand.

A woman's cervix can usually be found in the upper rear part of her vagina. It is easily felt if she is on all fours or brings her legs to her chest. The cervix feels like a little dome of tissue that you can run your finger around. It may also have a small cleft in the middle, like your chin. Some women may enjoy it if you carefully stimulate the area surrounding the cervix. Others won't. Cervical sensitivity can vary with a woman's menstrual cycle; massaging it may release some blood if she is close to her period.

☂The perineum is the groin's version of a demilitarized zone. It separates the anus and vagina. Push into the surface with your fingertips and see what she says. (A woman's perineum is much shorter than a man's.)

☂The ring of the anus contains a multitude of nerve endings. Women and men who don't have aesthetic problems with anal stimulation might enjoy an exploration of their rectal area. You may find that one part of the anus is more sensitive than other parts. Putting a finger on it might generate a deep sense of pleasure. Be careful about going from a woman's rectum to her vulva without first washing your hands.

☂While lying next to your partner, rest your arm across her body with your fingers on her vulva. Separate her labia with your first and third fingers and stroke between her inner lips with your middle finger, bringing lubrication up from the bottom of her vaginal opening. Also, some women like to have their vulvas tapped with fingers, and some even like to be lightly slapped on the genitals. Ask first!

☂A woman's pubic bone can be an excellent perch for a tired hand whose fingers are playing with the lips and folds below.

☂Place a well-lubricated hand between your partner's legs with your fingertips resting below her vulva but not touching her anus. Pull your hand all the way up to her stomach, with your fingertips gently separating her labia with each stroke. Then do the same thing with your other hand, alternating strokes.

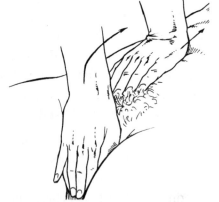

Massaging the Mons

The mons pubis is the fleshy mound at the top of the vulva just above where the lips begin to open. It usually has hair on it. It's easy to ignore the mons and head straight for the clitoris, yet some women masturbate by put-

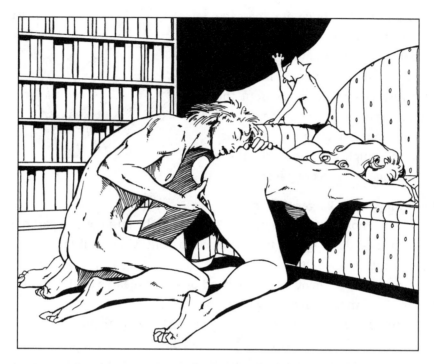

*Some women enjoy being touched from behind,
when they are lying on their stomach or are on all fours
or while they are leaning over something.*

ting fingertip pressure on the mons and making a circular or back-and-forth motion with it. Some women enjoy it when a partner kneads the mons or taps on it with his fingertips.

Or you can try pushing the palm of your hand against the mons and make a circular motion with it. If you are trying to amplify sensation, you might pull up on the mons with one hand while gently tugging on the inner lips with the fingers of the other.

The Lip Part of Erotic Massage

To massage the outer lips, clasp each lip with a lubricated thumb and forefinger. Then run your fingers from the lower to upper part of the lips, as though you were tracing one side of a parenthesis.

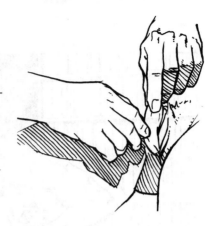

Another form of genital massage is done by holding a lubricated inner lip between your thumb and forefinger. While squeezing just a little, pull your fingers straight away from the woman's body. Your fingers will end up in the air an inch or two above her body, as though you had pulled them off the edge of a sheet of paper.

Dry Humping vs. Finger Fucking

There's no reason why a woman shouldn't lube up a favorite part of her lover's body and rub against it with her vulva. Some women like to do this on a man's back, thigh or hip.

Some women enjoy using the head of a sweetheart's penis for masturbating. This can be invigorating for both partners.

There's also a form of dry humping where the woman presses the lips of her vulva over the penis like a bun over a hot dog. She then moves her hips up and down, rubbing her clitoris along the shaft of the penis. The penis never goes inside of her vagina as it would if this were intercourse. This form of dry humping was invented by Eve after she discovered that doing what the Devil had taught her to do with Adam's penis resulted in unwanted pregnancies.

Even if the male doesn't ejaculate, unwanted sex germs can be passed on, or the woman can get pregnant from such activity. You can greatly diminish these risks if the man is wearing a condom that is well-lubricated.

If getting pregnant or sex germs aren't a consideration, some women like to use a man's ejaculate as a lubricant to masturbate with. This might be fun to do when he comes first. She might add saliva or her own lube.

The Extra-Sensitive Clit

Some women have a clitoris that is super-sensitive to touch. Even the most sensitive of lovers would feel at odds with it. This kind of clitoris is not particularly forgiving. Make sure the woman is highly aroused before your fingers go near her clit, and be mindful of how quickly it can go from being sensitive to totally numbing out. Also, try to become a master of indirect stimulation. It might be better if you caress her crotch when she's wearing blue jeans or underwear than when she's naked. Some women masturbate with their fingers over their underwear rather than inside.

Agony vs. Ecstasy

We recently had to take a friend to the emergency room. From another part of the ER, a young man was moaning in excruciating pain. He would pepper his moans with an occasional "Oh God." If you had changed contexts and heard these same moans coming from a bedroom window, you would have smiled in envy, sure he was receiving the mother of all blowjobs.

How is it that pain and sexual pleasure can sound identical? They certainly don't feel the same, not for most of us anyway. The sounds we make when our bodies are spinning out of control are similar, whether we are spinning toward ecstasy or agony.

This is why it can be difficult for a partner to know when you are expressing pleasure as opposed to pain. It's up to you to help your partner learn the difference.

What Did You Discover?

It will take time to explore a woman's genitals. Maybe you will find one special place to focus on, or maybe ten. You might want to stimulate these spots while having intercourse or oral sex. Experiment with different positions that will help you take advantage of what you have discovered. Or try stimulating an outer spot with your tongue while using your fingers to reach a spot that's deeper inside. The sensations won't necessarily change the course of humanity, but the overall effect can be pleasing.

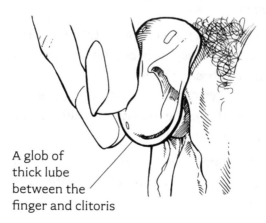

A glob of thick lube between the finger and clitoris

Never fear trying a glob of thick lube on the tip of the clitoris. This can be a helpful way to approach a clitoris that is hypersensitive. [Inspired by the "Illustrated Guide To Extended Massive Orgasm" by Steve and Vera Bodansky.]

Why Is Aquatic Sex Dry Sex?

Many couples find it sensual to feel each other up in the shower, hot tub, or bath. You would think this would be plenty wet. However, water washes away natural lubrication. To grope with your fingers in a hot tub, keep a plastic squeeze bottle of vegetable oil or silicone based lube next to the tub. Lube the outside of your genitals before getting into the water. This will help keep your genitals slick and slippery during aquatic hand play. For intercourse while submerged, try silicone-based lube, but be very careful with how slippery silicone-based lube can be if it drips on the floor inside a shower, bathroom, or beside a hot tub.

Here are two advancements in hydrotechnology that have helped take the fingers out of aquatic fucking:

Hand-Held Shower Head: If you don't have one of these, consider getting one. It shouldn't take more than fifteen minutes to install, unless your plumbing is really rusty. Hop in the shower and try out the various settings. When you hold the shower head point-blank against the skin, it causes the water to bubble somewhat like the jet on a hot tub. This might feel good. Don't point a focused jet of water directly into a vagina, as it might force air inside the body, which can be dangerous.

Different brands of hand-held shower heads create different kinds of spray. Some might be perfect for sexual stimulation, others not so. You can find them for under $35. They often go on sale.

Some men enjoy the feeling of the spray against the side of the scrotum. This might be one of those sexual experiences where the line between pleasure and pain is a fine but pleasant one.

Jets in the Hot Tub: If you haven't tried the jets of a hot tub for masturbation, what are you waiting for? Also, you might check with your hot-tub repair person about fitting an extension hose on one of the massage jets so you can direct the flow precisely where you want without having to sit in an uncomfortable position. Tell him it is for your grandfather's hydrotherapy. Cut the air to the jets so it won't get into the vagina.

Waterproof Vibrators: There are waterproof vibrators. These have only one conceivable purpose, yet the box shows a woman in a tub using the point of the vibrator against the side of her neck!

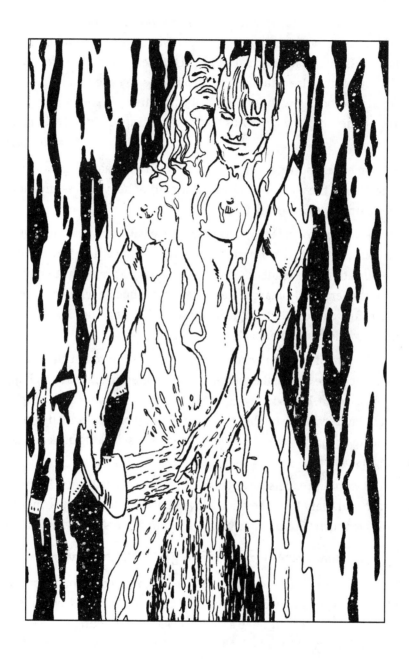

Winding Down

"The first time I felt a woman's vagina was with my first love. We were taking things very slowly, and when I would ask if I could go down her pants, the answer was no. I respected her wishes and we always did something else, usually making out. One day she finally told me I could proceed below the waistline. It was warm and wet and very soft. The wetness of her vagina was the most exciting feeling I'd ever had."

male age 25

For some men, putting their fingers between a woman's legs is a moment of magic. There's the woman's warmth, the start of her wetness, and how her body sometimes tenses and squirms.

While you are considering new ways to pleasure your partner's genitals, keep in mind there are other parts of a woman's body where touch produces intense sensation. One reader reports his lover has an area on the small of her back that is so erotically charged her knees nearly buckle when he caresses it. He once nearly caused her to orgasm in the middle of a busy hardware store by caressing this part of her back.

The fingers of another reader are so sensitive to touch that getting a manicure feels like a sexual experience. And sometimes, sensation happens purely by accident, like when you have been stroking those special spots on her body, playfully caressing her thighs or tugging on her inner lips, and suddenly, an orgasm just sneaks up on her. You were just kicking back and letting your fingers play.

Some women readers have complained that their lovers do the same thing each and every time they make love. It never hurts to experiment with new ways to touch your partner, both with your fingers and with your heart.

Reader's Advice on Playing with Their Vulvas

"I would first tell him to approach slowly. Having someone just dive straight towards where they think my clitoris is becomes overwhelming. I like to be teased, I like a slow and sensual working up to where they think my clitoris is. If they are totally in the wrong area (just because it's hard doesn't mean it's my clit!) I have no qualms about giving directions." *female age 22*

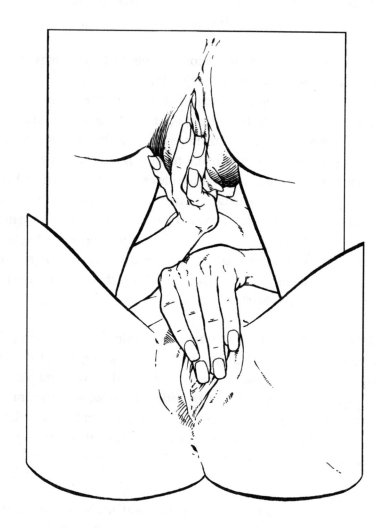

"Wait until I'm really turned on and I'm practically shoving your hand down my pants. Then, gently play around and see what I respond to. Once you've found my spot, start out slowly with only a little pressure. Don't focus exclusively on the spot, because that gets annoying, and it makes me less sensitive. As I get more turned on (which you can tell through body language like hip thrusting and my vocalizations), increase the speed but not the pressure." *female age 22*

"There's no point in approaching my vulva and clit unless I'm aroused. Touching me there is not the way to arouse me." *female age 23*

"Always get your fingers wet before touching where there isn't thick hair. Never, ever touch my clit dry. It hurts! Go ahead and play with my pubic hair. I keep it trimmed, but it means that every time you brush it, it sends a ripple of sensation through me. When I start arching up towards you, slip your finger just inside my outer lips and press gently, with a little circling motion. If I spread my legs more, please touch me! You should probably re-wet your fingers, either at my vagina (if I'm wet enough), or with some lube, or with your own saliva. I love being teased. Run your fingers along the edge of the inner lips, with just a little pressure. When I start moving against your fingers, caress my clit. Just barely touch me, that feels best. Again, that finger has to be very, very wet. In a very short while I'll be calling your name and God's!" *female age 20*

"The key word is GENTLE. At least in the beginning. Caress the pubic hair, then you could slightly penetrate with a finger near the vaginal opening. Gently move your hand forward till you find the clitoris. Never directly stimulate the clitoris, it's way too sensitive. Instead, position your finger(s) on top of the hood and gently manipulate it side to side. Be sure no matter what you are doing that there is plenty of lubrication, either from my natural supply or from a bottle."

female age 35

"Before you even think about coming near me with your fingers, please make sure that they are smooth. Long nails aren't fun, neither are sandpaper hands. I know that many men are very rough with their own members, but I do not need that. You'd be surprised what the lightest touch can accomplish. There is no need to "grind" your fingers into me. And please, when you find a pace that has me moaning, don't decide to switch to a different pace. That gets annoying."

female age 20

Reader's Advice on Fingers in Their Vaginas

"I like a finger in there, but please, don't dig for China." *female age 48*

"I like it if he inserts one finger until the opening relaxes, then adds a second finger. When I begin to breathe faster, he should start flexing his fingers." *female age 32*

"When I am sufficiently wet, I enjoy two fingers. I like it when he puts them in gradually and 'fucks' me with them gently. But no fingernails and no rushing!" *female age 35*

"Start with one finger, then go up from there. To find the G-spot, put your thumb over my clitoris, then insert your first finger into my vagina and feel for the rough spot on the upper wall. Rub this spot!!!"
female age 26

"I don't necessarily care for fingers in my vagina. I'd rather have a penis in there." *female age 43*

"I like him to rub the entrance of my vagina in a circular fashion, but don't like a finger all of the way inside." *female age 30*

"I like to wait until I can't stand it and beg him to put his fingers inside of me." *female age 25*

A College Sex Educator's Advice about the Clitoris

"When talking to guys about sensitivity in the clitoris, I compare it to the head of the penis right after ejaculation. The head can become so super sensitive that you don't want any direct contact. You can continue to stroke the shaft but stay away from the head. That's how it can be for a woman's clitoris when you first touch it."

Resources

We have videos on the clitoris at: *www.GuideToGettingItOn.com/videos/*

The Pleasure Mechanics DVD: *Guide To Fingering: How to Touch a Woman for Fabulous Foreplay & Powerful Orgasms*. This could be the most productive twenty minutes anyone who hopes to please a woman with his or her fingers could ever spend. There is nothing pornographic about the DVDs from The Pleasure Mechanics, but what you'll learn from their videos will make women think you're the hottest lover on the planet. Also, excellent for couples to watch together. You can order this from The Pleasure Mechanics: www.PleasureMechanics.com.

There are also excellent erotic massage videos at the New School of Erotic Touch: www.EroticMassage.com. This site is dedicated to different ways of stimulating and massaging people's genitals and rear ends. It is not porn and there is lots of nudity. They have many videos on vulva and penis massage.

Here's a finger-fucking resource that the author of *The Guide* found fascinating, but a female reviewer who he asked to look it over hated it (to put it mildly).

This DVD series appears to have been made by a pod of mostly humorless persons, consisting of five or six women and one man. Even their name is a bit unusual: "The Welcomed Consensus." They have devoted years to learning how to stimulate the clitoris, seemingly with the one man's finger. Their website is www.Welcomed.com. In the first DVD of their *Deliberate Orgasm Collection*, the members appear to be wearing uniforms from the original *Star Trek*. The fourth tape has the stiffest, slowest, and perhaps most awkward introduction of any how-to video in history. And if a bikini shaver ever got close to these womens' abundant mountains of *au natural* crotch hair, its bearings would cease in horror. When one of the women said, "Can you move your finger up just a hair?" the possibilities boggled the mind.

What Paul found fascinating was purely anatomical—how these women's vulvas changed with arousal, and how they pulsed for twenty minutes at a time. He thought it showed something that might be highly instructive. The finger-under-the-clitoral-hood illustration from earlier in this chapter shows what The Welcomed Consensus does.

16

Nipples, Nipples, Nipples

While the title of this chapter is eye catching, it should have been "breasts, breasts, breasts," or "nipples/breasts, nipples/breasts, nipples/breasts." That's because for many women, the part of their breast they prefer having kissed and caressed is between the neck and nipples as opposed to just their nipples. Plastic surgeons discovered this when they were doing studies on sensation in women's breasts.

There's also the implication that only women like breast and nipple stimulation. However, a study on nipple/breast stimulation found that 52% of males enjoy tender kisses and caresses of their nipples. Another 25% of the males were probably too manly to admit they enjoyed it, or unable to allow themselves to ask a partner to do it. Men seem to have similar variations in nipple and chest sensitivity as women do. Some men get an erection when their nipples are caressed. Some find it enhances their orgasm if a partner sucks on or caresses a nipple at the same time that they are coming.

One woman might find it heavenly when a lover barely breathes on her nipples, but convulses in pain if he is the slightest bit rough. So her partner learns to traverse her tender nipples like a butterfly and becomes a master at the art of subtle stimulation. Another woman wants her lover to handle her nipples with authority and doesn't find it erotic until his lips latch on like an industrial vacuum cleaner. Some women's breasts become more sensitive during certain parts of their menstrual cycle, especially if they are taking birth-control pills. Know your lover's body and be sensitive to the ebb and flow of what feels good and when. And don't assume it's the nipple that does the trick when it might be the area a couple of inches above, below, or to the side of the nipple.

Another thing to consider has to do with deeper meanings. To some women, whenever lips go near their nipples they automatically feel maternal. Every sparkle of sexuality drains out their toes. So be sure to talk to your partner about whether she gets turned on or off by nipple and breast play, or if she'd rather you be focusing your efforts elsewhere.

Six Facts about Breasts

In case you were wondering how much women's breasts weigh, the answer is approximately half a pound for each cup size. So if a woman has a B cup, each breast will weigh a pound, for a C cup, it's a pound and a half, and for a D cup, the breast will weigh close to two pounds. Most women's breasts weigh between 2 and 4 pounds total.

The breasts of younger women are primarily made up of glandular tissue and not much fat. That's why they tend to be so firm. As women get older, the breast lobes are replaced by more and more fat, and so the breasts become softer.

A woman's hormones influence almost every aspect of her breasts, especially the glands inside. This is why it's perfectly normal for women's breasts to change in consistency and sensitivity from week to week.

More than 90% of women have breasts that are asymmetrical, which means one is different from the other in size, shape or position on the chest. It's usually the left breast that's larger, and in almost 25% of women, the larger breast is at least one cup size bigger than the other.

Over the course of a woman's lifetime, her breast size will change up to six or seven times.

And if you are interested in inter-species breast trivia, the rabbit has 8 nipples and the rat has 12 nipples.

A Very Helpful Take on Breasts

Here are some women's perspectives on their breasts as reported to Meema Spadola in her wonderful book, *Breasts—Our Most Public Private Parts*, Wildcat Canyon Press:

From Elaine: "My preferences vary constantly. What feels pleasurable one moment can feel annoying the next. Sometimes I hit sensory overload and can barely stand to have my breasts touched."

Cecilia says, "My nipples are very sensitive and I could be aroused almost to the point of orgasm just by touching them, but only very gently, almost not at all." At the other end of the spectrum is Heather, who prefers a firm touch that includes clothespins and biting.

And there is Carrie, who was known as the girl with the big boobs. "Guys were sometimes more attracted to my boobs than to me." One day when Carrie was wearing a large rain slicker which hid her breasts behind a wall of

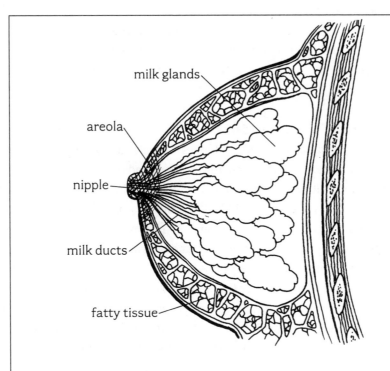

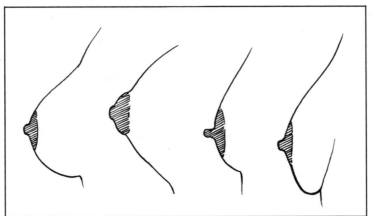

The breast is made up of glands, ducts, and surrounding fat. In younger women, the proportion of fat in the breast is usually lower. It tends to increase with age. It is the fat that gives the breast its unique size and shape. It is completely normal for breasts to feel lumpy.

thick yellow plastic, she met a man from out of town, and they seemed to hit it off. They talked on the phone and emailed for the first year of their relationship, with him never knowing that her bras were the size of saddlebags. Assured that he liked all of her and not just her mammaries, Carrie eventually married the man.

One woman reports, "When a man touches my breasts, I feel a little removed from the whole experience—as if he's on a date with my breasts." Another woman says, "My boyfriend loves to suck on my nipples, but sometimes I get this sense that he is focusing on them and tuning me out, and I can feel a wave of resentment, almost jealousy, when he latches onto my breasts." A third woman says, "I would feel like I had this 180-pound baby in my arms, and occasionally he'd fall asleep there sucking my breasts. I'm sure he thought he was giving me great pleasure, but it just didn't do it for me."

There are women who describe their breasts as being "a place of warmth and love," and "without breast stimulation, sex is purely physical with no emotional component." Another perspective comes from Scarlet, with 38DD breasts, who says, "I can't wait to take my clothes off in bed because I know that men will get excited; they always want to suck on my breasts. They think that I get incredibly turned on by it, but my breasts aren't as sensitive as men expect. Honestly, I could be balancing my checkbook while they're doing it. It's really not a big deal. But I do get turned on seeing them getting very turned on."

Finally, Ms. Spadola quotes a woman who has had sex with both men and women: "The men didn't seem to grasp that twisting them like radio dials does not work. They treated my breasts as something separate from my body. Women seem to know instinctively what to do with breasts. Women sense that there are times when you want your breasts to be touched, and times you don't. It didn't seem to occur to the men I was with that there might be mental and cultural baggage wrapped up there."

How Women Can Let Men Know What They Want

Even if your guy has a big hairy chest, tell him you are going to touch and kiss his "breasts" the same way you like to have yours kissed, and then do it. If there are times when you like it to be gentle, tell him, "This is what I like when I say *gentle*." If there are times when you like it extra-rough, let him know what you mean when you say *rough*. If you like your nipples tugged, show him exactly how and for how long. And don't get all bent out of shape if he requires refresher lessons. The learning process is not nearly as straightforward as you might think.

Techniques for Happy Breasts

There is no "one-size-fits-all" bra, and there are no sets of breast-stimulation tips and techniques that will work for everyone. Here are a few to pick and choose from. Many of these techniques focus on the nipples. If this doesn't work for your partner, find out what parts of her neck and chest do bring her pleasure when you kiss and caress them.

Size vs. Performance As with a clitoris or penis, the sensitivity of a breast has nothing to do with its size. Small ones can be like lightning rods, while big ones might not be sensitive at all.

Making the Nipple Taut When a woman is aroused, place your fingers on each side of the nipple, not quite touching the nipple but around the perimeter of it. Push down lightly and slide your fingers apart. This will make the nipple taut. Some people find that taut nipples are more sensitive.

In and Out Pucker up your lips and use them to make a gasket around the nipple. Then suck in and out without breaking the seal—so the nipple feels alternating currents of vacuum and pressure. This method also works well on earlobes and the clitoris. However, if you are sucking earlobes in this way, be sure that earrings are removed first. As for jewelry in the nipples or clitoris, discuss suction limits with your partner lest one of her favorite gold loops or bars ends up in the bottom of your stomach.

Five-Finger Breast Grab This works best if the breast and your hand are lubricated with massage oil. Rest your hand over the breast with your fingertips spread open. As you lift your hand, let your fingertips caress their way up the sides of the breasts until they are clasping the tip of the nipple. Pull on the nipple just a little or a lot, depending on what your partner likes and her level of arousal.

Nipple Between Your Index & Middle Fingers The ability to do this will depend upon the size and shape of the nipple. Cup your hand over the breast in such a way that the tip of the nipple rests in the space between your middle finger and index (or other) finger. Squeeze the fingers together so that when you lift your hand the nipple follows, pulling the rest of the breast up with it.

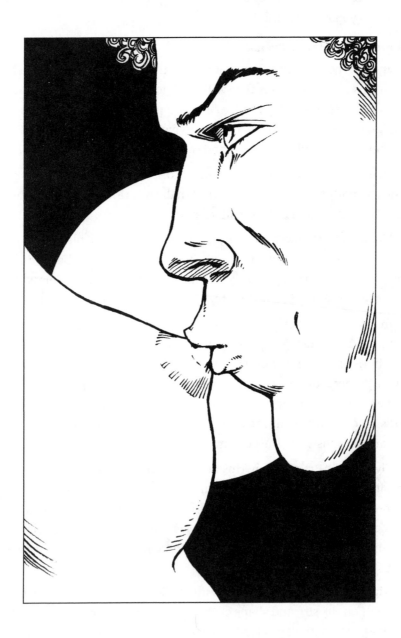

Nipple and Penis Some women find it arousing when a man caresses their nipples with the head of his penis or by pulling his foreskin up around the nipple. If he pulls apart the opening of his penis, he can sometimes stick the tip of an erect nipple into it.

The Whole Enchilada Find out if your partner wants you to lick or suck on the entire breast and not just the nipple, and remember to alternate breasts.

Hand and Mouth She probably has two breasts and you only have one mouth. So your partner might like it if your fingers are caressing one breast while your lips are tending to the other, or perhaps she would prefer your hand to be caressing some other part of her body. Ask.

Variations in Sensitivity & Menstrual Effects Sometimes one breast or nipple is more sensitive than the other. Find out if your lover would like you to spend more time on the sensitive side. Also, breast sensitivity can change with a woman's monthly cycle or if she's taking the pill.

Different Temperatures An ice cube in the mouth can be a rousing way to greet a partner's breasts. Or for nipples that are already cold, drinking something warm just before licking or sucking them can feel exquisite.

Playful Plate All kinds of fruits, dessert foods, and certain liquors can be served on chests, abdomens, backs, and other body parts with pleasing results. But do what you can to keep sugars out of the vagina.

Getting to Watch Some partners find it erotic to watch a woman play with her own nipples and breasts. So if you are a woman who enjoys playing with her breasts, there's no point in keeping it a secret.

Hard-Nipple Alert

Let's say you are playing with your partner's nipples and they get hard. Is this a good sign? Sometimes yes, sometimes no. Until you learn more about your partner's body, don't assume that hard nipples mean happy nipples. Nipples can get hard from unpleasant stimuli such as roughness, abrasion, and cold—so be sure to ask your partner if he or she likes what you are doing. Also be aware that what a person wants in terms of nipple play can vary with their state of sexual arousal.

Dads and Their Daughters' Growing Breasts

Growing breasts come between dads and their teenage daughters. For instance, one of a daughter's fondest childhood memories can be of wrestling and rough-housing with her dad. But suddenly, much of the physical intimacy can stop when her chest develops and it makes him feel uncomfortable.

Hopefully, dads will understand the huge loss this can pose to their daughters. They can gradually transform the physical closeness into involvement in other ways—with everything from playing catch to taking their daughter someplace special or fun each week or out to lunch. The important thing is to maintain the intimacy which is so important to many daughters and dads while moving the physical relationship into a realm that's more age-appropriate.

Readers' Comments

"Kissing my breast depends upon my mood. Sometimes I like being touched gently with fingertips and then gentle circles of a tongue followed by a very light sucking on the nipples." *female age 27*

"Most of the sensitivity is in the nipple, but there are good feelings from having the whole breast caressed and sucked. Swirling your tongue around the nipple is good. Sucking the nipple is great! Biting the nipple is a MAJOR no-no." *female age 34*

"Depending on how aroused I am, I like to be sucked hard and even gently bitten on the nipple." *female age 45*

"There doesn't seem to be any logical pattern or reason behind it, but sometimes even touching the breast area can hurt. Other times, pretty much anything is okay." *female age 32*

"I had to have a breast biopsy last year for a lump. I had not thought of my breasts as pretty before. They have always seemed too small compared to what all the boys were paying attention to. With a gain in self-esteem and self-respect and with the help of my current boyfriend, I've found that I really do think of my breasts in a whole new way, especially after going through the experience of surgery. My lump was benign, but it made me think about myself in a new way and what I really have to appreciate." *female age 20*

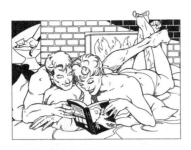

Dear Paul,

My boyfriend wants me to lactate for him. I am not pregnant nor have I ever been and I don't know how to lactate. I don't know if it's safe or if it is going to turn me into a hormonal wreck. If you have any advice or know any books I would be really grateful.

Madonna in Montana

Dear Madonna,

For starters, what you are asking about is different from the breast play that some couples enjoy during lovemaking. You are talking about a situation where your breasts would be lactating and your boyfriend would be nursing on them two to four times a day, seven days a week. If he missed a nursing, you would need to pump or express the milk from your breasts. This wouldn't be a problem if you were also donating breast milk to infants, which is becoming a cottage industry in a number of countries.

Adult couples who nurse refer to it as an "Adult Nursing Relationship." It usually begins after the woman has had a baby. The father may have started nursing alongside junior, or maybe mom encouraged him to take over once the baby was weaned. There are adult couples who keep nursing for years. The child could be graduating from high school, and dad might still be sucking milk from mom's breasts.

Having to nurse so often might cause even the most eager of couples to abandon the concept. However, couples who continue this kind of nursing seem to cherish the added closeness and shared dependency. Not only is one partner dependent on the other for milk, but she is dependent on him to relieve her swollen mammaries. The woman's milk will often let down at the sight or sound of her partner, just as a nursing mother's breasts will let down when she sees or hears her hungry infant cry.

There are two ways that someone who hasn't been pregnant can try to jump-start her non-nursing breasts. These methods have been pioneered by adoptive moms who are trying to breast feed their adopted infants. One method involves the use of drugs to trick your body into thinking you were pregnant and have given birth. The other involves seriously intense sucking on the part of your partner, several times a day for several weeks. Even then there is no guarantee he'll be sporting a milk mustache.

If this did work, your breasts would probably get bigger, so you would need to buy new bras and blouses. As for the potential of getting stretch marks, I don't think it would be any different than with mothers who nurse infants.

Also, you would need to supplement your intake of calories and calcium just as a nursing mother does. Otherwise, your body might start robbing your bones of the extra calcium that your breasts need to produce milk. And if your boyfriend didn't cut calories in other ways, he'd probably start to get fat.

As for the safety and impact of all this on your body—women have been nursing babies since the beginning of time, but would nursing an adult partner have the same impact on your body as nursing a baby? I don't know of any studies on this.

17
Balls, Balls, Balls

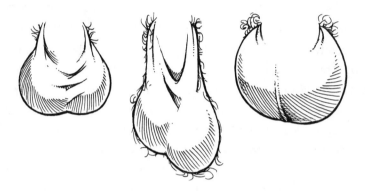

Balls usually take a back seat to the penis. One reason is the pleasure a man gets from his testicles is more subtle than the pleasure he gets from his penis. But just because the pleasure is subtle doesn't mean it should be ignored. As one reader comments, "When my wife caresses my testicles, it's one part excitement, two parts relaxation, and six parts bliss. I didn't appreciate this when I was twenty, but I enjoy it now as much as oral sex. The sensation is different, but satisfying."

A Few Facts about the Testicles

Testicles are far more rugged than you might think. You can squeeze or pull them with no problem, and they can bang against a lover's thighs with impunity. But pop them with a simple flick of a finger and you might have to peel their owner off the ceiling.

Testicles should feel a bit like hard-boiled eggs without the shell, but they won't be that big unless your lover is related to a racehorse.

When a man is highly aroused or is just about to come, his scrotum and testicles will pull up to hug the shaft of the penis. In some men this is so extreme you'll wonder where his testicles went.

The Scrotum

The scrotum surrounds the testicles. It's a thin layer of skin that is lined with muscles. People mistakenly think of the scrotum as a sack that holds the testicles in place. They believe if the scrotum were opened up, the testicles would fall out. This is not true. The testicles are held in place by the spermatic cords which suspend them from the lower abdomen.

The spermatic cords contain the cremaster muscles and connective tissue as well as arteries, veins, nerves and various tubes. You can remove the entire scrotum and the spermatic cords will still hold the testicles in place.

The scrotum is lined with a layer of smooth muscle which allows it to pucker up. This helps move the testicles closer to the body when they are too cold, and farther from it when they are too hot. However, the scrotum doesn't appear to do the major lifting. That's the job of the cremaster muscles, which lift the testicles close to the body when a man is highly aroused and ready to ejaculate. They can also reel them in when a man is frightened. While it's been assumed that the scrotum and cremaster muscles raise and lower the testicles to keep them cooler than the rest of the body, this might be an oversimplification. Debate continues.

The scrotum starts off in the womb as part of the same embryonic tissue as the labia majora or large lips of the female genitals. If the fetus is a boy, nature creates the scrotum by zipping up the two lips that would otherwise become the labia majora. This is why the scrotum has a seam running up the middle. It's where the two labia fused together to make a scrotum. Fused or not, the skin on the scrotum has the same kind of sweat and oil-producing glands, hair follicles and nerve endings as the labia majora. It should feel the same as the labia majora when it is caressed by a lover's fingers or mouth.

What's Inside a Ball?

Technically, the testicles are glands that produce testosterone and sperm. One is often bigger than the other, and one hangs lower. Each testicle is a factory. Sperm are produced in the tubules, stored and aged in the epididymis, and sent up into the abdomen through the vas deferens. Contrary to what you might think, sperm don't go straight from the testicles into the penis. Instead, they travel up into the pelvis to a place behind the bladder. That's where they make the connection with a tube that draws them in

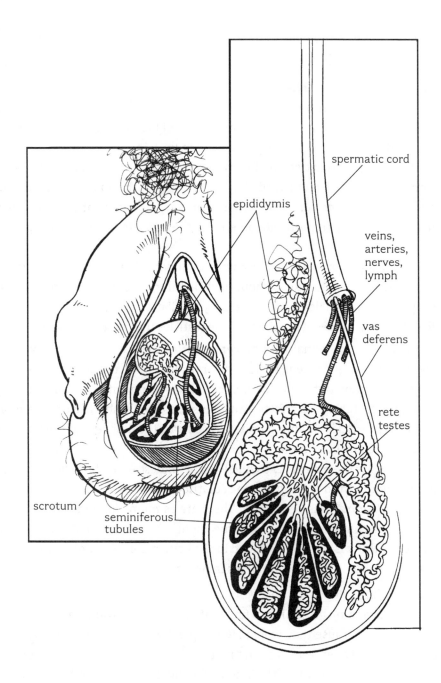

epididymis

spermatic cord

veins,
arteries,
nerves,
lymph

vas
deferens

rete
testes

scrotum

seminiferous
tubules

Ball Plumbing

through the prostate gland. From there, they eventually shoot out through the penis during ejaculation.

An Undescended Testicle

The medical term for undescended testicles is "cryptorchidism," which is Greek for "hidden gonad." One way to get hidden gonads is to go surfing during the winter; another way is to be born with them.

Contrary to what seems logical, the testicles in the male fetus don't form between the legs. Instead, they develop inside the abdomen and do not descend into his scrotum until a month or two before the baby is born. They make the journey from the abdomen into the scrotum through the inguinal canal.

Almost 3.5% of males are born with an undescended testicle. This testicle often descends on its own without medical intervention, so that by one year of age, only 1% of males (1 out of 100 or 150) still have an undescended testicle. In 90% of these cases, it's just one of the testicles that is undescended.

If the testicle remains undescended after the boy reaches one year of age, the current practice is to treat it surgically. This is often done as an out-patient operation. Attempts to coax the testicle down with hormone therapy have unacceptable side effects. Any gains are usually short-lived. The problem with a testicle remaining undescended past the first year of age is that it tends to become infertile.

If you are the parents of a child with an undescended testicle, be sure to get a second or third opinion from a pediatric urologist. As Dr. Joseph Dwoskin, a urologist from Texas Tech, says, "There are as many opinions about testes as there are physicians who examine them." It is also important to make sure everything is well documented in the boy's medical records. This will be invaluable should there be problems in ten or twenty years.

Late-Breaking News

Physicians are beginning to find that some guys who are sterile as adults got that way because they were playing sports without a cup and took a significant hit between the legs. Any man or boy who is involved in a contact sport should wear a cup. Ditto if he is playing catcher in baseball or goalie in most sports. The downside of wearing a cup is the discomfort, the upside is they can make you look really well hung. Fortunately, there are way nicer cups than most department stores and sporting-goods chain stores carry. Check out the Shock Doc cups at www.shockdoctor.com and the Spider Flex cup at www.sawsports.com.

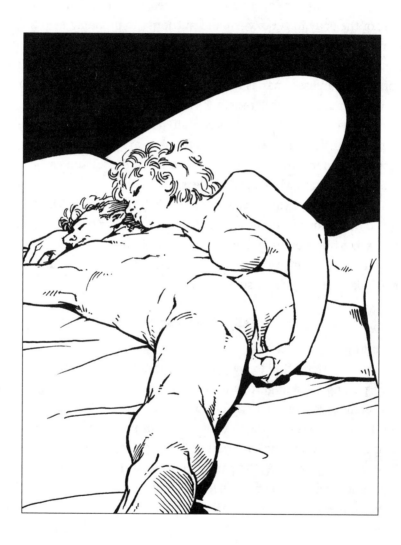

A Varicocele

Fifteen percent of young men have a condition in their scrotum called a varicocele. This is when the veins that exit a testicle become enlarged. While most guys never know they have a varicocele, in some cases it can get large enough to feel like a small clumpy sack of worms above one of the testicles.

How does a varicocele form? Testicles need a constant flow of blood from the rest of the body to get oxygen and nutrients, to probably help them stay cool, and to distribute the testosterone they make to the rest of the body. This means the blood that's leaving the testicles has to drain upward, against the pull of gravity, unless a man is lying down. (Varicoceles go away when a guy lies down because the uphill resistance is gone.)

The veins leaving the testicles contain gates or valves to help keep the blood flowing up hill from the testicles to the heart and to prevent backflow. If these valves don't function well, the downward pressure can cause the veins to widen. That's what a varicocele is.

More than 90% of varicoceles occur above the left testicle. This is because the blood that drains from the left testicle encounters more resistance when it returns into the body than the blood in the right testicle. Varicoceles can be associated with infertility. So while varicoceles usually cause no problems, if you think you have one, be sure to have it checked out.

Testicle Pleasure

Ball Tending

If you are attempting to give your partner's testicles a satisfying caress, start by placing your fingertips on the sides of his scrotum and caressing lightly. Let his verbal feedback guide you. You might also try resting the palm of your hand over his penis with your fingertips pointing down. Experiment with lightly massaging the back part of the scrotum, where it attaches to his body. As your fingers move, the part of your wrist that's resting on his penis will move as well. This should give his penis pleasure, which might mix nicely with the more subtle sensations that your fingertips are providing his testicles.

Intercourse Extra

You can handle a man's testicles during intercourse from some positions, such as the reverse cowgirl where you are on top facing his feet. Different rear-entry positions may also allow you to reach between your legs and caress his testicles. Experiment and see what both of you and both of them like best.

The Exquisite Brush-Off

Have your partner spread his legs and gently brush his inner thighs, testicles, penis, and abdomen with a soft makeup brush or an artist's brush. Doing repeated circles around the scrotum can feel especially nice. The sensation is subtle, somewhere between a feather and a fingertip. It can feel relaxing and exciting at the same time. If you enjoy taking control, you can always tie him up first. Don't limit your strokes to just his genitals. If you're lucky, he'll grab the brush and return the favor.

Perineum: Taint, Gooch or Grundle

There is a patch of anatomical real estate between the testicles and rectum which is often ignored but has the potential for sensation. It is called the perineum. (Women have one, too.) Tantric and Hindu types get excited about this particular area and regard it with the same kind of awe that we Westerners do the reset button on a computer or gaming console. Place your fingertips on this area with just enough pressure so the skin moves over the tissue beneath it. Experiment and see what feels best.

Another Kind of Tenderness

Don't hesitate to reach between your partner's legs and cup or cradle his

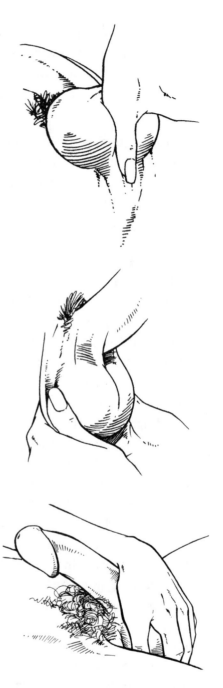

There are many ways to caress testicles. Here are three of them.

genitals at nonsexual times, like when watching TV or while falling asleep. Some men will find this to be extremely thoughtful and caring. For others it will be too arousing or unwelcome.

Cancer of the Testicles

The term "cancer of the testicles" is a misnomer. It should be cancer of the testicle (singular), given how it's usually only one testicle that gets the cancer. The good news is we only need one testicle to be fertile and to have a perfectly normal sex drive. The reason for having the other testicle is for back-up or pocket pool.

Anyone with testicles can get testicular cancer, but it is more likely to affect younger men, particularly men between the ages of 15 and 35. It is curable 97% of the time if detected early enough. Considering the testicles are hanging out and easily examined, you would think it is almost always detected early. But the last thing most guys between the ages of 15 and 35 think about is getting cancer. Cancer is something that happens to people your parents' age, so it is beyond the average male's consciousness to check every month for lumps or changes in texture.

Another problem is that a lot of men would rather sit naked on a fence-post than call the doctor's office and say, "I'm concerned about my testicle, and I'd like you to check it out." So they wait until the cancer has spread before getting care. This isn't good, since some forms of testicular cancer can double in size in fewer than thirty days, and you won't feel a bit of pain as it is happening. It would be easier if cancer of the testicles usually caused pain. If that were the case, most men would go to the doctor immediately. But cancer of the testicle usually doesn't hurt.

A third roadblock in detecting cancer of the testicles is the meaning we attach to testicles, as in the term "He's got balls!" On a symbolic level, it's a big thing when a guy loses a ball. Most of us would rather deny the possibility.

In spite of the way men feel about their own testicles, women are not necessarily enamored by them. (You don't want to know how some women describe scrotums on our sex survey.) So unless you've been caught cheating on them, most women would want you to be healthy with one testicle rather than dead with two. In fact, some guys who have lost a testicle to cancer play the cancer card quite effectively. Far from being put off by the idea of a scrotum with only one ball in it, women are sometimes curious.

Partners and Symptoms

Cancer of the testicles is one of the few cancers where it is often a partner who discovers the problem. This can be a lifesaver. Hopefully, women readers will learn how to examine their partner's testicles in the name of health as well as pleasure. They should insist he sees a healthcare provider if they find something that's worrisome.

The most common symptom to look for is a small lump or nodule on the side or sometimes the front of the testicle. It's usually not painful when you press on it. Another symptom is hardening of the testicle. While testicles can swell and shrink, it's time to get it checked when the entire testicle starts to lose its spongy texture. It's also important to see a healthcare provider if you are feeling unusual swelling in your scrotum. Less common symptoms include pain or discomfort in the testicles, back pain, swollen breasts (guy breasts), or a feeling of heaviness or unusual discomfort deep in your pelvis.

There are a number of things that can look like cancer of the testicles. One of these is a spermatocele. This is a sperm-filled cyst in the epididymis that feels like a smaller third ball. These are pretty common and usually aren't a problem unless they get really big. Most of the things you will find in a scrotum besides balls aren't cancer and can often be treated with antibiotics. So don't assume your doctor is going to present you with bad news.

It is wise to do a routine exam once a month. The best time is when the scrotum is warm and saggy, like after a hot shower. Don't do an exam when you have an erection, as erections can pull your testicles up. The **Ball Check** chart on the next two pages explains what to do.

The mother of all ball-cancer websites is Doug Bank's incredible Testicular Cancer Resource Center: tcrc.acor.org. See also Chapter 78: *Sex and Breast, Brain & Ball Cancer.*

A Note on Self Exams: While the medical community no longer recommends that men do monthly testicular exams, our cancer-of-the-testicles advisor suggests that men do monthly exams, and that their partners learn to do exams on them as well. If you examine the testicles every month, you will recognize what's normal and when there is a change. The problem is when men don't do the exams monthly and suddenly check their scrotum. They will sometimes freak because they're not used to what's there.

BALL CHECK!

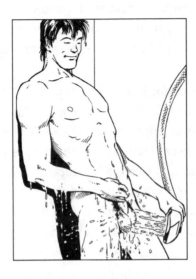

You need to do a ball check every 30 days or 10,000 strokes, whichever comes first.

The best time to check your testicles is after a warm shower, but not when you have an erection. An erection can raise your testicles and make them harder to examine.

One of the things you are looking for are changes, so it's important to know what your testicles usually feel like.

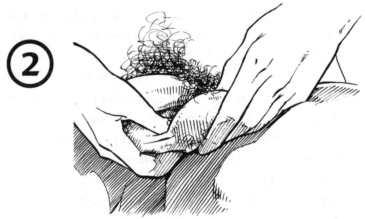

Use both hands. Grab a testicle. Roll it between your fingers. You are looking for any bumps or lumps. They can be smaller than a pea. Check the sides really well, and the top and bottom.

BALL NOTES If you ever get popped in the scrotum and the pain lasts for more than ten minutes, get it checked by a physician. If not treated quickly, testicle trauma can cause your huevos to become sterile. Also, one ball is often bigger than the other. Nature made them that way.

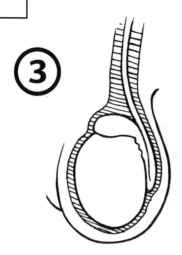

(3)

What You Are Feeling

When you feel your scrotum you may notice that there is more inside than just two testicles. There are a couple of spaghetti-like cords that attach to each testicle at the back, toward the top. They are called the epididymis. They form a structure that is shaped like a comma. These might be fuller if you haven't ejaculated in a while. It may feel a little strange, but check out your comma for any small nodes, lumps or changes since the last time you checked.

(4)

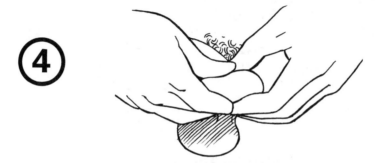

Squeeze that puppy. It should feel a bit spongy, although this can vary. Be aware if a testicle becomes extra firm or tender or starts to lose its spongy texture. Also note if the testicle is larger or smaller or heavier than it used to be.

(5) Grab your other testicle, and have at it.

(6) If either testicle has any nodes, bumps or lumps, take it to a physician for a checkup. Chances are, it is only a cyst or infection, but that needs attention, too.

(7) **CONGRATULATIONS!** You are done. Now go grab your favorite lube, click on some porn, and liberate a few million sperm.

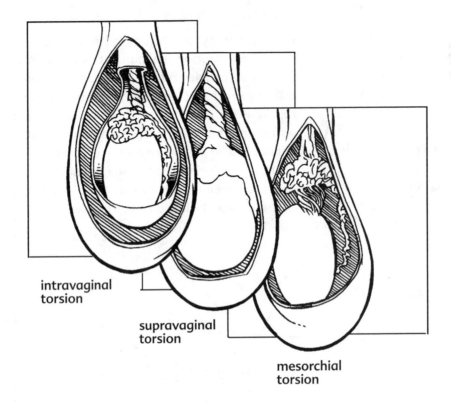

intravaginal
torsion

supravaginal
torsion

mesorchial
torsion

Testicular Torsion

Testicular torsion occurs when the testicle twists in the scrotum, causing the blood vessels in the spermatic cord to twist shut. It is very serious, and if emergency surgery is not performed within four to six hours, it is quite possible that the testicle will be lost. This is why any sudden or acute pain in the testicles that lasts for more than ten minutes should result in an immediate trip to the emergency room. The same is true for an excruciating pain that appears for a few minutes and then suddenly stops. Don't take a wait and see attitude, as it might be too late if you gambled wrong.

Torsion happens more often in teenagers, but adult males can get it as well. The potential for torsion is created when the testicle is not properly anchored in the scrotum. The three most common types of testicular torsion are illustrated above.

Twisted testicles are modeled after the illustrations in the excellent book *Imaging of the Scrotum*, by Hricak, Hamm & Kim, Raven Press.

18

The Prostate & The Male Pelvic Underground

One of the truly cool things about the prostate is that it is completely hidden. It is the one sex organ a guy doesn't have to worry about the size of when he's naked at the gym or when he is with a new lover. Prostates are measured in grams instead of inches, and a man has to be extremely neurotic before he'd worry about how his prostate stacks up against another guy's. (You'd need to be chewing on some seriously strong mushrooms before you would ever hear one woman say to another, "You won't believe the size of Brandon's prostate!")

Like the prostate, the seminal vesicles are important sex glands that are tucked inside a man's pelvis, but you don't hear as much about them because they rarely give a guy a hard time. The seminal vesicles sit on top of the prostate like a pair of rabbit ears on a 1960s television. They make up about 70% of semen. Without seminal vesicles and a prostate, ejaculation would be a non-event. The wad would be a few drops.

This chapter provides information on the two glands that make up 96% of the semen when a guy launches his load—and they are not his testicles.

The Prostate in Ancient Greek Mythology

You've probably heard how Zeus was the head of the Gods on Mount Olympus, and how he was a jealous man with paranoid tendencies. What you probably don't know is how the prostate gland came to be. To make a long story short, there was a rather peculiar god by the name of Prostateus whose saliva smelled like chlorine bleach. Zeus feared that Prostateus was scheming to overthrow him, so he asked his wife Hera to land Prostateus in the underworld near the River Styx. Hera didn't get the message quite right. She thought Zeus said to make Prostateus a gland by the river of shit.

To this day, you can still find Prostateus, who the Romans called Prostate, by sticking a finger about two inches up the male rectum. He'll be sitting just below the bladder, where Hera put him. If you reach up a little farther, you will find the two bota bags that Prostateus used to carry his wine in. They are now called the seminal vesicles.

From Marbles to Golf

Take any fourth-grade boy, and you can be pretty sure that his prostate is the size of a marble. If you take his dad, you're dealing with a prostate the size of a walnut, a small plum, or a golf ball.

If a fourth-grade boy jerks off, he'll produce only a drop or two of clear sticky fluid. While he can still enjoy the nice feeling of an orgasm, he won't start to ejaculate until puberty begins. Until then, his prostate and sleepy seminal vesicles are but a twinkle in the eye of his older, semen-producing self. It will take a jolt of testosterone from his teenage testicles to make his marble-sized prostate morph into a man-sized gland.

Geography of the Glands

The prostate is located between the bottom of the bladder and the start of the penis. The urethra (tube you pee through) runs through the prostate like the Mississippi runs through the heartland. The prostate wraps around the urethra like a donut around a straw, or your hand around your penis when your partner says, "Not tonight, dear."

The prostate is made up of smooth muscle fibers, connective tissue, small tubes, and clusters of glands that produce a clear fluid. If you find fruit metaphors helpful, the prostate is like a miniature orange, with a tough skin and pulpy insides. The fluid from the prostate makes up around 30% of each ejaculation. As a guy is starting to ejaculate, the muscle fibers in the prostate squeeze the fluid from the tiny glands into the urethra.

The seminal vesicles are about two inches long. They sit above the prostate on the side of the bladder. They are long and narrow like a pair of puffy rabbit ears. The seminal vesicles have special cells that make a gelatin-type of juice that puts the "thick" in semen. The seminal vesicles manufacture about 70% of the volume that's in each and every wad.

Note While the testicles are the master glands of the male pelvis, they contribute no more than 2% to 4% of each ejaculation. The testicles are hugely important when it comes to keeping a male looking like a man, but they don't produce much of his ejaculate.

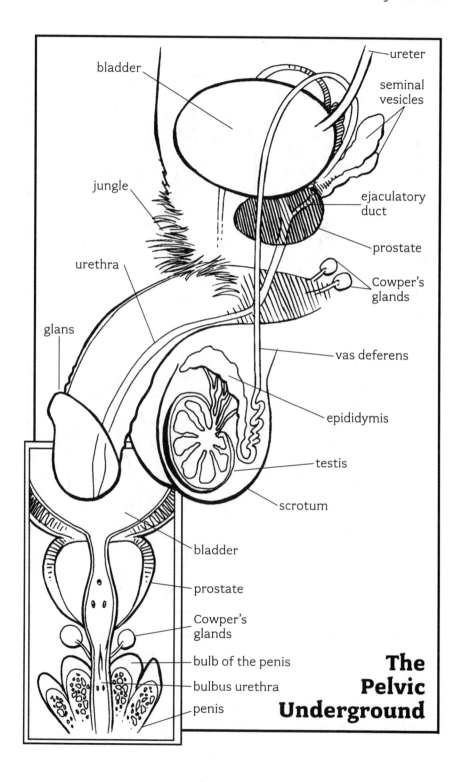

bladder

ureter

seminal vesicles

jungle

ejaculatory duct

prostate

urethra

Cowper's glands

glans

vas deferens

epididymis

testis

scrotum

bladder

prostate

Cowper's glands

bulb of the penis

bulbus urethra

penis

The Pelvic Underground

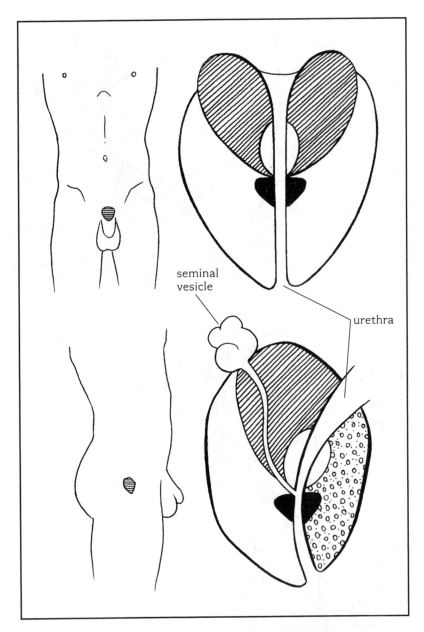

seminal
vesicle

urethra

Prostate Cut in Half—Front and Side Views

Some people think of the prostate as a lump. However, as you can see from this diagram, the prostate is a complex organ that has a number of different parts to it.

Why Girls Drip after Intercourse without a Condom

Did you ever wonder why ejaculate shoots out of the penis thick, but ends up dripping out of a woman's vagina as she tears out of bed and tries to get to work or class on time? The easiest way to find out why is to have a guy come in a glass. In a few minutes, the thick whitish cum in the glass will start changing into a thin watery fluid. If a woman who's had intercourse stands up when the ejaculate is in its thin-as-water state, it will drip. And drip.

How come? When a man is about to ejaculate and he reaches the point of no return, a couple of different things happen in his pelvis.

There's a collector part of the urethra that's located at the base of the penis. It is called the bulbus urethra. When a man is about to have an orgasm, the ingredients that make up semen collect in the bulbus urethra. These ingredients include a tiny squirt of sperm, a big squirt of gelatin juice from the seminal vesicles, and a medium-sized squirt of prostate fluid that contains an enzyme called PSA. All in all, semen has more than 300 ingredients.

When the bulbus urethra fills with the different ingredients that make up semen, the pressure seems to trigger the muscles around it to convulse. This sends the wad flying through the penis and out the end. Ejaculation!

As for explaining the trick in the glass, the key is the PSA from the prostate: when it mixes with the thick gelatin juice from the seminal vesicles it causes the gelatin juice to change its state from thick to thin. This makes the semen get watery. Scientists think this happens so the semen can more easily be sucked up into the woman's cervix. Evolutionists say it's so other males will smell semen dripping from her vagina and realize their sperm has been out-competed. Socialists say it's a capitalist plot to sell more tissue. No one really knows why.

Prostate Has the Right Name, But Not the Seminal Vesicles

The prostate was named around 300 B.C. by Herophilus, the father of anatomy. The word prostate supposedly means "guard of the bladder." The prostate glands that Herophilus studied were fresh and in working order, as he was allowed to do dissections on criminals who were being put to death. Herophilus deserves credit for disseminating correct information about the prostate. This was not the case for those who eventually found and named the seminal vesicles.

The name "seminal vesicles" implies they are containers that hold the semen. But the seminal vesicles aren't containers. They manufacture several ingredients that go into semen, but the seminal vesicles never see fully-mixed semen any more than an ice-cream machine sees a hot-fudge sundae.

Curiosity Will Not Kill the Prostate

Some people can read about the prostate and be perfectly content leaving well enough alone. Others will want to reach out and touch one. It probably depends on whether you view the prostate as a lump in a landfill or a diamond in the rough.

There are two ways to feel a prostate: one is by doing the type of prostate exam that a healthcare professional does. We advise against this, but if your goal is only curiosity instead of providing pleasure, go ahead. The other method is by doing a pleasurable prostate massage. There's an entire section on prostate pleasure at the end of this chapter.

If you are doing a DRE (digital rectal exam) like the one shown in the illustration on the next page, be sure to trim the nail on the finger you are using. Put on latex exam gloves (without powder), and slather a generous amount of lube like KY Jelly on your finger. Have the man bend over.

You don't want your finger to enter his anus at the same angle that an arrow does when you've shot it at a bull's eye. Instead, you want your finger to be against his anus like it is when your are putting it against your lips and going "Shhhhh!" This means the pad of your finger will be laying flat against his anus and your wrist will be against his scrotum or in that general area between his thighs.

As you are pushing the pad of your finger against his anus, it will momentarily relax. This is your opportunity to ease the pad of your well-lubed finger farther into the opening. Simply flick the tip around and in. During the flicking process, your finger will suddenly go from the "Shhhhh" direction (vertical) to the arrow in the bull's eye (horizontal). The quick flick can't really be seen because it happens as your finger is pushing into the anal opening. As long as you are gentle but firm there shouldn't be any need to peel the man off the ceiling or call an ambulance.

Slowly push your finger in a couple of inches and start to explore. The illustration on the next page should be an adequate guide. While the prostate

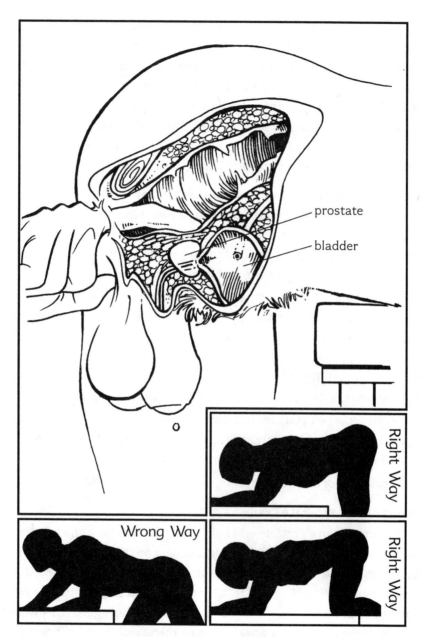

DRE—Digital Rectal Exam

The examiner can reach only about a third of the entire prostate. So she tries to check for symmetry in the lobes of the gland. To do this correctly, you need to be standing or squatting square, with your butt sticking up and out.

will be much bigger than the tip of your nose, the surface will probably feel a bit like it or like the padded part of your thumb as it meets your wrist.

If you explore the entire surface of the prostate from side to side, you might discover it has an indentation running down the center. Also, experiment with different levels of pressure. Be sure to get lots of feedback.

If a man is sufficiently able to contort himself, he should be able to feel his own prostate with his finger. But the notion of a man being able to do an accurate exam on his own prostate is kind of silly.

Prostate Play for Lovers vs. Prostate Treatment

It's one thing when you are exploring a lover's prostate. It's quite another when a guy is having prostate problems and a health care professional tries to do a prostate massage or milks fluid from it to study under a microscope. Looking at what causes prostate problems might help explain why.

One theory says that some types of prostate problems are caused by small pockets of infection that get trapped inside the gland. These pockets become surrounded with a hard material that encapsulates the infection. The purpose of a prostate massage is to push hard enough to burst these pockets of infection open. This requires a good deal of pressure that's not any more sexually arousing than breasts being squeezed during a mammogram.

However, when you are stimulating a man's prostate in a sexually exciting way, you are pushing only as firmly as he tells you to. There is no medical agenda, and the motions are based on your mutual pleasure.

See the end of this chapter for information about prostate massage.

Getting a Good Prostate Exam

Feeling a man's prostate will help you appreciate what an art it is to do a good prostate exam. A lot of physicians who are too embarrassed to do a good exam tend to stick a finger up a guy's rear with lightning speed, touch it long enough to say, "Tag, you're it," and yank their finger out. It's a wonder why they even bother; they aren't doing the patient any good. This would be the same thing as waving a wand over a woman's crotch and telling her she's had a pap smear.

One of the reasons why a "Tag, you're it" type of exam is useless is because on a really good day, the examiner is able to feel along the surface of only one-third of the entire prostate gland. He or she is trying to get a lot of information without being able to put a finger on most of it. Some of the things they are trying to determine are the size and symmetry of the gland, if there are lumps in it that might raise suspicions about cancer, and if it is spongy or hard.

Our medical consultant estimates he has done more than 35,000 prostate exams during his career in urology. He says a thorough prostate exam takes time and concentration. He tends to close his eyes once his finger reaches gland zero so he can focus better on the limited amount of information he is receiving. For him to feel like he's done a good job, he has the man stand or kneel square with his butt pointing up in the air.

So here you've got two grown ups, one with his finger up the other's butt, both have their eyes closed, and each is hoping that when it's over, the one with the finger can give the one with the prostate a big thumbs-up.

While a DRE isn't going to provide any answers by itself, it is one piece of information that might be helpful in ruling out conditions like BPH, prostatitis, and cancer. Yikes — BPH, prostatitis and cancer?

Trouble in the Pelvic Underground

A gland that has to spend its entire life next to a guy's rectum is going to get uppity every now and then. We're talking about life without parole inside a human porta-potty. So if the gland is going to revolt, what are its options? Its most immediate targets are the bladder and the urethra. With a little enlargement here and there, the prostate can nearly cripple a man's ability to do everything from peeing in a straight stream to making him drip for a long time afterward. It can cause such an urgency to urinate that he can't hold it for more than a couple of minutes and it can make him wake up four times a night. It can also interfere with his ability to ejaculate without pain, to fully empty his bladder, or to even walk or sit without discomfort.

Most prostates get bigger as a man gets older, yet there's no room for expansion. As you can see from the illustration on the next page, if the gland grows one way it's into your bladder, the other way it's up your rectum. Or the prostate might not feel enlarged, but the growth is on the inside of the gland in the central zone, where it can push against the urethra and clamp it shut.

If this weren't bad enough, the prostate is one of the most understudied parts of the human body. Scientifically valid studies on the prostate are few

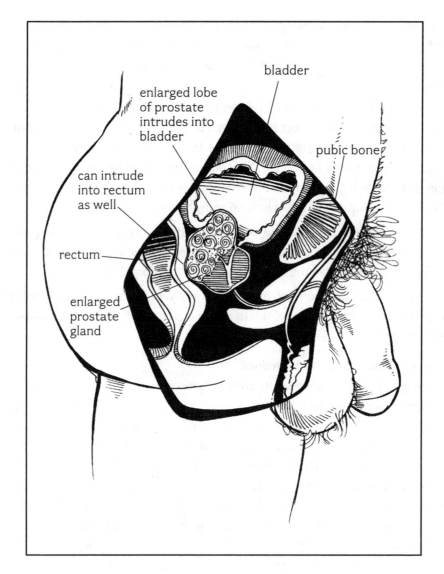

When the Posterior Lobe of the Prostate Pushes into the Bladder

This is what it looks like when a lobe of the prostate swells and pushes into the floor of the bladder. It can cause intense bladder discomfort. When a man tries to urinate, this enlarged lobe can push against the opening of the urethra and block the flow.

and far between. Although prostate cancer is the third-most-common kind of cancer men get, there isn't a huge amount of science to guide physicians.

Half of all men will at sometime have BPH or prostatitis, yet treatment remains more of an art than a science. While studies are now being done, it will be years before there is a decent body of findings to help health care practitioners make quick and accurate decisions.

Prostatitis—A Young Man's Disease

Prostatitis is a syndrome that can include pain in the pelvis, painful ejaculation, pain with erections, an array of urination problems, and pain with life in general. Some men say it feels like they've got a golf ball up their butt."

Prostatitis is often described as a young man's disease, yet it can pummel the pelvis of any man at any age. It can be caused by anything from an infection to chronic tension in the pelvis, although infection is found in less than 10% of all cases of prostatitis. To quote an article in the *Journal of Urology*, prostatitis is a syndrome that is "poorly defined, poorly understood, poorly treated, and bothersome." Or to quote our prostate expert, "Prostatitis is a young guy's disease that is not diagnosed properly and is not treated properly."

If you've got a sudden, acute attack of pain in your pelvis, get yourself to a physician as soon as possible. This kind of prostatitis can usually be treated successfully. If you have chronic prostate problems, educate yourself about prostatitis. A good source of information is www.prostatitis.org. Then, after you have an idea of just how many theories there are and how complex the problem can be, find a good urologist. The prostatitis.org website usually keeps a list of urologists with whom people have had positive experiences.

Since chronic prostatitis tends to wax and wane, a lot of men take several courses of antibiotics, thinking that the antibiotics helped it improve the last time around. This is not a good idea. You need to approach chronic prostatitis with patience and intelligence. A shot gun approach is not wise.

Regarding sexual practices and prostate health, there aren't any studies to offer guidance. Having anal sex without a condom (barebacking) makes the man who inserts vulnerable to prostatitis because E. coli can cause prostatitis, and there are abundant legions of E. coli in our rectums. There are also concerns that couples who are having vaginal intercourse can be passing some prostate infections back and forth, so if you have prostate problems, you need to let your urologist know about your sexual practices.

BPH (Benign Prostatic Hyperplasia)—Middle-Age or Older

Let's say you are getting close to 50 and you notice that the wall doesn't shake anymore when you are peeing at a urinal. Or maybe you don't make it through the night like you used to. This could be due to a prostate that is getting larger as you are getting older.

It is called BPH when your prostate gland is enlarged and physicians don't think you have cancer. The symptoms can range from mild to severe. One of the fascinating things about BPH is that the prostate can be greatly enlarged in a man who experiences no troubling symptoms, or it can be completely normal in size but the man is going through hell. In the latter case, the swelling might be on the inside of the prostate, clamping the urethra shut.

Although BPH and prostatitis are supposed to be two different things, a man who is under 40 is likely to be given the diagnosis of prostatitis while a

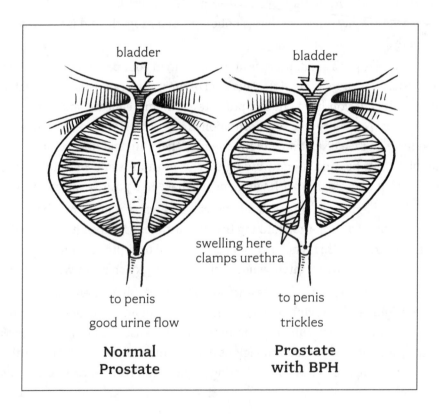

bladder

bladder

swelling here
clamps urethra

to penis

to penis

good urine flow

trickles

**Normal
Prostate**

**Prostate
with BPH**

man who is over 50 is likely to be given the diagnosis of BPH, even if they have the exact same symptoms.

Prostate Cancer

It has been estimated that half of all grown men have an early form of prostate cancer called microcarcinoma. It usually stays where it is and you never know it is there. When this kind of cancer does grow, it often remains inside the prostate and is not aggressive. However, some forms of prostate cancer can be very aggressive. The challenge is in knowing which is which.

Prostate cancer is sometimes diagnosed on a wing and a prayer. One of the big challenges with prostate cancer is deciding when to treat it aggressively and when to take a "wait and watch" attitude.

One test that can possibly indicate the presence of prostate cancer is called the PSA test. PSA is the enzyme that makes a guy's ejaculate go from thick to watery. When the level of PSA in the bloodstream starts to rise, it might be due to cancer of the prostate. On the other hand, BPH can also cause the PSA level to rise, and some men who have prostate cancer show no rise in their PSA level at all.

At this point, some groups are recommending against doing routine PSA tests. PSA tests can often result in a wild goose chase and sometimes do more harm than good. If you have reason for concern, check with your doctor. Researchers are trying to find ways to improve the PSA tests. Some of the things they are looking into include free vs. total PSA, PSA density in the interior part of the prostate that surrounds the urethra, PSA velocity and PSA doubling time.

Here are just a few prostate cancer suggestions:

💡 Newton Malerman, author of a book on prostate cancer, says: "If you are diagnosed with prostate cancer or any other serious illness, take someone with you to your doctor's appointments. My wife was able to ask much clearer and tougher questions than I was. If you are single, or your spouse or partner is too emotional about what's happening, take a trusted friend or family member... If you are treated to a rough digital exam, find another urologist. The procedure is not too unpleasant if the doctor has a gentle touch."

💡Explore several websites. Some of your best help will come from the posts of men who have been through it before you. However, be aware of which companies contribute funding to the websites you are searching. It is unlikely that these companies will tolerate posts that question wisdom of taking their products.

💡If you have cancer or BPH and if surgery or radiation is being suggested, ask if it will cause incontinence, impotence, a shorter penis, dry ejaculations or if you will squirt urine when you ejaculate. Also inquire about vacuum pumping your penis after surgery. Some urologists recommend it.

A Healthy Prostate Diet?

Long-term studies on diet, prostate irritation and prostate cancer are just starting to come in. Check with your healthcare professional about what foods might help and which to avoid. Smoking definitely causes bladder cancer, and it causes men with prostatitis to have worse symptoms.

Prostate Massage for Pleasure

Prostate play should never feel like a rectal exam from a healthcare provider. If a healthcare provider took the time to caress and massage your anus like a lover should before sticking a finger up it, he or she would probably lose their license. Or they would experience a massive decrease in billable hours due to how much extra time is involved. And they would probably be so popular it would take months to schedule an appointment.

The following tips are from Charlie Glickman's excellent book *The Ultimate Guide to Prostate Pleasure: A Guide for Men and Their Partners* and from a video called *A Guide For Prostate Massage* from The Pleasure Mechanics.

💡Lube up your fingers with massage oil.

💡Begin with external massage just below the testicles in the perineal area. Glide a well-lubricated finger around the outside of the anal opening, making circles with it. Spend several minutes doing this, allowing your finger to make friends with it. Don't try any penetration until the opening becomes relaxed.

💡Don't push your finger into the anus. If you've massaged the outside for long enough, the anal sphincters will relax and allow easy insertion of the finger. Gradually increase the pressure, but don't push your finger farther in than feels comfortable for the man.

💡 Sometimes all that's necessary is putting your finger in a quarter or half of an inch. Massage there and call it a day if going further in is not pleasurable.

💡 The sphincter muscles are like two small donuts that sit above the anal opening. If your finger encounters resistance when it reaches the sphincters, stop there. It means the man is not relaxed enough to go farther.

💡 Once you reach the prostate, you might try a "come here" motion. Also try moving your finger in circles around the prostate. It should never feel painful or uncomfortable for your partner. Then try gliding your finger from the outer edge to the center of the prostate.

💡 Some men experience prostate stimulation as being midway between the sensation of needing to pee and having an orgasm. Men who enjoy prostate stimulation sometimes describe it as providing wavelike sensations through their entire pelvis and body. Orgasms that occur when the prostate is being stimulated can sometimes last longer and result in prolonged sensation.

💡 When you are ready to stop, let your finger glide out slowly; never pull it out quickly.

💡 Once you get the prostate simulation down, you might try stimulating his penis with a well-lubed hand at the same time you are stimulating his prostate with a finger from your other hand. You may need to go easier on the penis stimulation, as it might be more sensitive due to the simultaneous prostate stimulation.

💡 The prostate will swell as the man becomes more aroused. You'll be able to feel this with your finger.

💡 The prostate especially swells right before ejaculation. You should be able to feel ejaculation-related swelling with your finger.

💡 Some men find that direct prostate stimulation results in a super intense orgasm, while others find it's too much or it dulls the feeling of orgasm. They might prefer to avoid prostate stimulation altogether, or that you just push against the rim of the anus with a finger.

☀Regarding positions for prostate massage, there's face up and face down. Try each one and see what works best for both of you.

☀For men who want to stimulate their own prostates, an S-shaped lucite sex toy (Crystal Wand) or a special butt plug might help. Charlie Glickman's prostate massage book has a lot of information about different devices for prostate stimulation. For instance, the surface area of a dildo is larger than that of a finger. This results in a different sensation on the prostate than a finger. Some men prefer the sensation of a dildo on their prostate more than a finger, others like the greater precision that finger massage offers.

Highly Recommended Resources for Prostate Massage and Pleasure:

The Ultimate Guide to Prostate Pleasure: A Guide for Men and Their Partners by Charlie Glickman, Clies Press, 2013. A very thoughtful and well-written look at this hidden but important part of male sexuality. Highly recommended for any man or couple who wants to explore the prostate and its potential for extra sexual pleasure.

A Guide For Prostate Massage from The Pleasure Mechanics. This brief video which is only twenty minutes long is one of the best resources you'll find on prostate pleasure. Couples will feel very comfortable watching it together, and it will give you a wealth of helpful information that you can't find in a book. Visit The Pleasure Mechanics: www.PleasureMechanics.com.

Resources for Prostatitis and BHP: Be sure to visit the extremely thorough and competent website of the Prostatitis organization: www.prostatitis.org.

Thanks: A very special thanks to Dr. Joe Marzucco, formerly of the Portland Kaiser Urology Department and now a sex therapist in private practice in Portland, Oregon. Thanks also to John Schulman, a sex educator in Corvallis, Oregon, who helps students learn how to do prostate exams.

19
Doing Yourself
In Your Partner's Presence

Some women have never seen a man masturbate, and some men have never seen a woman masturbate in real life. Yet plenty of us would find it erotic to watch a partner do it. That's what this chapter is about.

Many of us have the fantasy that once we get into a relationship, we won't be playing with ourselves anymore. In some cases, that's how it is for the first couple of months or years. You either don't have the urge to masturbate because you're having enough sex with your partner, or you can't remember why you used to do it so often. In other relationships, which can be just as satisfying, you don't really stop masturbating. And some women report that they start masturbating more once they are in a satisfying sexual relationship.

While there are times when masturbation is something you will prefer to do alone, there are other times when doing it with or in front of a partner can be extremely satisfying.

Masturbating in front of a partner can sometimes take a lot of trust. That's because masturbation tends to be more self-disclosing than other types of sex. On our sex survey, the vast majority of people say they would rather be walked in on while they are having sex with a partner than when they are masturbating.

Masturbation can also leave you feeling vulnerable if your partner finds you doing it: "Oh, hi, honey, I was just sitting here jerking off."

Being open about it can help expand sexual enjoyment for both partners. Here are nine reasons why:

💡 There is often something erotic and even forbidden about seeing your partner masturbate. This is just as true for women watching men as for men watching women.

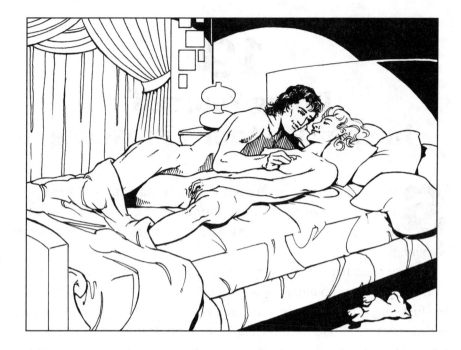

💡 If your partner can see how you please yourself, it might help him or her understand more about pleasing you.

💡 Orgasms from masturbation can be more intense than other kinds of orgasm. It might increase the level of intimacy in your relationship if you can ask your partner to hold you while you get yourself off.

💡 Masturbating together is an excellent way to share intense sexual feelings without the risk of unwanted pregnancy or STIs.

💡 Although the sex you have with your partner can be really satisfying, masturbating is the only way some people can have an orgasm.

💡 There are times when people feel like doing it solo. If this is an accepted part of your relationship, you won't have to hide or feel weird when you want to control your own orgasmic destiny.

💡 People often have unreal expectations that a partner can satisfy all of their sexual urges. There will be many times when one of you is in the mood and the other isn't. There may also be times when your partner is so pleasantly drained by what you have just done (oral sex, genital massage, etc.) that he or she curls up and falls asleep on the spot. If the two of you are comfortable about it, the spent one can hold the horny one while he or she masturbates, or you can masturbate while your partner conks out.

🔆 When you do masturbate in each other's presence, don't forget that a partner's pleasure might be greatly enhanced with a special assist on your part. A man might enjoy it if his partner caresses his testicles, chest or neck while he masturbates, and a woman might find it delightful if her partner caresses her neck, shoulders or breasts or whispers sweet or nasty things into her ears while she masturbates. The possibilities abound.

🔆 Summers in the East, South, and Midwest are sometimes so miserably hot and muggy that the last thing you'll want to do is hug an equally hot and sweaty partner. Masturbating together is one way you can share sexual pleasure without full-body contact.

A Difficult Conversation?

Perhaps you would like to talk to your partner about masturbation, but aren't sure how to bring it up. Or maybe you discovered him or her doing it, and you feel jealous or worried that your partner isn't satisfied with you.

One way of approaching it might be to ask your partner if he or she would hold you while you gave yourself an orgasm. A lot of lovers would find this to be a turn-on, and it would help make the subject of masturbation safe for conversation. Eventually, you might ask your partner if he or she does it in addition to the sex that the two of you have together.

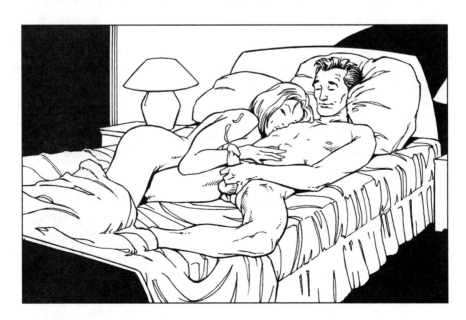

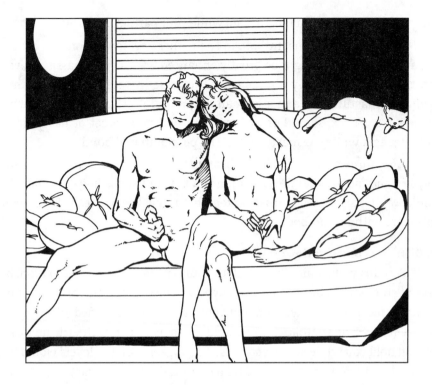

Readers' Comments

"I wish he would do it in front of me more often. I've even named his penis Squeegy Loueegy." *female age 37*

"I never realized it was possible for a guy to be turned on by seeing a woman touching herself. Needless to say, once I figured this out about him, I put on a good show." *female age 45*

"It took a while for us to get comfortable with it, but I like to watch my husband stroke his penis. He enjoys watching me, too. I often masturbate as part of our loveplay because I like stimulation in more places at once than two hands are capable of doing." *female age 47*

"During intercourse one of us always has to touch me so I can have an orgasm, so in that respect, he's seen me do it. And we both chat about how we masturbate when we are alone sometimes." *female age 30*

"Masturbation is the act in my life that keeps me sane. My wife even helps me sometimes." *male age 38*

"I masturbate in front of my husband, mostly with a vibrator. I still find it a bit embarrassing." *female age 35*

"I masturbate at least once a day. My lover loves it when I masturbate with him or beside him. He thinks it's one of life's great mysteries. I like to watch him masturbate, though sometimes it makes me jealous. I'd like him to take the time and attention he spends on himself and use it on me." *female age 24*

"I masturbate regularly because in the fourteen years that I have been sexually active I have never received an orgasm from intercourse. The only way I can come is from a vibrator or by my husband performing oral sex on me. Sometimes I masturbate privately, other times in front of my husband right after intercourse." *female age 35*

"I masturbate several times a week, and if she doesn't know after twenty-five years, well, I'd be surprised." *male age 48*

"Sometimes, you just want to come and not have intercourse with your partner. It makes sense because you know how to make yourself get off better and faster than anybody else. You might also get to know yourself and discover new techniques." *female age 26*

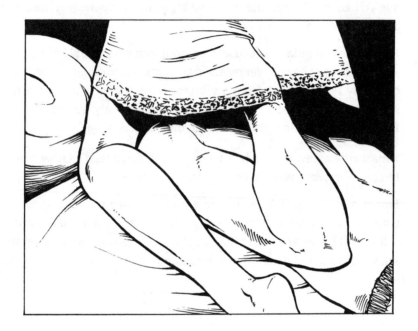

For an even better look at the wonders of sex:

www.GuideToGettingItOn.com

CHAPTER

20
Oral Sex
Vulvas & Honeypots

It's a funny thing about oral sex, at least when you are a guy on the giving end. The woman you are giving oral sex to sometimes disappears. All that's left is a twitching, moaning protoplasm which only partially resembles the person who was there a few moments ago. You are pretty much alone. After it's over, you might want to ask, "Hey, where did you go?" but you learn not to because she will usually just give you a big smile and want to curl up in your arms,[1] or maybe she'll want to have intercourse.

You would think a chapter on giving a woman oral sex would be straightforward: place tongue on detonator (clitoris), start licking or sucking, and wait for the explosion or implosion to occur. Instead, this is one of the more difficult subjects to write about. If you doubt that, consider some of the answers we've received from women about receiving oral sex:

"I hate it when a guy sucks on my clit"

"I can't get off unless he sucks on my clit"

"I'm more sensitive on the right side of my clit"

"My clit is omni dimensional, left side, right side, it doesn't matter"

"I want him to lick from bottom to top with a flat tongue"

"I need him to flick the tip of his tongue from side to side, hard and fast"

"I love it when he fucks me with his tongue"

"I hate it when he fucks me with his tongue, that's what his penis is for"

"I like his mouth on my whole vulva, like he's nursing on it"

"I want him to focus on my clit, anything else is a waste"

---

[1] A female reader says that when she is receiving oral sex, she isn't as aware of her partner's presence, so it's easier to let her fantasies run wild. She wouldn't necessarily want to tell him "where she went," since her fantasy might have involved someone else.

"Women are so much better at this than men"

"I'm bisexual, and the best oral sex I've gotten is from men"

"I love it when he pushes a wet finger into my asshole just before I come"

"He better not touch my ass when he's giving me oral or it's over"

Anyone who can predict the exact type of oral sex a new lover will want deserves *The Congressional Medal of Muff Diving*. One lover might have a clit that's so sensitive anything beyond butterfly kisses will push her from ecstasy to agony. Keeping your head stationary with a wet mouth and light suction might be best. Another lover may have a sleepy clit that needs the oral equivalent of a demolition derby. And then there are women who enjoy oral sex but let other things get in the way:

"I worry I take too long"

"I don't like his face being down there; I'm sure I smell"

"There's no way he can enjoy doing it"

"I can't relax; it makes me feel too vulnerable"

"I so much prefer intercourse!"

So instead of going insane by trying to write the perfect chapter on giving a woman oral sex, the best way to approach the subject was to provide an array of basics. *Give your partner a pen or high lighter and ask her to highlight the parts of the chapter that are relevant to her puss and your mouth.* Better yet if she'll make notes for you in the margins.

This type of approach will help prevent the oral-sex version of being benched, e.g. when she pulls your head up before your mission is accomplished. Involving her in this way will give her a clear signal that you want to learn. She might not have gotten that from her former partners.

Does She Want Your Penis or Your Mouth?

We have asked hundreds of women survey takers if they had to choose between receiving oral sex and intercourse, which would it be. No one anticipated that a large majority would say intercourse, hand's down, even if they have orgasms more reliably when receiving oral sex. The deciding factor was usually intimacy over orgasms. However, for a lot of women the best of both worlds is having intercourse after they've had an orgasm from oral sex. That takes the orgasm onus off of intercourse and allows them to focus on the closeness of intercourse and the full body sensations. Some women enjoy it

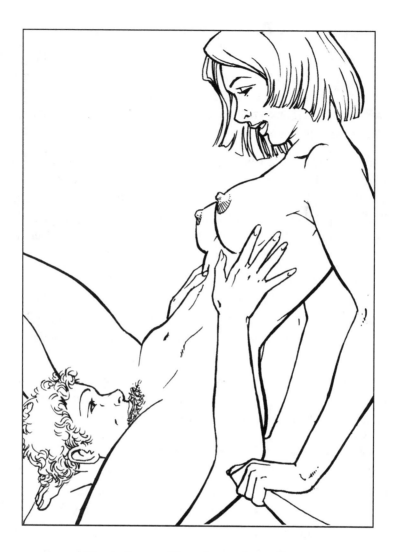

when a partner will mix it up with oral sex, then intercourse, then oral sex, and he finishes off with his penis inside of her.

Of the women who were not comfortable receiving oral sex, about half were concerned with the way they might taste, smell, or how their labia look. Some worried they take too long and it's asking too much of a partner to keeping doing it for what they perceived was an eternity. Other women couldn't believe a partner would enjoy having his face between their legs, and some said they can never come that way.

There are also women who don't have aesthetic concerns or partner worries. They just don't like having oral sex.

Oral Sex in Real Life vs. Oral Sex in Porn[1]

"I have a lot of hang-ups about oral sex because I think the guy wants to get out of there as soon as possible. So I need to be reassured you really enjoy it. The orgasm I have with oral sex is the most wonderful, but it often takes a long time and would try the patience of anyone." *female age 38*

"The least amount of time I give a woman oral sex is about 30 to 45 minutes. From my experience, women don't start to relax until about 10 to 15 minutes into it. Then they go to a stage of comfort. It also depends on the amount of build-up and foreplay and the existing relationship you have. The more foreplay and better the relationship, the quicker the comfort level is reached." *male age 33*

Plenty of women need thirty to forty-five minutes or longer of oral sex before they can orgasm. This is very different from what happens in porn, where oral sex seldom lasts for more than a minute. So a woman who needs actual oral sex instead of the nonsense they show in porn may worry there is something wrong with her, or she may be concerned she's taking too long.

If that's a concern for your partner, assure her you'll surface when you stop enjoying what you're doing. But be aware it's not unusual for a woman to need a half-an hour, and sometimes much longer.

When a Woman Doesn't Like Her Own Body

Some women don't like their bodies and are uncomfortable when a man has a close-up view. If this is the case, it might help ease your partner's mind to do oral sex with the lights out. On the other hand, if your partner is looking for an excuse to feel bad about herself, she will assume you turned the lights out because you find her body ugly. It never hurts to talk about this.

If she worries her genitals smell, one solution is to do oral sex when the two of you are in the shower or right after a shower. That could her feel she is clean enough for you to enjoy going down on her, and sometimes it is nice to give a partner oral sex when she or he has just had a shower.

---

[1] There's a well known porn actress who cannot orgasm in real life unless she receives forty-five minutes of focused oral sex. Yet in hundreds of porn movies, she pretends to easily orgasm from intercourse and oral sex. Porn gives an incredibly distorted view of oral sex.

How Being Aroused Can Help Her Feel Less Modest or Inhibited

Given the mixed messages women receive about their bodies and sexuality, it's not surprising a woman might let modesty or shame get in the way of allowing a partner to go down on her. Fortunately, inhibition tends to decrease as sexual arousal goes up. So while a partner may let negative feelings keep you from giving her oral sex before she's highly aroused, she might be more open to it and even encouraging after she has become aroused.

Giving Up Control and The Need for Reassurance

When receiving oral sex, a woman needs to give up control. While this won't be a problem for most women, others will struggle with turning the reins over to a partner. This can especially be an issue for women who have experienced sexual abuse. If that's the case, be sure to listen carefully to her concerns. If you can't come up with a way to progress that is mutually acceptable, do not push the issue.

Whatever the reason for a lover's concern, reassure her that you'll stop whenever she asks you to. And if she asks you to stop, stop that very moment. You'll always have time to discuss it later.

The Way Women Taste

Most carpet munchers know that some vulvas taste great, others less so. Beyond that, men are fairly useless when it comes to discussing genital taste. Lesbian and bisexual women, however, will talk your ear off about the subject of how women taste:

> "One woman who I loved going down on suddenly began tasting different—not nearly as good. As it turned out, she had started taking vitamin pills. It was never a problem if she took herbs, but vitamin pills would ruin the way she tasted."

> "A former girlfriend was a tennis pro. Sometimes she would play tennis for a few hours and I could go down on her without her taking a shower and she would still taste sweet. There are other women whom I have gone down on right after we showered, and they still didn't taste good. In making my own inquiries, I found that the sweeter tasting women didn't eat red meat."

> "I watch my diet carefully, but I have to admit, the sweetest, best-tasting lover I ever had was a meat-eating, beer-drinking dietary disaster."

So much for consensus. For a thought from the cleanest lesbian in all of Hackensack, New Jersey:

> "Some women spend more time filing their toenails than they do taking care of their pussies. When I'm in the shower, I always separate the lips of my vulva and wash between them. I'm also careful about little bad-tasting pieces of gunk that collect under my clitoral hood. These are what uncircumcised males get under their foreskin if they don't pull it back and clean it."

A Q-tip dipped in mineral oil works well to get rid of "little pieces of gunk" that stick under the clitoral hood. *For more about taste and smell, please see Chapter 47: Vulva Care–Keeping Your Kitty Happy.*

Learning to Listen: Getting Your Muff-Diving Mojo Going

One of the goals of oral sex is to help your partner achieve a degree of pleasure when she's not able to speak coherently. This is what happens during higher states of sexual arousal. Certain parts of the brain appear to shut down. This can take away a woman's ability to conceptualize what's going on or to give you helpful feedback. Ordinarily, she would know what direction your tongue is moving across her clitoris. But as she becomes highly aroused, she might not be able to tell. She just knows it feels good.

So you're left having to interpret what her sounds and body movements mean. They can be anything but straightforward. If a sign reader had to make sense out of a woman's hand motions when she's tugging on your hair or ears during oral sex, he might think she was having seizures. (Actually, our neurological consultant believes that orgasmic states are not dissimilar from brain seizures; fortunately with more enjoyable results.)

So you'll want to learn what some of the following movements mean when you are giving a woman oral sex, since they will be your way of receiving directions from her:

Sudden flinching, convulsing or jolting

Hips arching

Hips bucking

Inner thighs quivering

Inner thighs squeezing your face

Crotch moving into your face

Crotch pulling away from your face

Body goes limp with occasional twitching

Body goes limp with no twitching

Her hand squeezing yours

Fingertips on the top or side of your head can also speak volumes, but their movements can be frantic and difficult to understand. The same is true with gasps and cries if she makes them. It's also important to be mindful of her breathing patterns.

Some of the things you might discuss with a lover after you've had oral sex a time or two are her signals for when she wants you to keep doing what you are doing without making any changes, as well as when she wants you to make changes. Also, if you are giving her oral sex and she says something like "harder," she might actually mean faster, or vice versa. So there's no point in getting frustrated or angry if it seems like she's not being clear. You've been doing something right if she's not able to string words together with much coherence.

Cunnilingus Catastrophe #1 — Avoid the Porn Model

Like so much of porn, what's done on the screen should stay on the screen. The porn version of muff diving is an abomination that's created for the sole purpose of providing camera access to the woman's crotch.

Cunnilingus in porn is called "fence painting" because the person who is giving the oral sex sticks his or her tongue out as far as is humanly possible and makes licking stabs at the woman's puss. The entire event is over faster than a teenage boy on prom night. In real life, giving oral sex is more like wrapping your lips around a juicy peach, which is terrible for the camera. You should also plan to be at it from ten minutes to an hour.

Cunnilingus Catastrophe #2 — Taking the Direct Route

There's only one truly wrong way to arrive at a woman's crotch, and that's by going straight to it. This is why the term "muff diving"—as useful as it is—is so terribly wrong. Never, ever dive. Approach slowly with lips that meander and a tongue that teases. You should have already engaged your lover's other favorite hot spots before beginning your descent into the valley of your dreams. Your partner's entire vulva should be throbbing and moist before your lips make contact with it.

Cunnilingus Catastrophe #3 — When All Systems Are Not Aroused

A wet tongue is not an antidote for a dry puss. Fantasy, romance, teasing, kissing and caressing are your oral sex advance team. If your lover likes to walk on the wild side, add the occasional spanking, kink or rough sex if she enjoys that before going down on her. Remember, arousal first, before approaching a lover's clitoris.

Focus in Muff Diving vs Focus in Video Games

Nina Hartley, who has given oral sex to many women and men, says she sometimes struggles to keep focus when giving a woman oral sex. While it's doubtful Ms. Hartley is as good at gaming as she is at making porn, it might be instructive to consider the differences between muff diving and playing video games—especially when a number of this book's readers do both.

Video gaming is all fingers and thumbs; going down on a woman is all lips and tongue, with the occasional finger assist. Video gaming is a visual feast, but when you are giving a woman oral sex, the lights are often low or you'll have your eyes closed so you can be at one with the job at hand and with your partner's subtle cues.

Gaming invites you to lean into the action and sometimes go wild. Muff diving requires a calm, deliberate focus. With gaming, the better you do the more feedback the game gives you. With muff diving, the better you do, the more likely she'll fade off into her own space. Sometimes there will be hip-bucking feedback and cries of pleasure, but other times a woman's body goes into a state of suspended animation with occasional moans and twitches.

With muff diving, your joy is in helping your partner to drift into a world of pleasure. That's what you need to stay focused on. Once you get her there, you pretty much stop existing, which is its own special joy.

Positions for Giving a Woman Oral Sex

With time and experience, each couple will find which oral sex positions work best for them. For starters, it's hard to beat the classic missionary-style position, which many consider to be the default position. This is where the woman is on her back and the man is on his stomach with his face between her legs. This position allows her legs to flex comfortably, which helps her pelvis to tilt up for better access. Her thighs can be over his arms or shoulders, or under them.

A great thing about this position is how comfortable it is for the woman and how it doesn't interfere with her ability to take long, deep breaths. It's also a position where your bodies are both pointing in the same direction. This means your tongue has clear access to the tip and shaft of her clitoris. You will be licking in an upward direction, which works well if your partner likes you to retract her clitoral hood and 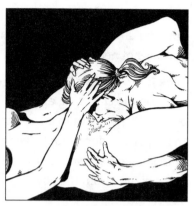 lick the underbelly of her clitoris. It also allows you to lightly suck on her clitoris or to wrap your mouth around her entire vulva if that's what she prefers.

A disadvantage of this position is your head is looking up, which causes your neck to bend backward. This can be very uncomfortable after awhile. A variation is when you are kneeling at the edge of the bed. This can allow your neck to be less bent, depending on how the two of you position yourselves.

Another comfortable position is the classic missionary but turned on your sides. This allows the man to rest his head on the inside of his partner's thigh. If she's a fan of wrestling, it lets her apply the ultimate head scissors. Some men love having a woman's thighs around their head, while others find it to be claustrophobic. One disadvantage of this position is a man doesn't have as much access or control as when her legs are spread apart. Some men will start off in the missionary position, when a woman's clit might be more sensitive and mouth and tongue control are critical. Then they ask the woman to roll on her side so they can get into a more comfortable sides position and keep going for as long as she likes.

Another oral-sex position is where your partner is sitting on your face. However the term "sitting on your face" is rife with deception. While it might look as if she is sitting on your face, the human face isn't the most comfortable object to sit on. As an alternative, she might want to stay on all fours, with you propping your head and upper body on pillows. This will give your face the necessary altitude to make the contact you need with her crotch.

A position that can be especially comfortable for a man's neck is when the woman is sitting in a chair or on a stool with him sitting or kneeling between her legs. (See the illustration on p. 289.)

Some couples enjoy a 69 alignment where his head is pointing in the opposite direction from hers. Unfortunately, the alignment of your face to her vulva is not necessarily optimal.

Lock Jaw & Tongue Cramping

Tongue cramping and jaw paralysis are common side effects of giving oral sex. These tend to occur moments before the woman blurts out, "There, that's perfect, don't stop!" Being able to continue when every ligament and muscle fiber from your neck up is screaming for mercy is what separates the oral-sex men from the boys.

Protect Your Neck—You are not a Crash-Test Dummy

If your neck is in a strange position or angle, you won't have the stamina to do a good job. Make sure your neck is comfortable. Always assume you may be in this position for longer than anticipated. Sometimes much longer.

A strategically placed pillow under your partner's bum can provide better access to her clitoris. It can raise her pelvis so the angle of your neck isn't as severe and it can help increase the sensation in her clitoris. Don't hesitate to put a pillow under your head if it makes you more comfortable. And if chronic oral sex-related neck pain is an issue, try it with her sitting in a chair.

With experience, you will discover which positions do and don't land you in traction. Do not suffer in silence. Discuss this with your partner so you can find positions that are mutually pleasing. That way you'll be able to give her more of what she likes. And don't hesitate to give your mouth a breather by gently replacing the tip of your tongue with the tip of your wet finger.

Also, it is not unheard of for a woman in the heat of oral passion to grab a man's skull and yank it one way or another with enough force to cause whiplash. If she grinds your face into her crotch with a nose-flattening swoosh, she probably wants you to up the tempo or pressure a bit. But don't let your tongue go full throttle, because this might cause her to whip your head in the opposite direction. Learning to shift tongue-gears gradually can add years to the life of your neck.

The Thermal Envelope of a Woman's Crotch

Besides porn, the second worst source of information on how to give oral sex is the movies. When you see an actor with his face between a woman's legs in the movies, his head is almost always covered by sheets or a blanket.

This might be fine if your partner's crotch could double as a home for penguins. But once a woman begins to feel sexually excited, the heat signature between her legs increases. This means you will start sweating like a pig if you put a blanket over your head while giving a woman oral sex. It will help ruin what should be an enjoyable experience. So be sure there is plenty of air circulating around your face and head.

Avoiding Beard Burn

When discussing oral sex, one thing that women often complain about is men's beards. Their advice: grow a full beard or keep your face clean-shaven. Grunge is not good on a woman's thighs. Five o'clock shadow is killer.

If you are the kind of guy who grows a five o'clock shadow ten minutes after shaving, find a favorite set of towels and drape one over each of your partner's legs, like mechanics do on the fenders of cars when they are working on the engine. Talk to your partner about this and see if it would help.

On the Tip of Your Tongue

During oral sex, your tongue can be hard or soft. To understand the difference between a soft and a hard tongue, spend a few minutes licking the palm of your hand. This can be a good way to learn about subtle variations in oral-sex technique.

Notice how quickly the end of your tongue goes dry. So much for the fantasy that the human tongue is always wet. A dry tongue creates drag or friction. Nature did not create the clitoris with a high tolerance for friction.

This is why you'll need to coat your tongue with saliva before licking a woman's vulva. After a few minutes, saliva from your mouth should automatically run down your tongue and keep everything well-lubricated, but not at the start. (There's nothing wrong with keeping a bottle of water or good-tasting lube by your side.)

Try licking your hand again, but let your tongue go soft in a way that would cause you to slur your words if you were attempting to speak. You may need to push your hand closer to your face to accomplish this, since a soft tongue is not as long as a hard tongue. Some women will prefer a softer, more rounded tongue when you are licking the underbelly of the clitoris, given how it isn't insulated by the clitoral hood. Or, if she's highly aroused, she might want the tip of your tongue to feel like an arrowhead.

Oral Sex Cheat Sheet...

The Mons is a mound of tissue that's over the pubic bone and above the labia. You might massage the entire mons with your fingers before starting oral sex. Pushing the mons up with your fingers during oral sex can change the angle of the clitoris and give better access..

The Vestibule is the area between the inner labia. Chart this sensitive area with the tip of your tongue. If you grasp her clit between your tongue and top lip and gently nod or shake your head, it will stimulate the vestibule.

The Inner Labia or Lips can thicken and darken when a woman is sexually aroused. Some women will enjoy it if you suck on them or pull and tug them with your lips. You might also try tugging on them with your fingers while licking or sucking on a woman's clit.

A Vulva with Large Inner Lips

Taint or Perineum The space between the genitals and anus is much shorter in women than it is in men. While she can still find it very enjoyable if you lick this area, be careful not to dip your tongue into her anus and then back into her vulva. If you are going to rim, you should rim and only rim.

...Using Two Different Vulvas

The Outer Labia or Lips are made from the same type of skin that the scrotum is. Some women will enjoy it if you kiss, lick or suck on their labia. Try tugging them with your lips.

A Good Place to rest your upper lip when focusing on the clitoris.

The Clitoris should be an end point, not a place to start. It responds better after a woman is aroused. Some women like a gentle sucking or nursing motion on the clitoris, some a flicking with the tip of the tongue or circles around it, some prefer long licks with a flat broad tongue from the fourchette to the mons.

The Vagina is mostly sensitive around the opening. Try making circles around the opening with the tip of your tongue. If she likes you to thrust into it, you don't need to push your tongue in far. She won't feel much past the first inch.

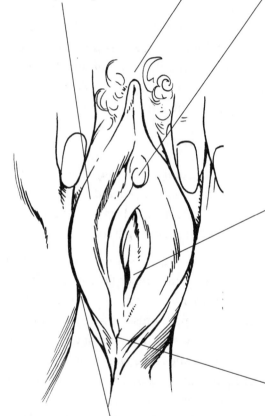

A Vulva with Large Outer Lips

Fourchette is where her lips come together at the bottom of the vulva. It's where some of the lubrication pools. This is another good area to massage with your fingers before using your mouth, then with the tip of your tongue or by pushing your mouth into it.

Furrows and Folds along the length of the vulva. Try running the tip your tongue up and down the furrow between the lips, and then between the outer lips and inner thigh.

Northern Route or Southern Route?

It rarely shows good form to begin oral sex by suddenly pouncing on your partner's clitoris. Instead, when she is on her back and is sexually aroused, start kissing around her stomach and work your way down, or start kissing the inside of her knees and work your way up.

With the stomach-down route, you might begin kissing the skin over the bones that stick out on the sides of her hips. You'll eventually move down to the crevice near her inner thigh. Then return to the hip bone on the other side, kiss circles around it, and work your way down.

With the knees-up route, start on the inside of one knee. Smother it with kisses. Work your way up her inner thighs with kisses until you reach her outer labia. Then move to her other knee and start smothering it with kisses. Work your way up her inner thigh until you reach ground zero.

By then, she will hopefully feel that life will stop if you don't begin giving her oral sex.

Ground Zero

Perhaps you are a total pro at giving oral sex, or maybe you know more about troll rogues than going down on a woman. Regardless of your experience, what follows is a blueprint for giving really good oral sex—as long as you get reliable feedback from the woman you are giving it to.

💡Oral sex tends to make your salivary glands sing. Instead of swallowing or letting it pool in your mouth, let your slobber flow wherever gravity wants to take it. That way, if your partner doesn't shave, you won't have to worry as much about pubic hairs wrapping themselves around your tonsils each time you try to swallow. Putting a towel under her rear will help to keep the mattress from turning into a lagoon, and some women will appreciate it if you push an edge of the towel against the area that's just below their vulva so the saliva doesn't trickle down their butt crack.

💡When a woman flexes her legs, her pelvis arches forward. This will provide access to give good oral sex. A lot of women will do this themselves by putting their legs over your shoulders, or by planting one or both feet on your shoulders. Some pull their legs up to their chest. You can also wrap your arms around the back of a woman's thighs and push them forward.

💡Some women provide all the oral access a man needs by simply spreading their legs. Or you may want to separate the outer labia with your fingers. This gives your mouth better access to the inner lips, and can sometimes feel like the difference between kissing a woman whose mouth is open versus one whose lips are closed. Some women will offer a helping hand by separating the lips themselves.

💡 Lavish the outer lips with licks and kisses. Then try running the tip of your tongue up and down the furrows between the outer and inner lips.

💡 The mons pubis is the mound of flesh that sits directly above the labia. It is where the bulk of the pubic hair grows. Pushing or pulling up the mons while doing oral sex can heighten the intensity for some women, and some might want you to nibble gently on the mons. If a woman doesn't shave, lightly tugging on her pubic hair can feel enjoyable.

💡 The inner lips of women's genitals tend to be longer around the vaginal opening. You might try clasping them between your fingers and tugging on them gently while your mouth is focused on the clitoris. A woman who is highly aroused may enjoy this, but be sure get feedback.

Her Clitoris

> "Don't immediately dive into the clitoris and stay there. Warm up by licking all of the vaginal area. Suck on the labia. Then turn your attention to the clitoris. I like my clitoris to be licked, flicked and sucked. Sometimes I get off faster if my partner licks lower on the clitoris, rather than at the top of the hood. It makes for a different kind of orgasm." *female age 25*

No matter how small your penis is, nobody should have trouble finding it. Not so with the clitoris. Some are in clear view, others play hide 'n' seek. Sometimes all it takes to expose the tip of the clitoris is a single finger to pull the hood up. Other times it takes both hands and a litany of prayer.

To find the tip with your tongue, separate the outer lips with your fingers. Make sure your tongue has plenty of saliva on it for lubrication. Take a long slow lick from the bottom to the top of the vulva where the big lips meet. Somewhere along the way you will most likely feel a small knob or slight protuberance. Find out from your partner if this is the tip of her clitoris. Have her explain to you exactly how she likes it licked, assuming she likes it licked.

As your partner becomes aroused, the tip of her clitoris will swell. Some swell predictably; others don't. This process can be challenging until you become familiar with the way her clitoris changes. You might learn to lick on a specific spot or location rather than being able to find her actual clitoris with your tongue. You might need to go on faith and past experience.

> "Gentle teasing brings me to an orgasm. I like him to start off gently, with light licks and kisses all over my vulva. I can't take too much pressure on my clitoris, though, and sometimes that ruins it for me."
>
> *female age 23*

You would think the surest way to arouse a woman would be to start at the tip of the clitoris, since that's where so much of the sensitivity can be. But this is not the way it usually works. For most women, you don't approach the clitoris until you have planted plenty of kisses in the surrounding area. With some women, you never touch the tip at all, while others might want you to throw a lip lock on the tip of the clitoris. It depends on how aroused your partner is, and on how sensitive her clitoris is.

Some women enjoy it if you kiss their vulva in the same way you do their mouth. Some crave a gentle nursing action on the clitoris. Some like it if you flick the tip of your tongue over the clitoris in a sideways direction; others prefer an up-and-down motion as though you were rapidly turning a light switch on and off. Some enjoy a circular motion. These motions may seem awkward at first, but you'll get the hang of it. Also, some women will want you to speed up or change locations as their arousal grows, while others prefer a constant motion from start to finish.

When it comes to the clitoris, less is sometimes more. Stay simple and steady unless she advises to the contrary. Your partner might have a favorite side of her clitoris where she wants you to lick. To help improve access to the favored side, she might try flexing one leg while the other lies flat and a bit to the side. Other women have an ambidexterous clitoris that welcomes an approach from any side.

The clitoris sometimes disappears soon before orgasm. No one knows why. With input from your partner you will learn how to respond; in the meantime, when a clitoris disappears, you might try giving a little suck to pull it back out.

After learning more about your partner's responses, you might experiment by puckering your lips around her clitoris and making a light vacuum. You can then push the clitoris in and out of your mouth either with your tongue or by reversing the suction every couple of seconds.

Your partner's clitoris or the area around it may begin to pulse once she is highly aroused. This is probably an indication to stay your course without changing the speed, tempo or rhythm. Problems start when you assume she'll love it even more if you double the tempo or do it harder.

The contractions of orgasm are said to happen less than once a second. Some people say the best way to stimulate a woman's clitoris is to use strokes that are in synchrony with the contractions. Good luck making that one work.

Some women prefer to receive different kinds of stimulation depending on the time of the month. At one point in her menstrual cycle you might avoid the tip or glans, but two weeks later you can lick the tip silly. It's nothing you're going to learn in a one-night stand.

The Clit Requires Precision

If you're focusing on other parts of the vulva besides your partner's clit, or if you have most of her vulva in your mouth, you don't need to be as careful with your movements. But when you're mostly focused on your partner's clit, precision and focus can be the key. As Nina Hartley says, "With women, millimeters mean everything."

Landscape Mode vs. Portrait Mode

Most men can do side-to-side flicking longer and better than they can do up and down flicking. Rapid up-and-down flicking will often bring out your tongue's inner spaz. If rapid up-and-down flicking is what your partner wants, you might experiment with turning your head to the side, eg from portrait mode to landscape mode. With your head turned sideways, she might experience your side-to-side flicking as up-and-down flicking.

One Change at a Time

Once you've isolated her clitoris and know it's really her clitoris, you'll want to go slow and easy. If you make changes, try only one new thing at a time. Wait for your partner's reaction before making further changes.

For instance, if you want to speed up, don't speed up and change direction at the same time. Otherwise, you won't know what worked. What if speeding up was what she needed, but when you changed direction your tongue lost contact with an important bundle of nerves? There's no way you'll know which change worked and which set you back if you attempt more than one at a time.

Passive Sucking While Your Partner Controls the Movement

With some women, it works well to only apply pressure or to pull a light vacuum with your mouth but nothing more. Let her move her hips back and forth or up and down. All it takes is less than an inch up and down or side to side for her to achieve a very pleasing effect.

This can work especially well if you aren't sure what to do, or if the two of you aren't able to get into a good rhythm. Let her provide the movement.

The Urinary Meatus

Using terms like "urinary meatus" or "the area around her peehole" can cause an aesthetic flat tire. However, the part of a woman's vulva between her clitoris and vagina which contains the urinary meatus is definitely worth exploring with the tip of your tongue. For some women its stimulation might be the difference between good oral sex and great oral sex. If you have aesthetic problems with this notion, think about what your lover gets when she is sucking on the head of your penis—one great big urinary meatus. Also keep in mind that urine is more sanitary than the human mouth. Kissing her down here is usually more hygienic than kissing her on the mouth.

Her Vagina

The opening of the vagina is in the lower half of a woman's vulva. A man might occasionally feel compelled to stick his tongue far into his lover's vagina. But reaching far inside a woman's vagina can cause your tongue to cramp, and she's not likely to notice because the nerves that register touch only go in as far as the first inch.

Some women may treasure a finger or two inside the vagina during oral sex, but usually not until they have reached higher levels of arousal. Some might like a thumb pushing down on the floor of the vagina. As for what to do with your fingers once they are inside, some women like them to stay perfectly still while others will enjoy it if you twist, jiggle or thrust your fingers in and out. Also, there might be special spots in her vagina that your partner enjoys having stimulated.

The inner part of a woman's vagina often balloons open when sexually aroused. Some women enjoy having this filled up. A dildo works well for this, and some couples find that inserting a dildo during oral sex can be a turn-on. Also, a woman might fantasize about having one man's penis inside her vagina at the same time that another man is licking her clitoris. Using a dildo

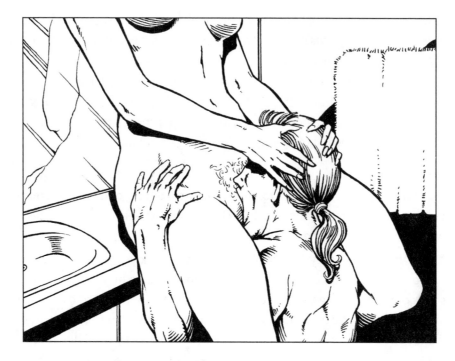

while receiving oral sex can help satisfy this fantasy unless a threesome is in play or a second lover is handy. (There are even oral sex dildos that strap on a guy's chin. It looks like a trip to the orthodontist that went very wrong.)

All of Her in Your Mouth

One maneuver is to open your mouth wide, put your top lip just above your partner's clitoris, and your bottom lip at the lower end of her vulva. Then push your face in and begin to suck all of her into your mouth. Ease up on the suction a few seconds later, then keep repeating. The emphasis is on gentle suction, unless she wants you to amp it up.

If She Starts Bucking

It's not unusual for woman who is receiving oral sex to start bucking her hips with pleasure when she is having an orgasm. This kind of motion can knock a guy off her mound.

A response that some women appreciate is as follows: Wrap your arms around her thighs from behind, as in the illustration above. Put your hands firmly on her hip bones. The female hip bones provide a perfect handle and were probably put there for this very purpose. Flex your arms so that she has to lift the weight of your upper body in order to buck. This shouldn't hurt her and will keep her pelvis still enough so you can give her more of what's causing her to buck in the first place.

However, don't let yourself think that orgasmic histrionics mean a woman is receiving more pleasure than one who is mostly still during orgasm. A woman who orgasms quietly may be having a more intense experience than a woman who is expending energy doing a porn-star imitation.

Ass Play during Oral

When a woman is about to have an orgasm during oral sex, a finger tip gently inserted into her anus can launch a cascade of pleasure, or it can be the worst thing you could possibly do.

If you decide to try this, there is no need to stick your finger in very far. Just putting pressure on the rim around a lover's anus might light up thousands of nerve endings. A variation is to insert a well-lubricated butt plug or vibrator in your partner's rear while doing oral sex. Or your partner might want you to firmly squeeze her butt cheeks, but stay away from her anus.

You can always go for a triple play: lips on her clitoris, one finger in her vagina and one up her rear, although a lot of women will find this to be over stimulating and not in a good way.

If She Has Vulva Jewelry or You Have a Tongue Piercing

Genital piercings can be an important player in oral sex if you learn how to use them correctly. Experiment with sucking her clit into your mouth and flicking the jewelry with your tongue. Her response may depend on how close to a nerve bundle the piercing lies. With the proper feedback, you'll learn exactly how to use a woman's genital jewelry to provide her with exceptional oral sex. But be careful about the jewelry coming apart. It's not the kind of thing you want the doctors in the emergency room to be fishing out of your stomach. (For tips on giving oral sex when you have a tongue piercing, please see the Chapter 43: *Piercings and Tattoos*.

Mixing Up Oral and Intercourse

Some couples enjoy it when a guy goes down on a woman for several minutes, then they have intercourse for a few more minutes, then he goes back down on her, then they have more intercourse. In other words, don't assume there's a rule book here that anyone needs to follow. Figure out what works best for the two of you and enjoy it.

It Ain't Over until It's Over, or She Pulls Your Head Away

Just because you think your lover has had an orgasm, there is no reason to come up for air. Keep doing exactly what you're doing until she relieves you from duty with the oral-sex sentries: her hands. Do not leave your post until instructed by lefty and righty pulling on your head.

Keep in mind, though, that the slightest movement can feel abrasive after a woman has had an orgasm. So be respectful if she wants you to slow it to a crawl or call it quits.

When you are with a partner long enough, you will learn the best post-orgasm protocol. She may want you to lay off for a minute or two, then gently rev it up. Or she may want you to surface and put your penis where your mouth has been.

Fun at The Y—Oral Odds'n'Ends

🔦Find out if your partner likes you to play with her breasts or other body parts while you are going down on her. One reader loves her partner to squeeze her toes when she is receiving oral sex—it can be the difference between coming or not for her.

🔦Here's a game suggested in *Ultimate Kiss*. Bring your lover to the edge of orgasm with oral sex and then pull your mouth away for a count of fifty. Then bring her to the edge again and pull your mouth away for twenty-five seconds. Then bring her to the edge and pull your mouth away for ten seconds. Do this once more, pausing for just a few seconds. Be sure to explain this game beforehand. One female reader says this game can work equally well when you are finger fucking.

🔦It can be fun to give a woman oral sex when she is still wearing her panties or a bikini bottom. Start with your lips on her inner thighs, work them up to her vulva, and then sneak your tongue under the material. Some women might like it if you blow warm moist air through the front panel of their underwear. But never blow air directly into a woman's vagina.

🔦Consider pulling your lover's panties off with your teeth. But be careful not to leave holes or rip the material, given how lingerie can cost an arm and a leg; it's best that she not remember you as the one who destroyed her favorite undies. Then again, the memory might bring a smile.

It is difficult to do oral sex when a woman is standing. The access is too limited. Think nothing of crawling under her dress while she is standing to plant tender kisses in places where other guys only dream of touching, but she'll need to sit or lie down to enjoy your oral finest.

After she is highly aroused, place the tip of your tongue on the side or bottom of her clitoris. Then push the tip of a small vibrator on the other side of your tongue.

Separate the outer lips with your fingers and lay your tongue flat against her vaginal opening at the lowest part of her vulva. Take a slow, long, wet lick that lasts for about thirty seconds. This way, her clit gets a slow protracted licking as your tongue creeps up her vulva.

Some women like enough pillows under their rear end that their entire body is on an incline with their crotch angled up in the air. This provides great access, a wonderful view, and your neck won't cramp as much.

A more subtle way of making your tongue vibrate is to hum while placing it on your partner's clitoris. A well-hummed aria can push some women into orbit. Others will start laughing hysterically.

On a hot muggy day, ice cubes can spice up any kind of sex play. During the cold of winter, sipping a warm drink before kissing a woman's vulva can leave her with warm and sensual feelings.

There are swings that are great for doing oral sex. They can be hung from a door jamb or ceiling rafter. The swing spreads the woman's legs and places her at the perfect height for a man to give her oral sex while he is sitting upright. An added benefit is his neck stays straight. Beware: many swings are poorly made and uncomfortable. You'll need to shell out a lot for a good one.

For special celebrations, some couples report pouring champagne into a woman's vagina when her legs are elevated. (Vamosa?) Her partner then licks out the champagne, although this is not recommended for men in twelve-step programs or for women whose vaginal tissue might become irritated. (The sugar in the champagne can cause a yeast infection, and who knows what harm the alcohol will do.) An extremely dry champagne with low residual sugar might be preferable, and even then, her gynecologist might cringe at the thought. Avoid putting cold duck in a woman's crotch, although a goose on her rear is often welcome.

🔆 Some women have a problem with being kissed on the face after being kissed on the crotch. If that's the case in your household, consider keeping a wet washcloth handy. Run it across your face before kissing above after kissing below.

Safety Note: It can be very sexy to blow warm moist air over your lover's vulva, but very dangerous to blow air into her vagina. Never lock your lips on your partner's vulva and blow air into it.

Female Fluid Flow

Some women expel fluid from their vulva around the time they have an orgasm. One female reader who gushes says that her male partner finds it exciting. If your partner gushes and you have a problem with it, take solace in knowing that she's at least having an orgasm.

Those Damn Dental Dams

Several years ago, someone decided the way to safely go down on a woman was to spread a latex dental dam over her crotch. Why not just use neoprene or Naugahyde?

First of all, you have no clue what you're licking. And then there's the texture problem. Try whipping your tongue back and forth over latex. No matter how much slobber you throw on it, your tongue drags and your RPM rating tanks. Some people find Saran Wrap to be a more satisfactory barrier. You can see through it, it doesn't slow your tongue action, and you can always re-use it afterward to cover a casserole.

Maintaining a Hard-On While Giving Oral Sex

If a guy is giving his lover oral sex, it might be nice if he kept doing it long enough to get her off. But once he feels his hard-on starting to go, a man will sometimes surface from between a woman's legs and try to have intercourse before it's "too late." Otherwise he feels unmanly about his penis going soft.

So why does a man sometimes lose his erection while going down on a woman? Doing oral sex requires the kind of concentration that isn't always conducive to maintaining an erection. There is also mouth and neck fatigue. Whatever the cause, it's not unusual for a man to lose his erection when he is going down on a woman, but not because he is unhappy or unexcited.

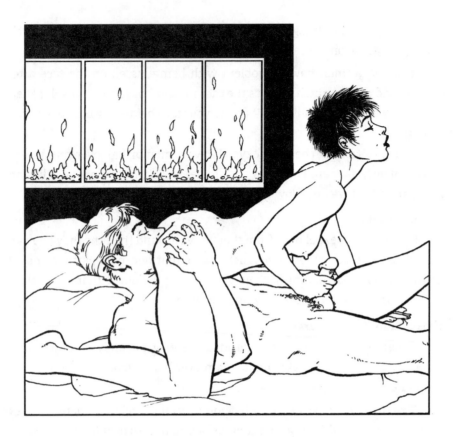

There are men where it's instant wood when tongue meets thigh and it remains that way no matter what. But you'd think a woman would be more interested in the quality of the oral sex than whether her partner has a boner.

Things a Woman Can Do to Help a Partner Who Is Going Down on Her

Tugging on Your Bush If you have pubic hair, take a moment to tug on your bush before a man goes down. You'll pull out loose hairs that would end up sticking to the back of his throat.

Trimming Your Triangle A woman who shaves or waxes shouldn't hesitate to put her lover in charge of muff maintenance and coiffure. Many men find this a joyful duty.

Labia Laundering Separating the labia and washing between them once a day will help to keep your genitals clean and tasty. Douching isn't necessary nor advisable, and avoid soap that is scented or is too alkaline. See *Chapter 47: Vulva Care–Keeping Your Kitty Happy.*

Not Helpful A guy might be having a wonderful time kissing and caressing his partner's genitals when she suddenly pulls him up because she's decided that he surely can't be enjoying something "as gross as that." If a woman fears her genitals don't taste good, she should ask her partner. And if she feels there is something bad about her genitals, she should tell her partner lest he feels hurt by her rejecting behavior. Perhaps his reassurance will be helpful. But if it's something that genuinely makes her feel uncomfortable, then he shouldn't keep trying to do it.

Feedback As long as it's done with sensitivity, most men will appreciate a woman's suggestions about giving her oral pleasure. If a man's ego is so fragile he can't handle the input, perhaps he would do better with a mindless partner who has no input to give. If you aren't equal partners in sex, you aren't equal partners, period. Is that what you want?

Playing with Yourself Don't hesitate to reach down and masturbate while your partner is doing oral sex. If you want him to keep licking while you are stimulating your clitoris, be sure to let him know.

Humor Next to bathing, humor is the most important sex aid there is. Try not to forget this.

Oral Sex during Her Period

Some couples are fine with oral sex while the woman is having her period; others wait a few days until the flow has stopped. Here are some solutions if you want the action but not the extra nutrition:

Instead, The Keeper, Diva Cup These are tampon alternatives that collect menstrual flow inside the vagina. They work well for oral sex during your period. Pop one in before oral sex and it will catch most if not all of the flow. These are not for birth control.

Tampons A woman who is having her period can insert a tampon before a man goes down on her. The tampon will usually catch most of the flow. She must take the tampon out if intercourse is going to follow.

Diaphragm Some women get a diaphragm for the sole purpose of having sex during their periods. The diaphragm becomes a barrier that traps the menstrual flow. Some couples use the diaphragm for oral sex but not for intercourse, since period flow can help make intercourse better.

Plastic Wrap A simple way of dodging menstrual flow is by putting plastic wrap over the woman's vulva before going down on her.

STI NOTE Little if anything is known about the risks of HIV transmission when doing oral sex on a woman who is having her period, but it is a way to give and get hepatitis. Never give a partner unprotected oral sex if you have a canker sore or active oral herpes in your mouth, or if your partner has a herpes outbreak on his or her genitals.

Sixty-Nine

69 is when a man does oral sex on a woman at the same time she does oral sex on him. Some couples enjoy 69 as their favorite way of having sex. However, there are plenty of couples who enjoy oral sex but don't necessarily like doing 69. That's because when a person is on the receiving end of oral sex, he or she might want to kick back and not have to worry about getting the other person off. 69 should be avoided if either partner involuntarily clenches his or her jaw when having an orgasm.

Readers' Comments

"Get a good rhythm going. Don't suck or lick too hard on the head of the clit. Also, either be smooth-shaved or have a beard, but no in-between. Beard burn really kills down there!" *female age 45*

"Stubble on the face is not welcome in tender areas down below." *female age 48*

"Please quit when I say so; it gets really tender and ticklish after I come." *female age 43*

"Lick around the area of the clitoris, not directly on it, until I am more aroused and then only part of the time." *female age 35*

"Start out slowly, working around the outer area with your tongue. Don't just push in. Do a lot of gentle rubbing and caressing on the insides of the leg. Gradually probe the vulva with your tongue. Develop a rhythm and keep going until I come." *female age 32*

"If my partner's tongue gets tired, he uses his finger and sometimes it feels the same." *female age 25*

"I like a man to first shave me smooth, then gently kiss and finger me." *female age 34*

"It's great when he puts a finger into my rear while giving me oral sex. It makes for quite the explosion!" *female age 38*

21
Oral Sex
Popsicles & Penises

Some women enjoy giving a man oral sex. It can give them a feeling of power and control over their partner's body. It can also provide feelings of intimacy and closeness that can be both soothing and exciting. Other women don't find anything special about it, but will go down on a guy if he enjoys it. And some women would rather suck on a rusty pipe than let their lips stray south of a man's beltline.

Whatever your preference, this chapter offers tips and techniques about giving oral sex to the male of the species. It starts with a candid discussion about male ejaculate and then offers techniques for giving splendid blowjobs. It also includes suggestions for the man who is receiving oral sex—things he can do to help make it a good experience for his partner and himself.

When Gay Guys Blow

Women often get the feeling they need to swallow a guy's ejaculate in order to give a truly fine blowjob. If this were true, you'd think it would apply just as much in the gay community, where the giver of the blowjob knows exactly what it feels like to receive a blowjob. But that's not true. Gay guys don't always swallow when giving blowjobs. As one gay male reader says, "No way am I going to do all that work getting a partner to come and not watch him ejaculate. Besides, I don't exactly love the taste."

You might love swallowing. But do it only because you want to and not because there's some *Emily Post of Blowjobs* who says it has to be.

To Swallow or Not to Swallow—That Is the Question

Considering what happens if you suck on a penis for long enough, a woman who gives oral sex eventually has to decide if she wants to swallow ejaculate. While some women don't mind swallowing, others find it weird. For some women the salient factors are how they feel about the guy and how they feel within the relationship. For others, it's the taste and texture.

Different guys come in different flavors. As a female reader states: "My current lover tastes great, I like swallowing his ejaculate. But when my former boyfriend came, it felt like battery acid in the back of my mouth." Another reader comments that she has no problem with the taste or texture of male ejaculate, but that it sometimes upsets her stomach. A British sex expert with a Margaret Thatcher-like voice says that male ejaculate is an acquired taste, like swallowing raw oysters. She says it's nothing to get worked up over. We're not so sure, given how nobody around here likes swallowing raw oysters. As for the smell of male ejaculate, it's like a weak solution of Clorox—original scent rather than Lemon Fresh or Spring Rain. It also smells like alfalfa sprouts. For more on taste, texture, smell and volume, see Chapter 6: *Semen Confidential.*

Who knows what to advise about swallowing male ejaculate, except that a man shouldn't push the issue unless he is willing to swallow a mouthful of his own, although the actual amount is closer to a teaspoonful. Suggestions for how to give a really good blowjob without swallowing are listed later in this chapter.

To Swallow or Not to Swallow: Hormonal Considerations

Women sometimes wonder if they are going to get a dose of male hormones when they swallow male ejaculate. While the testicles produce the lion's share of male hormone, this goes directly into a man's bloodstream and not into his semen. You don't need to worry about sprouting a beard or growing a big Adam's apple from swallowing your partner's cum. And the only way you will gain weight from male ejaculate is if it makes you pregnant.

Regarding the issue of health, ejaculate from a healthy guy has fewer germs than saliva. It seldom causes an allergic reaction. The main health concern about male sex fluids is whether the man has a sexually transmitted infection. For more on STIs, see Chapter 52: *Gnarly Sex Germs.*

Have an Understanding

The important thing to remember about giving a blowjob is that no matter what you are doing down there, it is going to feel pretty wonderful to your partner. So lighten up, loosen up, stare his one-eyed snake in the scrotum and say, "Listen here, you strange thing, this lady's the one with the teeth, so behave yourself and do as I say!" Giving a good blow job is about being in charge. Enjoy it and have fun calling the shots.

Quick & Easy

Going down on a man isn't as much a mystery as going down on a woman, given how the penis is pretty much in your face. The childhood experience of sucking on popsicles will give you an idea of how to begin. However, popsicle-sucking does not make for an excellent blowjob.

There are many different kinds of blowjobs. Some women like to include lots of kissing and licking; others mainly suck on the penis. Using your hands while giving oral sex adds an extra dimension. We discuss it all in the pages that follow.

Blow Jobs in Porn vs. Real Life

Have you ever noticed that porn actresses never gag when giving blow jobs? Maybe that's why they go to porn acting school. Or maybe they've had the nerves that cause the gag reflex surgically removed. Whatever the case, blowjobs in porn often seem like they are more about humiliating or objectifying women than they are about sexual pleasure.

As for a man who wants to ram his penis down a woman's throat like they do in porn, why not find a girlfriend who is a porn actress? Although it's quite possible even she won't want to do that at home.

Gag Prevention

Here are four suggestions to keep yourself from being gagged while giving a blowjob, but the most important suggestion is the first:

Tell Him! If he thrusts and it gags you, let him know. Women who gag when giving oral sex seldom tell their partner about it. So if gagging is a concern, tell your partner the two of you need to work on it, because you enjoy giving him blowjobs except for the gagging part. Be specific! If a little thrusting is OK, help him recognize the difference between good and painful thrusting.

Fist on Shaft Make a fist around the shaft of your lover's penis, with your little finger resting on his pubic bone. This will give you four knuckles' worth of washer or buffer. If your man has an average-sized penis, there should be no way he can gag you. If your man is luckier than most, use two hands instead of one, as you would when swinging a baseball bat. As an added benefit, keeping your fingers around the shaft allows you to pump the foreskin or pull it taut. More on why you might want to do that later.

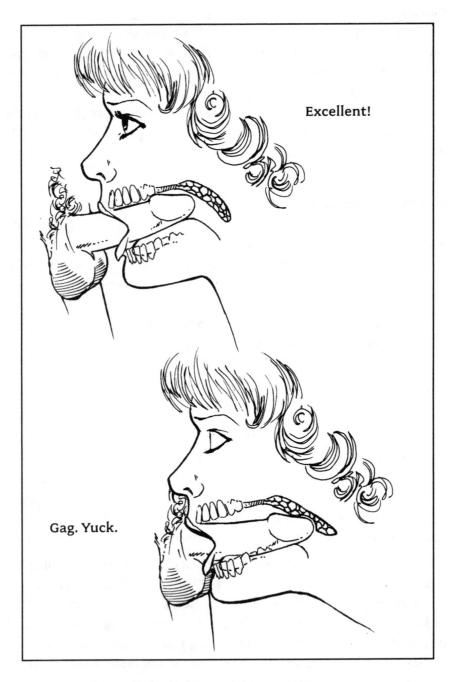

Inspired by illustrations from Violet Blue's "The Ultimate Guide To Fellatio" 2nd edition

On His Back Some guys thrust involuntarily when they come. To deal with this, keep your partner on his back and position your body between his legs. When he is close to coming, keep both of your hands around the base of his penis and your forearms flat against his pelvis. The weight of your body distributed against his pelvic region will help discourage any unwanted thrusting. If he does thrust, his pelvis will pull you up along with his penis.

Grab Him By the Balls Clamp your thumb and forefinger together around the upper part of the man's scrotum where it attaches to his groin. This will place the testicles in the palm of your hand. Some men find this pleasurable, especially if the woman gently pulls downward. If he thrusts more than you want, increase the downward pull.

Positions

A highly effective position for doing oral sex is to place yourself between your partner's legs, facing his body. This gives your tongue direct access to the most sensitive parts of his penis and scrotum, and the angle minimizes the tendency of the head of the penis to bang against your molars. It's a comfortable position for most women, and it lets a man watch you giving him head, which some men find to be a turn-on. Another variation is to sit, kneel or crouch in front of your partner while he is standing or sitting.

Some couples like the woman to straddle the guy's chest. She faces southward as she would if the couple were doing 69. This can be particularly nice for the man if staring at his sweetheart's crotch and rear end provides an extra turn-on. But it places her mouth in a poor position to give his penis maximum stimulation. It puts her tongue in contact with the back side of the penis (that part that faces his stomach), which isn't as sensitive as the front.

In the positions mentioned so far, the guy lies still, and the woman provides the up-and-down motion. Another way of doing a blowjob is where the woman keeps her head still, and the man moves his penis in and out of her mouth. The fancy term for this that nobody but priests ever use is "irrumation," which is Latin for "altar boy, hold still!"

The position the woman sometimes takes in irrumation or "face-fucking" is on her back with her head propped up on a pillow. The man sits astride her upper body and gently thrusts his penis in her mouth. The woman lets her partner do some of the work and she has good access to his testicles and rear end, or she can easily masturbate while she's blowing him. The couple can also alternate penis thrusting with French kissing. On the other hand, some women become bored or feel claustrophobic giving a blowjob with the guy on top, or they fear that the man might be rough or thrust too deep. Putting your hand around the shaft of his penis while he thrusts will greatly decrease any chance that he might thrust too deep.

A position some couples enjoy is where they lie on their sides facing each other, but her face is level with his crotch and her chest is closer to his knees. That way, she can lay her head on a pillow while giving him oral sex.

Deep-Throat Myth

You wouldn't stick an entire popsicle down your throat, so why try it with a guy's dick? Truly great blowjobs have nothing to do with deep-throating a man. Deep-throating is more of a novelty than something that makes a penis feel great. If your man insists that you deep-throat him, go to the market and buy a vegetable that's the same size as his erect penis. Hand it to him and ask, "How would it feel if someone shoved this thing down your throat?"

Don't confuse a penis with the tips of a clitoris and assume every square centimeter is packed with thousands of nerve endings. As was said in the porn film *How to Perform Fellatio:* "The most sensitive part of the penis is the top part, so stop wasting your time on the bottom," and the male actor who uttered this profound statement had a penis with a great deal of bottom part.

The Most Sensitive Parts of the Penis

The average penis has parts that are sensitive and other parts that are mostly for show. The part of the penis you will want to focus on is a sensitive nickel-sized area called the frenulum. It's just below the head on the side of the penis that's away from his body when he has an erection. Many men can be brought to orgasm by stimulating this area alone. (See the illustration on page 309.)

For some guys, especially those who are uncircumcised, the head might be really sensitive. Find out how he likes you to suck or lick the head before and after he has an orgasm. *The head of the penis can become painfully sensitive after orgasm. Ask him about this.*

The seam of the penis that runs from the scrotum to the head usually responds to tender kisses, as does the entire scrotum.

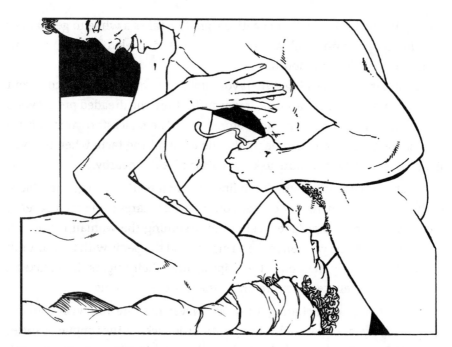

This position is also good for deep-throating your partner if that's what you want to do. Position your body so you are lying on your back with your head over the edge of the bed. or you are on top of him in a 69. These positions will help to straighten the pathway down your throat. They are better for deep-throating but not nearly as good for regular blowjobs..

Blow-Job Basics

Here are several tips and techniques for giving a really good blowjob.

Slobber People who are neat freaks often try to swallow all of their own drool when giving blowjobs. This can result in near drowning. Let gravity carry your saliva down a lover's penis. You can also use it as a lubricant for pumping the bottom part of the penis with one hand while doing the upper part by mouth. Don't hesitate to place a towel under your partner's rear or to wedge one behind his testicles; that way there won't be a big wet spot on the mattress, couch or seat of the plane or bus.

If It's Still Soft Some women enjoy sucking on a soft penis and feeling it grow inside their mouth. Just because it's soft doesn't mean that each kiss, lick and suck won't feel exquisite. One of the few times when a man can be totally passive and feel no need to perform sexually is while he is receiving a blowjob. Don't assume it's a negative sign if he takes a while to get hard or if he doesn't get hard at all. A man can still have a lovely time with his soft penis when it is in your mouth.

Lubrication for Licking When you first lick a man's genitals, coat your lips and tongue with extra saliva. If you suffer from the dreaded pre-blowjob dry mouth, try sucking on a mint beforehand to help kickstart your salivary glands. The mint might also help take the edge off the taste when his wad hits your buds. Never hesitate to keep a glass of water nearby.

Teeth Some women wrap their lips over their teeth when giving a blowjob, given how the mere hint of teeth on the penis scares some men. A set of sexy choppers can sometimes feel erotic, assuming the woman is not in a pit-bull mood. Some women make a ring around the penis with their thumb and forefinger. They then push their lips against their fingers. This makes a gasket that can help keep your teeth off the shaft of the penis.

Little Kisses & Flickering Tongues Never hesitate to lavish a man's genitals or any other part of his body with little flicks of the tongue or sweet kisses. The kisses not only feel nice, but allow you to rest your jaw without having to yell "Intermission!" It usually works better if the area you are flicking your tongue over is already lubricated with saliva or massage oil, so get it good and wet first.

Twisting Your Head Twisting your head when going up and down (in a corkscrew pattern) provides the penis with a higher level of stimulation.

Twisting Your Head, and Your Tongue on the Frenulum (for the experienced) While on the upstroke, put the tip of your tongue under the ridge of the penis head. Not only does your tongue press against the sensitive frenulum while your head is twisting, but the tip of your tongue adds extra stimulation to the sensitive ridge below the glans.

A Shirley Temple You can lick the penis with the pointed end of your tongue, or you can soften your tongue and give it a long flat lick that covers more real estate. The latter is called a "Shirley Temple" because it's similar to the way a person licks a big lollipop.

The Long Lick Nature left a seam on the penis that runs from just below the head to halfway down the scrotum. Never hesitate to take a long, wet lick from beneath your partner's testicles all the way to the tip of his penis, along the length of the seam.

If Your Partner Isn't Circumcised #1 Without retracting his foreskin, stick the tip of your tongue inside his foreskin and run it in a circle around the head of his penis. You can pull the foreskin up with your fingertips as your tongue does circles between it and the glans.

If Your Partner Isn't Circumcised #2 By varying the level of vacuum in your mouth, see if you can make the foreskin come up and down as you bob your head.

If Your Partner Isn't Circumcised #3 A most excellent conversation to have with a man about his foreskin is at what point he wants you to retract it (pull the extra yardage down the shaft so the head is bare).

Making the Foreskin Taut This applies as much to men who are circumcised as for those who aren't: Wrap your thumb and forefinger around the shaft of the penis an inch or so above the scrotum. Then pull it down to the scrotum. This makes the skin tighter on the penis and usually increases the sensitivity in the upper part of the penis. It might also help him to come sooner if he seems to be taking forever. If he isn't circumcised, you may need to start higher up the shaft before pulling the foreskin down.

Pumping the Shaft While your lips are focusing on the upper part of the penis, there's no reason why you can't be pumping the bottom part of the shaft with your hand or fingers. Let your saliva flow down the shaft, lubricating it and your hand. Then start pumping. Some women synchronize the shaft pumping with their head bobbing, so their hand follows just beneath their lips at all times.

The Vacuum (Hoover Fellatis) Some men like it if you draw a slight vacuum with your mouth. One way to draw a vacuum is to take as much of the penis in your mouth as feels comfortable. Then make a seal around the shaft with your lips, and suck some of the air out of your mouth. Then, as you pull your head back, a vacuum is created.

Man Nipples Some guys have nipples that are highly sensitive. Caressing them with your finger while doing oral sex might add to the man's pleasure. Experiment and seek feedback.

Inner Thighs and Other Places The inner thighs of both men and women can be extremely sensitive. There's no reason why you can't alternate a blowjob with licking and sucking on your partner's inner thighs, or caress them with a free hand.

Fingers in His Mouth When you are blowing him, you might try sticking your fingers in his mouth. Some men find this to be erotic.

Perineum (between the Testicles and Rear End) There is an area behind the testicles called the perineum that is often overlooked but has the potential for good feelings. Licking this area can light some men up. Gentle finger massage down there can also add a little extra to oral sex.

The Blow Hole It might be fun to explore the slit in the head of his penis with the tip of your tongue.

Rear End Some men welcome a finger on or up the anus when receiving oral sex. (See the illustration on page 371.) There are men who say their most intense orgasms are when a woman gives them oral sex while putting a finger on their prostate. Other men hate this sort of thing. Also, a small vibrator up the rear might catch some men's attention, and some men enjoy rimming (oral-anal contact) that alternates with oral sex.

Visual Assist There are plenty of men who enjoy watching a woman give them head. Some women might be offended by the notion, thinking it has something to do with submission. The chances are that the man is way too appreciative to be thinking about gender-power issues when you are giving him a blowjob. In her video on how to give blowjobs, porn star Nina Hartley comments, "It took me a long time to be able to do a blowjob in the light and not get embarrassed." She apparently got over it.

Oral Intermission If your mouth gets tired, do your partner by hand for a while, or run your hair over his genitals. Or if you feel like playing with yourself, let him watch you do that. Some women give their best blowjobs when they are just as turned on as their partners. Don't be afraid to let him know about it if you are turned on. It may help speed things up.

Tap & Hum It may enhance the feeling of a blowjob if you occasionally hum or tap the shaft of the penis when the head and frenulum are in your mouth.

Hot, Cold, Etc. Don't hesitate to suck on ice cubes to make your mouth cold, or drink hot liquids to make it extra-warm before and during oral sex.

Going Down after Intercourse Some women enjoy giving blowjobs after intercourse. They find it erotic to suck on a penis after it has been inside of them.

A Little Help from Your Friends If you have a friend who is more experienced at giving blowjobs, consider asking her or him for pointers, but keep in mind that you will soon be evolving your own style. What you do will also vary depending on the man you are doing it with.

Finger Action

Using your fingers is as important to blowjobs as it is to sign language. At the same time that your mouth is on your partner's penis, try caressing his testicles. The part of his penis that runs under his scrotum might also respond nicely to fingertip massage while you are giving him oral sex. Massaging this area with your free hand can substantially increase the sensation. (See the illustration on page 191.) If you make hand play a normal part of oral sex, he's not as likely to notice when your mouth needs a rest.

Cojones by Mouth

"I love my boyfriend's testicles. I like taking them into my mouth one at a time and sucking on them. The skin on the sack is really soft and feels great in my mouth." *female age 23*

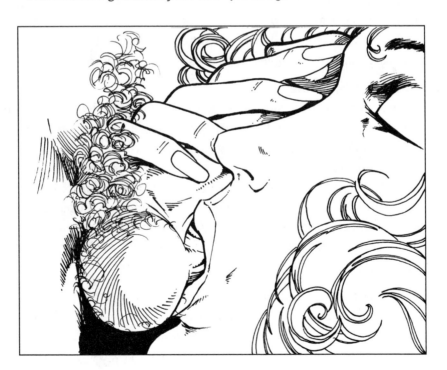

Some men will be highly appreciative if you take one or both of their testicles in your mouth. Don't fear doing this. Just go slowly the first couple of times until you get the hang of it. The skin around the testicles (scrotum) also loves being licked and kissed. The sensitivity of the scrotum has been compared to the lips of a woman's genitals. If he doesn't have an erection, you might be able to fit his testicles in your mouth as well as his penis.

Right before He Comes

There might be certain things that you can do just before a man starts to come that will increase his pleasure. Some women wrap a hand around the bottom part of the penis so the entire shaft feels like it's inside a vagina. Others place their fingertips along the seam on the front side of the penis and apply a bit of pressure. They might be able to feel the ejaculate surge through the penis when they do this. Some men appreciate it if you increase the vacuum in your mouth as they are about to come, but be careful about sucking the ejaculate into your sinuses when it surges out. Some men enjoy it if you hold or caress their testicles or massage the part of the shaft that's beneath them. Since this is a highly individual matter, let him know that you would like to experiment and seek his feedback.

An experienced prostitute who consulted on this chapter said a number of men like to have their nipples pinched as they are about to come.

Learn When He's Coming

If you know the right signs to look for, you can often learn when your man is about to come. This will give you options to get your mouth out of the line of fire if you don't want to swallow.

Until you learn his body's signs, ask him to tell you when he's about to ejaculate. You might notice that his penis starts to swell and contort just before it spurts. You can feel this in your mouth. A hand over the testicles may be a good source of information, as testicle tend to draw closer to the body when a man is about to ejaculate. Also, his buns or abs might tighten up or his hips might give a thrust when coming is inevitable.

Oral Sex with Men of Size

Oral sex may be problematic if your man's penis is on the enormous side. Never fear. The illustration on the following page shows how you can give great oral sex without having to dislocate your jaw. Use your hands to pump the shaft while focusing your lips on the frenulum.

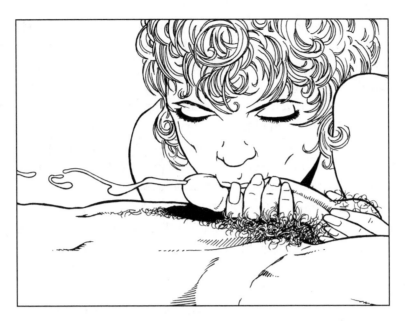

**An Effective Way To Get Him Off Orally When You Don't Want
To Swallow Or When It's Too Large to Fit in Your Mouth**

*This feels so good that a lot of guys won't be able to tell you aren't swallow-
ing unless they are actually looking. The trick is to focus your lip action on
the sensitive frenulum area while cradling the penis with your hand. This
area is just beneath the head of the penis. Use lots of saliva and put plenty
of tongue into it—almost like you are French kissing this part of his penis.
Occasionally fill your hand with your hot steamy breath.*

If You Don't Like the Way He Tastes

If you know you're not going to swallow, keep a hand around the base of
his penis while you are sucking on the upper half. As the signs of ejaculation
present themselves, free your mouth from the line of fire, slide your hand up
the shaft, to just below the head, and start pumping for Old Glory.

Be sure your grip is firm and pump fast and furious. This is no time for
a gentle touch. And don't stop pumping just because he starts to ejaculate.
Keep stroking until you have milked out the lasts drops of ooze.

Here are some other suggestions that you might find helpful:

Toothpaste, Mints, or Sweet Liquor Sticking a dab of toothpaste in your
mouth before inserting a penis can improve the taste greatly. Or try sucking

on a mint beforehand. The flavor of blowjobs can also be enhanced by sipping on your favorite sherry or liquor, unless you are a confirmed whiskey or Scotch drinker. Or you might try glazing his yam with things like honey, jam or whipped cream. Champagne blowjobs can be fun, although they can result in nasty hangovers. If you enjoy experimenting with minty liquors such as creme de menthe, do a small test patch on the side of the penis beforehand. While a little menthol on the skin can feel great, especially when you blow on it, too much can burn. It takes a few minutes for the full intensity of the burn to peak, so wait before declaring your test a success.

Slobber and Punt When Old Faithful is about ready to blow, start to mobilize a pool of slobber in your mouth. When he comes, let the floodgates loose. The saliva will help thin the ejaculate, making it run out of your mouth faster. And don't worry about the mess. The more goo and slime running down the shaft, the better.

To the Rear If you are going to swallow but want to decrease the taste, place his penis as far back in your mouth as you can while still being comfortable. Then start swallowing fast. Unless he comes in buckets, this can help decrease the amount of ejaculate that hits your taste buds.

Sublingual Ejaculation This tip is in the excellent book *Tricks—125 Ways to Make Good Sex Better* by Jay Wiseman. When it feels like a man is close to coming, put your tongue over the head of his penis. He won't know the difference, but the first splash will hit the underside of your tongue where there aren't any taste buds.

Let Him Help Some guys won't mind finishing themselves off with their own hand if you have taken the time and energy to give them a really good blowjob. It might be a special treat if you kiss or suck on their testicles while they pump themselves to orgasm.

Bag It There are flavored condoms specifically for blow jobs. But never use the same condom for intercourse, as it's easy to make tiny rips in it with your teeth, without he or you ever knowing.

Jewelry on Your Tongue or On His Penis?

If you have jewelry on your tongue, experiment with ways of focusing it on certain parts of his penis for an added effect. If he has jewelry on his penis, explore ways of using your tongue or mouth on it that are pleasurable. For more on sex with piercings, see Chapter 43: *Tattoos and Piercings*.

Putting a Condom on with Your Lips

An experienced partner can slip a condom over a man's penis with her mouth and he will never know it is there. This suggests the problems some men have with wearing condoms might be mental. (What else is new?)

In her book *The Ultimate Guide To Fellatio,* Violet Blue suggests you wet your lips and put the unrolled condom up to your mouth. Pull just enough vacuum to suck the reservoir tip of the condom into your mouth a bit. This should hold the rest of the condom, which is still rolled up, against your lips. Bend over the penis and pop the unrolled part over the head. Then walk the unrolled part down the shaft either with your lips or fingers. You might want to practice on a banana.

A key to this is getting flavored condoms. Condom lube tastes absolutely awful, as do spermicides. Be sure to check the consumer reviews, as some flavored condoms taste pretty bad.

Also, if you don't mind the taste of the lubricant, the condoms made of polyurethane might transmit the warmth of your mouth better, and the warmth is one of the things that feels extra nice about receiving a blowjob.

WARNING! Do not use the same condom for intercourse that you use for a blowjob. Your teeth are probably making micro tears in the condom, which will make it ineffective for birth control.

Dealing with Condom Balkers

Here are two approaches to consider if you want a man to use a condom while blowing him but he balks.

1. In a loud and clear voice, say, "Forget it, Charlie! If you think it tastes THAT great, suck on it yourself." Although he probably would if he could, and has maybe even tried a couple of times.

2. Try making the whole process of oral sex more fun and pleasurable for both of you. If he knows oral sex is going to be lots of fun, putting a condom on won't be such a big deal. You might hawk a small wad of spit on the head of his penis right before putting the condom on. This will help the sensations translate through the condom better. If you are really prepared, use a drop or two of water-based lube on his penis or put it in the condom before rolling it on. Once you have rolled the condom over the penis, squish the lube around the entire head. This will make it feel better.

While He's Coming, and Afterward

If you keep his penis in your mouth while he is coming, find out what he wants you to do while he's in the process of ejaculating. Does he want you to suck harder, suck less, pump his shaft with your other hand?

Then try to get a sense of how soon after your partner ejaculates the head of his penis becomes extra sensitive. For some men, the head of the penis can become painfully sensitive. Does he want you to keep his penis in your mouth, but to slow the action? Or maybe he's got callouses on it and he wants you to keep going as if nothing happened. The only way to learn this is from experience and plenty of helpful feedback on his part.

Clearing the Pipes After He Comes

When a man is masturbating, soon after he comes he might push into the hidden part of the penis that's between his testicles to push out any remaining semen. It's the equivalent of wagging his penis after he pees.

You might ask him about it. Perhaps he can show you how to do it, assuming it's what he does.

Lasting Shorter vs. Lasting Longer

"Why is it when you are giving men head, they take forever to come, but are so much faster when having intercourse?" *female age 29*

During vaginal intercourse, most guys make an effort to last as long as their partners want, sometimes successfully. While this might be a noble gesture during intercourse, it is not appreciated nearly as much during oral sex. So a man shouldn't try to hold back his climax to show what a stud he is.

If your partner is one of those lucky guys who can pretty much orgasm at will, you and he might devise a signal for when you'd like him to come.

What If He Doesn't Come?

This is where one woman's blessing is another woman's curse. More guys than you think don't come from oral sex no matter how great your blowjob. If he doesn't come from oral sex, you and he will need to settle on how long the blowjob should last. You will also need reassurance from him about how good the blowjob feels, and that he's simply wired in a way that this isn't how he has an orgasm. He probably loves your blowjob every bit as much as a man who can orgasm from it, and he needs to let you know.

Pre-Cum Jitters

Some women who are giving oral sex experience a brief paralysis or mini-dread right before their partner ejaculates. If this keeps happening, try to talk to your partner about it. Maybe he can give you early warning before he's going to come so you can stop sucking and start pumping by hand. Maybe it will help to put a condom on his penis before giving him a blowjob, Or perhaps you can switch into the position that was illustrated earlier in the chapter for giving a no-swallow blowjob.

His Hands on Your Head

Men will often put their hands on a woman's head when she is giving oral sex. For most guys, this is a loving gesture which can also be used to let a partner know what feels good and what doesn't. However, some men will put their hands on a woman's head in an attempt to forcibly push it down onto the penis. This is rude, and you need to tell him to stop.

Counterpoint: One woman says, "It can be particularly exciting when a man pushes my head down on his penis. But I would never have sex with a man who I didn't love going down on. Also, you make a joke out of it when a woman grabs a man's head and pulls it into her crotch in the other chapter, but call it assault when a man does this to a woman. You present a double standard that says we women are either more fragile than men or more easily offended when it comes to sex."

Research Findings

One of the more interesting articles about the hazards of oral sex was by a group of dentists and published in a medical journal (Bellizi, Krakow and Plack, *Military Medicine* 145 (1980):787—honest, his name is Dr. Plack and he's a dentist). The article is titled "Soft Palate Trauma Associated with Fellatio."

The article tells about the daughter of an officer who was taken to the base hospital because she discovered a black-and-blue blotch in the back of her mouth. Several dentists eventually converged on the mystery blotch, trying to discover its origin. After eliminating all other possibilities, the dentists asked the officer dad to leave the room and then popped the big question: "Gotta boyfriend?"

In the back of the mouth near where the tonsils hang is a highly vascularized mass of tissue (vascularized means lots of small blood vessels). An erect penis hitting against this sensitive tissue can cause a bruise.

This isn't a common injury. It goes away like any other bruise, but it is a reminder that the woman, and not the man, should control the level of movement during a blowjob. It's fine if she wants a lover to thrust in and out of her mouth, but the choice needs to be hers.

Ejaculate-Related Sinus Infections

When some women give blowjobs, they like to create a slight to moderate vacuum around their lover's penis. Men who enjoy this kind of sensation find it to be heavenly. However, a problem can occur when a man comes with the head of his penis in the back part of a woman's vacuum-pulling mouth. The vacuum can sometimes draw ejaculate up into the woman's sinus cavities, creating what might be a cum-related sinus infection. If this is the case, the woman and her partner need to work on keeping the head of his penis in the middle part of her mouth when he is coming. Another solution is for him to wear a condom.

Things a Guy Can Do to Help a Woman Who Is Trying to Give Him Oral Sex

To help a partner give you the best blowjobs, it's important to explore and give each other feedback. It might also help to read this chapter with your partner.

Smelly Balls Based on thousands of sex surveys, the number one complaint women have about giving guys oral sex is smelly balls. Whether you are going out on a first date or have been married for twenty years, if you want to receive oral sex: #1: Shower at least once a day; #2: Don't wear the same underwear for more than one day without washing them; #3 If everyone including the dog and cat runs out of the room when you take your shoes off, use foot powder or foot spray. #4: While not particularly popular with the organic crowd, deodorant can be a wonderful thing. #5: Brush and floss your teeth often, as kissing often precedes and follows a blowjob. #6: If you wear cologne, ask your partner how she likes the smell of it, as well as how much you should use. Some guys smell great from just bathing alone, or she might like you marinated with a citrus or spice.

Uncut? If you haven't noticed by now, this Guide abhors circumcision. However, all good things have their downsides, and smegma is one of the downsides of having a healthy, intact penis. Why not establish a pre-blowjob routine where you go to the bathroom, retract your foreskin, and tidy up a bit around it?

Pube Tug Tug on your pubic hair ahead of time so you'll pull out the strays that might end up in her mouth.

He Who Gives, Gets A fine way to get great oral sex is to give great oral sex. This assumes you are okay giving each other oral sex.

Avoid Arrogance Don't assume that a woman automatically wants to suck on your penis. Never take blowjobs for granted, and be thankful whenever you get one, even if your partner loves doing it. Tell her how good it feels. Also, it never hurts to ask yourself, "What have I done lately to deserve a blowjob?" Did you give your partner a long lingering body massage? Did you help her with a project she's been struggling with? Did you do your share of the housework? Did you respond kindly in a situation where most men would have been jerks? Are you a loving partner and good friend?

Talk Is Not Cheap The best oral sex requires a doer who is willing to accept helpful feedback and a receiver who is willing to give it.

Attitude Never, ever cop an attitude such as "My last girlfriend blew me really well. Why can't you?" There are reasons why you aren't with your last girlfriend. With enough mutual caring, love and experimentation, the chances are good you will soon be receiving oral sex, but don't expect it to happen magically.

The Deep-Throat Fantasy A throat is not a vagina. If a woman gags on your penis, do you really think she's going to be excited about putting it in her mouth again?

When Is Asking for Oral Sex Okay?

Every once in a while you might have a horrible day and are in desperate need of a blowjob lest you totally fall apart. If you don't abuse the privilege and have a loving partner who hasn't had an equally hideous day, it could be fine to ask or beg for a blowjob. However, it's rarely a good idea to routinely ask for oral sex. Few women take well to being pestered for blowjobs. Talk to your partner about whether it's okay to ask for oral sex, and if so, under what circumstances.

Improving the Way Your Ejaculate Tastes

It is certainly possible that ejaculate, like cow's milk, can take on flavors of what the beast eats, including its favorite vices. Unfortunately, there is no science to guide us on this matter. It could just be urban myth.

It has been said that dairy products make ejaculate taste bad, but not nearly as bad as asparagus. Curry is a spice of interest. Smoking and/or drinking coffee might cause ejaculate to taste strong or bitter. Perhaps Starbucks can formulate a new blend and call it "Sweet Wad."

Some people claim that vegetarians, both male and female, taste better than their carnivore brethren. However, it is likely this is just propaganda from cows and chickens.

One woman said that her partner's ejaculate tasted good unless he was under a lot of stress at work. Then it would start tasting bad. Perhaps adrenalin and hormones associated with stress might cause semen to taste funky.

Drugs are another possible culprit. Whether it's over-the-counter drugs such as antihistamines, prescription drugs, or recreational drugs like speed, people claim that drugs can taint the way semen tastes.

One common suggestion for improving the taste of male ejaculate is to eat sweet fruit such as pineapple and apples. The sugar in the fruit is supposed to give semen a sweet taste. Perhaps this is just folklore. But if this is what a partner asks you to do before giving more blowjobs, most guys would become the pineapple industry's best friend. If your partner is willing to be the taster, why not experiment with different combinations of food? Does ingesting a little cinnamon make a difference in the way you taste? What happens if you drink less coffee or eat less broccoli or garlic?

If you've eliminated the assumed culprits and your partner has had experience with other men and still says your ejaculate is extremely bitter, consider seeing a urologist to screen out the possibility of an infection in your prostate gland. Although you might not be feeling pain, it's still possible to have an infection. It might be embarrassing to call a doctor's office and say, "Stormy says my cum tastes bitter." So why not tell the receptionist or nurse that you'd like to rule out a prostate or urinary-tract infection. Then tell the physician the real reason once you see him or her in private. Under no circumstances should you take antibiotics unless tests have been done and show a problem. Antibiotics are not breath mints for your penis.

Readers' Comments

"I am certain that women would give more blowjobs if they didn't feel like they had to swallow." *female age 43*

"Cum is not a gourmet treat, but not unpleasant. I'd rather be eating mocha-chip ice cream, but getting there isn't half as much fun. My partner's orgasm is often a total turn-on for me, and occasionally just a relief that the blowjob is now over with." *female age 47*

"If he smells bad down there, it's a turn-off for me." *female age 34*

"If I'm in the mood it's really sensual. If I'm not it's like a job." *fem, 43*

"It is a major power trip for me if he comes in my mouth. I like knowing I have the ability to take this big strong man and turn him into a sack of Jello." *female age 37*

"I used to tell my partner that I was semen-intolerant." *female age 26*

"I like running my tongue around the head and sliding it in and out of my mouth. I like to take his penis in my mouth as far as possible and rub my tongue on the underside of it, pushing the head into the roof of my mouth. It seems to drive him crazy." *female age 37*

"More than anything it feels so good because I am in control." *fem, 43*

"When it comes to blowjobs, let the lucky son of a bitch treat you like a queen, honey, because you are." *female age 48*

"I never was very good at blowjobs until I had a lover who had a small penis. Then I felt comfortable with him in my mouth." *female age 34*

"It feels very sensual if he lets me take it at my own pace. I think the penis has the most wonderful velvety skin." *female age 38*

"I like to give head, so I don't need much persuasion. I get really wet from giving someone that kind of pleasure, and I always feel so powerful when I do it." *female age 23*

"I only like it if I can keep the hair out of my mouth. I enjoy it only because I know he enjoys it so much." *female age 35*

"I like it. I especially like the little leaks before he comes. I think cum has an interesting taste, sort of fizzy." *female age 38*

"I have discovered that we both find it erotic to have him come on my face or on my breasts when I give him head. I don't care for the taste of his semen." *female age 22*

"I really don't like it when he comes in my mouth. I kind of gag on it."
female age 26

"It's fun to suck on a limp penis until it hardens." *female age 37*

"One thing that's really neat about sucking on a guy's cock is watching it change shape and color and get harder. You're right up there in the front row. You don't get that with intercourse." *female age 42*

"I've observed that not all guys come as much; some have very little, and others lots and lots." *female age 27*

"Never forget to caress and tickle the balls." *female age 44*

"My mouth and hand work as a team. As I pull away with my mouth, I twist my hand almost like a corkscrew." *female age 26*

"I love to give head, but I hate to feel pressured into doing it. Also, remember what goes around comes around. If I'm the only one going down, I'll be less likely to do so again." *female age 26*

"Please don't do it like they do in the porno flicks, where the girl just about bobs her head off. Not a turn-on." *male age 46*

"Don't be fooled by the name. Blowing has nothing to do with it."
male age 26

CHAPTER
22
Condoms
For The Ride of Your Life

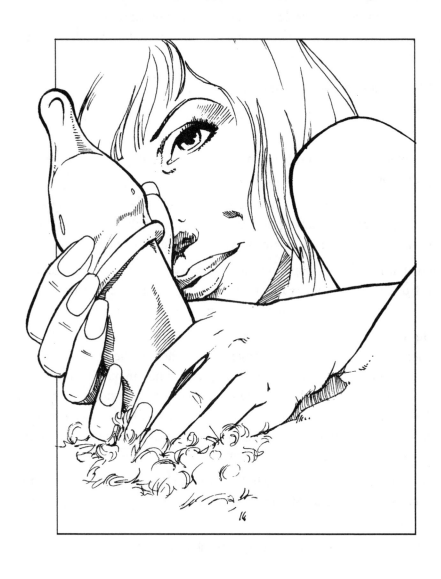

Besides the seriously hot illustration on the preceding page, there's not much that's sexy about condoms except for the sex that follows after you put one on. Condoms are next to athletic cups and bicycle helmets on the scale of things you should us but don't want to. If it weren't for unwanted pregnancies and sexually transmitted infections, you wouldn't see a word about condoms in this book.

So from the start, *The Guide* is being more honest with you about condoms than most books. So hopefully you can trust that what follows about condoms is honest and true.

Making Condom Use Sexy — It Can Be Done!

"It would really help if I could finger her while she put the condom on me." *male age 24*

Few lovers talk about ways to help each other stay aroused when putting on a condom. Here are some possibilities:

Anticipation: Slip a condom into your partner's pocket followed by a welcome kiss, fingertips rubbing over the front of his or her pants, and a few words about what you are looking forward to once the condom is on.

Masturbating: Some women find it arousing to watch a guy put on a condom and stroke himself. Or if a man finds it arousing to watch his partner masturbate, he can watch her warming herself up while he's putting the condom on.

While Giving or Receiving Oral Sex: If giving a woman oral sex makes her partner hard, the couple can arrange their bodies so she can put the condom on him while his face is between her legs. Or he can put the condom on while she kisses his testicles, but she should avoid getting saliva on the base of the penis where the condom needs to grip. **NOTE:** Putting on a condom with your mouth or lips is a bad idea unless it's just being used for oral sex, as it's easy to leave tiny nicks in the condom with your teeth.

Talking Dirty: If the couple finds talking dirty to be arousing, she can be telling him what she wants him to do with his penis as she's putting the condom on it.

Grinding: She can rub her vulva against his thigh as he is putting the condom on his penis.

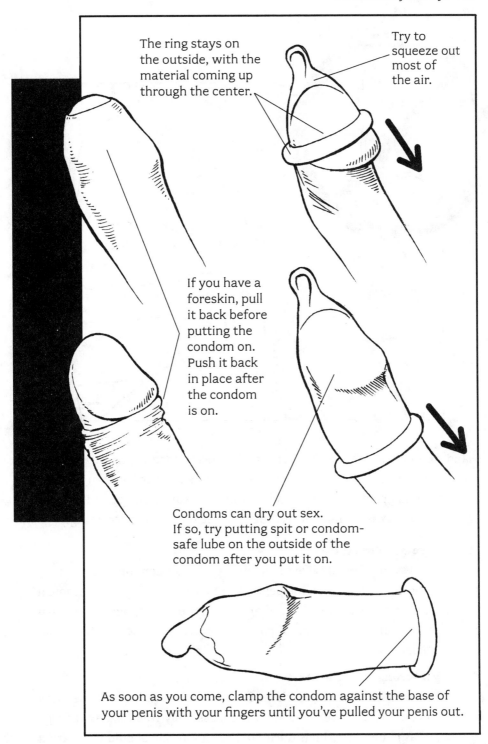

The ring stays on the outside, with the material coming up through the center.

Try to squeeze out most of the air.

If you have a foreskin, pull it back before putting the condom on. Push it back in place after the condom is on.

Condoms can dry out sex. If so, try putting spit or condom-safe lube on the outside of the condom after you put it on.

As soon as you come, clamp the condom against the base of your penis with your fingers until you've pulled your penis out.

For the Ride of Your Life!

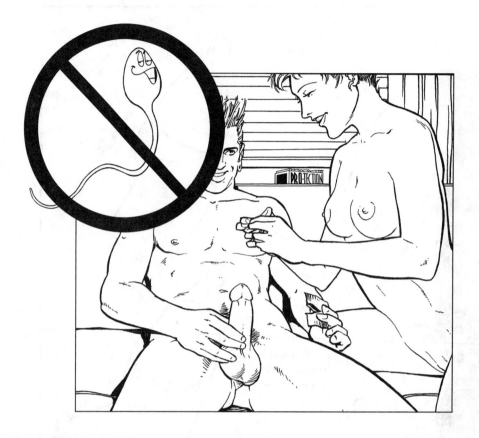

Hand Action: She caresses his penis and testicles, then opens the condom package but puts it down and strokes and caresses some more, then puts the condom on his penis. Keep in mind that precum can have sperm in it, and can transport sexually transmitted infections, so deal with it accordingly.

When a Woman Puts It On

A lot of women would like to try putting the condom on, but feel awkward asking. If she rolls it on his penis, putting on a condom can become a turn-on for both partners instead of an interruption. Also, when a woman puts a condom on a man, it's an important signal that the sex is consensual and mutual.

Getting It Wrong from the Start

When a question about condoms for men who are uncircumcised was posted on a listserve for sex educators, the mass reply was, "Get extra-large condoms," as if any guy who is uncut and has a foreskin should be wearing condoms that are extra-large. Can you imagine if a woman posted a question about her bra causing her discomfort and the fashion experts replied, "Buy the biggest bra you possibly can!" Instead, they would ask for more information about her specific problem. Unfortunately, when it comes to condoms, even sex educators can still be in the dark ages.

Penises come in different sizes and shapes. Fortunately, condom companies make condoms that come in different sizes and shapes, from snug to condoms that are extra-baggy around the head. The condoms that have the extra headroom fit snugly around the base of the penis, but the top bags out. This lets the head of the penis slosh around inside the condom, which can feel really nice.

Part of your job as a couple is to explore and find condoms that work best for the two of you. Visit www.GuideToGettingItOn.com for links to many different online condom sampler packs (enter "sampler" in the search box). Once you find a couple of favorite brands, stock up on them.

If You Are a Woman Who Doesn't Like the Feel of Condoms

We've been surprised at how many of the women who take our sex survey say they don't like the feel of condoms. So if you notice it feels different when a partner is wearing a condom, you are not alone. This is why it's important for women to weigh in on the matter of which condoms to buy.

Also be aware that condoms are not the most effective method of birth control. If the sole reason you are using them is for contraception, you might consider more effective methods like the IUD. But if there's any possibility that you could possibly get HIV, use condoms no matter what, in addition to a more effective method of birth control.

Need Extra Large Condoms? Some Do, Most Don't

At least 10% to 20% of men need bigger sized condoms. So if you need a bigger size condoms, there are several choices on the market. The following account from a reader explains what can happen when a guy who needs a bigger condom isn't using one:

> "The one traumatic thing about sex with my first partner in high school was using a condom. I'm on the larger side. The first time I tried to use a condom, it was so tight I could barely get it on and it felt like a tourniquet at the base of my penis. It was awful and I

couldn't keep an erection with one on. Unfortunately, I'd read that the whole "the condom's too small" excuse is not valid because someone once squeezed 17 oranges into a condom so it's silly that a guy can't fit into one. So of course I was convinced that something was wrong with me. I kept trying, and once broke two condoms while trying to get them on! I didn't even know that they made large condoms at the time—all I knew was that if I tried to use any condom, sex would end in disaster. All they needed to say was, 'Larger condoms are available for those who need them' and my adolescence would have been a lot less stressful." *male age 26*

While it's easy to blow up a condom to the size of a watermelon, that doesn't mean you can roll a condom over a watermelon. When you first start to unroll a condom, you are dealing with a thick ring of condom material that doesn't stretch much at all. It's only when a condom is fully unrolled that it stretches to obscene proportions. Even then, some guys prefer condoms that are baggy around the head.

If the reason you are buying condoms the size of a circus tent is to impress your friends or a partner, the truth is going to come out once your pants are down. And if you don't need the extra large size, the condom is more likely to slip off during intercourse.

Lubing Protocol

When you are wearing a condom, you are putting a waterproof barrier between two body parts which nature designed to share fluids. To help compensate, some couples add lubrication to the outside of the condom. This helps to make up for the loss of natural lubrication.

For increased sensation, you might also try putting a dab of saliva or a small amount of lube on the head of the penis before you put the condom on. After you've rolled the condom down the shaft, smush the condom material around the head so you are spreading out the lube. This will allow the head of the penis to slip and slide inside the condom during intercourse. (Some condoms now come with lube already on the inside.) Make sure the lower part of the penis is dry and has no lube on it. If you are putting a condom on right after receiving oral sex, be sure the shaft of the penis is dry so the condom won't slip off during intercourse.

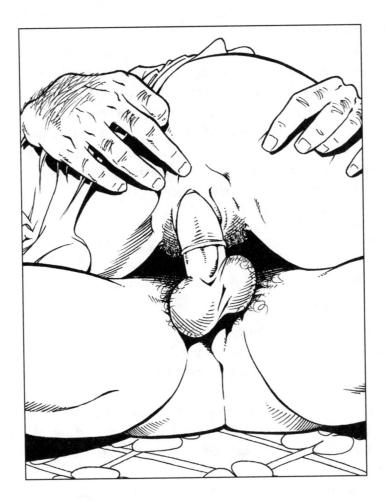

Lube and Condom Compatibility

Unless you are using a condom that's made of polyurethane like the Trojan Supra, be sure the lube is compatible with latex. If the lube doesn't say "safe for use with latex condoms," don't use it.

Marathon Sex and Rough Sex

Condoms will usually dry out during marathon sex, so lube up accordingly. However, after you've applied lube, try adding water instead to rehydrate the lube in order to avoid having a gunky, glue-like mess. Intense thrusting shouldn't cause a condom to break. Condoms are not fragile as long as you are wearing the right size and are using lube if you need it. So don't think you need to go gentle if both of you prefer a rougher ride.

Foreskin Wedgies?

Condoms work fine for the vast majority of men with foreskins. However, if you are uncut and are having condom-related problems, you might retract your foreskin if you can and put a drop or two of lube on the head of your penis before putting the condom on. Then, after you roll the condom on, work the foreskin back and forth over the head of your penis with your fingers to get the lube all smushed around. A condom with a baggy head or more headroom might help as well. Some men who are uncut find relief when their partner uses the female condom.

Tying Condoms Off

Be sure to take a condom off as soon as you pull your penis out, and tie off the end of it. Semen liquefies or becomes watery in a few minutes, and will run out the end of the condom if you don't tie it off.

Reasons Why Condoms Break

One of the most common reasons why condoms break is from damage due to blunt puncture. That's when the condom material gathers more tightly around the head of the penis with each thrust, until the penis bursts through the condom.

If you feel a condom tightening around your penis, pull out right away and make sure that the condom material hasn't stretched over the head of your penis. If it has, assume that damage has been done to the condom material, and put on a new condom.

Another reason why condoms break is when couples use lubrication that is not safe with latex condoms. Make sure any lube you use with latex condoms states on the container that it is safe to use with latex condoms.

Do not use Vaseline, petroleum jelly, or hand creams or lotions like Nivea, Johnson's Baby Oil, Vaseline Intensive Care, Corn Huskers, or Jergens to lubricate a latex condom. These will quickly rot the latex.

If your penis is of the jumbo variety, try out the various magnum or maximum sizes. If your penis doesn't cast the widest shadow in town, get a condom that's snugger fitting.

Teeth, nails and jewelry can cause tiny nicks in condoms. Do not open condom packages with knives, scissors or your teeth. And check the date on the package of condoms. Latex does not last forever.

Reservoir Tips May Be Irrelevant

Some condom brands make a big deal about having reservoir tips to hold a man's ejaculate. There are a couple of problems with this concept. The first is that most reservoir tips hold about 2.9 ml. of ejaculate. While half of all guys produce 2.9 ml. or less, there's still another 50% of men who produce more than 2.9 ml., which means their tips runneth over.

The other problem with reservoir tips is the assumption that they really do hold the fluid. Reservoir tip or not, try to squish the air out the end of the condom before rolling it down the shaft of your penis.

Do You Need To Leave Extra Material at the End?

Conventional wisdom advises to leave an extra half of an inch at the end of the condom before rolling it over the head of the penis. But there has never been any science to say whether this is good or bad. So the best advice is to follow the instructions that come with the brand of condoms you are using.

If a Condom Doesn't Come Out When You Do

For a condom that doesn't come out with the penis it rode in on, take solace in knowing there's no place for it to go. The condom might play a mean game of hide'n'seek behind the woman's cervix, but that's about it.

The first step in finding a jettisoned condom is to wash your hands and make sure your nails are well-trimmed. The woman might try lying on her back with her knees up, like when she's at a gynecologist's. This is no time for modesty: the farther apart her legs, the better. Explore her vagina with your index finger. If lube is necessary, use just a little. Extra lube might make it difficult to grab the condom. If you don't have lube, try spit.

If female sexual anatomy is one of life's great mysteries for you, see the illustrations in Chapter 7: *What's Inside a Girl*. Look at how the cervix is located at the far end of the vagina on the roof of it. It might feel like the tip of your nose. Try exploring the space in the back of the cervix with your finger. If the condom is there, try to dislodge it and edge it into a more accessible part of your partner's vagina.

Once you have a good handle on where the condom is, you might try inserting your index and middle fingers in the hopes of snagging the rim of the condom between your fingertips which will act like pincers or tongs.

Condoms are stretchy, so pull it out by the rim slowly but firmly. If your partner clamps down when you are trying to insert two fingers, go slowly and gently. Her vagina is not going to implode if you take an extra ten minutes searching for the buried latex treasure.

If you have any questions or concerns, call your doctor or visit an emergency room. If you were using the condom for birth control, the operative words are "Emergency Contraception," "Plan B," "Ella," or "a Copper IUD." For condoms that get lost during anal sex, see Chapter 24: *Anal Sex: Up Your Bum.*

What to do if a Condom Breaks

If you were using a condom for birth control and discover that it has broken while in service, immediately take emergency contraception. Ella and Plan B are two different pills used for emergency contraception that can be very effective in preventing pregnancy if you take them right away.

In the meantime, do not inject birth control foam or jelly into the vagina. The pressure might push the ejaculate up into the cervix. The same is true for douching. Wash your external genitals and pee. And if you honestly think that douching with Pepsi, Coke or Mountain Dew is going to do anything but prove you're not the bright bulb on the planet, nothing this book has to say is going to count for much.

Who Brings the Condom? Reasons for Mistrust

Researchers have found that males don't always trust the condoms that females supply. One fear is that a woman may have poked a hole in it if she wants to get pregnant. A second concern is that she may have had it in her purse since she was in junior high. Women sometimes mistrust male-supplied condoms as well: How old is that puppy? Did he have it in the same pocket with three jump drives and his car keys?

These problems can be greatly reduced if the two of you talk about it first and perhaps order condoms online or buy them in a store together.

Resources

For an outrageously large list of links for condom sampler packs, visit www.GuideToGettingItOn.com and enter "sampler" in the search box.

23
Intercourse
Horizontal Jogging

Intercourse can mean different things. It can be an intensely private and delicious act. People can use it to honor and expand their relationship at the same time they are doing fun things with their bodies. It can be a way to get off, a commodity for making money, and a means for achieving protection or status. It's the only way some people make physical contact with another human being. It is also what couples do when they want to create new life.

Dick, Laura & Craig

To learn more about the role of intercourse in sex, we have invaded the privacy of three young adults, Dick, Craig, and Laura. Laura used to go out with Dick, and now she's involved with Craig. Here are their stories:

DICK

Dick is a very nice-looking guy who won his fraternity's "Mr. All-America" title two years in a row. Dick has a nice job, a nice social manner, drives a nice sports car, wears nice clothes, has nice biceps, triceps, and pecs, and goes out with nice women. Since this is a book about sex, you might as well know that Dick has a tree trunk of a penis that stays rock hard from dusk to dawn. A former girlfriend referred to it as "the sentry."

CRAIG

Craig is the same age as Dick. Craig is a sports writer. Craig is no longer eligible for the Mr. All-America contest. During a football game a few years ago, Craig went airborne to catch an overthrown pass. On the way down he got sandwiched between two spearing linebackers. Craig's spinal cord snapped, and he hasn't been able to walk or have an erection since.

LAURA

Laura is a fine young woman who just left a big corporation to form her own company that makes sporting gear. Laura's had sex with both Dick and Craig. Let's see what Laura has to say about these two different men.

"Dick's the kind of guy that many American women have been raised to worship. Parading him around your friends or taking him home to your parents would win you the female equivalent of the Breeder's Cup. I've always really enjoyed sex, and until recently I could never understand why a woman would want to fake an orgasm. But it didn't take too many nights with Dick before I started faking orgasms. There was Dick, Mr. Right Stuff, making picture-perfect love. I didn't want him to think there was something wrong with me since I couldn't get into it like he was, so I started faking orgasms."

"Craig is nowhere near as perfect as Dick, but he has a great sense of humor and he is genuine. Craig is able to laugh at himself, which Dick never could. Craig has taken the time to learn exactly how to kiss, touch, and caress me, and the sex I have with him is great. When I'm with Craig I don't need to fake a thing."

"This may not seem relevant to your question about sex, but I work in a male-dominated business. I have to think like a guy from morning to night. Sometimes it leaves me feeling alien from my femininity. With Craig it's easy to find it back again. Craig never wakes me up at 3 a.m. with a hard-on poking in my back, but he feels just as masculine as Dick. With a lot of guys there's a huge difference between how they treat you in bed and how they treat you the rest of time; with Craig that's not the case. Maybe that's another reason why sex is so nice with him, even if it's not intercourse."

Okay, so here we have Dick, more functional than a Sidewinder missile. He fulfills everybody's definition of what a sexual athlete should be. Then we have Craig, who redefines the term *sexually dysfunctional.* If Craig had the same erection failure but no spinal-cord injury, therapists would collect a small fortune trying to make him "normal." At the very least, they would have him taking boner pills like they were M&Ms. And probably other medications, as well.

And finally, there is Laura, a woman who enjoys sex a great deal. She is telling us that the man who can't get it up is a more satisfying lover than Mr. Erectus Perfectus.

In telling you about Laura, Dick and Craig, the intent was not to dump on intercourse. Intercourse, when it's good, can be one of the sweetest things there is. What this book is dumping on is the assumption that intercourse is good just because it's intercourse and that a man is a man because he can

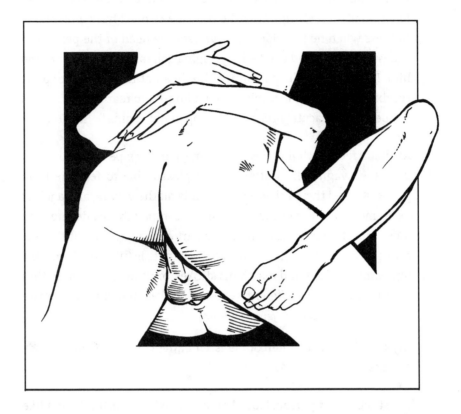

get hard and fuck, or that a woman is a woman because she can get wet and fuck him back.

What Does It Feel Like When You Have Intercourse?

"Oh God—It's like describing the universe. It feels like I might explode and can't wait to but at same time want it to last forever. Breathless, hot, turned on in the extreme. I want to engulf and squeeze his penis, get it in me as much as possible. I love the connection of it."

female age 48

"When his penis first enters me I want to feel every inch of it because it is exquisite. I feel like I need it inside me and I don't know if I can describe that. The actual sensations of his penis sliding in and out of me are sometimes over-powered by the pleasure I feel all over my body, so I don't necessarily concentrate on the intercourse."

female age 23

"As he enters me I feel myself spreading open to accommodate him. Emotionally it feels right that he is inside of me. I have a feeling of fullness when he is inside me. I can feel the head of the penis as it slides in and out and can feel my vagina collapse or expand around him. If he plunges deep I can feel the head of the penis bump my cervix, a not altogether unpleasant feeling. From rear entry I can feel the penis more acutely rubbing the top of my vagina." *female age 37*

"At first I feel the light pressure of my partner's penis against my unopened vagina. It is often deeply pleasurable to feel the head penetrate, and then a slow, smooth slide all the way in, and a jolt of excitement when my lover's penis is completely inside me. The most sensation is around the outer part of the vagina, but there is also a pleasurable feeling of fullness when he is fully inside me. My hips want to move and match his strokes, or create my own rhythm for him to match. Different types of strokes and rhythms create different sensations." *female age 47*

"My favorite part of intercourse is when he comes; his entire body stiffens." *female age 55*

"I'm strictly a clit person. I love having sex with men, but I don't like intercourse." *female age 36*

"The first thrust is the most vivid for me. I like to slowly slide down his cock and feel it go up me. I love it when he is trying to hold back from coming; I can feel him get more swollen and hard and I get very excited when I feel that. It actually is the time when my vagina gets the most pleasure from intercourse." *female age 23*

"It depends on how sexually excited I am and whether I'm in the mood or if I'm just doing it because he wants to. If I'm into it, it's like ecstasy!" *female age 43*

"I enjoy the pumping and grinding a great deal. I love it when we are rubbing our pelvic bones together and when the penis is in deep."
female age 21

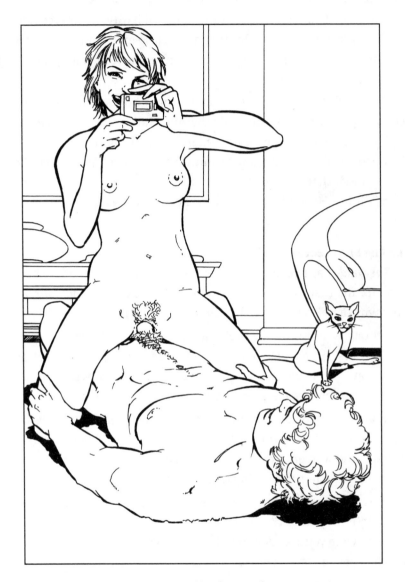

This family moment was inspired by photographer Trevor Watson.

"It feels different every time. Sometimes it is very satisfying. Sometimes it hurts inside my vagina if I'm not lubricated enough. And sometimes when his penis hits my G-spot it takes my breath away!"

female age 34

At the Start—New Relationship or New to Intercourse

For a lot of couples it takes time and familiarity for intercourse to get that sloppy-intimate-erotic edge that makes it so much fun. This means intercourse won't necessarily knock your socks off at the start. It may not even feel as good as masturbation.

Also, each partner brings his or her own hopes and expectations, as well as physical anatomy and body rhythms. Patience can be a virtue. Some couples who are having dynamite intercourse during the fifth year of their relationship had lousy intercourse during the first year. And even if the sex is great at the start, there will likely be periods in any relationship when sexual desire falls flat. Hopefully you will continue to grow as a couple during those times.

Your First Intercourse

The Guide has a separate chapter for people who are about to have intercourse for the first time: Chapter 40: *Bye Bye V-Card—Losing Your Virginity*. Here's why there's a separate chapter for your first intercourse:

On our own sex survey, we've asked hundreds of women to compare how their first intercourse felt with how it feels now. While most of these women say it feels great now, it is an unusual woman who says she cherished her first intercourse, even if it was in a loving relationship.

In another study on first intercourse that included 659 college students, researchers found that while 79% of the men reported they had an orgasm, only 7% of the women reported having an orgasm. Males had far more overall pleasure than females during their first intercourse.

The mean age for first intercourse was 16½ years, although those who waited until they were 17 or older reported having a better experience than those who were younger. A year or two of added life experience can go a long way when you are only 15 or 16.

Both males and females reported more pleasure if they had intercourse for the first time in a more serious or long-term relationship than in a casual or brief one. People who used alcohol during their first intercourse (about 30% of the total) reported significantly less pleasure and more guilt than those who did it sober. Those who used contraception reported more pleasure than those who didn't.

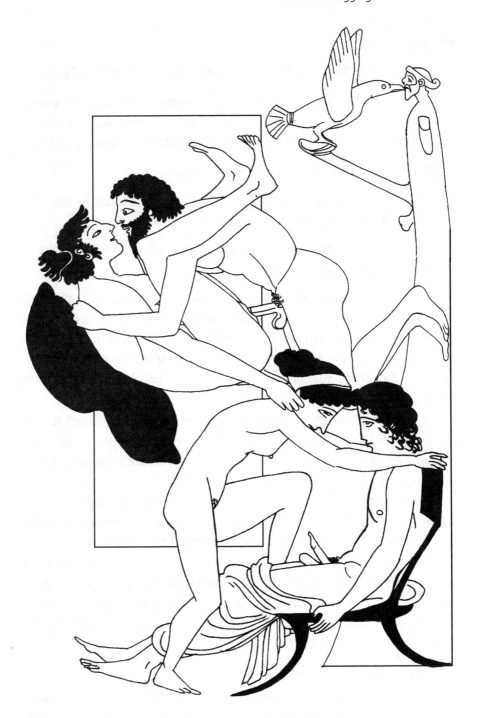

Intercourse in the old days.

Who Sticks It In?

"I generally prefer to put it in; otherwise we seem to miss a lot." *fem, 32*

"I like to put his penis in me because it seems no matter how many times we have had sex, he still misses a little bit when aiming. Also, I find it exciting to hold him while he thrusts into my vagina." *female 23*

"It's really whoever grabs ahold first." *female age 36*

"He prefers to put it in, because if I do, he thinks I think he doesn't know where in the heck that hole is." *female age 38*

"She always does. No matter how many years we've been doing this, I still manage to miss!" *male age 43*

This may seem like a dumb thing, but the issue of who sticks the penis into the vagina can sometimes be significant. A rule of thumb is that either the woman, or the woman and man together, should stick it in the first few times. That's because only a woman knows when she is ready to have a penis inside, and all those years of inserting tampons have taught her exactly where the head of a penis needs to go.

Some women might be shy about grabbing a penis and guiding it in for a landing. This kind of reticence is silly but understandable. Once your penis-to-vagina guidance system is up and running, all bets are off regarding who puts the penis in.

Whoever puts it in needs to make sure the woman truly wants it and her vagina is wet enough to take it. If not, more kissing and caressing or a bit of spit or sex lube are in order. (See Chapter 12: *Sex Lubes—A New Look.*)

If you are using water-based lube and it starts to dry out, a drop or two of water or saliva will give it new life, while more lube will just gum things up. The women at Good Vibrations suggest keeping a water pistol handy for just this purpose, although women without humor will find this offensive, and wives of NRA members should be careful not to grab the Glock by mistake.

The First Thrust

In reading the sex survey responses of our women readers, an amazing pattern emerged. A large number of women said the part of intercourse they like best is the first stroke. For a lot women, it seems like the first stroke is a

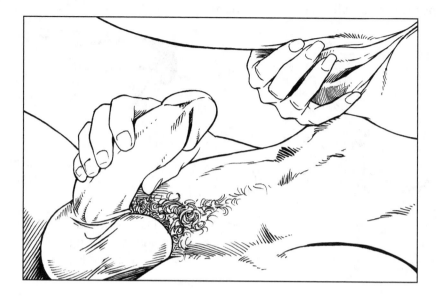

near religious experience, assuming they were fully aroused and eager for the thrusting to begin.

If you are a man, do not hesitate to ask your partner how she likes you to do your first stroke. Does she like you to start by teasing her with a series of short little thrusts, going in only an inch or two? Or does she like one big straightforward glide for the gold?

Legs Bent or Straight, Open or Closed

The biggest variable in the physics of intercourse is often the position of the woman's legs—whether they are straight or bent, open or closed, over your shoulders or in your face. When a woman's legs are straight, penetration is not as deep, but the tip of her clitoris might receive more stimulation. When a woman bends her legs and brings her knees closer to her chest, the penetration is deeper. This can be nice if she likes more pressure in the back of her vagina.

If a woman's legs are together or closed, the penis is hugged more snugly. This might offer better clitoral stimulation, because the extra snugness may push the inner labia more tightly against the shaft of the penis as it goes in and out. If a woman's legs are open or apart, there is greater skin-to-skin contact between her vulva and the man's genitals. This can also result in more bouncing-testicle action if he is on top.

Each couple's anatomy is different, so it's not possible to say which positions will be best.

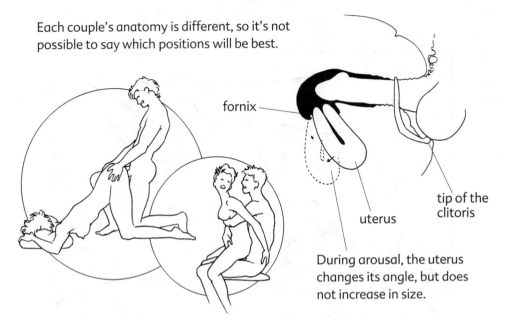

fornix

uterus

tip of the clitoris

During arousal, the uterus changes its angle, but does not increase in size.

Some couples enjoy intercourse with one leg straight and the other flexed. And many women stimulate their clitoris with their fingers during intercourse. Some push their clitoris against a partner's penis as it strokes in and out.

Some women keep their legs straight and together while flexing their thighs to help achieve an orgasm.

Legs Bent or Straight, Anatomical Consideration

A woman's decision to keep her legs straight or bent might vary with the length and thickness of her partner's penis. A woman whose partner has a really long penis may find she gets poked in the cervix if she opens and bends her legs during intercourse, while a woman whose partner has a short penis might prefer the feeling of deeper penetration that bent knees allow. (Sex books these days don't use the term "short penis." Instead, they say a penis that isn't overly long. This is meant to protect the allegedly fragile male ego, yet we hate to think today's male is so fragile that he can't say "I've got a short one" without experiencing a crisis of character. As for the sentiment expressed by the 20 Fingers song *Don't Want No Short Dick Man*, making peace with body parts is discussed in Chapter 84: *Techno Breasts & Weenie Angst*. For consolation, when a woman is highly aroused, her genitals usually puff up, which can make for a tighter fit.)

The male's pubic bone can push or grind against the clitoris in the missionary position, adding stimulation.

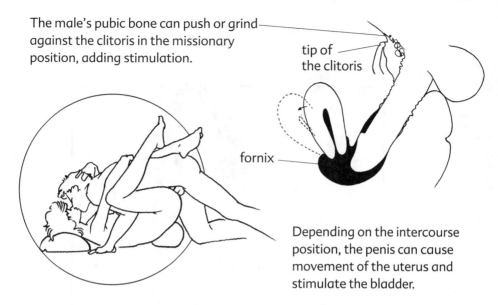

tip of the clitoris

fornix

Depending on the intercourse position, the penis can cause movement of the uterus and stimulate the bladder.

A Fix for When a Woman Feels Pain Due to Deep Penetration

There can be times during intercourse when a penis collides with the cervix, leaving a woman feeling like she's been punched in the stomach. Any woman who is experiencing sexual pain should consult with a gynecologist. But if it's determined the pain is from a penis hitting her cervix, there are things you might consider.

It's not necessarily the biggest, baddest or longest penis that will cause this kind of problem. Sometimes it's an average sized penis. While adding lube might help, it might make things worse. Waiting until a woman is more highly aroused before starting intercourse may help, because an aroused cervix raises up, hopefully taking itself out of the line of fire.

Some couples find it helps to try positions that discourage deep penetration, like rear entry when a woman is laying on her stomach or rear entry when she's on her side with her body straight. Or, she might do better on top.

You can also jerry rig a donut or gasket to go around the base of the penis to decrease the depth of thrusting. One type of sleeve that a number of couples recommend is called a "universal silicone sleeve for a penis pump." While using this sleeve during intercourse was not its intended purpose, it supposedly works well. Or, you might get a masturbation sleeve called "Maven" by Vibratex. Cut an inch or more off the end of it to make a donut-

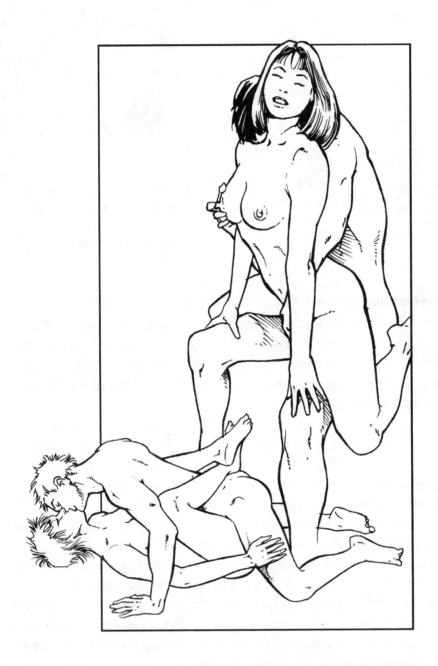

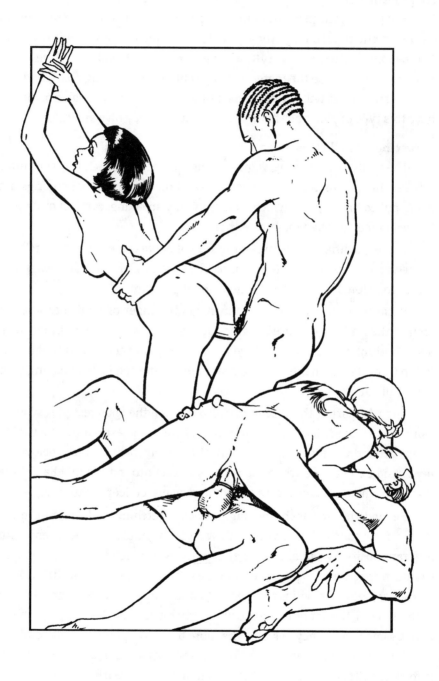

shaped ring that you can slide onto the base of the penis before intercourse. This will prevent the penis from thrusting too deep, and the extra pressure of the Maven material on the woman's clitoris can provide a welcome dividend. The people at **www.SexualityResources.com** recommend the Maven over other sleeves because the material can be cut without falling apart, and it is not so snug that it will act like a cock ring. Many of their female customers have this type of pain and this is the one solution they rave about.

Thrusting — Shallow vs. Deep

The walls of a woman's vagina change shape with each thrust of intercourse. This means that with each stroke, thousands of nerve endings are being pulled and tugged, which, neurologically speaking, can feel quite nice. (It doesn't feel half-bad for guys, either.)

There is a difference between the kind of nerve receptors in the first part of the vagina versus those in the back. The first inch of a woman's vagina is sensitive to touch. After that, it's more about pressure.

Because of its sensitivity to touch, gentle finger or penis-head action around the rim of an aroused vagina can be a nice way to begin intercourse. Shallow thrusting allows the ridge around the penis head to stimulate this first part of the vagina. The art is in not pulling out too far and having your penis fall out.

The first part of the vagina can also become the snuggest part when a woman is aroused. So with shallow thrusts, the snuggest part of the vagina wraps around the most sensitive part of the penis, which is just below the head. And exception is when the penis is thicker around the middle or base than at the head, in which case a woman may prefer deeper thrusts.

Beyond the first inch, the vagina feels stretching and pressure more than it feels touch. This is where it's wise for a couple to experiment with different positions and angles. They can discover which parts of a woman's vagina respond best to pressure from the head of his penis. While the classic missionary position will work best for some couples, others might do well with some of the more exotic positions they show in Cosmo. (A problem with Cosmo is how they describe the more bizarre or gymnastically difficult positions as being "advanced" or "for experts"—as if the missionary position is for losers. This is like criticizing a woman who is wearing a classic black dress for being unadventurous or plain.)

Deeper thrusting offers its own advantages: 1.) Deep thrusting can position a man's pubic bone to make better contact with a woman's clitoris. 2.) Deeper thrusting may allow the penis to pull on the labia minora (inner lips) longer with each stroke, providing more indirect stimulation to the clitoris. 3.) As she approaches orgasm, a woman may find it pleasurable to have a penis or penis-like object filling her vagina.

Learning with His Fingers

A good way for a man to learn about his partner's vagina is with his fingers as well as with his penis. This will give him a better understanding of what needs to be done with his penis. (As one female reader says, "It wouldn't hurt for women to know this about themselves.")

Battering Ram or Pleasure Wand? Mosh Pit or Symphony?

Some men use a penis as a battering ram, believing women enjoy being slammed during intercourse. Other men, perhaps a bit more sensitive or experienced, realize there are different thrusting rhythms that can help make intercourse feel more symphonic than heavy metal. Maybe she will like it slow at the start but strong at the end.

An excellent way to find out what works best during intercourse is when the woman is on top. That way a man can feel how she moves up and down on his penis and what parts of her vagina she focuses the head on. Does she move up and down on it repeatedly, or does she keep the penis deep inside and rub her clitoris on his pubic bone? Does she like to rub her clitoris or breasts with her fingers while a penis is inside her vagina, or would this be an unwelcome distraction? Where does she like to look, and what does she do with her mouth? Does she change the rhythm and speed, or does she keep it constant?

The Tantric Police Talk Thrust

Some Tantric and Oriental sex masters caution against constant deep thrusting during intercourse. They believe that the vagina does best with a ratio of five to nine shallow thrusts to every deep thrust. This is an interesting observation, given how they don't allow women to be monks and they don't allow them to enter business meetings unless it's to bring tea. But they have no shortage of suggestions for pleasing them sexually. If you are following the nine-shallow-for-every-one-deep thrust dictum, increase the ratio to

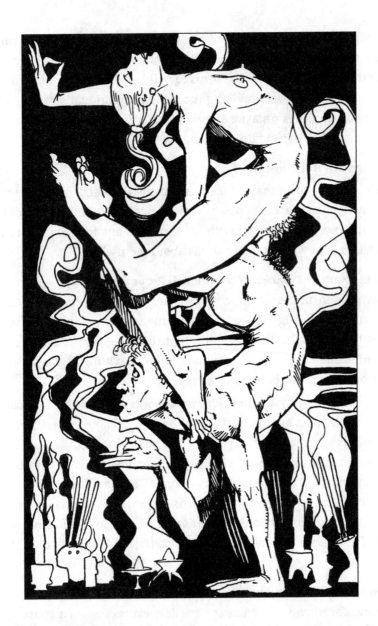

two deep for every four shallow as she becomes more aroused, or live dangerously and go for one shallow to one deep.

Mixing up the thrusting between shallow and deep is certainly something to experiment with. But if your partner starts threatening you with grief if you don't knock off the shallow stuff, you can safely assume she wasn't an Asian princess in a past life.

Intercourse as Your Private Language

If you are feeling terminally reflective, it might be helpful to think of intercourse as two separate acts: the thrusting part and the orgasm part. If the sole purpose of thrusting is to achieve orgasm, then intercourse might not have much emotional depth to it. That's because it is during the thrusting part of intercourse (before orgasm) when feelings of love, friendship and gratitude are often shared.

Most couples have a variety of thrusting modes—hot and furious, fun and playful, giggly, tearful, passionate, powerful, passive, and maybe even angry. This becomes part of the private language that lovers share.

Popping Out

During orgasm, the vagina can sometimes contract enough to expel a penis. When asked about this, most women advise, "Push it back in!"

Thrustless in Seattle

Some couples don't thrust at all during intercourse, but move their entire bodies in sync. Or the man might do a circular motion with his penis or pelvic bone grinding against the woman's vulva. Some couples occasionally stay really still during intercourse and try to coordinate their breathing. One partner breathes in at the moment the other breathes out.

You don't have to be a yoga master to achieve peak experiences with breathing instead of thrusting. You don't even need to meditate or stand on your head while chanting mysterious incantations. All you need to do is be in sync with each other.

Another way of enjoying intercourse without thrusting is to play "squeezing genitals." This is based upon the anatomical fact that when the male squeezes or contracts his erect penis it momentarily changes diameter, and when the woman squeezes her vagina it hugs the penis—sometimes snugly and with memorable results. To play "squeezing genitals," partners alternate squeezing their genitals. This doesn't require a particularly high I.Q. or a daring sense of adventure.

Riding High — Tom Landry Remembered

Each year a new book comes out that promises to reinvent the wheel sexually. One book talked about a radical "new" way of having intercourse. The couple starts by assuming the missionary position with the man on top.

Right before the thrusting begins, Mr. Top makes a quick shift toward the head of the bed, like the Cowboys used to do at the line of scrimmage before the set call, back when they were America's team and Tom Landry was coach. (Many of you weren't born then. Landry was one of the all-time greats.)

During the quick shift, the male pushes his entire body a couple of inches forward over the head of the woman. This puts him in the position of being able to say, "Honey, your roots are showing something awful," or "Time for a new weave." This new position also brings the man's penis in more direct contact with the woman's clitoris, assuming it doesn't cause his penis to snap off between the down-and-set-calls.

There is no in-out thrusting in this new form of intercourse. The couple simply moves their hips back and forth in synchrony. This intercourse position attempts to maximize clitoral stimulation by making the man ride high. Men who are sensitive lovers figured this one out long ago, although an occasional man may have had the knowledge forced upon him by a rambunctious lover who rode so low that she made him wonder if his penis would survive the night. Her riding low is the equivalent of his riding high.

Nasty Reflections

Watching your genitals at work or play during intercourse can be an awesome way to pass time. There are several positions that allow one or both partners to watch the vagina erotically swallowing the penis and then easing it back out. A good-sized hand mirror can offer a nice view of genital play until one of you accidentally kicks it over. Also, try using the magnifying side of the mirror. It will make you look huge! A woman reader comments: "That's a frightening thought."

Some couples like to use a phone instead of a mirror and shoot a video of themselves when having intercourse.

Kissing When Thrusting — Size vs. Intent

There's nothing nicer than kissing passionately when your genitals are locked in a loving embrace, but this isn't possible for some couples. If a woman is 5'1" and her partner is 6'4", there is no way her tongue is going to play inside his mouth when they are having intercourse.

This is one of the reasons why it is impossible to make recommendations regarding intercourse positions. Different couples come in different sizes. Some positions will feel better for lovers who are relatively the same height and of proportional weight, while those positions might be a disaster when a partner is really short and the other is really tall. Likewise, certain positions will feel better or worse depending on the size and angle of your respective genitals. Some positions that feel best during the first part of a woman's menstrual cycle might not be the best during the later part of her cycle. And that's just physical differences. You also need to factor in each partner's psychological needs.

Intercourse When Standing

To get an idea of how seldom couples have intercourse while standing and being face-to-face, you might do a search of websites where amateur couples post clips of themselves having sex. You'll find the only time couples have intercourse while standing is when it's rear entry and the woman is able to lean forward on a piece of furniture or some sort of railing.

One of the problems with intercourse while standing and being face-to-face—or "undies-down/skirt-up sex" as one of the women's magazines calls it—is that it can feel like a workout at the gym. Trying to thrust while bending your knees into a good angle can be tiring.

Leaning against a wall can help, and some women say it works best for them if they can keep one leg firmly planted on the ground while tucking the other around a partner's waist. That way, she doesn't have to worry about him dropping her, and having the other leg up can improve the angle and amount of stimulation. He can reach under it and help her hold it up.

In the Shower

You'd think that having intercourse in the shower would be as easy as shampooing your hair. Not so. While taking showers with a lover can be fun and incredibly sexy, having intercourse in the shower is a different matter. The first concern is slipping, so if you're going to have intercourse in the shower, make sure you've got a non-slip shower mat or put down some gripper fishies. You'll also want to install grab bars. Shower grab bars are easy to find, but reviewers usually don't rate them for their sex worthiness.

Although water is wet, it washes away natural lubrication. So you might want to keep a bottle of sex lube in the shower. Silicone-based sex lubes can be great for having sex in water because they don't wash off, but one little drop on the shower floor can make it treacherously slick. We're talking one thrust shy of a fractured femur. So if you are using silicone lube, consider putting it on before you get into the shower.

As for what position to use for shower sex, some couples find rear entry with the woman leaning forward can be the most practical. Or you might consider doing what a lot of couples do: enjoy showering together before or after you have intercourse.

Signaling

Sex seldom works well when one partner is too passive or inhibited to let the other partner know what feels good and what doesn't. Fortunately, signaling during intercourse doesn't need to include words, because hands on a partner's hips or rear end can be great rudders—as long as the partner with the hips is hip to his partner's hands.

To Come or Not to Come...

People have this notion that women who have orgasms during intercourse come by thrusting alone. Some do, some don't. Most women need help from either their or their partner's fingers.

"I come faster sometimes when he's inside me, but I always have to rub my clit to climax." *female age 25*

"I rarely have orgasms with intercourse, unless I'm playing with myself at the time. The best way for me is oral sex or using a vibrator." *female age 36*

"I don't usually have orgasms during intercourse. In a very open relationship, I can have an orgasm after intercourse by manually stimulating my clitoris or by rubbing myself on his flaccid penis." *female age 26*

"I usually have them with intercourse if my husband is rubbing my clitoris or using a vibrator while he is thrusting. Sometimes when I am really excited, I can have one just with thrusting." *female age 35*

When Is Intercourse a Success?

Most books imply that intercourse is a success if you give each other orgasms and a failure if you don't. Hardly. A woman can love the feelings she gets from intercourse, both emotional and physical, but still not have orgasms from it.

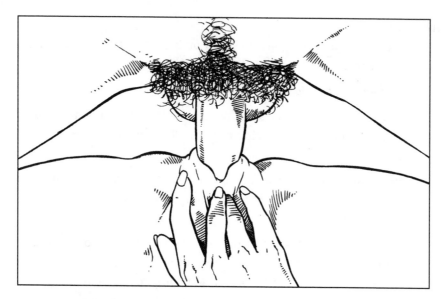

*Of the five thousand women who have taken our sex survey,
the VAST majority either need finger stimulation on their clit or they
grind their clitoris into the pubic bone of their partner in order to have
orgasms during intercourse. Few have orgasms from thrusting alone.*

Intercourse needs to convey certain feelings between partners that are too primal for words alone. These feelings rest on the boundary between body and soul and are transmitted from one person to another in many different ways. If orgasm is part of that process, fine, but having an orgasm is no guarantee that anything special has taken place. It's possible to have intercourse with no orgasm and experience it as wonderful or enchanting.

When is intercourse a success? Intercourse seems successful when it leaves you feeling more solid, less grumpy, more able to face the day, and less afraid of the world when it's an overwhelming place. Intercourse is successful when it makes you feel more whole or wholesome and secure. It's a success when it's fun or satisfying and leaves you with a smile.

When is intercourse a failure? This book's criterion for failure is waking up at three or four in the morning, looking at the person who's sleeping next to you and thinking "I wish I were home in my own bed, ALONE." This can be a particularly nasty dilemma if you are married or living together. Intercourse that conveys less pleasure than when someone leaves you a free hour on a parking meter is not necessarily worth having.

After Intercourse — The Drip Factor

Unless a guy is wearing a condom or pulls out and ejaculates to the side, he usually leaves semen inside a woman's vagina during intercourse.

So where does the ejaculate go?

"Runs down your leg," says one female reader. "It usually drips out," replies another. "Like water in a cup that's turned upside down," says a third.

This might not be a problem if you are going to sleep, except for the wet spot on the mattress, but what if you had intercourse in the morning or at lunchtime?

"You can usually get it out in the shower" was one response, while another woman said, "Not true. It tends to drain out at its own pace, and all the showering in the world isn't going to hasten it along."

What if you already took a shower or don't want to take another shower just then?

"Sometimes I'll wear a panty liner," said one woman, "but it's not worth a tampon."

All of the women said they know of other women who douche right after intercourse even when they have sex at bedtime. Most thought this was silly and unnecessary. As one woman said,

"It's not dirty; I put the stuff in my mouth!" Another woman said, "I don't have sex with a man unless I really care about him. I find the occasional dripping to be a sweet and sometimes exciting reminder that he's been here."

As for why the ejaculate goes in thick but drips out thin, you will find the answer in Chapter 6: *Semen Confidential.*

Top Dog

It has been said that people who always need to be on top during intercourse are insecure, while people who have it more together are happy to switch off. If this is true, then intercourse is no different from life in general. What's probably more true is the couple has tried it both ways and likes it better with one or the other of them on top.

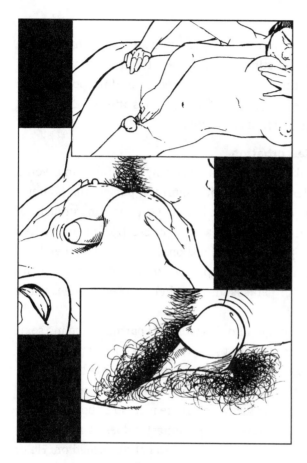

Intercourse between the thighs, breasts, and femoral intercourse, where the penis slides between the lips of the vulva without going into the vagina.

Also, feminists claim that intercourse usually follows a prostitute model of sex—once the male comes, the sex is over. If that's true in your relationship, a workaround is in order. Work on ways to help the woman get her share of pleasure before the man comes.

On Not Pulling Out

Staying inside your lover after the thrusting is done can sometimes feel magical. Since most men lose their erections after coming, the two of you need to keep the fading member in while getting comfortable enough to stay in each other's arms. Some couples like to fall asleep this way. The desire to stay inside your partner after ejaculation is one of the downsides of using a condom. A man who is wearing a condom needs to pull out soon after he's come. Otherwise he might leave the condom inside his partner.

Missed the Train Again

Men who have trouble coming tend to pump faster during intercourse, hoping this will provide extra stimulation to help them ejaculate. This is a bad idea. The rapid thrusting desensitizes the penis, and it's possible the female partner won't be able to walk right for a few days afterward. For more information, see Chapter 54: *Delayed Ejaculation.*

Passive Intercourse vs. Masturbation

Let's say a woman wakes up at 5:00 a.m., horny as can be, and would like to have intercourse. Her partner is not a morning person and is pretty much comatose until noon. Assuming he's not an early-morning grouch, he might allow her to stimulate his penis to a point of erection, or maybe he's already got an early-morning (REM-state) hard-on. The couple can then have intercourse in a position where he can be passive while she is active, or she massages her clitoris while his penis is inside of her. In a sense, she is using his penis as a dildo.

Or let's say it's nearly midnight and this woman's partner is feeling sexually amped, but she is pretty much dead to the world. She doesn't mind it if he uses her vagina for intercourse, but doesn't want to have to fake being into it. So she rolls on her side and allows him to have rear-entry intercourse.

Why didn't the horny partner just masturbate instead of bothering the one who is zoned out? Sometimes a partner honestly doesn't mind being "used" for sex as long as he or she isn't expected to get all turned on. He or she might even enjoy the other's pleasure. However, it is essential that the passive partner feels comfortable saying, "Naw, not now," and the horny partner is willing to masturbate instead. *As for having sex with a partner who is passed out or asleep and is not able to give consent, this would be sexual assault. Please read Chapter 13: Consent.*

What's the Frequency, Dan?

When it comes to frequency of intercourse, people who ask, "What's normal?" usually aren't asking the right question. If you are in a relationship, good questions to be asking are, "Do we have intercourse as often as each of us likes?" "Do we have intercourse more often than one or both of us likes?" The reason these questions are more important than, "What's normal?" is because the only thing that matters about sex is what feels best for you—whether it's three times a day or three times a decade.

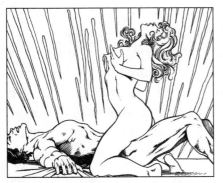

Warning! This can hurt you. Really.

Intercourse injuries can cause a penis to forever bend in a strange way. Most of these injuries occur when a woman is on top. When using this position, the woman should be well-lubricated and she might restrict her up-and-down motion. This helps decrease instances where she sits down on the penis at a funny angle, or when it comes out on the upstroke and gets crunched on the downstroke instead of sliding in the way it's supposed to. Putting a pillow under the man's rear end can help make his pelvic bone more accessible. His partner might enjoy grinding against his pelvic bone for extra stimulation instead of using his penis like a pogo stick. She might also try squeezing his penis, as if she is peeing and trying to stop the flow.

"Vaginal Wind"

When you ask women what's your most embarrassing moment during sex, many will say it's when they've had a vaginal fart. The official term for this is "vaginal flatulence," although this type of acoustical event is more commonly known as a queef, beaver burp, muff music, or a fanny fart when the woman is British.

As for the mechanics, think of the vagina as a bagpipe between a woman' legs. Air can collect in the vagina during intercourse and then belch out. This can also happen during exercise or even yoga. When a vagina burps air and a penis is not involved, the medical name is "vaginal wind."

Because there is no way a woman can contract the opening of her vagina to modulate the outflow of air, vaginal flatulence will sound more like a fog horn or tuba than a tea kettle. Some women are able to produce vaginal flatulence on command, with the adeptness of middle schoolers in a burping contest. Unlike gas coming from the rear end, vaginal flatulence shouldn't smell because the vagina is simply spitting out air that's accumulated inside of it rather than acting as a portal for foul winds. So if vaginal flatulence smells badly or is accompanied by discomfort other than from embarrassment, a woman should consult with a gynecologist.

Pillow Power

Never underestimate the power of a pillow under the small of the back or rear end of the partner who is on the bottom. Changing the angle of the hips can change a person's experience of intercourse. Experiment to find what placement might be good for you. If you like intercourse from the rear, keep a lookout for the perfect bigger pillow that will provide support and raise the woman's rear end to an angle that is comfortable and inviting. You might try bolsters and different kinds of cushions, including wedges with waterproof covers made specifically for sex.

Environment

If intercourse is seeming a bit stale, it might help to scout out new locations. While it never hurts to try a resort on a tropical island or a four-star hotel in Europe, most of us will need to consider other possibilities:

The Kitchen Always a fine place for intercourse until you have kids. Once the kids reach school age, the kitchen is game for an occasional nooner.

The Yard It's a shame to spend the time and money making the grass grow and never have sex on it—although local ordinances may disagree.

In Front of the Fireplace There's nothing quite like doing it in front of the fireplace, until they deliver wet pine instead of seasoned oak and a slew of hissing, burning embers showers your naked bodies.

In Water Hot tubs, bathtubs, pools, and other large bodies of water can be great places for people to do all sorts of nasty things. But intercourse in water provides its own unique hazard because water washes away natural lubrication. Why hot tub manufacturers don't include samples of silicone-based lubes is beyond us. Another solution is to bury the penis inside the vagina while both sets of organs are outside the water. To help facilitate underwater hand play and sexual groping, coat your genitals with something oily while they are still dry-docked.

Sex at the Office Sex at the office often has elements of risk and mischievous fun. A reader from Los Angeles is a commercial-real-estate agent who has keys to some of the finest high-rise buildings in the city. When he and his GF want a dramatic change of scenery, they visit the upper floors.

Candlelight The standby for erotic ambiance is candlelight. Make sure candle wax doesn't drip on your carpet. (A reader kindly comments: fold up a paper towel a few times and place it over the cooled wax on the carpet. Then put a warm to hot iron on top of the towel. It will melt the wax into the towel and the carpet is wax-free!)

Extra Odds'N'Ends

💡Some couples enjoy the sensations when the woman uses a vibrator during intercourse. This can work in any number of positions, or you can get artsy and try doing it like the couple in Chapter 26: *Oscillator, Generator, Vibrator, Dildo.*

💡A woman who is on top and facing a man's feet can watch his penis go in and out of her vagina, especially with a mirror. She can also reach forward and play with his testicles or toes.

💡Rear-entry positions allow the head of the penis to focus on different parts of the vagina than missionary positions do. Rear entry also provides extra padding, which can be welcome if one or both of you is really bony.

💡Rather than thrusting, some couples find that rocking back and forth with a penis inside feels pleasant.

💡Some couples take an intercourse break to have oral sex; some do oral sex afterward.

💡Rather than inserting the penis inside a woman's vagina, some couples enjoy a lubricated penis moving between her labia, like a hot dog going back and forth through a bun. The ridge around the head of the penis glides back and forth over the clitoris.

💡In the highly recommended book *Tricks - More Than 125 Ways to Make Good Sex Better,* Jay Wiseman suggests having the man lie on his back and the woman places a pair of her panties over his penis. The penis sticks through a leg hole, with the panties draping down over his testicles and between his legs. The couple has intercourse with the woman on top. If the panties are silky or rayon-like, the material might stimulate him with each stroke.

💡Some couples find a well-trimmed and freshly bathed big toe to be a fun penis substitute. Also, a heel that's jiggled back and forth can be used to stimulate a woman's genitals.

☀ There are couples who like to gently bite each other's shoulders or run their teeth along each other's skin while having intercourse. This works best when the skin is well-lubricated.

☀ Some lovers prefer the feeling of intercourse after a woman has had an orgasm rather than before.

☀ Women might not lubricate very well for the first couple of months following pregnancy, especially when she is nursing.

☀ Extra lubrication may be necessary if the woman is using drugs such as antihistamines, alcohol, or pot, and if the man is wearing a condom.

☀ Why not try feeding each other while having intercourse? That's what nature created papaya for.

☀ Some couples enjoy a finger, thumb, vibrator, or butt plug on or in each other's anus during intercourse.

☀ Most sex stores sell rings that fit over a man's penis and provide extra stimulation to the woman's clitoris when she rubs up against his pubic bone. There are also vibrating cock rings, and vibrators in harnesses that can be strapped over the clitoris for use during intercourse.

☀ Positions where you are sitting up might allow more blood to pool in the pelvic region, which could help some men get better erections and women receive more vaginal engorgement. These include positions where the man sits on a chair and the woman sits in his lap, wrapping her legs around his waist, or where he sits in the chair and she sits on his lap but facing away from him.

Betty On Intercourse

What better way to wind down a chapter on intercourse than with a few passages from Betty Dodson's book *Sex for One?* These refer to what transpired during Ms. Dodson's sex groups for women.

On Pretending You're a Guy during Intercourse "One amusing and informative exercise was called "Running a Sexual Encounter." It involved reversing sex roles with the women on top. We made believe that our clitorises were penetrating imaginary lovers, and we had to do all the thrusting. I would set the egg timer for three minutes, a little longer than the Kinsey national average. As the fucking began, I would participate and at the same time comment on everyone's technique. 'Keep your arms straight; don't crush your lover. You're too high up; your clitoris just fell out. Don't stop moving, you'll lose your erection. Don't move so fast; you'll come too soon. And don't forget to whisper sweet things in your lover's ear between all those passionate kisses."

"Watching the egg timer, I coordinated my theatrical orgasm with the ding of the bell, frantically thrusting for the last ten seconds. Then, falling flat on my imaginary lover, I muttered, 'Was it good for you?' and promptly began snoring loudly. It was always hysterically funny. Panting and exhausted, the women all exclaimed, 'How do men do it?' Complaints included tired arms, lower-back pain, and stiff hip joints. Most of the women had fallen out long before the bell went off. After that, there was always more empathy for men, and the women showed an increased interest in other positions for lovemaking."

Odds & Ends "Some of the women talked about experiencing pain with deep thrusting intercourse, while others claimed to want a hard fuck. In my youth, I'd confused hard pounding intercourse with passion, and experienced internal soreness afterward.... While I enjoyed a strong fuck when we were two equal energies in sync, I also loved the slow intense fuck."

"Another problem the women complained of was lack of lubrication and the pain of dry intercourse. Some women felt inadequate if they weren't wet with passion. My experience varied; sometimes I lubricated when I wasn't even thinking about sex. Other times I could be dry even though I felt sexually aroused..."

On Orgasms "Some women had good orgasms with oral sex but not with intercourse. Others could come with intercourse but couldn't get off alone. Still others were having orgasms with themselves but not with a partner. All of the orgasmic women agreed on one thing: Their experiences of orgasm varied greatly from one orgasm to the next."   —From *Sex for One* by Betty Dodson, Harmony Books.

Readers' Comments

Some of your favorite intercourse positions?

"My favorite position is doggy style, with me on my hands and knees, and him behind me. I like this best for two reasons: my vagina is tighter this way, and I can easily rub my clitoris and have an orgasm. I also love to sit on a guy while he is sitting up. This just feels wonderful. Our bodies are so close." *female age 26*

"Good old missionary, with me on the bottom and him on top!"
female age 32

"One of my favorite positions is sitting in his lap in a chair. He can kiss my neck or armpits, which drives me nuts, and I can move freely. If we are on the bed, I can also lie back and touch my clit if I want."
female age 38

"My favorite position is sitting on top of him. That way I can stroke my clitoris or I can watch him do it." *female age 43*

"I like it best when we're doing it doggy style and I hold the vibrator and rub my clit with it. The sensation is wonderful!" *female age 25*

"I enjoy having him on top but recently discovered that if we lie on our sides with me in front and I throw my upper leg over his, he can enter me from behind and it's very exciting." *female age 45*

"I like to bend over a table and have my partner insert his penis from behind. We get great penetration this way, and he is also able to hit something in there that makes me feel really good!" *female age 34*

"I like to be on my back with my legs up while he is on his knees entering me and rubbing my clitoris. We started using this position when I was pregnant and I still like it best." *female age 35*

What do you like the most, and least, about intercourse?

"Worst part—the big wet spot. Best part—making the big wet spot."
female age 27

"It is wonderful when we first start having intercourse and I love the cuddling after. I don't like how, if you don't clean up afterward, the ejaculate runs out of you (sometimes cold) and drips down your butt onto the sheets." *female age 30*

"I like it when he first inserts his penis into my vagina the best. The thing I like least about sex is having to really work for a long time to get him to orgasm when he's had too much to drink." *female age 34*

"I like the beginning the most and orgasm, of course. If somebody takes too long, the middle gets dull." *female age 25*

"The first moments of penetration are the best. The wet spot on the bed, the worst." *female age 44*

"The part I like best is when my man spends a long time getting me hot until I want him so badly I can't wait and he finally sinks his penis into me. It's such a relief to finally be joined together. I like it least when he enters too soon and comes too fast and says, 'I'm sorry' when I had my hopes up for more." *female age 38*

"I love feeling him on top of me, kissing and caressing, and I love the feeling of his penis inside me. The part I don't like is the mess." *fem 35*

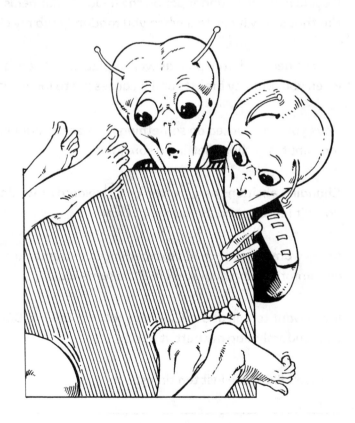

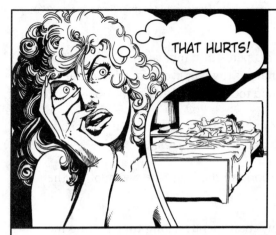

THAT HURTS!

This is what hurts when we have sex.

Women readers say men don't realize how much sex can hurt. They think porn is partly to blame, because women in porn never have pain, or feel embarrassed or humiliated. And when they do, the men get off on it. So here are conversation starters for couples.

—Check any boxes that apply.—

☐ If my vagina were ready for your penis the minute you get hard, we'd dispense with the kissing and conversation. Oh wait, what kissing and conversation?

☐ I would never use sandpaper on the head of your penis. But that's how it can feel when you randomly rub my clitoris.

☐ Nipples get hard from pain as well as pleasure. There are times when you grab my breasts and it causes me to jolt in pain.

☐ Have you ever sucked on something the size of your penis for ten minutes without getting a sore jaw?

☐ Changing positions as ☐ often or ☐ seldom as we do doesn't feel as good as you might think.

☐ Many women say they have experienced extreme pain or discomfort during anal sex. I feel the same way.

☐ If you want to talk about kink, let's talk about kink. But when you randomly slap my butt, it hurts!

☐ If I didn't like it the last ten times...

☐ Has anyone ever hit the back of your throat with an erect penis? Yet you want it to go deeper down my throat?

☐ A facial? What if I collected your semen and dripped it in your eyes or smeared it on your face and chest?

☐ Has anyone tried to sneak a penis up your ass when you were having sex? I could always buy a dildo and help you experience what that feels like.

☐ It would be more exciting for me if you were ☐ more or ☐ less take-charge in bed.

☐ There's a difference between being assertive and having rough sex. Rough sex hurts. If I want rough sex, I will ask you for it.

☐ Please don't assume it feels good just because you read about it online or saw it on Pornhub. Talk to me about it first.

☐ Would you be okay if I rammed a finger up your butt every time you ram a finger into my vagina?

☐ If you'll wait for me to tell you when I am ready for you to _____ it will end up being more fun for both us.

☐ _____
_____

☐ _____
_____

If you experience pain every time you have sex, please see Chapter 56: *Damn That Hurts! When Sex Is Painful.*

Top Notch Resources: It's explicit, hot and excellent, showing real-life couples: Jamye Waxman's *101 Positions for Lovers*. A DVD from Adam and Eve.

Fun, funny and perceptive—Sadie Allison's *Ride 'Em Cowgirl! Sex Position Secrets For Better Bucking*, Tickle Kitty.

24

Anal Sex—Up Your Bum

"I grew up in the country. We had neighbors, Amos Wheatley and his wife. One night while washing dishes, Mrs. Wheatley told my mother that she let Amos 'use the other hole.' Then they had a baby girl, and I heard my father comment that Amos must have got it right at least once. Sometime later, Amos, who was uneasy about the expense of having a new baby, told my father he'd rather have had a team of horses. My father said, 'Isn't that expecting rather a lot of Mrs. Wheatley?'"

—The recollections of a 71-year-old woman, as told to Julia Hutton in her *Good Sex: Real Stories from Real People,* Cleis Press.

Some couples would rather drink goat sweat than try anal sex; others enjoy an occasional rear-end soiree. Whether you are straight, gay or somewhere in between, the chances are good that at some point in your life you might try anal sex.

Please be aware this Guide couldn't care less whether you do or don't practice anal sex, but it does have a few suggestions in case curiosity nips you in the rear.

For those of you who have been watching too much porn—where the rectum is the new vagina—consider the responses about anal sex from thousands of sexually-amped people who have taken our sex survey. Based on their answers, less than 10% of straight couples have anal intercourse on a regular basis. And "on a regular basis" might be once or twice a month, if that. On the other hand, some women have their strongest orgasms when anal stimulation is part of the mix, and some men find a finger on the prostate to be a welcome sensation.

Also, there are other forms of anal play besides putting a penis inside a rectum. These include finger tips, tongues and sex toys. You'll be hard-pressed to find a part of the body that has more nerve endings than the anus.

In Butt Play, What's Good for the Goose...

It's only fair that if a guy wants to stick his penis up a woman's rear end, she should be able to stick something of comparable size up his. Plus, it should help him become a more sensitive anal lover.

Vegetables aren't a good idea; you don't want a vegetable breaking off inside your partner's rectum. Use a dedicated anal toy or butt plug.

Anal Massage

If someone says they had sex last night, we assume they had vaginal intercourse. When you add the modifier "anal" in front of the word sex, we assume it was a penis up a partner's bum.

Yet one of the nicest forms of anal pleasure comes from anal massage, where a penis is not inserted into the anus. The anus is alive with nerve endings. A well-lubed finger or thumb massaging the anal opening or massaging the nerves further up the rectum can bring subtle but enjoyable waves of pleasure.

> "I hate admitting this, but I like it when Dave wets one of his fingers and slides it into my anus. It is a huge turn-on, and there are times when it makes me orgasm. The only problem is pulling out. It always hurts coming out and usually throws off my bowel movements for the next few hours. It feels like I have to go...." *female age 26*

> "When Erica is all worked up, she sometimes really likes me to massage her anus. When I slip a lubricated finger inside her, it is often the thing that puts her over the edge. If I have a finger inside her vagina and one in her anus, she reacts very well to the sandwiching of the wall when I press the two together. Other times, she really hates it when I touch her there. I can never quite guess when it's going to be a green light." *male age 25*

What Can Brown Do For You?

Some people like anal sex because it's forbidden. Some men have anal sex as a way of getting work in the entertainment industry. Some women have anal sex who would like a partner's penis inside of their vagina but can't because of chronic pain. But the most obvious reason why people have anal sex is because they enjoy the experience.

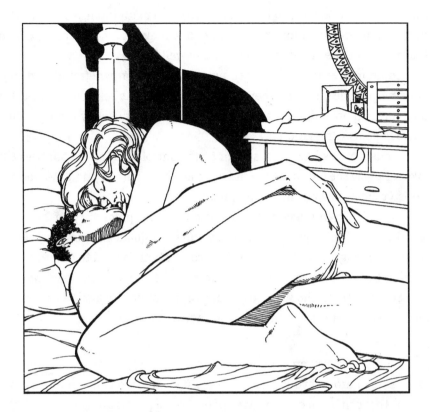

"Anal sex helps me feel a whole different part of my vagina and vulva. The fact that it is so tight and kind of nasty is a turn-on to me too."

female age 23

"My wife asks for anal intercourse on occasion, usually late at night when she is very aroused and her inhibitions are down." *male age 41*

"I can come from anal intercourse, but not from vaginal intercourse."

female age 32

"Both of us like it. I will sometimes put a finger in her anus while we are having intercourse. It's very exciting for her, and I can feel my penis through the wall, which I find to be very erotic." *male age 39*

Some people believe the only reason women have anal sex is to please a male partner. Not a single woman in our survey who has anal sex mentioned anything about pleasing a partner. Each one said she did it because she liked the way it feels. Some women report getting an extra intense orgasm when they stimulate their clitoris at the same time they are having anal sex. Some find anal sex to be emotionally intense, as well.

Some men enjoy having their anus massaged or penetrated, and some have memorable orgasms when their prostate gland is being stimulated. Few men have an orgasm from anal stimulation alone. It usually requires simultaneous penis stimulation.

Some couples have anal sex for birth control, such as in countries that take seriously the Catholic Church's opposition to contraception. (Maybe anal sex isn't what the Vatican had in mind.)

Is anal sex an effective means of preventing pregnancy, or can ejaculate run out of the anus and into the vagina? Pregnancies from anal sex are common enough that the term "splash conception" is used to describe them. Perhaps this is how people with anal-retentive personalities are conceived.

Some women who want to remain virgins might try anal sex as an alternative to intercourse that involves the vagina.

Rimming

Rimming is a slang word for kissing ass, literally. It means sticking your tongue up or around your partner's anus. It's not a good idea to rim just anyone, as that can be an effective way of getting hepatitis and parasites.

However, by the time a couple has been together for a couple of years, they pretty much share the same anal flora. This means you probably won't get anything more from licking your partner's anus than you would from licking your own.

Mother Nature & The Human Backside

When Mother Nature designed the female body she gave it a vagina that's rough, tough and durable. She made the walls of the vagina so they would stretch, swell, lubricate and straighten out at times of sexual excitement. This allows objects of desire to slide in and out with a fair amount of ease and enjoyment.

Nature was working from a different set of blueprints when she built the rectum. The rectum's main purpose is for elimination rather than romance. As a result, the walls of the rectum don't stretch and lubricate, although they comfortably fit objects that are even larger than a penis on a regular basis.

The rectum includes a pair of pugnacious sphincter muscles that guard the gates of your anus. These muscular rings were designed to facilitate outgoing rather than incoming objects, although they can be taught to yield in either direction. The anal sphincters are two of the most important muscles in the human body if you plan on living and working in the vicinity of other human beings.

Reports that anal sex will damage the rectum are not backed up by science as long as you are using lots of lube, your sphincters are relaxed, and you aren't using crystal meth or anything that might numb your bum.

A Brief Summary of the Structure & Function of the Human Rectum from the Time of Cro-Magnon Man Until the Founding of Ancient Greece

If you consider the history of the human rectum, say from the time of Cro-Magnon man until the founding of ancient Greece, its sole purpose was to hold things in. It wasn't until the ancient Greeks invented sodomy that our bums became multipurpose. (In giving credit where credit is due, the Old Testament may have had an interest in the subject of anal sex that possibly predated the Greeks. At the very least, one of the early Biblical plagues visited upon the Egyptians apparently included hemorrhoids.)

Thanks to the inventiveness of the ancient Greeks, we now have things in our lives like politicians, lawyers, doctors and anal sex. The only one of these that should never cause you any pain is anal sex. If it does, you are doing it wrong, according to psychologist Jack Morin, who wrote the bible on the subject, called *Anal Pleasure and Health, 4rd ed.*, Down There Press (2010).

The key to pleasurable anal sex is training the anal sphincter muscles to open for incoming objects. One set of these muscles is under conscious control. It's what people use to maintain their dignity when waiting to use the bathroom. The second set of sphincters is a total free agent. It automatically closes whenever something pushes against it. To have comfortable anal sex, the second set of sphincters must be taught how to relax when you ask.

Popular Culture Historical Note When Jack Morin published the first edition of his *Anal Pleasure* book, it was such a taboo subject that few bookstores stocked it. Now, a few decades later, Jack's book has been joined by several others. It's no longer unusual to see butt-sex books on bookstore shelves.

The next sections have been written as if the male is doing the inserting and the female is receiving. Far be it from this Guide to say how it is in your relationships. (Pegging, or the insertion of a dildo into the male butt by a female partner, may not be as popular as blogging, but it's not totally uncommon.)

Four Key Elements

There were originally three keys to anal insertion: relaxation, feedback and lube. The difference between anal pleasure and pain is having generous amounts of all three. Trust has now been added to safe sex guidelines as well.

Even the toughest of condoms can tear if the anus isn't relaxed. So the goal is to be turned on and relaxed as opposed to turned on and tense.

The Right Chemistry

"I truly hated anal sex the two times I had tried it before. But I agreed to do it with my new boyfriend, and it feels incredible with him! Am I weird, or are there any other women who enjoy anal sex?"

female age 28

We posted this reader's question on our sex survey and found a surprising number of women who said they'd had a similar experience. Many said the keys for them were feeling totally relaxed with their partner and being exceptionally horny.

Even a finger on your anus can be annoying if trust and arousal are missing, while a reasonably-sized penis can feel fine when you are relaxed and ready.

Learning the Difference between 'Strange' and 'Pain'

When experimenting with anal play, you'll want to learn the difference between sensations that are unusual or strange versus those that are painful. When you or a partner first start groping inside your anus, it might feel strange. With time and experience, the initial strange feeling can evolve into sexual pleasure. Or, it might continue to feel strange. You never know how your brain will translate the sensations until you are in the throes of sexual passion and desire.

If the sensations are painful as opposed to strange, back off and try to figure out what's causing the pain. Don't explore again until you have come up with ways to prevent the pain. There should be no pain in anal sex.

Nail Alert

When it comes to the rectum, jagged finger nails are weapons of mass destruction. Make sure your fingernails are trimmed and your hands are washed.

Practice and Preparation—By Yourself

The best way to prepare for anal sex is in the shower, for a couple of weeks before you do it with a partner. Try inserting your finger up your bum. Think of it as a rectal rover. Its job is to provide you with information about the geology of your anus. With each successive shower, you will learn more, and you will be teaching your anal sphincters to relax.

Another thing you might try is to masturbate with an anal toy or finger in your rear. This will help you get used to new sensations that involve both your front and rear, or two parts of the nervous system instead of one.

Practice and Preparation—With a Partner

Psychologist Jack Morin suggested the following technique for teaching your rectum to relax: Each night for a week or two, one partner lubes up a clean finger and gently inserts it in the other partner's rear, pushing very softly and slowly. This should encourage trust and relaxation.

Rectal expert Erik Mainard—known as the Avatar of Ass—encourages a gentle massage of the anus and suggests angling the finger slightly upward toward the tailbone, since that is how the rectum curves. He says to push in slowly and only as the resistance eases. This should feel good for the receiver; otherwise the person who is inserting the finger is rushing it or violating your comfort zone, in addition to violating your anus.

One way to help relax the anal area is for the receiver to push down as though she were trying to move her bowels. In addition to relaxing the sphincters, this adds a bit of suspense to the exercise. However, anal purists say that with the help of a patient, caring partner, one needn't trick the sphincters into relaxing. And even though only one partner might be inserting a penis, each should experiment with fingering the other's rear. This will help build knowledge and trust, or bum-bonding.

The receiver needs to feel comfortable with finger penetration before trying any unnatural acts. It is not until the sphincters learn to relax that anal sex will feel comfortable, and if it doesn't feel comfortable, you shouldn't be doing it. If there is any discomfort other than a feeling of fullness, which shouldn't be painful, spend an extra week doing the finger exercises or give up the concept of anal intercourse.

Swabbing the Decks of the Hershey Highway

Some people prefer to give themselves a quick enema ("short shot") with a bulb syringe or a prepared store-bought solution before having anal sex. Others will equate this with removing the patina from the Statue of Liberty Keep in mind that the rectum is not usually a storage space for poop. It is the toll booth between the colon and the toilet. A good soaping in the shower should make most anuses sparkle.

If you decide to give yourself an enema, do it an hour or so before sex. A bulb syringe with water should do the trick. Follow the instructions on the box. Do not use a Fleet or Fleet-like enema for sex, as it contains a laxative. Empty it and fill it with clean tap water. Make sure it's not too cold, unless you enjoy giving yourself cramps. For more cleaning options, see Tristan Taormino's *The Ultimate Guide to Anal Sex for Women,* 2nd ed. Cleis Press.

Simultaneous Clit Play

Women frequently find that clitoral stimulation helps take anal sex from being nothing to write home about to something that can feel good. The two of you need to talk about ways of helping the woman's clitoris get plenty of attention while you are doing anal play. This can range from using your fingers to using a vibrator.

Anal Play Combined with Other Kinds of Sex Play

"I like to have my anus stimulated when I'm receiving oral sex. I like to have one finger inserted, but it doesn't have to be very far, just past the sphincter will do. And rather than sliding all the way in and out, it is better if there is just a slight tugging movement. It adds one more sensation to the myriad of sensations involved in oral sex." *female age 37*

"My boyfriend likes me to rub a finger on his anus while I give him oral sex. Gentle pressure and a rotating finger add a lot to his pleasure."
female age 23

Some couples enjoy adding a finger or butt plug on or up the anus during handjobs, oral sex and vaginal intercourse. You will need to decide if you

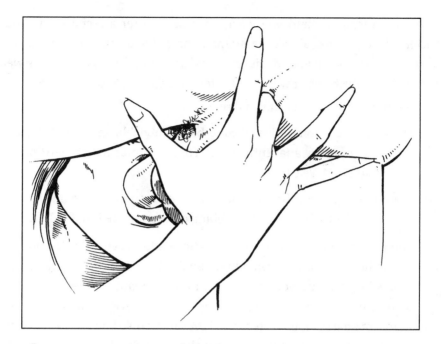

want the finger or toy to move in and out, or to stay put to stimulate the prostate or give a sense of fullness. Lube and a glove can make a finger glide nicely, and keep anything that has touched an anus out of a vagina.

Playin' the Back Nine? Bag It

Straight or gay, single or married, monogamous or orgy-inclined, you are always wise to use a condom when having anal intercourse. Women's chances of getting HIV are 17 times higher when they are having anal intercourse than vaginal. While avoiding HIV and AIDS is the most important reason to use condoms during anal sex, there are other concerns as well.

Fluids deposited in the rectum are absorbed more easily into the body than fluids deposited in the vagina. A woman's colon is going to slurp up male ejaculate that's been deposited in her rear end. How her immune system will respond is anyone's guess. If you put a condom on the penis, you've eliminated a potential source of concern. And both of our prostate consultants balk the thought of sticking an unbagged penis up a rectum, even if it belongs to a wife of twenty years. That's because the same bacteria that are prevalent in the rectum can cause a prostate infection (prostatitis). They can also cause vaginal infections when a penis goes from an anus to a vagina.

No matter how hard you wash your penis after a rectal rendezvous, bacteria-laden chunks of feces can remain inside the urinary opening. So not only should you wash your penis after anal sex, but try to take a leak as well. This will help flush out unwelcome bacteria that's inside your urethra.

For more on condoms and anal sex:

Using latex condoms with silicone-based lube Silicone lube is the lube of choice for many anal enthusiasts. For more information, See Chapter 12: *Sex Lubes—A New Look.*

Condoms Without Ribs Don't used ribbed or studded condoms for anal sex; the extra friction from the ribbing on the surface is not helpful.

Female Condoms Some anal sex aficionados have been trumpeting the value of the female condom for anal intercourse. You might see if it works for you. Plus, you can leave it in if you want to take an intermission, or need to go shopping or something. However, using female condoms for anal sex has not received FDA sanction, so beware. Experienced users recommend that you take out the inner ring before inserting the female condom in the rectum.

Sex Toys and Condoms: It's best to put a new condom on any sex toys that go into the rectum and to wash the toy afterward. If you have favorite toys for butt play, dedicate them for that purpose only so they never see the inside of a vagina.

What Porn Leaves Out

In her book, *The Ultimate Guide to Anal Sex for Women*, Tristan Taormino warns that porn leaves out the most important parts of anal sex. Porn actors don't have anal sex without lots of preparation and anal foreplay—none of which is shown in porn. So when you are watching gonzo porn classics such as *Bongwater Butt Babes*, don't for a moment try to replicate it in real life. (See our video *Reality Check: Porn and Anal Sex* on the website for *The Guide* at www.GuideToGettingItOn.com.)

In Slow—Out Slow

No matter what you are putting inside a rectum, it needs to go in slowly and come out slowly. Few people have difficulty grasping the idea that incoming objects need to be inserted slowly. But they don't realize that things being

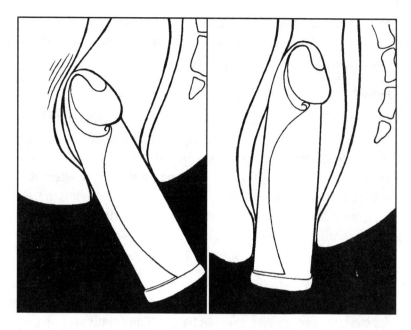

Unlike the vagina, the rectum curves. So you will want to experiment with positions that will help straighten out the rectal curves. Otherwise, a penis might rear-end the walls of the rectum.

pulled out of a rectum need to be removed slowly. It doesn't matter if it's a finger, penis or butt plug. Otherwise, extreme discomfort and even damage might result.

Butt Plugs

Butt plugs are dildo-like toys made specifically for the rear end. They are wide in the middle and have narrow bases that flare out to keep them from getting lost in the rectum. This is a hazard that should not be taken lightly. Objects that are lost in the rectum often require Emergency Room assistance.

Butt plugs come in many different sizes, and some even vibrate. Because of their unique shape, people use butt plugs to give their rear ends a feeling of fullness. Butt plugs don't work well for thrusting.

If you are looking for sex toys, do research on which ones are best for anal play. If you plan to use a sex toy for both vaginal and anal recreation, get a separate one for each port of entry. Having dedicated sex toys helps decrease the chance that fecal matter will get into the vagina.

Sex toys vary greatly in price. Some are made from funky or dangerous materials. Find a reputable source. If a sex toy has a porous surface, be sure to use a condom on it, as it might otherwise collect fecal matter.

Pegging or "Bend Over Boyfriend"

"My boyfriend of five years actually made the suggestion that I penetrate him anally. I lubricated the finger with the shortest nail on it and slowly slid it into his anus. He enjoyed it so much that he asked for two fingers and then three. While doing this, I also alternated sucking and manually pumping his cock with my other hand. He had a mind-blowing orgasm. He tells me it's the kind you feel deep down to your toes.... I'm now looking for a strap-on that stimulates me as well as him!" *female age 40*

Some people believe only gay men enjoy anal stimulation. Yet straight men have rectums that are every bit as sensitive as those of gay men. While plenty of straight men would rather not have a dildo or butt plug up their rear, other manly guys enjoy the feeling. There are even straight adult video series titled *Bend Over Boyfriend* and *Babes Ballin' Boys*.

As for penetrating male partners anally, fingers that are well lubricated work incredibly well. Some women will use a dildo. Some even wear a dildo harness and propel it with their hips. A dildo harness looks somewhat like an athletic supporter. It holds the dildo in the same position as a man's erect penis. This allows the woman to thrust in and out, more or less. Learning how to use a dildo in a harness is an acquired art that takes time, patience, and practice. (If a harness is what you'd like, there are different kinds of dildo harnesses, including some that that strap to your thigh.)

When it comes to sex play, a man's anal sphincters need just as much practice and preparation as a woman's.

Prostate Stimulation

The only time most straight men get anal stimulation is during a physical exam, and this is more like a drive-by than an attempt to provide pleasure. Men who are curious about feeling their own prostate and who have a finger as long as ET's can do so by inserting a finger up their anus. Pressing on the prostate will probably cause a dull, subtle sensation in the penis. Some men find the physical contortions needed to reach their own prostate can ruin the

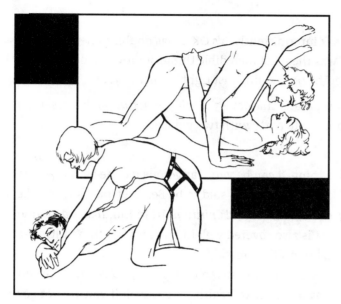

Positions for anal intercourse are the same as with vaginal intercourse. Some are more intimate and allow for the couple to kiss, while others provide better access to the clitoris or penis.

moment. To avoid this, you can purchase specially curved sex toys that help a guy to stimulate his prostate.

For more on stimulating the prostate gland, see Chapter 18: *The Prostate & The Male Pelvic Underground.*

Toy Precautions

Rectums are hungry orifices. Make sure that anything that goes up them is firmly anchored on the outside of the body so it can't get sucked up inside. Dildos or butt plugs with flared bases are best for anal play. Otherwise, you may need the assistance of an emergency-room crew to get them out.

Anything inserted into the rectum must be smooth with no points or ridges.

Anal beads resemble worry beads, but each bead is held in place on the string so it doesn't slide. While anal beads can be used to count your worries on, people usually stick them up their butt. They are slowly pulled out, often at the point of orgasm, which can make for a super-charged orgasm. Anal beads can be as small as mothballs or as big as golf balls. If the beads are plastic and have sharp blow-mold edges, file them down first. Also, it is wise to encase anal beads in a condom before inserting. That's because they are very difficult to clean.

Double Penetration

"I have had anal sex intermittently. It's OK. I was double penetrated twice and *THAT* was the most incredible thing, but it was a dangerous science to get the positioning just right." *female age 28*

The Guide has a separate Chapter 45 *Double Penetration*. It's essential reading if you are planning to party with two penises.

Anal Fisting

Yes, there is such a thing. It can be very dangerous if done by the inexperienced. The best book on the subject is said to be Bert Herrman's *Trust: The Hand Book—A Guide to the Sensual and Spiritual Art of Handballing,* Alamo Square Press. The subject is also covered well in Tristan Taormino's *Ultimate Guide to Anal Sex, 2nd edition,* Cleis Press.

It never hurts to check with a physician first, perhaps one who is recommended by your local gay and lesbian health center. Even if you are not gay, an LGBT center is more likely to know about the practice and will send you to a more fisting-friendly practitioner. There are also organized groups of fisters in large cities who sometimes offer talks and demonstrations.

When a Condom Gets Lost in the Dungeon of Doom?

According to the excellent book *Sex Disasters,* a condom lost up your rectum can go farther up than your partner can reach with his or her fingers. Not to worry, it will most likely come out the next time you have a bowel movement. However, if you are worried you will die from a condom up your crapper, call your healthcare provider or visit an ER.

As for a sex toy lost up your bum, this is a different story. Do not try to reach up and grab it, as you are likely to shove it farther up. If you can't squat and push it out, seek medical attention. Depending on the object, this can be a very serious situation.

Precautions for Anal Sex—A Recap

💡 Straight or gay, married or in transition—if you are doing anal intercourse, use a condom and LOTS of condom-friendly lube.

💡 Do not put anything up your rectum that has sharp edges or can break. Make sure that your nails are well-trimmed.

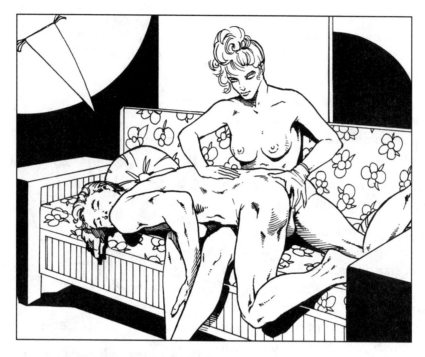

Using the forefinger instead of the middle finger allows for a deeper probe. If you use a middle finger, the knuckles on the index and ring fingers act as governors. They prevent it from going very deep.

💡 Use only sex toys that were designed for anal sex play.

💡 Make sure that anything about to go up your rectum is clean and well-lubricated. You may need to re-apply the lube often. That's because the rectum was designed to absorb fluids back into the body.

💡 Positions for anal intercourse are similar to those used with vaginal intercourse. Feeback is important. Discuss which positions and angles feel best with your partner.

💡 Remove anything you have placed in the rectum very slowly. This includes a penis.

💡 Don't stick a finger, penis or other object directly into a vagina when it's just been up an anus. Wash it first with soap and water.

💡 People who have anal intercourse should occasionally get a rectal swab done to check for sexually transmitted infections.

💡 Never, ever have anal sex unless your rectum is in 100% good health. Do not attempt anal sex if it is painful.

💡 Try not to hold your breath. Breathing deeply will help you relax.

💡 Once you get a finger, penis, or sex toy inside your partner's rear end, don't start thrusting with it. Leave it in place and gently start making circular motions. If and when your partner wants you to start thrusting, pull out slowly and add more lube. Then start thrusting slowly.

💡 Using a latex glove helps fingers slide in more smoothly. Using a condom helps a penis slide in more smoothly.

💡 Don't have anal sex when you are drugged or drunk. Your rear end is more easily damaged by sloppy sex than other parts of your body. Anal sex requires that the driver as well as the passenger be alert and sober.

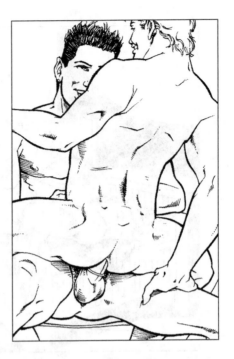

These young lads want to remind you to use condoms with anal sex, even if you are married and straight as a road through Kansas. Condoms help protect the prostate from infections, and they protect your bum from getting dangerous STIs.

💡 Do not use lubes like *Anal Ease* that numb your butt. This is the equivalent of unhooking the fire alarms in your home because you sometimes burn the toast.

💡 If you have medical questions about anal sex but are not comfortable speaking to your healthcare provider, call your local free clinic, LGBT center, or national sex hot line. If they can't answer the question, they should be able to find you a healthcare provider who you will be comfortable speaking to.

Anal Recreation Resources

See our video *Reality Check: Porn and Anal Sex* on the book's website at www.GuideToGettingItOn.com.

You won't find a better 25-minute video on anal sex than the *Guide To Anal Play for Women* by The Pleasure Mechanics. This video is HIGHLY recommended for any couple who is interested in anal stimulation. Their *Guide to Prostate Massage* is equally as good. Find out more on their website at www. PleasureMechanics.com.

Jack Morin's *Anal Pleasure and Health, A Guide for Men, Women and Couples*, 4th revised edition, Down There Press, (2010). Now in its 4th edition, many people that if you are having anal sex, this is one of THE books you should read. Individual who are having anal problems will also find *Anal Pleasure and Health* to be helpful. This book really does get you thinking about your anus in a different way, and if you have any kind of stress-related anal problem (especially hemorrhoids), reading it will be more than worthwhile.

Tristan Taormino's Ultimate Guide to Anal Sex for Women, 2nd edition, Cleis Press. This book is just as informative for men as for women. Tristan Taormino's infectious zeal and her zest for life and sex provide a welcome backdrop to all things anal. An excellent resource, well-organized and easy to read. Tristan is also the author of *The Anal Sex Position Guide: The Best Positions for Easy, Exciting, Mind-Blowing Pleasure* from Quiver.

The Ultimate Guide to Prostate Pleasure: A Guide for Men and Their Partners by Charlie Glickman, Clies Press, (2013). A very thoughtful and well-written look at this hidden but important part of male sexuality. Highly recommended for any man or couple who wants to explore the prostate and its potential for extra sexual pleasure.

Tickle My Tush: Mild-to-Wild Analplay Adventures for Everybooty, Tickle Kitty Press, (2012). Sadie Allison is one of the best "how-to sex" writers today. Her books achieve a rare combination of being fun, helpful and reader friendly.

For that little extra when playing with yourself,
visit the book's website:

www.GuideToGettingItOn.com

25
Playing with Yourself

Before the 1960s, people who wrote books on sex stated with an almost religious fervor that playing with yourself (masturbation) was a bad thing to do. Today, people who write books on sex speak with the same kind of religious fervor, only now they say that playing with yourself is a good thing to do.

It doesn't seem as though anything has changed. That's because none of the experts are asking you what you want to do. When it comes to the question of whether you should or shouldn't be masturbating, this book doesn't have any answers. It's your hand and your pants; if you want to stick one into the other, that's totally up to you.

What we can tell you is that as teenagers we felt certain that masturbation was an adolescent thing, something people get over when they become adults. That never happened.

There are times when people masturbate a lot, and times when they hardly do it at all; times when it feels great, and times when it's a letdown. But during those times when the world doesn't seem like such a nice place, masturbation can usually be counted on to help take some of the edge off. It also helps ease the transition between wakefulness and sleep. And contrary to what you might think, it will sometimes play an important role in relationships even when the sex between you and your partner is wonderful.

Some people find their bodies simply work better if they have an orgasm every day or two, with masturbation being a natural way to help this happen. Sometimes, you might find you get into a certain state of mind where you need to masturbate to relax enough to get your work done.

Whatever the motivation, if you are going to get yourself off by hand, why not try to get the most out of it? That is the focus of this chapter.

Wanking Protocol—When You Have A Roommate

Even if they're not particularly horny, a lot of people masturbate in bed at night to help turn their brains off. This can be especially necessary when you've had a full or stressful day and you need as much sleep as possible. Lying there awake just makes you feel more stressed.

Firing up a 30-amp vibrator or humping your teddy bear until his stuffing starts to explode is usually not a problem when you have your own room. But tender moments with yourself can be few and far between when you have a roommate. Add to this the fact that most of us would find it less embarrassing to be walked in on while we are having sex with a partner than when we are masturbating.

The usual solution is to wait quietly until your roommate is making sleeping noises. This is not as easy as it sounds, since your roommate is probably waiting for you to make sleeping noises as well. Fortunately, there are common-sense solutions they usually don't tell you about at your college orientation.

First, is to pull out your copy of *The Guide*, point to this page, and say to your roommate, "I wonder if we should talk about this?"

There are roommate situations where you'd rather be anally penetrated by a herd of buffaloes before talking about masturbation, but let's say your roommate is reasonable and has the same needs you do. So here are some solutions roommates in the past have found to be helpful. Some roommates are comfortable only adopting the first solution, others will whip it out together. It just depends.

 You agree to share with each other your class and work schedules, and if there is a change, you will notify your roommate, especially if a class was cancelled and you're returning early. A quick text, call or a long, loud series of knocks on the door accompanied by a thoughtful, "I can come back in ten minutes" shows consideration.

 You agree if you are leaving and won't be right back, to tell your roommate, "I'll be gone for at least ??? minutes." Don't come back before then unless it's totally necessary, in which case you'll knock loudly and wait to hear "Come in" before coming in.

 You agree that after the lights are out, it's fine to masturbate as long as you are reasonable about it. While it's usually impossible to be totally silent, one doesn't need to sound like a porn star, nor do you need to have porn blaring. (Even when you're using earbuds, porn can be annoying and distracting to roommates.)

 You agree it's okay to rub one out first thing in the morning while you are still in bed to help to tame a raging A.M. erection or to relieve a crippling case of sunrise horniness.

 You agree if one of you has a significant other at a different school or on a another planet, you will try to work out specific times when that person can be alone to message or be on the phone with his or her lover. That way, if they want to get themselves off while aided by the sound of their lover's voice or from the cam between his or her legs, there's no problem. However, this is a privilege that a less-than-sensitive roommate can easily abuse, so the one doing the phoning needs to be fair, reasonable and not overdue it.

 You agree if one of you is seeing a person who is abstinence-only to the extreme or not interested in sex—upon returning from an evening with this person, at least fifteen minutes of alone time will be provided in addition to heartfelt condolences.

Two things to avoid:

Masturbating while wearing earbuds or noise-cancelling cans, as you won't be able to hear your roommate's warning knock or keys in the door.

Never, ever masturbate in a bathroom stall unless it's in your own dorm and it's well understood that everyone does it. The problem with jerking off in a rest room stall is that it could be against the law and you could get busted if there's a sting operation going on. It doesn't matter if you have the stall door locked and are being discreet.

And finally:

Tissues and toilet paper remain the usual standbys for guys to masturbate into, although socks and dark-colored underwear are strong contenders.

For males who are wanking in the shower, do not leave a wad of your hair on the drain cover with chunks of clumpy spunk stuck to it. That's gross. Also, it's better to use hair conditioner for lube than soap, because soap can make your urethra burn. Unfortunately, while the conditioner may claim to add volume or thickness, your penis is not what they had in mind.

Vital Statistics on Fapping

The following was told to Harry Maurer by a young woman for his book *Sex: An Oral History,* Viking Press:

"My mother has a vibrator that my father gave her one year. When I used to come home from college, I knew where she kept the vibrator, and I knew they never used it, so I would put it into my room and use it for the vacation. One summer I came home and it wasn't there. I was going crazy, I'm really a vibrator addict. Finally I was just so horny I said, 'OK, Mom, sit down. Where's the vibrator?' She's like, 'What!' I said 'Look, here's the deal. I've been stealing your vibrator for three years, and I need it now.' She was blown away, but she goes into her room, comes back with the vibrator, and says, 'By the way, have you ever used the jet in the hot tub?'"

According to just about everyone who has ever researched the subject, somewhere between 80% and 95% of men eventually masturbate. Depending on whose statistics you look at, between 50% and 85% of women do it.

Contrary to what you might think, people don't masturbate any less as they get older. In fact, many people who are married or deeply involved in a sexual relationship still get themselves off by hand. Masturbation doesn't decrease a person's desire for shared sex. For some people, it increases it, and masturbate more when they are in a relationship rather than less.

How often do people masturbate? It varies from a couple of times a day to never. As for the number of orgasms per effort, researcher Thore Langfeldt interviewed children in Norway from kindergarten through high school. He found younger boys and girls could give themselves multiple orgasms when they masturbated. But as they got older, the boys started reporting fewer orgasms per attempt, while the girls reported more. This is a trend that continued with increased age and experience.

What the Sandman Knows about Masturbation

According to the Sandman, the most common time when people masturbate is at night before they go to sleep or before taking a nap.

Sometimes it feels good to masturbate after a workout. Plenty of people masturbate during a study break or when they have to spend long hours doing a paper or a project. It helps them to refocus. Some people masturbate before a date so they will be more intellectually present. Women sometimes masturbate during their periods to help relieve cramping, or before intercourse to help it feel better, or after. Some people wake up feeling horny. They might masturbate early in the morning, before having their Corn Flakes®.

Seriously Twisted Lunacy from Kellogg's of Battle Creek

Kellogg's Corn Flakes were created to give children more stamina so they wouldn't want to masturbate. John Harvey Kellogg, M.D., founder of the flake, believed that masturbation was "more immoral" than adultery. He called masturbation the "most heinous, revolting, and unnatural vice."

Kellogg proposed a six-point program for every American male that included taking cold enemas every day and wearing a wet girdle to bed at night to help prevent masturbation. His advice for parents whose children were caught masturbating included bandaging the genitals, covering them with cages and tying the child's hands together.

Dr. Kellogg, who was a prominent physician, recommended circumcision without anesthesia for boys who masturbated. He felt believed the pain would be a helpful punishment for the act that had been committed. Whatever foreskin was left should be sewn shut over the glans of the penis to keep the young man from having erections.

Kellogg was an interesting guy.

Dr. Kellogg's cereal is still known as "Kellogg's of Battle Creek." Battle Creek was the name of his mental asylum, where he served his special cold cereals to help keep the inmates from masturbating.

The finest medical minds of the day couldn't quite agree on the specific horrors that masturbation would cause. Some claimed it caused a man to become feeble, lackluster, feminized, impotent and to have underdeveloped genitals. Others claimed it had the opposite effect, turning young men into sex fiends who would have uncontrolled eruptions of lust and would blow the family fortune on prostitutes. Ads in popular papers promised to cure "the excesses of youth" and "underdeveloped genitals," which were what happened if you masturbated.

To keep Dr. Kellogg spinning in his grave, this book encourages its readers to occasionally masturbate while eating a bowl of Kellogg's Corn Flakes.

Men & Masturbation

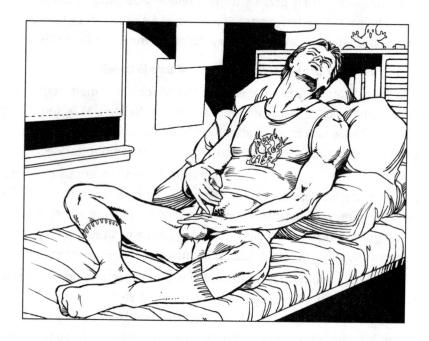

How Guys Learn

"When I was ten, an older friend showed me how to masturbate. He had a full ejaculation, but nothing came out of my penis. I believed technology could fix anything. So I decided to create a jack-off machine. Planning and building it kept me busy for days. But it didn't make anything more come out of my penis. Time, rather than technology, was the answer to that problem." *male age 45*

Males often learn to masturbate from friends, porn or a big brother. Or they learn on their own. That's because a teenager has to be pretty numb to himself to miss the connection between soaping his penis in the shower and the nice feelings that result. Also, when lying face down on a mattress with a hard-on, most guys are eventually compelled to hump or rub. More than other human organs, the penis pleads to be yanked, stroked and squeezed. (Anyone who has raised a daughter in a non-repressive environment might disagree, saying that girls can give their clitorises a pretty good work out.)

If they haven't seen porn before having their first ejaculation, some guys will experience concern or terror the first time they produce semen, e.g., "Oh no, I broke something!" or "I promise I'll never ever do it again! Just make it OK." Then they do it again the next day.

Today's pre-teen males who are raised on porn might have the opposite concern, "Mine doesn't squirt, what's with this?"

The Group Thing

"I can understand all sorts of things about guys' sexuality, except why they jerk off together. It seems so gay. Why do they do it?"
female age 23

Good question. The majority of men will tell you that they have never jerked off with another male. For those who have, it may have to do with the maturation process. Most young guys need little encouragement to take their pants off and explore. Getting naked can be so exciting for some boys they get hard-ons from that alone. It's also natural for boys to share experiences, whether it's checking out an abandoned house or cave or showing each other what you do with your dick. You would want to show your best friend the latest skateboard trick, so why wouldn't you want to jerk off together?

"When we became teens, some of us boys would get together for a masturbation meeting in the tree house, but it was more the thrill of something exciting and forbidden than anything else. *male, 26*

Plenty of men will say, "No way. You'd never catch me jerking off with another guy when I was a kid." Others will say, "Sure, that's how we did it."

Some males have circle jerks where they stand around and masturbate. There might be games connected with this, like who shoots the farthest or who comes the fastest (it's interesting how priorities change as you get older). It's even been said that some young men feel excluded until they have been allowed to beat off with members of the local gang.

The urge to beat off together seems to peak before high-school age and drops off significantly after that. However, there are some adult males who are straight and who enjoy masturbating together. This isn't as much of a contradiction in terms as it seems. Straight men enjoy watching other men ejaculate in porn. So it's okay to watch another guy's ejaculation if he's with a woman in porn, but not acceptable if it's two guys together?

The following answers to a survey in the newsletter *Sex & Health* help to summarize some of what's involved:

> "While partying with fraternity brothers, someone suggested a contest to see who could ejaculate the farthest. Each of the five of us took our turn in a tiled shower room. Surprisingly, the least endowed among us won!"

> "Sometimes when I'm camping with a couple of my buddies and our girlfriends are otherwise occupied, we get to joking about sex. We soon get so aroused that when one of us whips it out to pee, we start joking and the others whip theirs out, too. Then we just start stroking ourselves and talking about our favorite techniques. We don't touch each other, but we do comment on each other's members and may cheer one another on to climax. We're all good friends and have become much closer sharing our sexuality this way."

Sex & Health had a large male readership, with 95% of the men characterized themselves as totally straight. Most were married and many had children. Still, a number reported fantasizing about masturbating with other men, e.g., "Although I'm happily married with two children, I do sometimes fantasize about masturbating with friends. I've thought about asking one friend in particular, but I haven't had the nerve."

Guy Tricks—"First, Nuke a Jar of Miracle Whip, Then..."

> "I made a false pussy out of bicycle tire inner tubes, and it worked quite well. I have also used banana peels, watermelons, and a hole in a piece of wood." *male age 42*

Most men use their hands to jerk off with. Some do it dry and some add lubrication which includes saliva, soap, hair conditioner, Vaseline, vegetable oil, coconut oil, baby oil, baby oil gel, and anything else under the sun that can make their penis slick. (See Chapter 12: *Sex Lubes—A New View* for a list of products men use for masturbation.)

A lot of men masturbate in the shower. Hair conditioner works well for lube. If you must use soap, start each stroke by grabbing your penis around the base and pulling outward only. Soap is not a friend of the peehole.

Another way that men sometimes masturbate is by lubricating the inside of a condom with a water-based lube like KY. They slide a condom on their, wrap their fingers around it and pump away. A variation of this is to lube up the inside of a Baggie or plastic bag and put it between your pillows or mattress and box springs. You then get on your knees and hump the bag. Be careful not to get your mattress pregnant.

Banana peels can come in handy. If you are having trouble with the peel falling apart and condoms are plentiful, try putting a condom over the peel. If you make an artificial vagina and heat it in a microwave, be careful. Microwaves heat unevenly.

Foreskin Tricks for Men Who Are Uncut

Fill a turkey baster or syringe with warm water. Pull your foreskin over the head of your penis and crimp it with your fingers over the end of the turkey baster. As you gently squeeze the end of the turkey baster, the warm water fills your foreskin and causes it to balloon out. Then let go of the bulb and the baster sucks up the water. Keep repeating until you come.

Another unusual method is to keep the foreskin retracted. Tug the foreskin lightly by pulling it down toward your scrotum. This will cause it to become taut. Keep repeating this until you come. It will take a while, but might be pretty intense. (Thanks to JackinWorld.com for these suggestions.)

Rushin' Roulette (for Men)

Guys tend to rush themselves when they are masturbating. There are reasons for this.

 A man often wants to get to the heavy-duty pleasure part as soon as possible.

 There is the matter of privacy, or lack of it. The last thing most guys want is for someone to walk in on them when they are stroking, so they teach themselves to come quickly and quietly. (Privacy is often in short supply when you are growing up, and then later, when you have children of your own.)

 If a guy takes a really long shower, most everybody knows what he is doing. Also, the extra speed helps you finish before the hot water runs out.

Learning to Live in the Zone of Subtle Sensation

Taking extra time when masturbating might help a man learn about subtle sensations that he won't notice if he's always red-lining it. If he slows down as ejaculation approaches, he might discover a rush of feelings in his stomach, bladder, or rectum. Instead of going for the big squirt, he might try to back off a bit, teaching himself how to live in the zone of subtle sensation. If allowed to emerge slowly, pre-squirt feelings can be intense and last for long periods of time without becoming an actual ejaculation. Learning to stay with these feelings might help a man experience deeper levels of intimacy when he is with a partner.

Instead of reaching for his crotch each time he masturbates, a man might start by touching or massaging other parts of his body: scalp, face, neck, shoulders, chest, hands, feet, etc. This can be a way of reminding himself that sex is a full-body activity rather than something that just happens between his legs. (One female reader says this section should have been written for women as well as men.)

Intercourse Spoilers

Grip of Death Guys tend to grip themselves tightly when masturbating. Yet few vaginas come close to generating this kind of squeezing action. This might be why some men have more intense orgasms when they masturbate than during intercourse. You might try masturbating with a lighter grip, at least occasionally.

Face Down It has been said that men who always masturbate face down can have erection problems or trouble reaching an orgasm when trying to have sex with women. If you masturbate face down and are having and are having these kinds of problems, try to limit your jerking off to sunny side up. If you masturbate face down, have good erections and are able to come when you and your partner would like, have a good laugh over this section.

We have a video on the bizarre "No Fap" movement
at www.GuideToGettingItOn.com

Women & Masturbation

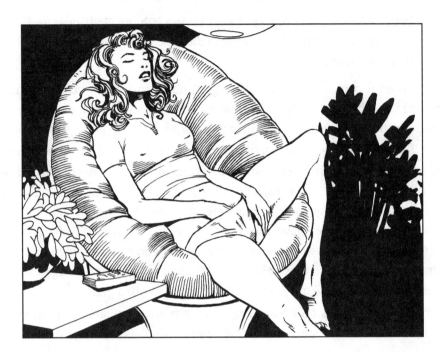

It is every bit as normal and natural for girls or women to masturbate as it is for boys or men. Unfortunately—and possibly do to the abomination of abstinence-based sex education—a number of young women today do not feel it is normal and natural for women to masturbate. This is both sad and incorrect. It is fine if you masturbate, and fine if you don't.

How Girls Learn

"It was my freshman year of high school. I was kissing this guy and was getting really turned on. He put his hand on my inner thigh and I was going crazy! This was my first heavy petting session. I didn't quite know what to make of it. When I got home, I went to the bathroom. My underwear was very wet. I went to touch myself and BAM!—instant orgasm! My very first. I've never had it that easy since." *female age 27*

"When I was young, climbing a flagpole always brought on such intense tingling feelings that I was only able to hold on tight and my legs would clamp around the pole. When the feelings subsided enough, I would resume climbing." *female age 37*

"When I had my first orgasm I kept saying, 'Oh my God!' over and over. I was really shocked because I didn't know I could do that to myself!" *female age 25*

When it comes to masturbation, girls don't do "show and tell" nearly as often as boys. They tend to learn about masturbation on their own or by reading about it or seeing women do it in porn.

Some women learn how to masturbate from the sensation they experience while bathing, from climbing trees, poles, or ropes, while on swings or when riding bicycles. Some learn by putting a pillow between their legs or by leaning up against the washing machine when it's on the spin cycle. It might also happen when they have a sex dream—the sensation is still alive in their genitals when they wake up and all they need to do is reach down and rub. One woman learned to masturbate by pushing a sanitary napkin against her vulva; another by stroking the shaft of her clitoris with a pencil.

The possibilities for discovering how to masturbate are too numerous to name, but here are some of the ways women readers say they do it now:

"Bathtub, vibrator, boyfriend's fingers (my own don't work). Electric toothbrush handle, my ex-husband's hammer (the handle), even celery once." *female age 26*

"I get the most intense orgasm by leaning on a hard surface like a counter and wiggling around till I come. I also use a dildo, and I use my fingers to massage my labia and clit, occasionally fingering my vagina." *female age 37*

"Occasionally I use my hands, but usually I use a running faucet before I take my bath." *female age 19*

"I rub my clit in a circular motion with my fingers or use a trusty old vibrator. I've tried putting things inside my vagina, but so far that's been a very neutral experience — I need my lover's hand or torso to be attached to what's going inside. Sometimes I gently rub my chest as I masturbate, or run a soft piece of cloth over my nipples."

female age 47

"I use a finger, then fingers." *female age 49*

"I do it while reading a book or having a fantasy. Usually I stimulate my clit directly with one or more fingers. Only rarely do I put anything inside my vagina, although I do like the feel of a tampon. I also like anal stimulation. That will make an orgasm more intense and more diffused." *female age 36*

It would require a database to list all of the ways that women masturbate. A lot of women use their fingers while lying on their backs or sitting in chairs. Some do it on their sides, or while lying face down so nobody can see what they are doing. Some women may even occasionally prefer to squat.

See Chapter 15: "The Zen of Finger Fucking" for a four-page spread on nine finger techniques women commonly use when they masturbate.

Men sometimes have the fantasy that a woman who is masturbating sticks her fingers inside her vagina. Some women do, but many don't. Instead, they might squeeze the lips of their vulva together or push against it in ways that create pressure rather than penetration. A woman who has responsive nipples may make nipple stimulation part of her masturbation.

Plenty of women use lubrication when they masturbate, either their own (vaginal or saliva) or store-bought. Lots like to use vibrators for masturbating, and some use dildos.

Bathtub Faucets

Some women like to masturbate by using the faucet in the bathtub. After they get the water temperature just right, they lie down in the tub and push their bum against the wall of the tub where the faucet comes out. It might help to have an inflatable pillow to put under their rear to get the angle just right. Some women say it works better if they spread their labia open with their fingers so the water cascades onto their awaiting clitoris.

Water Safety When masturbating with a water jet in a hot tub, sit back at a distance. The current might be stronger than you think, so approach slowly. Some women like to pull their labia apart; others don't. Do not get extremely close to the jet, and don't aim it up your vagina or rectum.

Additional Ways

There are women who can have an orgasm by doing stomach crunches (mini sit-ups). What an incentive for keeping your abs in shape! Other women get off by humping pillows or water bottles, swinging on swings, tugging on underwear, rubbing up against things, using peeled cucumbers, and riding a bike down bumpy roads. Some like to stimulate their anus, either by putting pressure on it or by sticking a finger or butt plug inside it. Some like to look in mirrors, some get turned on by wearing their boyfriend's shirt or underwear. Fill in your own blanks.

Straight to an Orgasm, or Making a Night of It?

"In my younger years, it usually took an hour or so before I had an orgasm. Now, if I'm especially hot, five minutes with a vibrator can do it, or about fifteen to twenty minutes by hand. Sometimes I like to keep things slow; I prolong it by starting and stopping. Other times, I just want to get off as fast as I can. Sometimes I masturbate, but not to orgasm. It feels good and relaxes me without wanting to come." *female age 47*

One woman might masturbate on and off for an entire evening, reaching between her legs every page or two while reading a book. Another woman might masturbate with the sole purpose of reaching a single, discrete orgasm, going from beginning to end without pause.

That's one of the really nice things about masturbation—especially women's masturbation. There are no rules for how it needs to be.

Women, Masturbation & Intercourse

While intercourse remains the most popular sex act for couples, far more men than women have orgasms from intercourse. A woman is much more likely to have an orgasm from masturbation than intercourse.

Even more interesting is that women who have orgasms during intercourse often need extra clitoris stimulation while their partner is thrusting. They usually do this with their fingers or by grinding their clitoris into a partner' pubic bone. While this is not technically masturbation, it is certainly masturbation adjacent.

Also, it's not unusual for a woman to masturbate before intercourse to help her genitals get more into it, or after intercourse because she wants more stimulation or enjoys the feeling. It is unfortunate that women often hide this and assume their partners wouldn't want to know. It seems like a sign of a good relationship when a woman feels free to finish what we aren't able to, or when we help her get started and she takes it from there.

Tennis Elbow? Say It Ain't So!

Tennis elbow is a form of tendonitis. A female physician suspects that some of her patients with tennis elbow did not get their tendonitis from playing tennis, but from the number-one repetitive finger motion that many women do: masturbation.

If you are a woman who is experiencing tendonitis or repetitive-stress syndrome in the arm you masturbate with, try using a vibrator for masturbation and see if the problem doesn't improve. Ditto for males who routinely masturbate their female partners.

Men with tennis elbow or tendonitis in the same arm they fap with might try switching methods, unless you are ambidexterous, then just switch arms. If you do it dry, use lube. The hand motion can be quite different. Or try using a masturbation sleeve or sex toy you can thrust into with your hips instead of using your arm.

Thigh High

A woman who contributes to the women's section at JackinWorld.com suggests women can teach themselves to come by squeezing their thighs together. She suggests you start by masturbating as you normally would, but press your thighs together when you start to have an orgasm. After a few weeks of doing this, masturbate to the point where you almost have an orgasm, but pull your fingers away at the last minute and try to finesse yourself into orgasm by squeezing your thighs together. Once you are able to do this successfully, start with the thigh-squeezing action a little earlier each time. Some women might prefer doing this with tight jeans on so they get an assist from the seam in front.

Girls, Their Horses & the Fifty-Minute Hour

"My first orgasm? I was riding my horse and I felt a strange sort of pleasure between my legs. I felt like I wanted it to stop so I could concentrate on my riding, but it felt so good." *female age 18*

"I was standing in the barn with my horse when I had a spontaneous orgasm. I gushed and everyone laughed at me for peeing in my pants. I was fourteen or so. I didn't discover masturbation until I was twenty, and then I thought orgasm was so incredible, I wanted one every day." *female age 37*

"My first orgasm ever was when I was riding a horse. I thought I was perverted and never told anyone. Then at a slumber party one of my close friends who also horseback rides admitted that she'd had a similar experience." *female age 18*

Having grown up close to livestock, your author knew from a young age that it was unwise for any man to come between a woman and her horse. But can you imagine his amazement years later when an occasional female patient would describe the euphoria she gleaned from the back of her favorite horse? It's information that's usually relayed in hushed tones of revelry and delight—warm, pleasing, primal sensations with one of nature's more magnificent creatures between her legs. Women rarely speak about their husbands or boyfriends with the kind of knowing sensitivity that is reserved for their favorite horse.

Fingers Over Your Panties or Inside?

When most women masturbate, they use their fingers most of the time. While most women who use their fingers make direct contact with their genitals, it's not unusual for women to masturbate with their fingers over their underwear.

Some say it reduces chafing to masturbate with their fingers outside of their underwear. Others say it helps because their clitoris is too sensitive. Some do it because that's how they first learned, and it feels best that way. And some women might do it as a compromise, telling themselves that masturbating with their fingers on the outside makes it not quite so dirty or nasty as truly touching themselves might.

Rub the Nub? Beat the Bush? Giving Girl-Masturbation a Name

There are numerous slang terms for male masturbation. This is not the case with female masturbation (Diddle? Jill off? She Bop? These are not universal terms). Since women don't usually masturbate together, they haven't needed to establish slang to convey what they are doing. It has only been during the last couple of decades that our society has openly acknowledged the existence of women's masturbation. Perhaps one of the women's magazines could have a contest...

The Limitations of a One-Grip Rhythm (for Both Sexes)

If you always use the exact same touch and rhythm when you masturbate, you might be teaching your body to expect that and only that. Given how it's difficult for someone else to do you in precisely the same way that you do yourself, you might consider occasionally mixing it up.

On Sucking Air (for Both Sexes)

Learning to breathe right is an essential part of being an athlete, unless your sport is billiards. It's no different with sex.

When you are having sex, be it solo or with a partner, you might occasionally pay attention to your breathing. Tantric types encourage taking long, slow, deep breaths where you imagine pulling the air all the way into your groin. This may help some people have a more intense experience.

Warnings

URETHRA SAFETY WHEN SOUNDING See "sounds" in the glossary. Some people, both men and women, are tempted to stick things up their urethra (pee hole) as a form of sex play. This is known as *urethral play* or *sounding*. If you don't know what you are doing, this can result in an embarrassing visit to an emergency room and maybe even require surgery. If you must try sounding, do lots of research on how to do it as safely as possible.

BUTTHOLE SAFETY Some men and women enjoy sticking things up their buttholes when they play. For info, please see Chapter 24: *Up Your Bum.*

BAGGING and EROTIC ASPHYXIATION Bagging or erotic asphyxiation is VERY DANGEROUS. Bagging is masturbating while chocking yourself. There is no safe way to do it. It is discussed in Chapter 46: *Kinky Corner.*

Give Porn a Rest!

Try not to sell your soul to the producers of porn by always using porn to masturbate with. Jerking off to your own fantasies that you have created in your mind is one of the nicer things in life. While porn will not damage most people, there's something wrong about always using the extreme visual input of porn for masturbation. Enjoy fapping to the images, fantasies and sexual scenarios that are your mind's own creations.

Readers' Comment Quiz

Guess which answers are men's and which are women's.

Have you ever needed to masturbate while away from home?

a. "I have done so occasionally in the car, while driving. Tricky, but doable."
    age 37

b. "I would pretty much masturbate anywhere if I could. I know it sounds silly, but when I am on the beach or catching a killer wave I get kind of horny." *age 23*

c. "Yes. Although never at my current job, I have masturbated at work."
    age 26

d. "Yes. I've masturbated driving in my car; the urge was just too great and I had to deal with it right then." *age 36*

e. "It has happened. I feel pressure like I'll go nuts if I don't get relief, and I'll sneak off." *age 38*

f. "Except for when I was on a long vacation, I've always been able to wait until I got home." *age 26*

g. "One time I was driving and I had a terrible urge, so I brought myself to orgasm. I've also done it at work once." *age 43*

h. "I was once on a long-distance bus trip and a teenage boy was next to me. I don't remember why, but I got very aroused, so I put my coat over me and masturbated while he slept." *age 45*

i. "While my partner lived in a different city, I would masturbate all the time. I would lock myself in the bathroom and put my feet on the wall while sitting on the toilet, with my legs bent and above my head. It was most satisfying this way." *age 37*

j. "I was using the computer at my brother's house when no one was home. While online, I was chatting to someone who was so hot that I had to masturbate to release enough tension so I could keep chatting." *age 27*

26

Oscillator, Generator Vibrator & Dildo

It used to be "sex toy" meant getting yourself a vibrator or dildo. Vibrators were one of the first electric machines created back in the 1800s. They have been a hit ever since. Other sex toys include sleeves for male masturbation, supplies for people who are into BDSM, toys for anal sex, harnesses, dildos in countless shapes and materials, and more.

While sex-toy aficionados will call this blasphemy, please remember there are lots of people who don't use sex toys and still have wonderfully fun sex lives. Plenty of women prefer their fingers to vibrators. And sex toy retailers might not appreciate this book's emphasis on sex toys that tap into your imagination rather than your pocketbook.

Instead of being a fluff piece in favor of sex toys, this chapter looks at what might—and might not—make a sex toy sexy. It covers sex toy safety and sex toy use in relationships. It describes how to size a dildo, and what to do when a partner might feel threatened by your vibrator or dildo.

Sex Toy Strategy, Part 1

Before investing money in the latest sex toy or getting your hopes up that the hype is real, why not think about what it is you want a sex toy to do for you? If you are trying to get a sex toy for a partner, what are some of the things that turn him or her on? If your gift doesn't resonate with a lover's fantasies, it will probably end up being just another buzzing piece of plastic or a suggestive *whatever* without any sexual oomph.

Another thing to ask yourself is, "Would my partner prefer flowers and the latest book by her favorite author?" "Would he like it better if I got him a new computer gizmo or brake cable for his mountain bike rather than this strange looking sex toy that he's supposed to stick up his ass?"

Let's say you are a woman who is trying to rev up her partner's interest. You could always buy him the latest vagina-like sex toy that he sticks his penis into. Forget that it might feel like the vagina of a dead woman. The websites that are selling it claim it's even better than blow-up dolls! Or you could take a smarter approach that's outlined in next section "Sex Toy Strategy, Part 2."

Over the years we have tried a $1200 sex-toy device that had nothing on a $30 vibrator. We also tried a $600 male masturbating device that made you appreciate how good your own hand feels. Just because it's supposed to be great doesn't mean it's great for you or your partner.

Sex Toy Strategy, Part 2

You might find that the perfect sex toy for your lover is one that you use on yourself. Perhaps he'll be turned on by watching you use it. Or make a deal with your partner: she selects a toy for you to use on her, and you select a toy for her to use on you. Then go shopping together. The neat thing about using toys in this way is they help you reveal new things about yourself to your partner, and vice versa. Sex can get boring when you think you know all there is to know about the person you are sleeping with.

Beware the Phthalates

Not long ago, Greenpeace issued a warning that sex toys put off a dangerous class of chemicals known as "phthalates." Did Greenpeace fear that schools of dildo-using dolphins were in danger? No. They were worried about humans. Very worried.

Phthalates have been linked to liver damage, kidney damage, lung damage, and damage to the developing testes in the fetus. Phthalates are added to plastics to increase their flexibility. They are used to create favorite sex-toy materials such as Cyberskin, Softskin and Futurotic. Phathalates put the jelly in jelly rubber sex toys.

Do not buy sex toys from dealers who are not highly reputable, or who won't certify their toys have no phthalate residues. Hard plastic toys usually do not contain phthalates, nor do 100% silicone toys or dildos made of glass or steel. The trouble with silicone is that it doesn't need to be 100% silicone to be called silicone. So you are at the mercy of the seller.

As for the "quick fix" of putting a condom between you and your phthalate-containing sex toy, the amount of phthalates in a number of sex toys has been described by researchers as being so high as to be "off the charts." A condom may decrease your exposure, but it won't eliminate it.

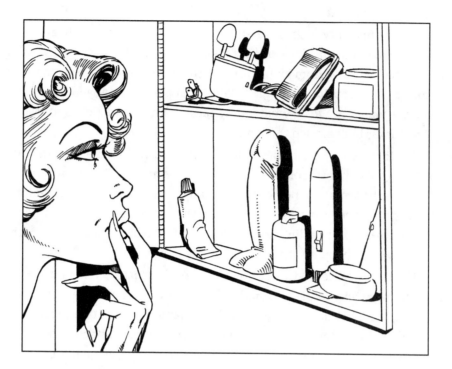

Books, DVDs & Websites

If you are going to get something sexy, why not search out some cool videos that the two of you could watch? Check out sites where the staff carefully reviews the videos and only carries what they consider to be the best.

There's a world of erotic books and literature that you and your partner can read together or to each other. Collections of short stories by competent writers abound. Some will get you going, others will fall short, but it's nowhere near as bleak as it used to be. A collection of erotic short stories might be the best sex toy you ever gave or got.

Another thing to consider is getting some of the wonderful how-to videos from The Pleasure Mechanics. These are some of the best how-to videos on sex we have ever seen. They are great for couples. We shudder to think how much more sexual pleasure there would be in the world if every eighteen-year-old were given these videos to watch. You can preview them at www.ThePleasureMechanics.com. Also visit www.erospirit.com, which is dedicated to sexual pleasure and has been for many years.

Creative & Low Cost

There are plenty of great sex-toy substitutes that cost hardly anything. You can make coupons that you give your partner. Each lists a special thing you are willing to do, from giving your partner a bath and full-body massage to things we can't print even in *The Guide*. Your partner gives you the coupon when she wants you to do what it describes. (Author Laura Corn's *101 Nights of Great Sex* is built around this concept.)

Another idea is for each of you to describe a scene that is a personal turn-on. Then go shopping for props to make the scene happen. For instance, if one of you has the fantasy of being stopped and frisked by an officer in uniform, you can go to a used-clothing store and buy the perfect uniform for acting out the scene, perhaps including handcuffs. If the fantasy concerns a visit to the doctor, do your shopping at a medical-supply house.

If you don't like that idea, try surprising your partner with a sex toy that's found at your local pet store. When your lover comes home, you can be standing there naked with your new dog collar around your neck; hand her the leash and say, "I'm yours for the night!" Don't forget to attach a bow to the collar, like they do at the fancy pet groomers, and hope she didn't bring her parents home for a surprise visit.

Penis and Breast Casting Kits—The Best Sex Toys Ever?

Consider making a mold and stunning sculpture of your partner's penis or breasts!

During this mostly magnificent and often hilarious sex-toy adventure, you will be creating an exact replica of your partner's penis. Imagine his excitement if you use the finished casting of his penis on yourself, or proudly place it on your bookshelf. (As for putting it on your desk at work, maybe not such a good idea. Then again...) It's also something to consider if he's about to be deployed, or you have a distance relationship.

What about making an art-quality casting of your partner's breasts or entire torso?

You can find kits that are specially designed to mold and make castings of the penis or breasts at www.artmolds.biz (.biz not .com). Under "Lifecasting Kits" look for the "Intimate Kit" and "My Breast Friends" or "Full Torso" kits The penis kit even includes skin and hair release cream—which could be the most important part!

Oscillators, Generators, Vibrators and Dildos

Some people claim the light bulb is the most important electrical invention of the last 130 years; others say it's the vibrator. The rest of this chapter is about vibrators and dildos. Its emphasis is on the use of these devices by couples as opposed to individuals, although many people use them for solo sex.

If what you want is a vibrator, dildo or butt plug, the people who work at reputable sex-toy stores try them out themselves and are pretty conscientious about what they will and won't sell.

Also, just because a lot is written in this chapter about vibrators, please don't view this as an endorsement for them. Fingers usually work just fine, and a lot of women prefer them.

Confusing Vibrators with Dildos

People often confuse the vibrator with the dildo, which is like confusing a rhino with a giraffe. Both are native to the bush, but that's where the similarities end.

Vibrators are valued for their buzzing properties and are usually rested on the surface of the genitals rather than placed inside them, although there are newer "rabbit" hybrids for both vibration and insertion.

Dildos are penis-shaped and are used as such. Most don't vibrate like a vibrator, but are made to be kept inside the vagina to give a feeling of fullness or to be thrust in and out. Women can also slide them up and down between the lips of their vulva, which can be a very satisfying way of stimulating the entire vulva including the lips and clitoris.

The common battery-operated plastic vibrator is sometimes thought of as a dildo. While some women use them as such, the vibrating part of these devices is usually located on the tip, which means a woman can't insert it deeply inside her vagina and expect it to keep her clitoris happy. These are also made of hard plastic. Some of them don't pack much of a wallop compared to the more adequately appointed AC models. Most of these novelty devices aren't in the same league as a well-made dildo or vibrator, although highly devoted users will disagree.

Some Men Worry

Most guys have no problem with a partner who uses sex toys; many find the situation a turn-on. However, some males worry their lover will start to prefer the vibrator or dildo to them. Some believe it means they aren't hung well enough or can't deliver the goods. This isn't necessarily true.

Some men are particularly confused when their partner says she loves having intercourse with them, but prefers a dildo that's bigger than they are. Because a woman totally controls the dildo play, she can go with tighter specs on a dildo than a real-life penis. Sex with a partner is more athletic, so she may prefer a penis that isn't as big as her dildo for actual lovemaking.

If he is a considerate, caring, real flesh-and-blood guy, most women will still want a real-life partner regardless of how often they fire up their magic wand. It's hard to have a meaningful conversation with a dildo, and no vibrator has ever played catch with the kids or gotten up in the middle of the night to feed the baby. Also, you can't cuddle up next to sex toys after you have an orgasm—not that you can with all men, either.

In purchasing a new vibrator or dildo, a woman who is in a relationship should consider making her partner part of the selection process. This way, her partner won't feel left out resentful or inadequate. On the other hand, good luck getting a guy to attend a sex-toy party.

Perhaps it might not hurt to show your partner this chapter, which encourages men to take pride in a woman's sex toys. It might also help to let him know that women who buy vibrators and dildos are often extremely happy with their flesh and blood sex partners.

Making Friends with Your Lover's Toys

There's no point in feeling at odds with your partner's vibrator or dildo. If you are a man and your partner orders a new sex toy, ask her to show you how she uses it. Hold her tight while she's getting herself off with it. If she has a vibrator, why not let her use it on you? Men might like the feel of a vibrator on their perineum (space behind their scrotum) better than on their penis.

Would your partner like to use her vibrator during intercourse? Some couples find the sensations during intercourse to be sensational.

It's even possible to combine vibrator play with oral sex. The man pushes a small battery-operated vibrator against the bottom of his tongue while the tip of his tongue is touching his partner's clitoris. Or you can place a dildo in her vagina or gently push it in and out of your lover's vagina while planting wet kisses on her clitoris. With plenty of feedback and a willingness to explore, you and a partner can have lots of fun with the right sex toys.

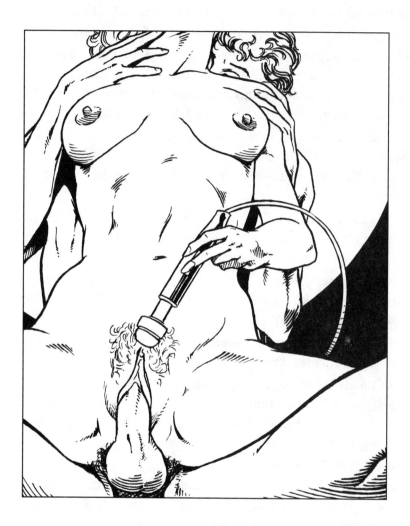

Vibrator Details

Here are some vibrator facts:

Coil vs. Wand When it comes to vibrators that plug into the wall, there are two different types: wandlike vibrators with longer bodies and large heads, and coil vibrators with compact heads. Each type delivers a unique sensation. Coil vibrators are smaller and very quiet. Their sensations tend to be more localized. The more popular wand vibrators are bigger and make a distinct humming noise. Newer models are rechargeable and will hum for up to an hour per charge. Some come with two heads instead of one.

Between the Lips vs. On the Clit: Women who use vibrators with a large head, such as the Magic Wand, often prefer to place the head between their labia near to the opening of their vagina as opposed to higher up on their clitoris. This helps vibrate the structures inside their pelvis, and saves the glans of the clitoris from a degree of stimulation that can be painful.

First-Time Users If you are new to a vibrator, use it on the lowest possible speed while you learn to navigate the head around your pubic bone. Some new users have bruised their pubic bones by placing the head of a vibrator on a bony pelvis.

Sensation Levels Some users like the sensations full blast; others like to muffle the vibrator with a towel or even a pillow. Some hold the vibrator in a way that allows their fingers to transfer the vibrations.

Hands Some vibrators strap on the back of your hand. Your fingers deliver the vibrations. These can be great fun to use, but they do tend to numb out your hand.

Fingers There are tiny vibrators that fit on your finger. They are incredibly small and almost unnoticeable.

No Hands Some women rest a vibrator between their legs so they can use their hands for other things such as holding a book, playing with their breasts if they enjoy breast stimulation, touching a partner's body, or channel surfing. There are special harnesses which can hold the head of a vibrator snugly between your legs.

Joni's Butterfly This is a small vibrator with built-in straps that hold it in place. It can be worn during intercourse, at work, on a date or wherever a woman might want to get a private buzz in a public place.

Positions Unlike men, vibrators are meant to be abused. Try different positions with it on top of you, you on top of it, and as you lie on your side.

Vibrator Vacations People sometimes worry a woman will become used to the vibrator and want only that. If you are concerned, take vibrator vacations for one week every month.

Attachments There are a number of vibrator attachments for both coil and wand vibrators. These can deliver a finger of vibration anywhere you want.

Vibrators and Airport Security

When viewed through X-ray, vibrators can resemble detonating devices on bombs. Airport security will make you open up purses, briefcases and suitcases that have vibrators in them. Resist informing them about what your vibrator does and doesn't detonate.

Vibrators and Men

Some boys learned that leaning their genitals into dad's hand-held vibrating sander could result in an easy orgasm. Just about anything around the house that vibrates will eventually find a young man leaning against it to see how it feels.

Given how many times the average male masturbates during his lifetime, it makes a certain amount of sense to try out a couple of sex toys made for that purpose. Some are interesting, most are disappointing. Many are nowhere near as convenient as using your own hand.

There is an attachment for certain types of vibrators called a come cup which fits over the head of the penis. (Be sure to lube up the cup first.) To make a come cup of your own, push the head of a vibrator against your hand as it is holding your penis. Some men wrap a vibrator with a towel and lean into it. The towel helps to muffle the sensation, so you're not left with a numb penis and no orgasm.

Dildos

Vibrators have become so socially acceptable that even Walmart and Target display them, although the boxes show women using them on their necks or calves. With dildos, there are fewer options for subterfuge and denial. Big stores would be hard-pressed to advertise that dildos help relax tense muscles, although they clearly do. And if people hear a woman say the word "dildo" in a public place, they are more likely to think that she is referring to a former lover or a politician than to an object that gives her pleasure.

After reading the next couple of pages, you won't be left in the dark about dildos, even if people often use them in the dark.

Dildo vs. Penis

The human penis, when fully anchored to the male crotch, imposes limitations upon a woman's sexual pleasure that the silicone dildo does not. A penis can't be radically flipped upside down without requiring a trip to the hospital for the man whose body it was attached to. There is also the matter of hardness: the male penis isn't always hard when a woman wants it hard, nor for as long as she might desire. And finally, a penis is not like a car that you can trade in every couple of years. Even if her partner's penis might not be the best size and shape to fit her psyche or anatomy, a married woman is pretty well glued to it till death or divorce. Fortunately a woman needn't ditch the man she loves because she prefers an SUV-type penis when nature gave him a Mini Cooper. She can purchase a dildo instead.

In Search of the Perfect Dildo

Dildos are made from a large variety of materials, including jade, acrylic, alabaster, latex, leather, glass, brass and wood. However, the most highly regarded dildo material is usually silicone. Silicone has a soft but firm texture with a smooth surface that is durable and easy to clean, although it doesn't stand up to cuts too well. The silicone material also warms up rather nicely, which is an added plus unless you like cold things in your vagina.

Since there is a fair amount of craftsmanship involved in producing a high-quality dildo, be sure to purchase dildos from places that carry only proven products and take pride in pleasing their customers. Check how long they've been in business and how well they support their products. As for dildo particulars, here are a few:

Getting the Right Size

The most important consideration in sizing a dildo is width or girth. One strategy for determining which width is best for you is suggested by the women at Good Vibrations. They say to buy different-sized zucchinis, carrots or cucumbers that have an inviting girth. Steam or nuke them for just a few seconds so they won't be cold, wash them, and put condoms over them. Add lubricant and try them in your vagina. Don't hesitate to use a vegetable peeler to fine tune the girth. When you find one that feels just right, cut it in two and measure the diameter, which will most likely be somewhere between one and two inches. If you are the one who will be inserting the dildo, order one that has the perfect sized width. However, if a partner will be doing the inserting, consider getting a dildo with a slightly smaller diameter. That's because a partner won't be as precise as you are, so a little room for forgiveness can come in handy.

As for length, a four- to five-inch-long dildo should be just right if you plan to keep it stationary inside your vagina, while a six- to eight-inch length might be easier to handle if you like thrusting.

Dildos are a bit like purses: some women have one favorite dildo; others have dildos of different shapes and sizes for every day of the week.

Expect to pay from $50 to $150 for a good-quality silicone dildo. For instance, rubber dildos have tiny divots in the surface which make them next to impossible to keep clean. You should always use a condom over them.

Shape and Lubrication

When it comes to dildos, there are plenty of variations within a basic theme. Some dildos are made to look like penises, complete with veins and testicles, some look like dolphins or bears, and some have ridges. Dildos also have different-sized heads. With a small amount of effort, you are likely to find the dildo of your dreams.

No matter how wet you might be, it's best to lubricate the dildo and yourself before inserting. You may need to add more as you go. If it's a silicone dildo, don't use silicone-based lube. It can melt the silicone toy.

Stationary vs. Movement and Possible Layering

Women don't necessarily use dildos for thrusting in and out. A woman might like a dildo to be stationary inside her vagina while she uses her fingers or a vibrator, or while a partner provides her with oral or anal attention. Or she might enjoy running the dildo up and down between her labia.

Cleaning

Dildos should be washed and dried after each use. If not properly cleaned, the porous surface of some dildos will grow microorganisms that are best not introduced or reintroduced into your body. If you are sharing sex toys, sterilize your dildo with hydrogen peroxide, rubbing alcohol or a light bleach solution (nine parts water to one part bleach).

If you use the dildo in your bum, be sure to wash it with soap and water before putting it into a vagina. Better yet, slap a condom on it before it goes up anyone's rear. Also, limit your anal play to dildos with a flanged end or use a butt plug which won't get lost up your rectum. *People who enjoy both anal and vaginal penetration are wise to have dedicated dildos for each orifice.*

Dildo Harnesses Dildos with a flared base can be worn in harnesses which make them appear like erect penises. With a moderate amount of skill and effort, the person wearing the harness and dildo can penetrate a partner. This can be disappointing, though, because the dildo isn't connected to the wearer's nervous system like a flesh-and-blood penis and she can't feel what the dildo is feeling. Nonetheless, there are straight and lesbian couples who enjoy using a dildo in a harness. The best harnesses are made of leather or nylon webbing. Harness construction and fastener application can be tricky; be sure to research the do's and don'ts of dildo-harness buying and wearing. Also, there are dildo harnesses that fit on the thigh. Users of these marvel at the utility and claim the human penis should have been attached to the thigh of the male rather than between his legs. There is even a dildo mounted on a beach ball that a person can bounce up and down on, and dildo harnesses that go on the chin.

Dildo Harnesses for Inner Wear Let's say you're trying to take the boredom out of shopping at the supermarket or you have a date and want to spice things up a bit. You can now do it with your favorite dildo inside your vagina and no one will ever know unless you want them to. That's because they make dildo harnesses that hold the dildo inside a woman's vagina so it won't pop out.

Doubles? A double dildo can be hand held or worn in a harness, with one end going up the wearer's vagina and the other end sticking out in front like a penis. There are a couple of highly rated double dildos on the market.

Double Penetration Some women like to be penetrated in both the front and the rear at the same time. In lieu of finding a second male for a threesome, the dildo can penetrate one gate while her partner fills the other.

Beware Of Gumby-Like Dildos Some dildos are embedded with wire rods to help keep whatever shape the person bends them into. Be aware that if the wire separates from the dildo material, it will become embedded in the wall of your vagina or rectum.

Menopause Masturbating with a dildo fully inserted might help some menopausal women without partners to keep their vaginas in good shape.

Suction Cups There are dildos with suction cups on the bottom so the woman can stick them on a wall or the floor while she moves her entire body

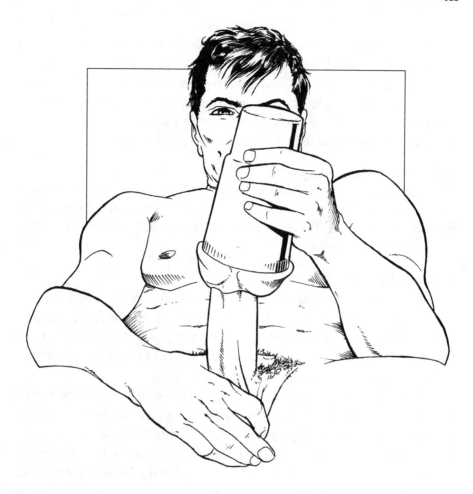

Man Toys

Male masturbation toys and sleeves come in all kinds of shapes and textures. Of those the staff at Goofy Foot Press have tested, none came close to using your hand and a few cents worth of lotion. There was a vagina substitute that's shaped like a big flashlight. Sticking your penis into cold mud would have been more fun and less of hassle to clean up. But these sell incredibly well and thousands of men enjoy using them. They are now making sleeves that warm up and the clean up isn't as much of a pain. If you get one, make sure it's phthalate free.

up and down or forward and backward while the dildo remains stationary. These can also be planted on the wall as decorations for your dorm room.

Dildos of Pegging Good Vibrations reports that about half of the dildo harnesses they sell are to heterosexual couples in which the woman wears the dildo to use for anal intercourse in her male partner's rear end. See Chapter 24: *Anal Sex—Up Your Bum* for illustrations and more information.

Sex-Toy Layering — Dildos & Vibrators

Some women use a vibrator on their clitoris while they have a dildo in their vagina. The dildo provides an internal fullness that creates a synchrony between the feelings in the clitoris and vagina, or it helps amplify the sexual sensations from the clitoris.

SEX-TOY LEGAL UPDATE

Less than ten years ago, the federal courts declared it is legal for Alabama to ban the sale of devices that are designed or marketed primarily for the stimulation of human genitals (Williams v. Morgan, Eleventh Circuit, February 14, 2007). While sodomy in the privacy of your home is now protected, you can't buy a sex toy in Alabama to save your soul.

However, our gynecology consultant offers a solution that won't get a Belle busted: "My new favorite item is a vibrating toothbrush. The vibration is a perfect frequency for clitoral stimulation. I remind my patients not to use the bristle side but the back side of the bristles. It travels great, is inexpensive, and doesn't threaten a man's masculinity..." [This disposable, battery-powered toothbrush she is referring to is from a well-known Oral hygiene company. It has bright, multi-colored bristles that Pulsate, and is usually less than $10 USD for a twin pack. You can find them wherever toothbrushes are sold!]

27
Fun with Your Foreskin

"Cut to the chase: I am an RN and have seen hundreds of uncircumcised males. No turn on. But when my most recent lover happened to be such it was so totally unexpected that my sexual arousal rate went up 200%. I am very turned on by stroking him to expose the head, kissing and licking it and then covering it again by pulling the foreskin back up. Sucking ever so gently with the skin covering the head gives him pleasure, but pulling it down near the base of his penis completely exposes him and his reaction is amazing. All it takes is tender gentle swirls to drive him crazy.... The wanton horny bitch that resides within myself has now been released and owes you all at the Goofy Foot Press gratitude and the author the best blow job ever!" *female age 27*

Drive south on I-5 until you reach the Corvallis exit, go west...

Medically speaking, routine circumcision in modern countries makes about as much sense as removing a child's eyelids or cutting out the labia of a baby girl. So why are so many American boys routinely circumcised?

During the 1880s, a few influential men like John Harvey Kellogg, physician and founder of a famous American cereal company, claimed that boys masturbate because the foreskin rubs on the head of the penis. Until that time, most American men were not circumcised. As a leading anti-masturbation fanatic, Dr. Kellogg believed that boys who were circumcised at birth would be less likely to masturbate. Swell guy that he was, Dr. Kellogg also recommended that girls who masturbate have their clitorises burned out with acid.

Dr. Kellogg's influence helped circumcision to become a routine operation in America—one that has lined the pockets of American physicians for more than a century. What's startling is that a number of today's proponents of circumcision are just as fanatical and irrational as Dr. Kellogg was.

There is clearly something about the foreskin that creates religious and medical fanaticism. Is it because the foreskin is attached to the genitals? Is it because so much money can be made from chopping it off? No one knows.

There is No Medical Need for Circumcision

America's medical establishment has tried to justify its hand in circumcision by saying that it prevents cancer of the penis, cancer of the cervix and now AIDS.

Cancer of the penis is extremely rare—more men get breast cancer. In Sweden, where few men are circumcised, cancer of the penis is just as rare as in the circumcision-happy United States. As for cervical cancer, women have no higher rate of cervical cancer who live in European countries where the men aren't circumcised.

The idea that circumcision is protective against HIV is the brainchild of pro-circumcision advocates in America. Until recently, a large majority of adult males in America have been circumcised, yet America has one of the highest rates of HIV infection in the industrialized world—higher than in a number of European countries where the vast majority of men are not circumcised. In the United States, blacks have the highest rate of circumcision, yet they also have the highest rate of heterosexually transmitted HIV. America itself has the highest rate of circumcision among the developed nations, yet the highest rate of heterosexually transmitted HIV. If circumcision decreased the spread of HIV by 8% to 60% as the pro-circumcision fanatics claim, America would have one of the lowest rates of heterosexually transmitted HIV, not one of the highest.

Perhaps the men in America weren't circumcised well enough. Maybe we need to be circumcised a second time!

Gold Standard or Fool's Gold?

Circumcision proponents frequently cite three studies from Africa as being the gold standard to bolster the case for circumcision. It's interesting that none of these studies were carried out in the United States. Perhaps that's

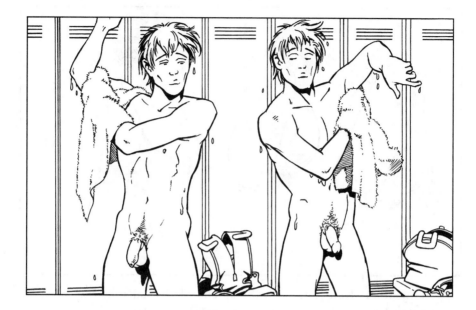

because it would not be as easy to hide poorly designed and poorly executed studies in America where there would be outside observers. The same is true for studies where there might be selection bias, lead-time bias, attrition bias and duration bias—effects that may have plagued the African circumcision studies.

If circumcision helps prevent the spread of HIV, how is it that men who are circumcised are more likely to have HIV than men who not circumcised in several countries in Africa? Competent analysis of the HIV data from Africa reaffirms that circumcision is not an effective means of preventing the spread of HIV:

> "Given what is known at the individual level, one would have expected HIV incidence or prevalence in circumcised groups of men to be consistently about 20% lower than in uncircumcised groups. This was not the case according to the results of this study. Until this discrepancy between demographic evidence and expectations from epidemiological evidence is resolved, is it wise to recommend mass circumcision? Once more, the dynamics of generalized HIV epidemics in Africa appear more complex than originally thought. Male circumcision appears only as a minor factor amid

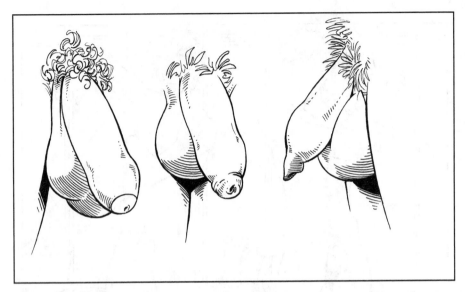

many others contributing to the spread of HIV, such as the complex web of social, cultural and economic interactions surrounding sexual behaviour, especially among adolescents and young adults."
"Long-term population effect of male circumcision in generalized HIV epidemics in sub-Saharan Africa," African Journal of AIDS Research [2008, 7(1): 1–8]

When pro-circumcision advocates get funding to carry out research, science appears to take a backseat to politics.

Studies Question the Effectiveness of Circumcision

Consider the findings from a study on circumcision and HIV infection done in the Caribbean that were published in the *Journal of Sexual Medicine*:

> "Circumcision did not confer significant protective benefit against STI/HIV infection. The findings suggest the need to apply caution in the use of circumcision as an HIV prevention strategy..."

The second article appeared a few days later in the *New York Times*:

> "Cholera Epidemic Envelops Coastal Slums in West Africa. In both countries, about two-thirds of the population lack toilets. Aid workers said the number of cases of the highly contagious disease continued to increase, particularly in Freetown, where most live in slums and children swim in polluted waters."

What, you might ask, do circumcision and the lack of sanitation have to do with each other? Millions of dollars are being spent to circumcise African males that could be spent on sewer systems in Africa that would truly save lives. Sanitation and water systems will make an important impact in the lives of Africans. Circumcision will not.

The Risks of Circumcising

For those of you who are concerned about your infant son's health, why not consider a danger that is more immediate than dubious studies from Africa? It is called Methicillin-resistant Staphylococcus aureus (MRSA). This infection can be a serious problem in newborn nurseries. Its most frequent infant victims are circumcised boys, although more research on this is needed. The infection gets into the body through the circumcision wound, and it can cause impetigo, staphylococcal scalded skin syndrome, bacteremia, cellulitis, pneumonia, arthritis, osteomyelitis, pustolosis, pyoderma, empyema, and sometimes death.

Why Do They Keep Doing It?

A physician in the US makes between $150 and $300 per circumcision. Doing one circumcision per day, five days per week, at a fee of $150 each for 46 out of 52 weeks a year nets a physician an extra $34,500 annually for a procedure that takes less than ten minutes. One circumcision a day at the higher rate brings in almost $70,000 a year. No wonder pediatricians and obstetricians have a history of fighting over who does the circumcisions!

Another reason for doing circumcisions is medical bias. Until recently, physicians in this country have had a long-standing bias that hysterectomies are good for women and circumcisions are good for men. Is this really true?

How They Do It

During male circumcision, physicians stick a prodding instrument into the foreskin to tear it away from the head of the penis. One-third to one-half of the skin on the penis is then cut off. Traditionally, male circumcisions have not been done with anesthesia. But even when anesthesia is used, there is still extreme pain from the raw scar on the penis.

Religious Considerations

Some people will say, "But circumcision is done for important religious and cultural reasons." The same is true for female circumcision, which we refer to as genital mutilation. Some people say this is being disrespectful of an important ritual in the Jewish faith. This is true. We are also disrespectful of the Catholic Church's ban on birth control and masturbation. If Jewish men want to be circumcised as an expression of their faith, why not let them wait until they are 18 years old and able to call the Mohel themselves? That would be a far greater expression of faith than having the end of your penis cut off when you are only a few days old and can't tell the Torah from a telephone book.

According to psychologist Ronald Goldman, Theodore Herzl, the founder of modern Zionism, did not allow his own son to be circumcised. Even Moses did not circumcise his son, and circumcision was not done during the forty-year period in the wilderness. It is quite possible that this custom arose out of the Egyptian practice to circumcise their Jewish slaves. Over time, this became a ritual or custom, and eventually became associated with the Covenant. The ultimate goal of circumcision, according to ancient rabbis and Jewish scholars from Philo to Maimonides, was to decrease sexual pleasure for both men and women. This would give men more time to study the Torah, and result in women receiving less sexual pleasure from a man who was circumcised.

In 1843, Reform-Movement leaders in Frankfurt, Germany started a mini-house revolt against circumcision. This group argued that 1) Circumcision had not always been practiced among Jews; 2) It was not commanded to Moses; 3) It's not unique among Jews, given how Muslims do it as well; 4) It is only discussed once in the Mosaic law and not repeated in Deuteronomy; and 5) There was no comparable practice for females. Perhaps the most interesting of all is for the first 2,000 years of the practice, only the tip of the foreskin was cut. This was called Milah. Only then, after the first 2,000 years of Milah, did they start whacking off the entire foreskin. Resource: *Questioning Circumcision—A Jewish Perspective* by Ronald Goldman, Ph.D., Vanguard.

For Parents—Foreskin Care

Do not try to retract the foreskin of a young boy unless there is a specific medical reason. During infancy and childhood, the inner surface of the foreskin is physically attached to the skin on the head of the penis. This protects the opening of the penis from irritation, infection and ulceration. Over time, the cells that attach these two surfaces together will start to dissolve on their own. By trying to retract the foreskin prematurely, you are ripping apart these delicate tissues that nature has "glued" together.

A young boy will often push his foreskin away from his body. As he gets older, he will begin to pull it toward his body. A number of males don't fully retract their foreskins until they are teenagers. This is normal and will usually happen without any coaxing or encouragement from mom and dad.

Parents do need to tell their teenage sons about cleanliness. They should explain that once a boy is able to retract his foreskin he should clean it every day in the shower. As for whether that daily cleaning should include soap, one of our urology-consultant physicians is himself uncircumcised. He is concerned that soaping the retracted foreskin daily might destroy the protective bacterial mantle and may result in foreskin odor. He suggests only soaping it a couple of times a week, while retracting it and washing it with water the other days of the week. Other healthcare providers recommend retracting the foreskin and washing it with soap every day.

Reader Comments

"I love the way his penis slides in and out of his foreskin when he's inside me. It not only stimulates me physically, but the thought of it also really turns me on while we are making love." *female age 30*

"I'd never even seen an uncircumcised penis until my current lover, but I've decided now that it's the best thing since sliced bread. The foreskin makes hand jobs 100 times better and easier because it slides over the penis so you don't need lube. I was kind of nervous about it at first but then I realized how stretchy the foreskin is even though it looks kinda fragile. For blow jobs, I pull the foreskin down to the base and massage it there and go to town." *female age 18*

"The only Jewish guy I ever slept with was also the only uncircumcised guy I ever slept with. He seemed to have more stamina than any of the others, but that might just be a coincidence." *female age 21*

"For a blow job, pull the foreskin up over the head and stick your tongue down inside of the opening and swirl it around."
female age 38

"Just ask the guy how he likes it. Some guys like you to pull the foreskin tight; others say this hurts." *female age 20*

"I use my foreskin to massage her clitoris. This might only be possible with a partner who has a larger-than-normal clitoris. You need to be able to get hold of it." *male age 65*

"Once my wife and I are ready for penetration, I roll my foreskin all the way shut. I press it gently against her labia while spreading them slightly, and push the glans in just a little. Then, I withdraw the glans back inside the foreskin, never exposing it to open air. What this does is spread her lubricant all over the first half of my penis. After several strokes like this, I am able to slip inside easily. Sometimes we find this so pleasurable that we continue a good long while before penetrating farther." *male age 38*

"A partner should know that the inside of a foreskin is where there is the most feeling, so gentle movement of it over a cockhead and down the shaft feels great. The best part of getting a blow job is what a tongue and mouth can do with that inside lining of a foreskin."
male age 59

"One thing I find particularly stimulating is to lubricate a finger or thumb, slip it between the foreskin and the head, and massage the glans. It feels really, really great." *male age 19*

"When did I first retract it? I was around ten. I would slowly pull it back every day in the shower. After about two weeks I was able to pull it all the way down." *male age 22*

"Letting the foreskin balloon is quite nice both when peeing and when enjoying the pool jets." *male age 37*

"I like to do the trick of clamping the end shut while peeing and making it swell up. Also, a similar and a more satisfying experience is to leave just a bit of the end open and put it under a strong flow of water so that the water flows in but has a place to get out."
male age 20

"My fiancee does all the foreskin movement for me. It's such a turn-on when she pulls it back and then returns it to normal. She does this with her mouth constantly while she gives me a blow job." *male 19*

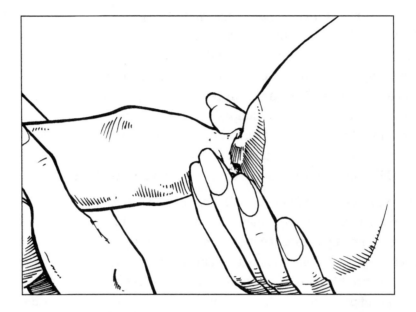

"There is nothing worse than cracking an erection in your pants and not being able to make it go away because your foreskin is retracted and the head of your cock keeps on rubbing on your pants." *male 18*

"The very tip of the foreskin (like the rim of a volcano) can be very, very sensitive when you're soft. A light, caressing finger running around the edge can feel electric… If she's giving you a handjob and her ring isn't tight around her finger, the flesh of the foreskin can get caught in between and pinch like hell. On the flip side, there's something pretty erotic about handjobs while she's wearing your engagement ring." *male age 23*

Foreskin Extras!

Is the recent circumcision campaign to help prevent the Spread of HIV in Africa backfiring? Any time special interest groups propose a simple solution to an extremely complex problem, run and take cover. Questions are now being asked about whether the drive to circumcise men in Africa might actually be causing HIV rates to increase rather than decrease. Until we have genuine data as opposed to supposition dressed up as "science," it's time to stop circumcising men in Africa and to spend the money and effort on the promotion and use of condoms to help prevent the spread of HIV. The same would be true for the rest of the world, including the United States.

A pleasant foreskin-related "bump" during intercourse? A small group of sexually-experienced female sex educators have reported they are able to experience a pleasant-feeling "bump" in the g-spot area with each thrust when they have intercourse with an uncircumcised man as opposed to one who has had his foreskin removed. This is most certainly not science, but it once again points in the direction that nature knew what she was doing for both men and women when she gave men a foreskin.

Resources:

National Organization of Circumcision Information Resource Centers
(Includes a list of foreskin-friendly physicians)
www.nocirc.org

Circumcision Resource Center
www.circumcision.org

Circumcision Information and Resource Pages
www.cirp.org

No Harm
www.noharmm.org

Doctors Opposing Circumcision (D.O.C.)
www.doctorsopposingcircumcision.org

THANKS to Marilyn Milos who founded the National Organization of Circumcision Information Resource Center.

28
Sex Fantasies

Given how sex fantasies are nearly universal, it's surprising we tend to be embarrassed about them. On the other hand, why bother fantasizing about things that everyone else approves of?

Some people have a single reliable sex fantasy that they go back to time and again. Others have a toolbox of scenes, scenarios and images that help get them off. Most people find it difficult to masturbate without a sexual fantasy, and many people fantasize during intercourse.

Some sex fantasies are highly scripted, others are little more than collages or fleeting images. Some fantasies are hardcore, others are more sensual than sexual. Some begin with sexual imagery, in fantasies, the sexual images evolve slowly.

The content of sex fantasies varies; some are sweet, kind and silly; others are weird, kinky and bizarre. Some are action-packed and exciting; others are quiet and etherial. Some sex fantasies are populated with past lovers, singers, people in uniforms, movie stars, teachers, priests, family members, total strangers and even furry friends from another species.

One of the more popular sex fantasies involves things you've done sexually with your current or a past partner.

Our fantasies get their fuel from the deepest recesses of our mind, and they can often be shaped by the culture we were raised in. In our fantasies, we can be very different from who we usually are or the person our friends and partners know us to be. We can also be active or passive, devil or angel.

There's nothing that says an obsessively neat surgeon can't have a fantasy of being masturbated by a pair of smelly feet, or a faithful and loving wife can't have rough sex with her husband's brother. Or maybe she fantasies about something more tame, like having her back rubbed. Things might get more interesting if you knew who was giving her the back rub, or maybe she's simply enjoying the sensations of having her back rubbed without any awareness of the context or who is doing it.

Fantasies of Rape

It is not unusual to have fantasies in which sex is forced, nor is it unusual to fantasize about sex with people in uniform. Consider the following passage from Betty Dodson's fine book, *Sex for One*, Harmony Books:

"A friend who considered herself a radical feminist got concerned that her sexual imagery wasn't politically correct because it wasn't 'feminist oriented.' I assured her that all fantasies were okay. Lots of people imagine scenes they never want to experience. I also pointed out that we can become addicted to a fantasy like anything else, and suggested she experiment with new ones. One of her new assertive fantasies is about moving her clitoris in and out of her lover's soft wet mouth while he's tied down. Whenever she gets stuck or is in a hurry, she brings out her old fantasy of being raped by five Irish cops and always reaches orgasm quickly."

Sometimes being raped in fantasy is a way to enjoy pleasure that would otherwise cause guilt. Sex that is out of your control keeps you from having to feel responsible for wanting it. It is also a way to feel sexually desired and valued, since the perpetrator would do anything to have you.

Why the Rape in "Rape Fantasy" Isn't Usually Rape

If you ask most women who have rape fantasies to describe the man who is "raping" them, you'll find he's not exactly what we picture when we think of a violent felon, unless the guy has been spending six hours a day in the prison weight room or reads Shakespeare to his cell mate.

The perpetrators in most "rape fantasies" are actors, musicians or bodice-ripping hunks—someone who the woman might want to have sex with anyway. Missing is the terror, violence, confusion, rage and disgust that makes rape RAPE. The woman is in control by virtue of who she has "raping" her or because she's the one scripting the scenario, while control is the last thing a woman who is being raped in real life has any of.

Even if the woman's rape fantasy involves her being degraded or humiliated, it doesn't make her fear men in real life like an actual rape often does. It doesn't make her afraid to go out of doors like having been raped in real life might.

No doubt, there are cultural, religious and perhaps biological reasons for why some women have sexual fantasies where they are "taken" by a man instead of the woman being the taker. But there are significant differences between that and the realities of an actual rape. These are usually fantasies of pseudo- or pretend-rape. Then again...

Fantasies of Real Rape

When it comes to sexuality, just when you think you know what you are talking about, someone will mercifully set you straight. When the author wrote something similar about rape in a post for *Psychology Today,* several woman agreed that this felt familiar. But then, a reader made the following comment:

> "This does not apply to me, and I am a woman with rape fantasies. I think there is such a thing as a true "rape fantasy," and that is what I have. My rape fantasies involve scenes of violent and degrading sex torture committed by men who disgust me, like an overweight and dirty old man, or a socially awkward and unattractive geek who masterminded a plan to imprison me and torture me with strange machines."

> "For me, there is a strong humiliation-pleasure connection. My own fantasies disturb me and give me fear, but they are the only thing that works for me sexually. I can't get off without them."

This is an important reminder of how complex sexuality can be, and how complex our sexual fantasies can be.

Men's vs. Women's Sex Fantasies

Young girls in our society are raised on videos and fashion magazines that highlight gorgeous female models—gorgeous if you don't take into account the degree of Photoshopping, or how many meals these women had to barf up to stay slim, or how much silicone they have surgically packed into their chests.

As girls look through these magazines, they often think about other women's bodies, particularly the ideal woman whom they hope to some-day become. Boys, on the other hand, often grow up fantasizing about doing things; for instance, being firemen, sports heroes, musicians, stuntmen and eventually stud lovers. Even when it comes to video games, boys are forever killing, bombing, shooting or building something.

Psychologist Karen Shanor believes that when women see an erect penis in their fantasies, they often relish it as a sign that the man finds them irresistible, as opposed to being in awe of the penis itself—although it's difficult to know what young women are thinking about when they see the perpetually erect penises in porn.

It could be that many young women learn to include men in their fantasies as an afterthought, with the fantasized male being little more than a woman retrofitted with a penis. Perhaps this is one reason why teenage girls so often fawn over androgynous male rock'n'roll singers, not that older women don't as well. (Teenage boys tend to look androgynous before puberty, so maybe the teen-girls' fantasies are right where they need to be in an age-appropriate sense.)

When a woman walks into a formal affair like a prom, the first thing she often notices is how the other women look and how she feels in comparison. The first thing a man notices is often the same thing: how the other women look. Men usually aren't concerned with how the other men look, unless they are actors or gay.

As focused as women sometimes are on other women, Shanor's theory does have its limitations. It doesn't explain why some women clearly prefer the sexual touch and feel of a man's body over that of a woman. It doesn't explain why a lot of women enjoy the way a penis feels when it's inside of their bodies, or why they might find a male's butt or shoulders to be sexy.

And when a woman is at a swim meet or water polo game, it's hard to believe her eyes don't focus on the front of the boys' Speedos, after checking out their abs, of course.

Your Lover's Sex Fantasies

Every once in a while, one partner will tell the other about his or her private sex fantasy. Stranger things have happened. But don't expect to see the fantasy plastered on a billboard surrounded by neon lights. Most of us are a little embarrassed by our sexual fantasies, sometimes with good reason. As a result, we don't reveal our fantasies in a way that's particularly direct, nor should we.

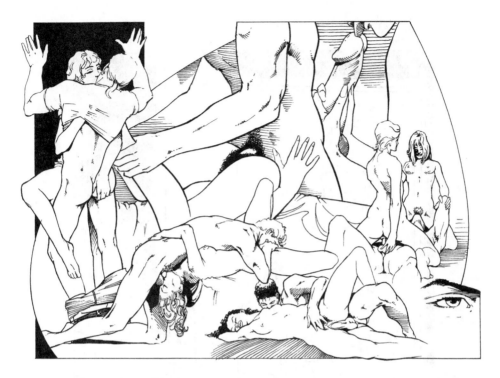

You Only Get One Chance

Let's say you are a guy and your sweetheart casually or jokingly makes an off-the-cuff statement that she likes seeing guys in jock straps. Boom, ball's in your court. If you have half a brain, and not many of us do, you won't laugh and tell her how much better you feel in boxers than wearing some old athletic supporter. Instead, you will consider buying about some new jocks, maybe in colors, maybe one with a cup, what the heck.

So there you are later that night, your sweetheart's warm familiar fingers are slowly popping the buttons on your blue jeans and bingo, she discovers that you are wearing an athletic supporter underneath! Before you know it, she's in sexual orbit and you are the happiest jock on your block! Or she might discover her fantasy was best when it was only imagined and that its erotic edge when acted out in reality.

To Share or Not To Share?

People occasionally have sexual fantasies about someone other than their partner. Sometimes it is prudent not to share these fantasies, e.g., "The reason I got so hot is because I pretended you were Mike." Other times your partner might find these fantasies very arousing.

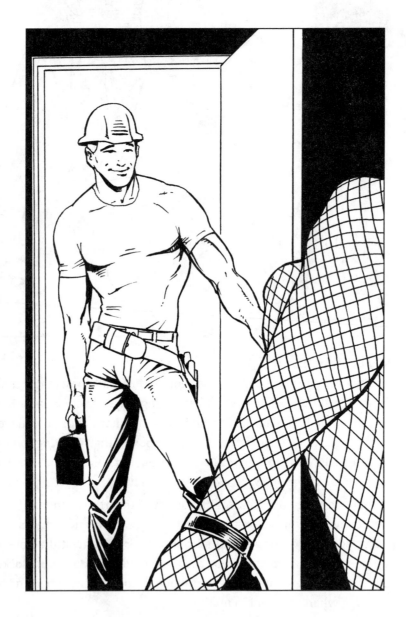

While it's great that you and your partner might be open to hearing each other's fantasies, this doesn't mean that you need to act them out. Sometimes you'll say, "That one doesn't work for me—let's look for something we can both get into!" When you do find the right fantasies that turn both of you on, acting them out together can be great fun.

Responsibility

Knowledge of your partner's fantasies is a trust that remains with you for life. This trust holds true even if you break up and otherwise find yourselves hating each other. No one forced you to be in a relationship with the person, so don't go blabbing personal stuff just to be hurtful. In the long run, it reflects badly upon you.

To put it another way, people who gossip about a current or former partner's sexuality are both shallow and deceitful. The laws of karma will someday haunt them, assuming there are laws of karma.

Readers' Comments

"At work I daydream a lot about sex and what it would be like with certain people that I am especially attracted to. Since I am about to get married, I sometimes feel bad thinking of others, but as long as you don't act on it, you're pretty much okay." *female age 30*

"As a working mother, I get sex and orgasms, but I rarely get romance, so that is what I fantasize about." *female age 36*

"My sexual fantasies always involve my current real life lover. We're making romantic love somewhere that is new to us, a beach, forest, remote island, in front of a fire in a cabin." *female age 34*

"I probably have similar fantasies to anyone who watches the Sci Fi channel too much." *male age 30*

"My fantasies don't play a huge part in my life, except that I get confused why I have fantasies about other girls when I love penises and my boyfriend very much." *female age 23*

"I had always fantasized about my girlfriend being totally naked with her legs spread apart when I came into the room. One day she actually did this! It was awesome!" *male age 21*

"I don't have any clearly defined fantasy. They are more fleeting feelings and don't affect my life much." *female age 38*

"My husband and I have been married for 10 years and still love to act out our fantasies. Last month he was a customs agent and I was trying to sneak something across the border. After he completely searched me, I had to bribe him with sexual favors until he let me go. Later, I was a physician and he the reluctant patient. Acting out your fantasies can be great fun, and it keeps your sex life young!"

female age 33

"I'd love to see my girlfriend get it on with another woman and I know it would be a turn-on to see her get it on with another guy, but I don't know if I could keep from getting jealous." *male age 39*

Have you ever had homosexual fantasies?

"I used to fantasize about women all of the time. Finally, I decided to give it a try and had sex with one of my best female friends, who is mostly heterosexual. It was fun and every now and then we play with one another. I have never developed an emotional attachment to her or any other woman, and I no longer fantasize about women."

female age 26

"I fantasize about being with another woman often, but I also fantasize about my boyfriend and Brad Pitt!" *female age 25*

"I am aroused by images of women with women; also by stories of multiple partners. On occasion, I use these fantasies to help me reach orgasm." *female age 32*

"I've had no fantasies or gay experiences, although I wonder sometimes if I could get turned on by another guy." *male age 30*

"Gay fantasies? I've never even considered being gay. I'm not gay. I swear it." *male age 22*

Thanks to Wendy Maltz for her astute and thoughtful article *Women's Sexual Fantasies* by Wendy Maltz and Suzie Bossfrom in *Private Thoughts: Exploring the Power of Women's Sexual Fantasies*, Booksurge.

29
The Fairy Pornmother

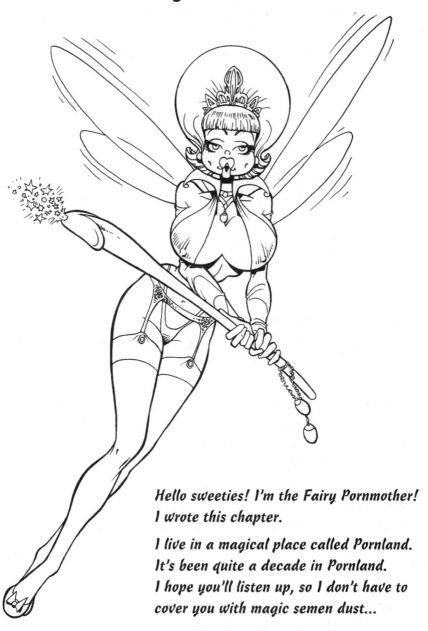

*Hello sweeties! I'm the Fairy Pornmother!
I wrote this chapter.*

*I live in a magical place called Pornland.
It's been quite a decade in Pornland.
I hope you'll listen up, so I don't have to
cover you with magic semen dust...*

Thank heaven for Viagra! What a wonderful vitamin. My actors couldn't manage without it. Have you taken yours today?

I'm sure you've got talent, but you can put it back in your pants. I'm not here to audition. The author of the *Guide To Getting It On* asked me to stop by and have a little talk. So I agreed to write this chapter and offer some perspective from an insider's POV.

For starters, nobody in Pornland ever dreamed so many people would take porn seriously. I mean, look at my titties! Look at my waist! My lips are purrrrfect! How many women really look like me?

And nobody in Pornland ever thought porn would be used as sex education. But given the lack of alternatives, I do get it. Porn may be over the top, but at least it doesn't try to make you feel bad for wanting to do what people have wanted to do since the beginning of time.

Here's the problem: it's not like those of us in Pornland are here because we're the best at making love. We may have the biggest love-making body parts, and we may last forever, but we're not the best.

We're really good at one thing: getting our freak on for the camera. We love it when people are watching us do things with our clothes off. But that's not making love.

Seriously, have you ever seen any of us kiss for half an hour? Have you ever seen any of us give each other massages or laugh and tease each other? None of that works for the camera. Imagine wanting to masturbate and landing on a website where couples do nothing but kiss? You'd hate us.

Pornland isn't like real life. We just pretend it is. There are no B-cup breasts or five-inch penises in Pornland. They're forbidden. We're all an exaggeration. We're here to sell you on porn. Click and stroke, click and stroke. We want you to be as excited about porn as a cat in a tuna factory. None of what we do is about making love. It's about getting you to click and stroke.

When's the last time you sat with your face two feet away from a partner' crotch the entire time you made love? When's the last time you made love to someone whose coochie had special makeup on it and a 400 watt spotlight shining between her legs? You haven't, because people don't do that. But it's what we do in Pornland. We're an amusement park of excess. We exaggerate everything. We have to. How else could a two-dimensional image get you to stick your hand in your pants?

To make you want to click and stroke, I have to hire actresses who can convince you they're having orgasms when a strange man with a penis the size of a Pringle's can is pounding them in ways that would cause most women pain. I have to hire actresses who won't throw up when I tell them to suck on a penis that's just been up their rear end. I have to hire actresses who don't mind being thrown around like rag dolls and can have sex in positions that would make Houdini cry uncle.

I have to hire actresses who will do things that cam girls and prostitutes won't. And I try to make you think it's normal, even if your wife or girlfriend won't do it either.

There's a lot of sex here in Pornland, but there aren't many real orgasms for the actresses. That's not why they're here. For a lot of these girls, it's their fifteen minutes of fame. It's about them getting to feel good about themselves because you're at home masturbating to them.

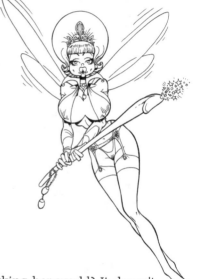

I understand that not all porn is from Pornland. There's a lot of amateur and homemade porn that people post online. But guess what? If their homemade porn doesn't look like what we produce in Pornland, you aren't going to watch it. You're not going to put up with some guy giving a woman oral sex for a half an hour while she's laying there looking like she took a handful of tranquilizers. Who cares if he's rocking her world? It doesn't matter unless the camera can make it look like he's rocking her world. And that would mean she would be in a position that isn't comfortable and he wouldn't really be giving her oral sex because we don't do that in Pornland. It blocks the camera's view of her goodies.

Even if all you're doing is watching the free tours, Pornland is making money each time you click. So it's in our interest to create a visual feast that you can't resist. We don't care if it has nothing to do with sex in real life. That's not why we're here. We're here to excite you without asking a single thing of you. Good luck making that work in real life!

We know you will habituate to anything that's even close to normal, so we provide you with extreme sex in the name of *diversity*. We keep upping the ante for what it takes you to get off, because we know the only place you'll be able to find anything close to that is with porn. No woman on the planet is going to do this stuff with you in real life. And even when you have sex with women in real life, we want you to be thinking about your favorite scenes from porn. That's because we're a business, and that's what businesses do.

If you watch porn occasionally, we like you. But if you watch it a lot, we own you. And that's what we're mostly about. We're not about making love and we're not about sex with a real-life partner. We don't care about that.

Ta ta!

Your Fairy Pornmother

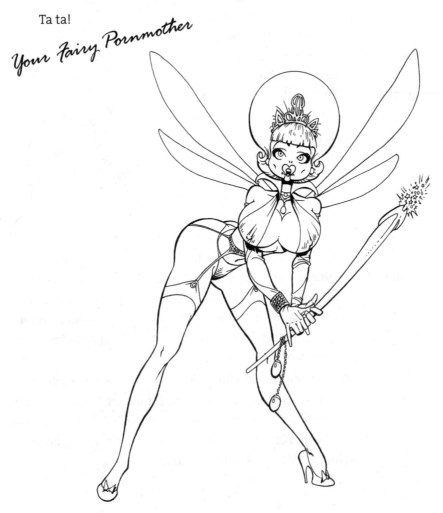

CHAPTER
30
Porndoggie's Dirty Dozen

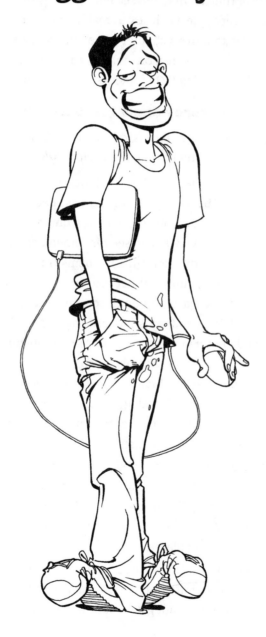

Most people understand the difference between sex in real life and sex in porn. They watch porn in moderation, and would far rather be with a real-life lover. They also understand that sex in porn starts at third base, while in real life, you seldom get to third base until you've spent lots of time on first and second.

Others, like Porndoggie, wish sex in real life were more like sex in porn. So when it was time to write a chapter on sex in porn, we interviewed Porndoggie. What follows are his reasons why sex in porn is better than sex in real life. The *Guide To Getting It On* provides a blow-by-blow analysis.

#1. Creampies and Money Shots (or 'Facials')

Porndoggie: *Creampies or facials, creampies or facials, I can't decide which represents a better use of a porn actor's talent.*

DEFINITION: Creampies and Money Shots involve a display of semen. The *creampie* has only been in porn for the past decade or so. It's where a man does a shallow ejaculation inside of a woman's vagina or anus, but quickly withdraws so the viewer can see his semen oozing out. The *facial* or *money shot* is when a porn actor pulls his penis from whatever part of an actress's body it's been in, aims it at her face, breasts, or wherever, and then strokes furiously until he ejaculates on the designated body part.

ANALYSIS: Facials or money shots are the hallmark of modern porn. Facials would rarely happen outside of BDSM relationships if it weren't for their popularity in porn, and creampies would never happen. Almost 95% of mainstream porn movies include facials or shots of men coming on their partner's bodies. A man with Porndoggie inclinations would not think he'd had sex unless he were able to give a woman a facial or a pearl necklace (which is coming on her neck or breasts).

REAL LIFE: We occasionally receive a sex survey from a woman who says it's really hot when a guy ejaculates on her face or breasts. However, most women do not enjoy this or only enjoy it due to the orgasmic bliss it brings their partners. Women who are insecure will tell a Porndoggie partner they are okay with it just to please him.

REAL LIFE SOLUTION: Do not assume your partner wants you to come on her face, breasts, belly, butt, or back. Do not attempt it unless she is genuinely excited about it, and do not get splooge in her eyes. It will burn.

#2. Anal Sex and ATM

Porndoggie: *While I think ATM is the coolest thing since anal bleaching, nothing hits the spot like good old-fashioned anal sex.*

DEFINITION: ATM or *ass-to-mouth* is a recent addition to mainstream porn. It involves a porn actor pulling his penis from an actress's rectum and placing it directly into her mouth without washing it first. It is referred to as ATM, A2M, or ATG if you are British (ass-to-gob). Sometimes, the actor will pull his penis from the rectum of one actress and place it into the mouth of another actress, or he might do "ass-to-pussy."

ANALYSIS: Anal sex dates back to the time of the ancients, but ATM is an invention of modern porn. It's porn's way of going the extra mile to get your view.

REAL LIFE: Anal sex requires trust, relaxation, lubrication, feedback, desire, and practice. None of these are ever shown in porn, where a porn actress's anus often sees as much action as her vagina.

As for ass-to-mouth, it is interesting that porn actresses never stick their fingers or dildos up the asses of male porn actors and then put them straight into the male actor's mouths. Perhaps that's because most straight men would find this horrifying.

It's possible the actresses who do ATM are simply damaged souls or they are so desperate to have a moment of recognition that they'll do things that not only degrade themselves but degrade women in general.

REAL LIFE SOLUTION: While we do hear from women who wish their partners would be more anally adventurous, do not assume all women are longing to have anal sex. Do not even inquire unless you've been together several times and have good sexual chemistry. If both of you want to experiment with anal sex, read the anal-sex chapter in this book as well other recommended texts. Go slowly and cautiously. That way, your chances of it being an enjoyable experience will go way up.

Trying to perform anal sex like they show in porn will assure it's a terrible experience. Ass-to-mouth should only be practiced by men who enjoy degrading women and by women who enjoy being degraded by men. Ass-to-pussy is a great way to get a vaginal infection.

See our video "Realty Check: Porn and Anal Sex" at GuideToGettingItOn.com

#3. Women Always Want Sex!

Porndoggie: *Porn actresses enjoy sex. The women in porn love sex way more than other women. And they know that porn actors have the skills to please them.*

ANALYSIS: In porn, having sex never depends on needing to invest in a relationship. There's no such thing as having a bad day, being angry, disappointed in your partner, or the need to respect and treat your partner well. No one ever feels tired or just wants to cuddle.

REAL LIFE: Women do not want sex 24/7 in real life.

#4. No Time Wasted on Foreplay

Porndoggie: *The reason women get tired of men is that men spend too much time trying to kiss them. Women want sex now.*

ANALYSIS: It's all about the penis in porn. No tender touching, no caressing, no passionate kissing, no running your fingertips through your partner's hair. Porn defines women as vaginas, mouths and rectums with breasts attached. Whatever the penis wants, the penis gets.

REAL LIFE: There are certainly times when a woman wants a man to get naked, hard, and inside of her without delay. But that's after she's already worked herself up. There are also many women who wish their partners were more take-charge in bed. But that doesn't mean they want sex the minute a man gets an erection.

REAL LIFE SOLUTION: The more time a man spends creating anticipation and erotic tension, the better. The same is true for kissing and caressing before a penis is ever part of the picture. Many women prefer at least 20 minutes of kissing and erotic play before a penis is involved. Also, read the *Guide To Getting It On* and other books on sex.

#5. You Never Need to Ask

Porndoggie: *Women don't respect a man who can't take charge. Women like a confident man who doesn't need to ask.*

ANALYSIS: The difference between being a confident lover and being a jerk is often lost in porn. "Asking" is relegated to the fringes of porn, such as when a submissive in BDSM says, "May I please kiss master's penis?" In porn, women want whatever men want, and it's the man's job to magically know how to please women.

REAL LIFE: In real life, a woman needs to say if she wants sex, and if so, what kind of sex she wants to have. That's called mutual consent. There's also the matter of learning about your partner. In her book on sex, porn actress Nina Hartley says a millimeter can make all the difference when it comes to the clitoris. How would you know without asking and receiving feedback?

REAL LIFE SOLUTION: If a man were able to read minds, wouldn't his time be better spent at a casino? For the rest of us, there is the reality that no two women respond in the exact same way. Nor will a woman necessarily respond on Friday as she did on Monday. Asking and seeking feedback are the cornerstones of being a good lover, except in porn.

#6. You Get to Fuck a Woman's Face

Porndoggie: *Women in porn enjoy a good face fucking. Most women find it comforting to have a penis in their mouths, delivered by a man who knows how to take control.*

ANALYSIS: In porn, the man often grabs the sides of a porn actress's head and thrusts his penis as far as he can down her throat. There is often a look of deadness or fear on the faces of porn actresses as this is happening.

REAL LIFE: Most women despise it when a man grabs their head and thrusts his penis down their throat. They say it feels like assault. It's way worse than going down on a man with smelly balls, which is number two on many women's lists of what they don't like about oral sex.

REAL LIFE SOLUTION: If you are lucky enough to be receiving oral sex, go out of your way to make sure your partner feels in complete control and never gags.

#7. Lots of Girl-on-Girl

Porndoggie: *What's better than watching a girl tongue another girl's pussy?*

ANALYSIS: When women are having sex with women, they usually aren't doing it for the pleasure of men, except for drunk college girls who are kissing and groping each other's breasts to up their status with college guys. In much of porn, the sex that women have with women is choreographed to fit a straight man's fantasy. (Lesbians with long nails; really?) Not many lesbians consider the sex that's shown in mainstream porn to actually be sex. In porn, the women usually end up sucking on a penis after they've had

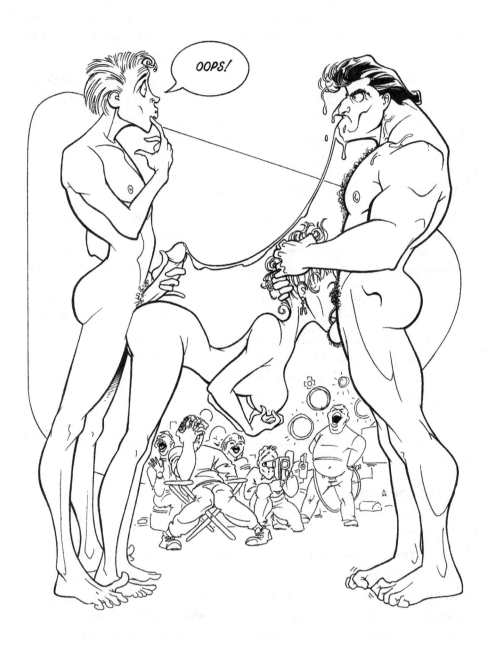

their token sex with another woman. And while straight porn often shows women having sex with women, if a man so much as touches another man's penis, the porn is called bisexual or gay.

REAL LIFE: If you are a woman who is interested in experimenting sexually with another woman, the sex that women have in straight porn is probably not your best guide.

REAL LIFE SOLUTION: The sex women have with each other in porn is often part of a threesome, with the male being the third. If this is something you are interested in exploring, try reading Chapter 44: *Threesomes.*

#8. Pussies without Flaps

Porndoggie: *Women in porn have the perfect pussies.*

ANALYSIS: Way more women want to be in porn than porn has room for. So porn producers are able to select women with smaller inner labia or women who have had labiaplasty. This has little to do with pleasure in real life, and everything to do with the camera.

REAL LIFE: It's highly unlikely that a guy is shining bright studio lights between his lover's legs and is staring at her crotch the entire time they are having sex. While some men might prefer women with inner labia that are less pronounced, others might prefer women with labia that are larger. Such is life. It might depend on how much time a man's face is between his partner's legs, although it's unlikely to be important then.

REAL LIFE SOLUTION: Labia come in all shapes and sizes. Inner labia get thicker when a woman is sexually aroused. They also have nerves that can feel delightful sensations when they are gently caressed and tugged. And if you are in an intercourse position where you can watch, it can be fun seeing more prominent inner labia hugging the sides of a penis as it goes in and out.

#9. Men Have Man-Sized Meat

Porndoggie: *If you have to look at another guy's dick, it might as well be a decent size. Plus, a thick dick leaves a nice gaping hole in a woman's pussy or ass for the camera to look into.*

ANALYSIS: Porn actor penis size falls in the top 1% to 10% of all men. Equally impressive is the control over erections and ejaculations that porn actors have, although drugs like Viagra often play a role.

REAL LIFE: Average penis size is around 5 to 5.5 inches when erect, give or take. The thickness varies. So does the shape, head size, color, angle of erection, ball size, and number of visible veins on the shaft. As for always having perfect erections, where does that happen in real life?

REAL LIFE SOLUTION: Most men who compare themselves to porn actors come up short. And most women who think their male partners should measure up to porn-actor dimensions will often be disappointed.

#10. You Get to Call Women Bitches and Whores

Porndoggie: *Women like it when you talk dirty to them!*

ANALYSIS: Women often like it when a partner tells them how hot they look, how much he wants them, how good it feels to be inside of them, that they give the best blow jobs ever, that their pussies smell sweet, that they've got great legs or breasts, that they're incredibly sexy, and that he'd die if he couldn't be with them. This is very different from calling them names.

REAL LIFE: There's a difference between talking dirty and being an ass.

REAL LIFE SOLUTION: By all means, say sexy things to her, but don't insult or demean her unless she tells you that sort of thing turns her on.

#11. Women Always Come

Porndoggie: *Women really get off in porn. You can tell.*

ANALYSIS: One of the reasons a lot of women don't like porn is they can tell the porn actresses are faking—faking being turned on, faking that it feels good, and faking orgasms. And how can a porn actress enjoy sex when everything from the positions she is in to the way she has to hold her legs apart is for the best camera angle?

REAL LIFE: In real life, women often need a good deal of time and specific types of stimulation to orgasm when they are with a partner. They also need to be highly aroused. None of this happens in porn. Most women in real life who have orgasms during intercourse either need fingers stimulating their clitoris while a partner is thrusting, or they grind their clitoris against their lover's pelvic bone. Good luck convincing a porn producer and cameraman to allow that. Couples who are making love in real life like to hug and feel each other's skin. In porn, skin-to-skin contact gets in the way of the camera's view of the woman's crotch.

REAL LIFE SOLUTION: Make sex about pleasure instead of orgasms and you'll be light years ahead! Never ask your partner if she came as a way of reassuring yourself that you are a great lover—it will seriously annoy her. Realize that a partner might be more aroused by your brushing her hair than by intercourse and you'll be on your way to having a great sex life. You'll see little of what matters in real relationships happening in porn. Which is probably the point of porn!

#12. You Can See Everything and It's Totally Intense

Porndoggie: *Not only do they have more kinds of sex in porn, but you get to see it all up close. Really up close.*

ANALYSIS: Porn offers much more visual variety than sex in real life. In addition to the close-ups and bright lights, porn actresses will often do things that prostitutes won't. That's because the only thing porn has to turn you on with besides the soundtrack (which a lot of people mute) is what you can see with your eyes. So everything about porn needs to push the limits visually. To help with this, the focus in porn will often ping pong between the woman's crotch and her face. Her expressions help reassure viewers that whatever is being done between her legs is giving her insane amounts of pleasure. Even amateur porn, which is supposed to be more life-like, is often an imitation of mainstream porn. Otherwise viewers would turn to something that's more explicit and has a faster pace.

REAL LIFE: How often are you staring between your partner's legs when you're making love? There's a massive difference between sitting in a chair and stroking your penis while watching porn and feeling your partner's entire body on top of yours—skin to skin—smelling her hair, and hearing her soft (or sometimes not so soft) moans. And what about having to prop yourself up on your elbows so you aren't putting too much pressure on her? You never need to deal with what when you are watching porn.

REAL LIFE SOLUTION: Watching porn can be fun, instructive, and hot. It can be a way to treat yourself when your partner is having her night out with her friends, or when you don't have a partner and it's just you and your fist. It can also be helpful to watch porn with a lover and have her tell you what parts she likes and what parts she doesn't like. But try to keep it in perspective, because it really is a much different experience than what happens when you are making love in real life.

Wait—It's a Baker's Dozen!

#13. No Condoms in Porn!

Porndoggie: *Porn actors get exams every month and don't need to worry about sexually transmitted infections. Plus they never get pregnant except for preggo porn and lactating porn.*

ANALYSIS: The porn industry has been fighting tooth and vagina against regulatory requirements that porn actors wear condoms. So it makes sense that the porn spin machine might want people to believe that the rate of sexually transmitted infections in porn is incredibly low because porn actors are supposed to test for sexually transmitted infections every 30 days. Yet according to a study in the *Journal of Sexually Transmitted Infections*, the incidence of chlamydia and gonorrhea among porn actors is much greater than in the general population. Also, female porn actors are more likely to have more reinfections than other women, which is a concern given how reinfections can impact a woman's reproductive system. The porn industry does not require porn actors to have tests for rectal or throat-related sexually transmitted infections, nor are porn actors tested for herpes, HPV, Trichomonas, hepatitis A, B, and C or bacterial vaginosis.

REAL LIFE: Read Chapter 52: *Gnarly Sex Germs*. Porn actors, like anyone else who is having casual sex, should be wearing condoms. They also need to be just as concerned about birth control as the rest of us.

REAL LIFE SOLUTION: A big advantage in staying home and watching porn is you don't need to worry about pregnancy and getting STIs. However, what you see in porn should never be generalized to sex in real life, where STIs are rampant and pregnancy is an ovulation away.

For Parents, please see
Chapter 64: How the Internet Killed the Plumber in Porn.

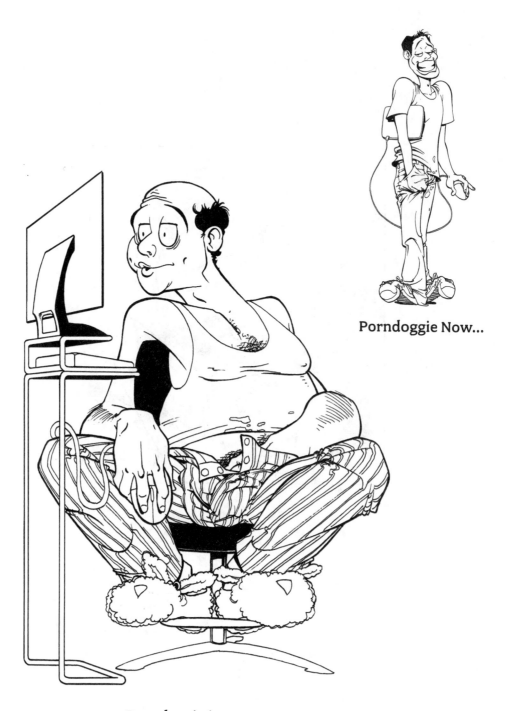

Porndoggie Now...

...Porndoggie in Twenty Years

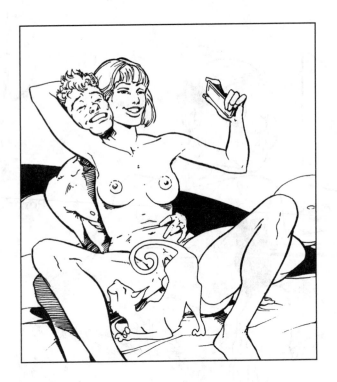

31

Casual Sex

> " Some of the best sex I ever had was with an unexpectedly talented stranger, and some of the most awkward sex I've ever had was with a boy I'd known for years and loved. Go figure." *female age 21*

There are at least two different kinds of sex — sex in an established relationship and casual sex. Casual sex can range from alcohol-aided sex with a stranger to sex with someone you know but don't want to have an exclusive relationship with.

This chapter is about casual sex, which is a vast subject that defies the armchair analysis that's been so popular in books and magazines. Six themes emerge in this chapter: the different types of casual sex, changes in dating and how we define peer groups, how the fingerprints of technology are all over your pants, the evolving sex roles of women, the omnipresent vapor of alcohol, and everything else. Early-morning thoughts such as "Who is this woman I'm sleeping with?" "What bed am I in?" and "Where are my panties?" are par for the casual-sex course.

Is casual sex something you should try? Realize that the following words of advice are coming from one of the more liberal books on the planet as opposed to an abstinence-only rant:

> *Some people are comfortable with casual sex, others aren't. What works for your friends might not work for you. If you decide to try casual sex, go slowly. Find what's best for you. Also, the luck of the draw can be a big factor in casual sex, both good and bad.*

NSA vs. FWB

Two very different forms of casual sex are sex with *No Strings Attached* and *Friends with Benefits*. Sex with no strings attached is as casual as casual sex gets. It often involves sex with a total stranger who you might have only met in the last hour. Or you may have been on each other's radar for weeks or months before opportunity knocked. NSA sex might be a one-night stand, or it may have its own jagged lifeline. The triggers can be many, but alcohol is often involved.

As for friends with benefits, there's a reason why it starts with the word "friends." It's usually with someone you know and it usually happens more than once. There's plenty of wiggle room when it comes to defining friends with benefits (aka "booty call" or "fuck buddy").

FWBs can just be for sex or it can include hanging out. It can be with an acquaintance who is maybe a Facebook friend but not someone you'd call when you need a real friend. It can also be with a good friend, which doesn't always end up as bad as you might think. There are situations where friends have sex and then stay friends after they stop having sex. There's no way to know how it's going to turn out ahead of time.

> "When I was involved in my hook-up relationship I would never call him up for a sober booty call. It was always when I was drunk and wanted sex. That is also how I knew there was no emotional attachment because I wasn't even interested in hanging out with the guy unless I had been drinking. He wasn't really my type. We didn't have much in common other than the sex." *female age 23*

> "He was a football player and wasn't someone I wanted to be in a relationship with. We didn't have a lot in common besides the sex. Most people didn't even know we were hooking up." *female age 22*

One problem with FWBs is that people who are in them seldom talk about their expectations or feelings. They don't talk with each other about their relationship, which is still a relationship of sorts even if it's not filled with "I love you's." FWB relationships more or less happen without much discussion.

Another form of casual sex is sex with an ex. If you are super horny or drowning in loneliness you might call an ex for sex. Or maybe you're both at a place where you realize the best thing about your relationship was the sex, so why not go for it. This might work. On the other hand, there are as many potential pitfalls in having sex with an ex as there are chapters in this book.

In short, friends-with-benefits sex can take on as many different forms as there are people who want to have it.

Motivations for Having Casual Sex

Casual sex can be limited to making out for an hour, or it can include intercourse, and sometimes oral or anal sex. It's about wanting more than you can get when you stay home and masturbate, but not always a lot more.

And it's more about excitement than emotional depth.

For men, there appears to be a few motivators. The penis tends to enjoy the feel of a warm and wet vagina, and there might be the joy of sexual conquest (which better be accompanied by mutual consent!) Or it could be that men get lonely and they need to be held and touched. But it's not always easy for a man to admit this, even to himself. Casual sex is a way for this vital contact to happen without a man feeling too vulnerable.

What are women's motivations? Casual sex can forestall worries about being trapped in a relationship. It can provide validation that a woman is sexually desirable, which can increase her self esteem. It can give women something to talk about with other women. And it's healthy and normal for a woman to want to know what different guys are like in bed—a curiosity that few women have been allowed free rein to explore until now. There might also be the occasional cross purposes, like having sex with a rival's boyfriend or rubbing it in an ex's face. But that's been a part of sex since the beginning of time.

Regret?

Researchers are starting to ask people if they regret their random or casual sex. If the sex was good or the person had fun, there are few regrets. Otherwise, it's not unusual to have regrets, especially if the expectations were high. Men can have regret as well as women, and there is frequently regret over not using condoms.

What researchers haven't asked people in these studies is if they have felt regret over any of their long term relationships. You do the math: one night of regret vs. months or years of regret. Regret over a one-night stand might be miniscule when compared to the regret about an unfortunate marriage. One might be an occasional nagging thought, while the other could be all consuming or the cause of a major depression.

Women's Satisfaction in Casual Sex—Cinderella Reconsidered

> "If you go into it knowing that it is just going to be a one-night stand then it is satisfying. If there was supposed to be more and it ends up without anything else, then it is disappointing." *female 22*

Women give men way more orgasms than they receive during one-night stands and casual sex. Yet almost as many women as men report being satisfied with sex during one night stands. How can this be?

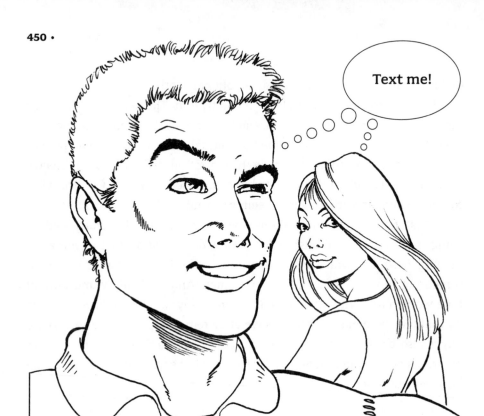

Perhaps we define sexual satisfaction differently for a casual one-night stand than we do in a more traditional relationship. The newness, excitement and risk of casual sex might make it feel better. Perhaps not having to invest as much effort or not worrying about what your partner thinks are big pluses. Alcohol can also make us remember a situation in a better light, and alcohol is often the lube that allows casual sex to occur.

Or maybe women have a more expansive definition of sexual satisfaction that reaches beyond the number of orgasms. Perhaps they are able to enjoy an imperfect quickie with an attractive stranger as much as having candle-lit sex with an adoring lover who wants to snuggle.

The increasing popularity of casual sex is forcing us to reconsider our beliefs about women's take on sex and love. Maybe all Cinderella wanted from the Prince was a good fuck. Or maybe she wanted him as a friend and lover, minus the castle, crown and demand to squeeze out a royal heir. When it comes to stories about love and sex, there are way more possible endings for women today than there were years ago. But the following account is not unusual either:

"The hook-up guy never, ever asked me how it was for me. He always quit after he finished and there was rarely foreplay. You could tell it was strictly sex. My boyfriend always asks how it was for me; he is always worried that he is not doing it good enough." *female age 21*

Gender Roles Keep Evolving

A 1950s conversation between a mom and her daughter who is a college senior:

Daughter: "Mom, it's awful. I'm really trying, but I can't find a guy."

Mom: "Don't worry, dear. Stay calm and focused. Men like women who have a good head on their shoulders. And your aunt just told me about a new bra that adds an entire cup size without looking fake. I'll get you one and have it in the mail by Friday."

A conversation today between a mom and her daughter who is a college senior:

Daughter: "Mom, Andrew and I have decided to get married!"

Mom: "But what about graduate school?"

For years, young women were supposed to keep their legs together until certain conditions were met, consisting of a relationship that was fully cemented. The words "engagement" or an engagement ring often had to be part of the deal before a guy got more than a handjob. It was her reputation vs. his wad.

Then, after the 1960s, parents started telling their daughters they could be anything they want to be. Girls were raised playing sports and were warned about burdening themselves too soon with kids and marriage. Magazines like *Cosmo* trumpeted the fact that girls get just as horny as guys. No other generation of women has been told so clearly that they should be proactive rather than passive when it comes to sexual pleasure.

So we've at least taken away some of old rules about relationships and marriage. As a result, women are just as likely to dive into a man's pants as he is into theirs. If a relationship happens, it happens, but the fact that a relationship is not part of the mix can make casual sex appealing to a lot of women as well as men. If anyone ends up being jealous or hurt, it's just as likely to be the guy.

The Double Standard — Without Sluts, There Would Be No Studs

"How many are too many? How much is too much? How assertive is too assertive? What is experimental vs. promiscuous? All of these questions are always there in the back of women's heads, and I don't think a lot of men realize that, or maybe they do and just don't care." *female age 22*

"The double standard still exists. If a guy sleeps with a lot of girls then all his friends think he's a player, but if a girl sleeps with too many guys she's a whore and no one wants to be her friend. I think girls have a lot more freedom sexually, but that doesn't mean the times have changed enough to have the girl start making every first move. I am kind of weird on this topic; I would never sleep with a guy who's had an outrageous number of women, but I also would not sleep with a guy who hasn't ever been with someone, not because of how they would be in bed but I just don't want to be someone's first because then they have to remember me forever."

female age 23

"I hear my guy friends saying, 'I hooked up with this girl last night' and then add a number to it. However, when a guy asks me how many people I have slept with, I am ashamed to say eight. I feel like it is so high. However, then when you ask a guy he will proudly say twenty." *female age 21*

The double standard still exists, but the distance between the goal posts is not as far as it was generations ago when virginity was still a commodity. The new ridiculously arbitrary question is how many men a woman can sleep with before she's slept with too many. One thing that hasn't changed is how it's women who are often the biggest enforcers of the double standard:

"Women who sleep around are very much put down by other women and men, but mostly put down by women. Men, on the other hand, are pressured and encouraged to sleep around."

female age 21

"Girls are also calling girls sluts. We don't like to be called it ourselves, but we use it to put down other women. It's a vicious cycle."

female age 22

Older Feminists Shake Their Heads in Disbelief

Some women assume that having casual sex is a sign of liberation. However, the old warhorse feminists might have some misgivings about this. It's not the lack of commitment that would bother them or the needing to drink before having sex. They would have sympathized and perhaps offered some ganja or suggested you ditch the dick altogether and try a little muff.

What would have made them crazy was the idea of hooking up with an anonymous guy when you didn't know how he voted in the last election. What if he was filling you up with his baby-making sperm but voted for politicians who want to end your freedom of choice and force you to have his child? What if he voted for politicians who are trying to shut down the Planned Parenthood clinic where you get your birth control?

When it comes to sexual freedom, being liberated means being able to make choices you are pleased with when you are sober, not ones you had to get drunk to make.

The Transformation of Dating

Dating underwent a huge transformation in the late 1800s and early 1900s. This was due in large part to massive changes in technology. (See more about this in Chapter 72: *Sex in the 1800s*.) Dating has undergone another transformation more recently, again due to changes in technology.

Another reason why dating has changed is that males and females are socializing more in mixed groups, so men and women don't have to go out on a formal date to get to know each other better. Group texts and Tweets announce where people will be hanging out. You show up hoping the person you are interested in will be there. Then, if you want to get together, you message him or her instead of calling and asking for a date. This protects males from the hurt of asking a woman out and being turned down.

There's also Facebook, which allows you to learn a great deal about someone without needing to speak with them. This can save time, but it can also be limiting. There can be a big difference between a person's life on FB and life in the real world. As more than one student has commented:

"There's your Facebook persona, your blog persona, your Tweet account... It's all about how you want people to view you. You can be anyone you want to be. But who do you really know? Most of your 'friends' have never met you."

Technology's Impact on Relationships Today

The author asked a college instructor who uses *The Guide* in her sex-ed courses about relationships and casual sex. She turned it over to her class, and a very lively two-hour discussion followed. As you will see, the students are no strangers to casual sex. If their thoughts about relationships were summed up in a few words, it would be "confusion," "too many options," "not wanting to commit" and "social media as a barrier."

In the students' words:

"We're impatient. We don't want to miss anything, so we don't take the time to really get to know anyone. We are always in 'go mode.' Maybe that's why we hook up. There's no energy left to do anything more complex."

"There are no rules anymore, at least not that anyone agrees on. There is no social code, everything is open to interpretation and it's all a gray haze."

"There is no more formal 'asking someone out.' Rather, they group text a bunch of people about possible plans for that night and see who shows up. That way, the guys don't have to ask one person out and face rejection. Plus, they don't want to limit their options. OPTIONS MUST STAY OPEN UNTIL THE LAST MINUTE!"

"Guys will google pick-up lines to text rather than trying to think on the spot. They also wonder, how soon do I text? If I call first am I coming on too strong? One male called a girl and she did not answer. He texted and she responded. She was afraid to talk on the cell. You meet, text and then see what happens."

"We are so used to communicating via text or social media that we are socially stunted when it comes to one-on-one."

"Texting is the easy way out. Plus, if you text, you can get help from friends on what to say, and how long to wait before you text back."

"This girl essentially asked me what I was doing this weekend. So I sent her a message via Facebook. She accepted, but during this pro-

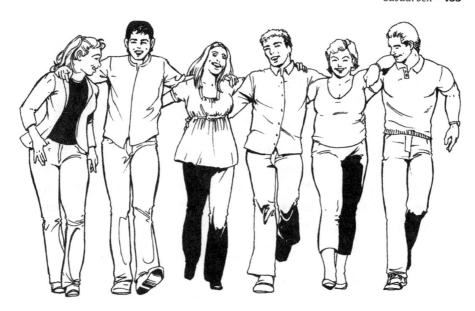

Peer Groups Today

cess I never once considered calling her. An abundance of secure choices have protected me from vulnerability: technology is the brick wall."

"We have a hard time committing. All of these strange, unclear relationships exist that have no formal rules. It seems we are just using each other to have sex. At the same time we do share mutual feelings of romance and passion, yet we do not call ourselves boyfriend/girlfriend in any aspect of the word. There might be someone better out there, which is constantly suggested by our friend count on Facebook. It scares us out of committing to someone who could be inferior to the next bidder."

"It's better to keep it simple and casual so it's easier to detach when the inevitable moving on occurs."

"I've had the stereotypical 'who is this girl next to me?' mornings. Although those have not been my best decisions, I've learned from each one. But some people get very confused. My most recent 'friends with benefits' relationship went spiraling into disaster when she got too clingy and tried acting like a long-term girlfriend. At the same time, I've found that girls are as likely to want sex-only relationships as guys."

"I've been with easier girls for random nights of sex, but there's nothing better than a girl who does not mind spending a Saturday night in the library studying. They tend to be more responsible, trustworthy, and able to have an intelligent conversation that does not include alcohol, drugs, blackout, and vomiting."

"I can't imagine calling seven girls and having insightful conversations with them all; however, I can imagine texting seven girls the same thing at once. This form of impersonal communication has replaced the art of conversation and serves as a way to avoid potentially stressful interaction."

"Relationships are complicated and the rules are puzzling. I have a hard time figuring them out. We have Facebook, Twitter, texting, IM, Skype, and iChat. Most of our communicating is done through a screen. There are hardly any face-to-face interactions, unless you are wasted at a party, and in most of those situations, you're looking for someone to hook up with that night."

"We're making up the rules as we go along, pretending we don't have feelings. We're sex-fueled young adults trying to figure out who we are by sleeping with as many people as we can."

"When trying to ask a girl out, I need to Facebook friend her. Once she accepts, I write her a comment about something that happened when we first met. If she responds in a positive way, I send her another comment saying we should meet up the next time both of us go out. If she responds with a yes, then I ask for her number and give her mine. After the numbers have been exchanged, I will text her during the evening of the day I plan on going out. She can then take this wherever she wants to: sex, kissing, just a hug at the door. If things go well, I ask her via text when I can see her again, because calling comes off too strong and can be seen as creepy. When I have tried calling or skipping one of these steps, I have failed. I believe this routine is somewhat messed up. The structure is flawed."

Starting with a Date vs. Casual Sex

Dating still occurs and is still important, especially for people who are getting near the dangerously old age of twenty-five, as they are getting their first full-time job or becoming more established in the working world. (If you are at that point in life, be sure to read Chapter 32: *Sex with a Coworker.*) There is also an in between kind of dating or "dating adjacent" that's a hazy area between dating and casual sex. It's where two people are checking each other out as possible relationship material. It's like an interview with your clothes off.

Dating is seldom as formal as it used to be, nor is it the major social event it once was. But in a world where people increasingly talk via texting and video messaging, dating can feel as stressful as ever. Not only do you have to make eye contact and use your tongues instead of your thumbs, but it's hard to edit before you press the "speak" button.

Dating Roles Remain the Same

> "Girls want to be on the same playing field as the boys, but when it comes to paying, asking out, approaching, calling and everything like that, a lot of girls still want the boys to be the initiator."
>
> *female age 22*

With dating, there are still well defined male-female roles, although they don't exactly scream at you like they used to. One defined role is that it's usually the guy who does the asking out, although that is often massaged and manipulated through interventions ranging from friends encouraging him to text her, to strategies where you "casually" run into each other.

Alcohol & Awkward, Horny & Excited—But Not "Abusive" or "Pain"

We interviewed a number of women for this chapter. The two words they used most often in describing casual sex were *alcohol* and *awkward,* but *horny* and *excited* were up there as well. In more than 25 pages of transcripts, *love* was used only twice, and that was regarding current boyfriends as opposed to former hooking-up partners. C*omfort, comforting* and *uncomfortable* were used often. *Abusive, unhappy,* and *pain* were not used at all. When it comes to casual sex, the kind of emotions the women value in a long-term relationship are not a big part of it—nor are the emotions they dread.

While much of the media coverage of casual sex ends with poignant accounts of how empty it can be and how hurt at least one of the partners ends up, that's not what the women who took our survey focused on.

"When you are not in a relationship and you want sex, you have casual sex. At times it can be satisfying sexually, but not emotionally. To have just casual sex you need to be able to separate the emotions. When I was involved in casual sex it was with the same guy, but there were no attachments. If one of us hooked up with someone else then the arrangement would be over. Now that I am in a committed relationship, I think that the sex with someone you know and are emotionally invested in is so much better. Knowing the person cares about you makes sex a lot more worthwhile." *female age 22*

Almost all of the women said that alcohol was their gasoline for hookup sex, but they didn't seem particularly concerned about it.

"I definitely think random hook-ups have more to do with alcohol than what is believed in the media." *female age 22*

"Alcohol plays a big role in hooking up. Many (including myself) have used the excuse 'I was drunk.' It's almost like a free pass." *female, 22*

"Alcohol is a huge influence on casual sex, especially for girls! I don't think I would ever hook up with a guy I didn't know unless I have the comfort of saying I was drunk at the time so I had an excuse in the morning." *female age 21*

"When I drink I want sex, so I knew I could get it from him. Drinking just makes sex more interesting to me because I am more open to trying things, and I am not worried about what I look like or how I am doing. I am more worried about my receiving sexual pleasure than anything else." *female age 22*

"You may think this person was attractive when drunk, but when you wake up the next morning and see him, you are like 'Whoa... I'm out of here.'" *female age 23*

"I see casual sex more when alcohol or substances are being used, especially in college. People don't think about what they are doing until the next morning when guilt settles in. I know this because, unfortunately it has happened to me and a lot of my friends." *fem. 23*

"Alcohol is more of an excuse than a reason sex happens. When I drink I act on my sexual needs more than when I am sober." *female age 22*

"Alcohol has a huge impact on my sexual activities. If I drink enough I have no moral rules with myself anymore. The next day I can wake up and make it okay by just saying, 'I was drunk.'" *female age 21*

"Alcohol is a big part of my life as a college student. I know it sounds like a crutch, but on the weekends, everyone I know is drinking."

female age 21

When it comes to casual sex, getting drunk allows women to act more like men. It's a testosterone patch in a can.

When we asked the women if they needed to hammer down a few Stolis before having sex with a boyfriend as opposed to someone they were hooking up with, you could hear the "Hell no!" loud and clear.

Casual Sex and Birth Control

Another college instructor from a rural area who uses *The Guide* in her sex-ed course sent in the following regarding her students:

"I'm concerned about some of our students using morning-after pills and abortions for birth control. They often hook up with guys and have unprotected sex. Their doctors prescribe them three months' worth of morning-after pills. Some of the young women use the pills as many as three times in a month. I am not certain what impact this type of use may have on their bodies. Additionally, some of the girls admitted to psychological challenges following abortions."

It's one thing to blame what you did last night on alcohol, but it's quite another to be having sex without a sound birth-control strategy in place. Please read Chapter 58: *Birth Control, Sperm vs. Egg* carefully. Also, emergency contraception is not meant to be used as regular birth control, although it can be taken several times a month without causing worrisome side effects for most women.

Men should be aware that the day when a man could easily skate out on paying child support is long gone. Paternity is not a difficult thing to prove with a simple DNA test. *Hopefully, today's women who are having casual sex know to get the information of the men they are having sex with, in case they become pregnant and need the dad's help, or if he turns out to be someone who commits sexual assault and the police are trying to find him. Having a record of his number or Twitter handle are important.*

Blow Jobs vs. Intercourse

Two of the last things you want from casual sex are unwanted pregnancies and sexually transmitted infections. This book would never suggest giving a guy a blowjob when you don't want to, but if it's something you are okay with and effective methods of birth control are not available, keep it in mind as an alternative to intercourse. It is impossible to become pregnant from giving a guy oral sex and your chances of getting a sexually transmitted infection are much lower than when you are having intercourse. Triple that for giving him a handjob. (Media hysteria about oral sex and oral cancer has been filled with misinformation. A woman's chances of being killed in a car accident are more than a million times greater than her chances of getting oral cancer from giving a guy a blow job before she's 60. She should be much more concerned about pregnancy and STIs like HIV. See Chapter 52: *Gnarly Sex Germs* for more information.)

Random Facts about Casual Sex

Oral Sex: Guys seldom go down on women during one-night stands. A woman is more likely to receive oral sex in a friends-with-benefits arrangement where her sexual pleasure is one of the motivators.

Was it consensual or forced? This is a very real concern for young women in casual sex situations, especially the Last-Virgin-Standing types who go to parties where there's a punch bowl of "jungle juice" or "panty dropping punch." Please read Chapter 13: *Consent*.

Orgasms: not all men have orgasms during casual sex. The estimate is 80% of men have orgasms during casual sex, while 20% of women might have orgasms. However, the women's orgasms count can go way up in a friends-with-benefits situation.

Cuddling: In spite of what you've heard, plenty of men and women want physical tenderness in casual sex that's more than just intercourse or oral sex. So men and women aren't always running out the door as soon as the last drop of semen hits the sheets.

Condoms: Using condoms not only helps prevent pregnancy and decreases your chances of getting most sexually transmitted infections, but it helps decrease morning-after regret.

More Responses From Our Female Survey Takers

"Hook-up sex cannot be with a guy you are wanting a relationship with. It has to be just for the sex."

"If I am at a party and meet a guy and I really like him and we start fooling around and he calls the next day well then great, let's hang out. Not because we fucked, but because I liked hanging out with him. It's always a scary possibility when you don't have sex in the beginning and you get into a relationship and your lover is horrible, then you're stuck in a bad-sex relationship and if we're being honest, sex is a huge part. For me, I like to meet the guy first, enjoy being with him and then sleep together, as scary as that is. Then I'll invest time and a relationship in him."

"For me casual sex can be uncomfortable or awkward. You don't know what to expect or what they expect. There is some excitement, but there is excitement in a relationship. You know what the person likes, what they are willing to try, and their comfort level."

"To me hooking up/one nighters are just that. Generally there are no feelings towards the person. If you're horny you call them up and have sex and that's about it. Alcohol is a huge factor. More than likely we will both be drinking with the same people at the same bar and then one thing leads to another and we are having sex."

"I think relationships are still the goal. It's just more relaxed on how we get to that point."

"I know people that were friends with their significant other and then started having sex. I also know people who have sex and then a relationship happens. I have tried both. I can't tell you which one is better. They both worked for me. I think it depends on the chemistry and how the two of you are."

"I still see relationships as a goal, but if you aren't near to finding someone to meet your goal, why not have fun until then?"

"I think that guys look at girls who sleep with them early in the relationship as slutty. If you sleep with a guy before you really know him he assumes that you do this with everyone. He is not considered unfit because of the double standard. It doesn't matter how many girls he has slept with, but it does matter how many guys a girl has slept with."

"I haven't met many men who don't want sex right away."

A Very Special Thanks to Dr. Dennis Waskul and his students at Minnesota State University, Mankato, to Janet Minehan and Marian Shapiro at Santa Barbara Community College, to Elaine Hatfield at the University of Hawai'i, to Justin Garcia at the Kinsey Institute, to Heather Flores at Madera and Clovis Community College Centers, California, and to Abigail Nitzel and Dr. Joan Chrisler of Connecticut College for some very thoughtful research done on Hooking-Up ("Hooking-Up versus Dating").

CHAPTER

32
Sex with a Co-Worker

The word "dating" is derived from the Latin phrase *ante eius toga datus in animao*. It means "get into a person's head before you get into his or her pants." This is an important concept when you are lusting for someone at work.

Work can be a great place to meet a partner. When you date someone you meet through work, you know what they look like, how they behave under stress and how they treat others. If they have a sense of humor, you'll know about it, and if they have a good work ethic, others will respect them. If someone at work has personality problems, their fellow workers will usually rat them out. These can be luxuries in the age of online dating when what you see is not necessarily what you get.

People you meet through work will often be geographically desirable, unless they're in the Omaha office and you're in Maine. You won't have to explain your company's quirks and culture to them, and there's a good chance you'll have each other's backs.

However, there can be a number of problems when you have sex with a co-worker, from relationship drama to company policy. This chapter's job is to walk you through that. Think of it as the missing section from your employee handbook—the one on negotiating the workplace environment when a fellow employees' legs are wrapped around yours while you are off the clock.

The Downside of Having Sex with a Co-Worker

Think about the social discomfort at work if one of you wants to take it further and the other doesn't. There can also be legal considerations when people in the same company are exchanging more than memos and platonic pleasantries. And when you are dating a co-worker, you're not just dating that person. If they belong to a close-knit group, you might as well be dating their entire department.

Another problem is when an employee uses work as a source of hook-ups and casual sex partners. This behavior almost always leads to workplace drama and can become highly disruptive. Casual sex among co-workers is one of the things employers dislike the most about co-worker dating.

Company Dating Policy

The vast majority of companies don't have a dating policy, but some do. You probably don't want to raise suspicion by calling your boss or HR and asking "What's our company's policy about dating co-workers?" But if your company does have a policy, it will probably be in your employee handbook.

Some companies have a policy that says it's not okay for a boss or supervisor to date a subordinate, or they can't work together in the same department. At some companies it's okay for co-workers to date, but if they get married, one of them has to transfer or get a job somewhere else.

In case you are wondering why a company would be concerned about sexual relationships among co-workers, consider the following:

Relationship-related workplace insanity: Companies don't want relationship issues in the workplace. They don't want their employees groping in front of the copy machine or hurling nasty barbs when a relationship starts to sour. They don't want things going on that will make other employees feel uncomfortable or angry.

Sexual harassment lawsuits: While these suits are not common, lawyers tend to come unglued when an boss or supervisor is dating an underling. What if the couple breaks up and the worker is denied a promotion? This can look like retaliation. There can also be a serious power differential. What if the worker feels he or she has to accept advances from higher-ups or else? This is why it can be wise for one of the parties to transfer into a different department when a supervisor is dating someone he or she supervises.

Preferential Treatment: Let's say Austin, who is a middle manager, is dating Brandi, who is an executive vice president. Stormy is another middle manager who is aware that Brandi and Austin are dating. So what happens when Austin, who is incredibly hard working and deserving of a promotion, gets a promotion that Stormy felt she should have had? Stormy can make a big stink about how Austin received preferential treatment due to Austin's relationship with Brandi. Even if nothing was underhanded or wrong, appearances can make a difference in the workplace.

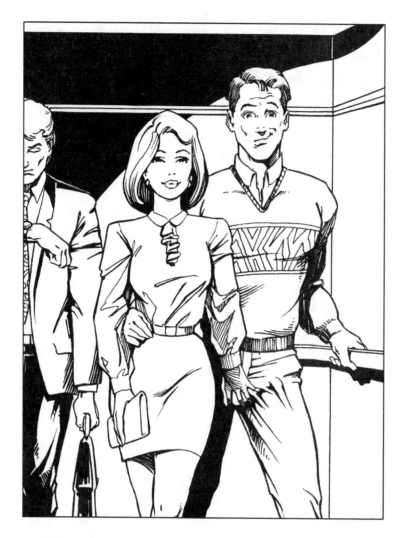

Company Adjacent

Work-related relationships can extend beyond your immediate co-workers. It might include dating a client, vendor, sales rep, consultant, or a patient. Does your company have a policy about this?

Dating In the Workplace vs. Casual Sex

You don't need to become the company virgin, but it won't help your career if you're known as the mailroom manwhore or the player from personnel. So if you are hot for a co-worker and value your job, put a lock on your fly or a latch on your labia until you've dated more than once or twice and have long-term potential. While marriage needn't be the goal, at the very least, you'll want to aspire to an exclusive and stable booty-buddy relationship. Otherwise, look elsewhere for a dating pool.

What Happens at Home Should Stay at Home

Normally, work can be a place of refuge during times of relationship drama. Try to keep it that way even if you are dating a co-worker. Talk to your lover about the importance of maintaining healthy boundaries between the two of you and your respective jobs. Create mutual strategies to achieve this early in your relationship.

PDA? NSFW!

Besides bringing relationship issues to work, the quickest way to get fired is to annoy co-workers with public displays of affection.

Even if you are in the safety of a locked supply room or have taken refuge in the furthest recesses of a warehouse, do not kiss, grope each other, or have sex at work. And while it might be perfectly normal to sext a lover who is working for another company, never sext a co-worker when either of you is at work. It's not smart and it's not worth the risk.

When you are at work, treat your lover the same as you would treat any other co-worker. Have an understanding about this. You have no idea how much better being discreet will work out for both of you.

When to Go Public

Never underestimate the power of pettiness in the workforce. When people get bored at work, there's no better way to pass time than with vicious gossip. This means that stealth is your friend.

Not that there's any research on this, but the longer you keep your relationship under wraps, the better. When you are first dating, try not to post photos of yourselves together on your Facebook page. And resist announcing "Ben from underwriting asked me out!" Give your relationship time to develop before telling your co-workers.

This might sound like overkill, but try making "an organizational chart" of co-workers who will be most affected when they learn you have become orgasm-bonded. This will help you evolve a more effective strategy of how to handle matters when your relationship status becomes known.

Once you are ready to let the cat out of the bag, plan who you are going to tell. Should you inform your supervisors first? If you have different supervisors, you should probably tell them on the same day so they find out about it directly from you. If you have the same supervisor, should you both be there to make the announcement?

If a co-worker pitches a fit because you've been dating another worker and haven't told him or her, how are you going to handle that? Perhaps it would help to explain that you wanted to make sure things would work out first, and that he or she is the first one you are telling.

Don't be surprised if everyone is aware of your secret. Still, most will appreciate how you've attempted to be professional about your "coupleness" at work. At the very least, being discreet will give your co-workers less ammo to say nasty things about you the moment your back is turned.

Extramarital Affairs at Work

One of the most damaging things you can do to your career is have an extramarital affair with a co-worker. You will be shocked to learn how many people will be affected if you are cheating on a partner with someone from work. Even if they don't like your spouse, cheating makes people squirm. Maybe it's because it reminds them of what their own spouse might be doing with someone else. Or maybe it just doesn't feel right morally.

If you and your spouse have an open relationship, it's not actually cheating. But good luck explaining that to your co-workers!

Breaking Up

Maybe you'll decide to take your relationship with a co-worker further than just dating. Or maybe there will come a point when one or both of you feels it's time to go your own ways.

Hopefully, if you split up, you'll be one of the rare couples that is able to remain friends. But even the most amicable of partings can be a challenge.

Something you might consider talking about at the start of your relationship is how the two of you would handle it at work if you split up. Unfortunately, there's no way to predict how you will feel or how you'll behave if your relationship falls on bad times.

Just as getting together may have impacted your fellow workers, your splitting up may impact them as well. You never want to pressure them into taking sides or make them feel uncomfortable when they are around either or both of you. As much as it might be tempting, do not diss your ex at work

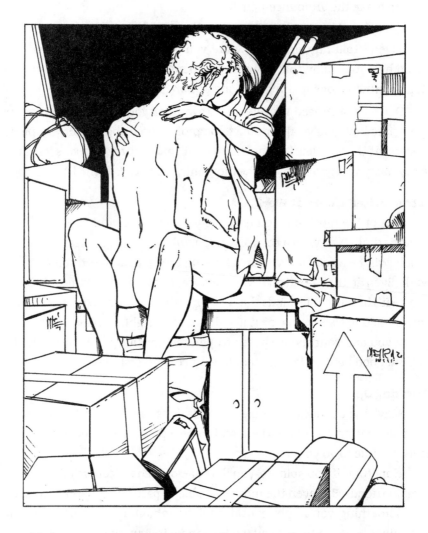

This is never a good idea. Keep all aspects of your relationship away from work, including quickies!

or with a co-worker. In addition to making you look petty, this will not help your career. If you are too hurt to act rationally, don't hesitate to see a therapist to help you keep it together.

A Human Resources Executive Weighs In

Here are the observations of a human resources professional with more than twenty years of experience. He believes that co-worker relationships are inevitable, given how much time workers spend together. However, the relationships don't always work out well.

> "Co-worker relationships are probably the most reoccurring cause of employee issues I have experienced. Typically the problems are worse when the relationship is in the end stages. However, I have seen a situation where the partners involved held senior positions and virtually destroyed a division when they were at the height of their relationship."

> "It's not unusual for workers to refuse to talk to or interact with anyone if it involves their ex. Essential information will stop flowing. Their friends become involved when things heat up and both sides jockey for position. Absenteeism will rise and one of the former partners will often quit or will be fired, especially if one continues to goad the other."

Hopefully you will take this to heart. With an awareness of how badly things can turn out, it's your job to keep the drama under control if you have sex with a co-worker.

Reader Comments

> "I have seen a lot of horrible office relationships! I have also seen a few great marriages stem from inner-office relationships. It's more common than I thought. I promised myself I would never date a co-worker. However, I have met some of my best friends here at work. And well, I broke my own rule and started dating one of my best friends who is a co-worker!"

> "My partner and I have been co-workers for almost six years. We met working on the same project. We continue to work together.

We have been lovers for almost four years and have lived together for two. Both our colleagues and our senior management are totally supportive. I totally enjoy working with someone I love and respect personally as well as professionally and it is a blessing to have a partner who is completely aware of and understands your work environment, stresses, etc."

"I had sex with one of my co-workers and it was fine. He was nice and the sex was good. Even when we stopped seeing each other we stayed friends and work was good for a long time. But I also had sex with my boss one summer and it went so badly that I lied and told him I had an STD when I eventually quit. He was mostly a jackass about it. I think that the sex basically made bad situations worse, and possibly made good situations better."

"I've had sex with co-workers on a couple of occasions, some have ended well and others haven't. Oddly, I've found its been the men in these scenarios that tended to get weird."

33

Sex When You Move Back Home

"Dear Paul,
I just graduated from college and had to move back home with my parents. Everyone says I need to get on with the next phase of my life, but I have no clue what that should be. I'm so depressed I don't even want to have sex. But if I did, I still wouldn't feel comfortable bringing a woman home to have sex here. I feel like I'm eleven instead of twenty two. Do you have any advice?

Mike from Manitoba

Dear Mike,

Like you, I moved back home with my parents after five years as an undergrad. I was depressed, dejected and had no clue what the future would bring. During my years at college, I had not been sheltered or lacking in initiative. I had ducked tear gas canisters from antiwar riots on my way to class and I'd worked long shifts in a mental hospital at night. I'd coached a winning woman's football team and had been on the staff in the dorms.

Yet when I moved back home with my parents, I had no idea how to be an adult in their household. I quickly returned to being the same son that I was when I was in high school, and they became the same parents. I eventually escaped by going to grad school.

It wasn't until later, after my dad became old and started to get dementia, that I could be the adult in his presence that I was in the rest of my life. And it wasn't until my mom could no longer manage on her own that I learned to be an adult in her presence.

I don't envy the task you have in changing your family dynamics. I totally sucked at it myself. And I understand how challenging it can be when the structure and safety net of college disappears.

Hopefully you'll find some of the things in this chapter to be helpful while you are ending one stage of your life and trying to begin another.

From Rusty Parent-Child Dynamics to Squeaky Bed Springs

If you want to have a sex life while living in your parent's home, you'll need to find a way to be an adult when you move back home. That's how parents begin to accept their children as sexual beings with sexual needs.

So the first part of this chapter is about getting your parents to see you as an adult. With some parents and some children, this won't be difficult. With others, it can be a challenge. But even if your parent-child dynamics get rearranged in all the right ways, you still might not feel comfortable having sex in your old room. And your parents might not feel comfortable when the child they used to read *Goodnight Moon* to is having sex with a lover whose name they hardly know.

The second part of this chapter is about the mechanics of having sex while under your parents roof—from how to quiet a bed with springs from hell to prepping your lover on what to say when they can no longer avoid having a conversation with your family members.

Boomer-What?

The media has invented the term "boomerang generation" to describe former college students who move back home. This is misleading, because when you toss a boomerang it comes back the same as when it left. That's not true for someone who left home at eighteen and comes back after years of answering to no one. Worse yet, before you left, it was as much your house as your parents. And when you had friends over, it was usually just friends and not someone you were going to have sex with, or not someone your parents knew you were having sex with.

So it's a different situation than the word "boomerang" implies. Expectations are different and adjustments need to be made.

You're Not the Only One Who Likes to Walk Around Naked

If you were an only child or the last of your siblings to leave home, your parents have now had a couple of years to walk around naked, get a little drunk, have sex in the kitchen and learn to cherish their privacy. (Where do you think your "walk-around-naked" and "I'm horny—let's fuck now" genes came from?)

Returning home might force your parents to give up some hard-earned freedom. Be sensitive to this and try to appreciate that they didn't have to let you move back home.

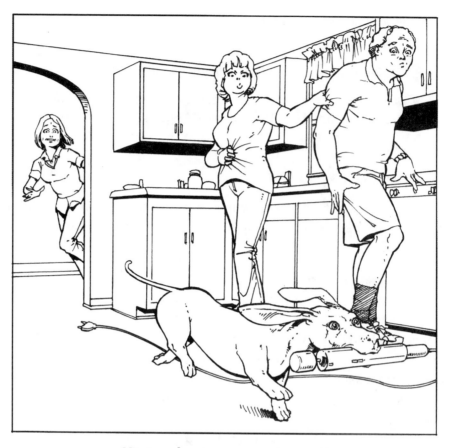

No more leaving your sex toys out!

Making Yourself a Grown-Up in Your Parents' Eyes

One way to be a responsible adult is to help pay your share of the expenses. But you probably wouldn't be moving back home if you could do that. So the next best thing is to calculate how many hours you'd have to work to pay your share of the rent, food, utilities, phone and Internet. Ask your parents what their expectations are of you and what you can do around the house to help make this work best for everyone. Here are just a few ways to earn parental respect and hopefully your sexual freedom when living at home:

- Help do the shopping
- Cook and do the dishes

- 💡 Be a work-out partner for unmotivated parents

- 💡 Clean the house and do the wash

- 💡 Garden, paint, run errands, and chauffeur siblings

- 💡 Do the bookkeeping for your parent's business, fix their website, or program their electronics and remotes

- 💡 Detail the car or help tutor a younger sibling

- 💡 Help your grandparents

It may be that your parents will never agree to you having sex with a partner in their home. But the way to give yourself the best chance is to be responsible and helpful.

Doing Yourself No Harm

The moment your parents have to start nagging you, you suddenly return to middle-school in their eyes. Middle school—wasn't that when sex meant your own hand in your own pants?

Statements like "Oh crap, I forgot to take out the garbage" or "Sorry, mom, I forgot to pick up Davy from baseball practice" will not cut it if you're trying to earn grown-up privileges. Being reliable will increase your standing in the eyes of most lovers as well.

Keep your parents updated about your plans and goals. Even if your chances of winning the lottery are better than landing a job, keep your family in the loop. It can be easy to lose hope. Sometimes, just making the effort to fake it can be important in making progress or moving forward.

Hot Water and Bandwidth — Two Things You Should Never Hog

Even if you always take a shower the first thing in the morning, you don't want your mom or dad taking a cold shower because of you. Nor does it matter if your younger brother drains every drop of hot water while jerking off in the shower. It's unlikely he gets to have a lover spend the night, while you're expecting a different set of rights.

What's true for hot water is also true for Internet bandwidth. Don't be downloading porn when your mom wants to watch a show on Hulu or your sister is streaming a movie. And as much as it might annoy you to cede bandwidth to younger siblings, it will not help your cause if they go whining to your mom or dad about how you are hogging the DSL.

Having Friends Over Now vs. Then

It's one thing if your parents offer your friends beer or wine, but your friends offering your parents alcohol or drugs might not go over so well. In some households, if your friends walk into your parents' house flashing twelve-packs of beer, it's no different than a terrorist walking into an airport with a bomb in his briefs. Double that if your friends bring acid, 'shrooms, hash or anything leafy, pill shaped, white or powdery that might cause surveillance by the feds.

Even if it's totally fine with your parents that you are having friends over, it's wise to ask ahead of time. It's different now than when you were in high school and everyone assumed your friends would crash at your place.

Social Before Sexual

When you were living on your own and you met someone new, you might have ended up at their place or yours for a night of sex. This doesn't work so well when you're living with your mom and dad.

The best solution is to first meet a potential new lover for coffee or lunch, or at a movie, sporting event, or museum. You won't believe how much you'll find out about a person when you are both sober and your clothes are on.

If you decide sex is a good next move, try making your first time at their place or at a hotel. Some hotels have a special day rate for this exact thing. They are known as hot-sheet hotels. Then, if you decide it's not going anywhere, you won't have to cash in one of your "here's-the-latest-person-I'm-sleeping-with" chips with your mom and dad. And if your new lover is a keeper but screams with wild abandon while having orgasms, you can discuss acoustic sensibilities before making love in your parents' home.

If your parents pester you mercilessly about meeting your new hookup, tell them you haven't decided if he or she is family worthy. Plus, if your family is a bit odd, delaying a bit avoids scaring away a perfectly good lover before he or she is more invested in you and is more likely to weather your family's unique habits.

Sharing Date Drama With Your Mama

It's one thing to be living hundreds of miles away from your mom and phone her in tears about how terribly your partner has been treating you.

That's what moms are for. It's quite another thing to have these kinds of conversations when you are living at home. How's your mom going to handle it when you invite the loser over the next day for make-up sex?

This sort of thing makes parents insane, especially dads with guns. So if you are experiencing less than domestic tranquility with a lover, consider not discussing it with your mom unless you need moral support.

Explaining Friends with Benefits

There might be times in life when you have a non-traditional relationship that consists of really good sex but nothing more. Unless you have the most sexually evolved parents on the planet, finding the right words to explain this type of casual-sex relationship to your mom and dad is beyond the scope of this book or any other.

On the other hand, is it possible your lover isn't someone you would want to admit to your family that you are spending naked time with? This might not have been so bad when all you had to deal with was the disgusted glares of your roommates. It could be that moving home will force you to set the bar a little higher when it comes to who you sleep with.

Facebook, Texting, Email and Sexting

It was one thing to be Facebook friends with your parents when you were twelve. But now? Even if you aren't FB friends with your family, the Internet is an open book. Once you move back home, don't put anything on it that you wouldn't want your mom or dad to see.

Nothing will piss off parents more than when your little brother hacks into your Twitter or email account and shows them your posts dissing them. If you don't want your family to know exactly what you are thinking, don't text it, email it or write it down.

Also, it is unwise to keep a lover's sexts for posterity or masturbation purposes. Assume your mom, dad, or siblings will find them. An upskirt photo from a lover is unlikely to increase your mom's opinion of her. And imagine having to face a lover's father after he found your dick pic to his daughter along with an explanation of what you're going to do to her in bed—while under his roof.

Younger Siblings

If the stork made a tragically late visit to your home and you have siblings in elementary school or younger, be sensitive to what an important figure you are in their eyes. Kids are always on the prowl for someone to look up to, and that might be you. When it comes to younger siblings, you are in the sometimes strange zone of being more of a parent than their brother or sister.

Siblings can also form strong attachments to your boyfriend or girlfriend, especially if your BF or GF is being extra nice to them. This is usually a good thing unless you decide to break up. It's also something to consider when it comes to bringing casual hookups home. Just like a single parent who is dating, you need to be sensitive about the impact that a revolving door of lovers will have on your siblings.

Kids tend to be curious, especially about anything having to do with sex. So it might be wise to put a lock on your door for when a lover is over. You don't want to risk having your third-grade sister or brother asking your mom, "Why does Amy have Trevor's penis in her mouth?"

Under no conditions should you ever give siblings in high school drugs or alcohol. Not only is this dumb, but you risk being charged with the criminal act of furnishing a minor with whatever you furnished.

Arriving with Pets

The difference between the family pets you grew up with and the one (hopefully it's one) you are moving back home with is that you and your pets are now guests.

In time, your family might grow to like your pet as much as they like you. Maybe more. But if your pet is so obnoxious that your former roommates tried to donate it for medical experimentation, you'll need to become super responsible. Pick up the pet's poop before it hits the ground, or make sure its litter box looks like the sand traps at the Pebble Beach Golf Course. If it's a dog, be sure it gets enough exercise and slap a no-bark collar on its neck if it won't stop barking.

Good luck if you've got a large dog that likes to occupy your dad's favorite chair or bares its teeth at your mom's yappy Poodle.

Strategic Room Choice for Better Sex

If sex in your parents' home is a possibility and you have a choice of rooms, place acoustic considerations at the top of your list. While you might love the room in the attic, think twice if it's directly above your parents' bed.

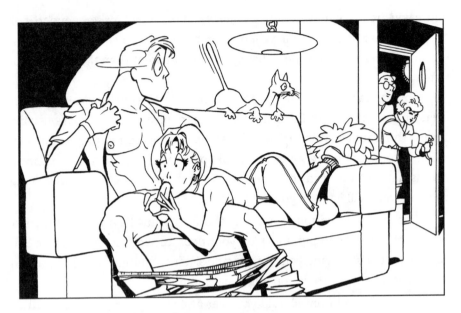

It's best not to have sex in family areas.

Even if it's smaller, a room at the opposite end of the hall from your mom and dad's bedroom might make for a better sex cave.

Another plus is having a separate entrance. This means you won't need to introduce hookups to your parents, which can save all kinds of embarrassment if you can't remember the hookup's name.

The ultimate situation is a guest house or a converted garage, but you already knew that.

Loud Music Is Not the Answer

Your mom to your younger sister: "What's Kyle doing?"

Your younger sister to your mom: "He just turned up the volume on Pandora, so he's probably having sex with Carrie."

Seriously, do you think that cranking up the volume is going to fool anyone? Turning up the music announces your fuck fest to the world. Instead, try pushing a towel against the bottom of the door if it leaks sound. It won't keep the smell of pot smoke from escaping, but it can shave a few decibels off cries of "Oh God, I'm coming!" and "Harder, Shawn, Harder!"

Vibrators

If you use a vibrator, try to find a model that doesn't shake the house off its foundation. If you are penniless, consider trying a famous-brand pulsating toothbrush that's battery powered and usually sells for around $8 to $10 for a twin pack. A lot of women say this micropulsating toothbrush vibrates at a perfect frequency and gets more off than the plaque on their teeth. (See Chapter 26: *Oscillator, Generator, Vibrator, Dildo.*)

Signals

Parents tend to worry about their children no matter how old they are. So it could be in everyone's better interest to work out a way of letting your parents know if you are coming home later than planned. Calling or texting are the usual standbys, but maybe something else that will work better, especially if it's late and you are worried about waking your parents. Turning off a specified light that they can see from their bedroom sometimes works, although there's not much point if the family dog starts howling the moment you open the door.

The Three Talks — "Barging In," "I'm an Adult Who Has Sex" and "How To Tell a Lover You Live at Home"

Moving home can be particularly traumatic if your parents and siblings are barging into your room at all hours of the day and night. If that's the case, you might try reminding your parents that you don't barge into their bedroom without knocking, but don't mention the reason is because you'd rather not see your parents doing something that might result in your needing years of therapy. Use a respectful tone when asking that they not enter your room without knocking unless the house is on fire or your dad is having a heart attack. Keep in mind that your parents are on solid ground to enter when necessary if your housekeeping habits are causing the rodent population in the neighborhood to double.

At some point, you may need to have the "I'm not a child anymore, I like sex!" talk with your mom and dad, but it's usually best to save it for a few months down the line after you've demonstrated how helpful, responsible and adult-like you are. One possible approach is to say "You did your job and did it well. You raised a responsible, caring young adult who, like other responsible caring young adults, has friends he or she spends the night with.

It's a normal, natural, biologically okay thing when you reach my age." Then see where it lands.

If you are embarrassed about living at home and are sheepish or apologetic when you tell a partner, then that's what the take-home message will be. But if you confidently explain that your parents are good people and you moved back home for good reasons, then that's probably how it will be received.

Not Being Able to Have Fights with Your Lover

Even the most perfect of lover has habits that will eventually get under your skin. That's why fights are necessary. But how do you have a good fight when your parents are in the next room?

It's a sad but true aspect of human nature that learning to have sex quietly is way easier than learning to have a good fight quietly. The same is true with texting: it's easy to text seductive messages, but good luck trying to text a fight! Finding a private place to have a fight can be as important as finding a private place to have sex.

Breaking Up

When you break up with a partner who has gotten to know your family, your family might react in one of two ways: with grief or sorrow, or with quiet cheers and high fives. If they genuinely liked your former partner, be sensitive to the impact that your break-up will have on your family.

Common Sense Considerations When Having Sex at Your Parents' Home

💡Don't ever flush spent condoms or period gear down the toilet. Condoms, tampons and sanitary napkins will cost your parents $300 or more in plumbing bills. You don't want to be around when the plumber tells your mom or dad what caused the backup in the line.

💡Unless you have a private bathroom, don't allow a partner to sneak out of your room naked or in their underwear. Sweats, pajamas, flannel nightgowns or robes that go below the knees are essentials if you or your partner need to leave the bedroom when not fully dressed.

💡It's your job to help your partners have good conversations with your parents, so have a list of family-socialization tips for new lovers. For example, "My mom had an affair with the tennis pro, so tennis is a sore subject with my dad," or "When my little brother isn't beating off to porn, he plays soccer and he's had some epic kills in World of Warcraft," or "The sewing stuff belongs to my dad, and the guns are my mom's."

Parents like to meet a partner who is respectful, helpful, at least somewhat engaging, and who doesn't try to sneak off into the bedroom without saying hello.

If you use the family car for sex, be sure to pack out what you pack in. Never leave a used condom, condom wrapper, intimate apparel, a roach, or anything else related to what you've been doing in the car. Semen stains and wet spots on the upholstery are especially bad.

Never bring a last-minute hookup home for sex. Only bring home sexual partners who you know and can trust.

When possible, schedule sex during parental time away.

Make no mistake about it, your family dog will find used condoms in the trash can. This is certain to cause a gross family moment. But at least the family dog has an excuse. It's not beyond some parents and siblings to check your trash for spent condoms. If this is a potential issue, create a secure place for used condoms that you can empty right before the garbage is picked up.

Never, ever have sex in your parent's bed.

Parents tend to hate it if you text at the dinner table or while having conversations with them. Once you move home, texting should be like masturbation—mostly done behind closed doors. This will make you seem more adult than your younger siblings or the children of your parents' friends.

If you are the athletic type when making love, try toning it down when your parents are home. While everyone in the house knows what's going on, there's no point in making the picture frames shake on the walls.

It's never good to leave wet spots or other spills on the mattress. Buy a mattress-pad cover that's waterproof. The better ones don't make crinkling sounds. Be sure to wash it and the sheets yourself.

Lubes that contain silicone can leave wicked stains on the sheets.

Get a big, soft, reddish-colored beach towel to put down on the bed before having period sex.

Noisy Beds—Signs of Studliness at College, Not So at Home

Intercourse can turn a bed into a battering ram. The entire bed will sway toward the foot with each out-thrust and toward the head with each in-thrust. If it's hitting the wall, try moving the bed away from the wall. If that doesn't work, stabilize it by cramming pillows or gasket-like material between the headboard and the wall.

A frequent culprit is the frame. If it's metal, consider putting oil on the rivets or where the pieces of the frame join together. If it's bolted together, undo the bolts and see if inserting plastic washers might help. If the bed has a headboard or footboard, check where the side rails connect to it. Tighten anything that can be tightened. Try shoving material in areas where metal might be rubbing against metal. Check the lateral or side-to-side support on the frame. You might need to add some boards or extra slats between the side rails.

If the box springs are a source of noise, make sure the mattress is centered on the box springs. You can also try putting a piece of foam or plywood between the mattress and box springs.

Squeaky box springs can be insidious and require surgery. If so, carefully remove the cloth cover on the bottom of the box spring. If you find a broken spring, cut it out. There are usually more springs than you need, so no one will be the wiser. If the springs are being held in place by screws, try tightening them. Lubricate squeaky springs with a spritz of WD-40 or vegetable oil, but be careful not to overspray and stain the fabric.

Don't ignore where the frame meets the floor. If that's a source of noise, put large rubber caster cups under the legs so there's insulation between the legs and the floor. Also, the floor boards might have become soft or squeaky in the area where the bed is located. If so, it's time to rearrange the furniture. If that fails, try putting the mattress on the floor or invest in a platform bed.

If you tormented your mattress mercilessly as a kid by jumping on it every day, it might be getting revenge on you now. If os, nothing short of a trip to the dump will do.

Moving Back Home When You Have Your Own Kids

This is such a complex topic it would require its own chapter. Be sure to do research on the kind of issues that can come up. Talk to your parents about what they expect of you, and what you should or shouldn't expect of them. Unless there are good reasons why you should no longer parent your kids, don't dump them on your parents.

If you are having casual sex, figure ways to do it away from home. Otherwise it will just confuse your children. And if your child is living with the other parent, no one will be impressed if you aren't involved in his or her life. Moving back home with your parents is not a free pass to be a deadbeat parent. One of the most difficult but important jobs in life is to be there for your children.

Moving Into a Multigenerational Home

The chances are good it won't be long before your grandparents need extra care. In some situations, this means they, too, will be moving in with your parents. It's not difficult to see how this can be overwhelming for your parents. Maybe you can help.

Having sex in a multi-generational home can be an extra challenge unless the house is large. On the other hand, it can be a helpful acoustical diversion if your grandparents snore loudly. Fortunately, there are many multi-generational households where it's one big happy family and everything manages to work out well.

Alternate Arrangements—Like Living in a Van

Since the first vans were created, surfers have lived in them for months on end if not longer. Living in a van is still possible in some locations, assuming you can join a gym or someone has a shower you can use. As for having sex in a van—why do you think vans were originally invented?

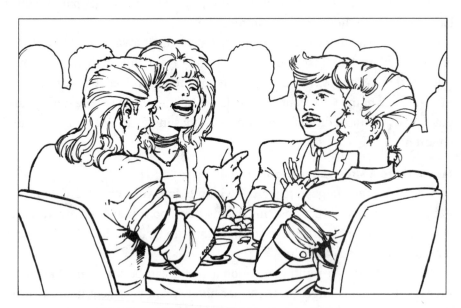

1980s — Friends Going Out to Dinner

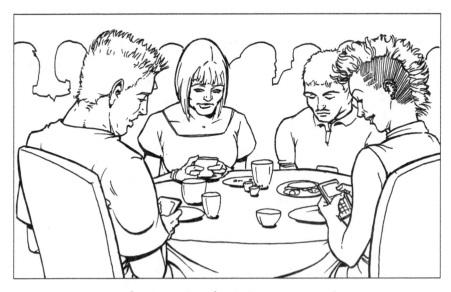

Today — Friends Going Out to Dinner

Phones can be a great way to keep in contact with friends and with your lover.
They can also undermine contact with friends and with your lover.

34

Talking To Your Partner About Sex

 Students will often say, 'Okay, so I know communication and feedback are so important, but I just don't know what to say or how to bring it up. So I end up not saying anything because I don't want to upset my partner or ruin the moment.'"

— from a college instructor who uses 'The Guide' in his sex ed courses

There's one way that dogs do it and one way that sheep do it. This is also true for elephants, lemurs and wildebeests. Unicorns need to be extra-careful when it comes to oral sex, and the female praying mantis eats her male sex partners—to death. But it's all programmed into the genes of each species. There's never any need for awkward conversations about sex except for humans.

Human brains are beefier, which means our minds have room for variation when it comes to sex. This wouldn't be so bad if we weren't the only animals who have sex indoors and in private. We could watch our neighbors do it, and have clues about what to do ourselves. Instead, we look at porn, and assume that porn is the right way to have sex—with guys magically knowing how to please women, and women up for anything that men want to do.

That's where books like this one come in. They try to shed light on the how-to part of sex. They offer tips and techniques for giving and receiving monster amounts of pleasure. But none of it is helpful if you aren't able to talk to your partner about sex. Because unlike the elephants, lemurs and wildebeests, we humans have different ways of getting off. So it's impossible for a sexual partner to know exactly how to please to us without conversation and feedback.

Give and Take

People assume that if both partners are sexually excited, then all they need to do is get naked and good sex will follow. If only it were that easy. Consider the following quote from a 29-year-old kindergarten teacher (Chris is her husband):

> "With Chris, I like having him in me, that warm good feeling. I've discovered I can ask for what I like, that there's nothing wrong with wanting your nipples pulled taut. I've learned that keeping a vibrator by the bed is not a crime. I've learned that Chris can come, and then I can come, and we can both enjoy watching each other come— as opposed to having this simultaneous orgasm that's supposed to move the world. If we have intercourse that's fine, if we don't that's fine. Sometimes we come home weary from work and it's, "what do you want? Do you want to masturbate? Do you think you can focus enough for intercourse?" It's negotiation, which I never thought it would be. I always thought it would be this mystical experience, but it's become a verbal experience."
>
> From Julia Hutton's *Good Sex,* Cleis Press

While some couples have good sex from the start, other couples take months and sometimes years to find a satisfying groove. Most couples report that their sexual desire for each other waxes and wanes, although sometimes it just wanes.

Shame between the Sheets

Guilt and shame are fascinating emotions. We become sloppy and unmotivated without them, yet with too much guilt and shame we can be at war with ourselves.

Plenty of us might do better in bed if we felt less guilt and shame about what turns us on sexually, assuming it does no harm to others. This is especially true for those who are too bashful to tell a partner what does and doesn't feel good.

Unfortunately, we get sex survey after sex survey from people who feel shame about their sexuality, and especially about masturbation or anything that's the slightest bit kinky. If that's the case for you, getting a reality check from a lover can sometimes be extremely helpful.

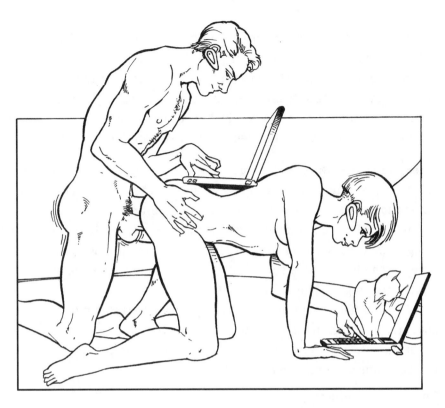

The way we connect keeps getting faster and easier. But the way we connect emotionally is still smoke signals and Morse Code. Matters of the heart require us to power down before we pucker up; to unplug before we unzip.

Naked & Tongue-Tied

Consider the following conversation between two people who are about to have intercourse together for the first time:

"Uh, should I...?"

"I guess."

"OK."

That's it. The intercourse begins. Fewer than ten words, most of them single-syllable. Grunting cavemen were probably more expressive. Then there's the prolific verbal exchange at the end of the event:

"That was really good."

"Me too."

While most of us aren't too ashamed to have sex, plenty of us approach critical mass when it comes to talking about sex. One problem has to do with the lack of a comfortable, shared vocabulary about sex. Many of us feel stuck between the rock of stiff Latin terminology and the hard place of sexual slang. For instance: "When I was giving you cunnilingus..." or "When I was eating out your pussy..." Neither feels particularly comfortable.

After Marriage — Grow or It May Die

Plenty of couples talk even less about sex after they've been married for a couple of years. Discussions about the interest rate on your credit cards or replacing the kitchen cabinets garner more excitement than finding new things that turn each of you on. Sexual desires become hidden, and we sometimes feel embarrassed or shy about mentioning things that we would have stayed up all night trying a few years earlier.

After a while, sex has no room to grow. "I don't want him to know THAT about me" becomes more powerful than "It might be exciting if he knew that about me!" Perhaps we have too much to lose if a partner disapproves, or maybe shame or humiliation get in the way.

Knowing vs. Asking

Imagine going to a restaurant where the chef served you whatever he or she felt like fixing instead of giving you a choice. Imagine a gardener who never asked, "How do you like your bushes trimmed?" Yet when it comes to sex, many of us assume that we know what our partner wants, or we clam up instead of giving feedback. Worse yet is the kind of attitude that is reflected in the following advice that *Teen Magazine* gave to its millions of girl readers:

> "When you're French kissing, it helps to let the guy take the lead. Part your lips gently, and let him explore your mouth with his tongue."

Teen's smooch advice gives the impression that guys come out of the womb knowing how to French kiss. Don't the editors of *Teen* realize that the average American male's preparation for sex is jerking off to whatever comes up after hitting the "free tour" button on porn sites?

And why are guys always supposed to know what to do? Why aren't men and women encouraged to explore sex together, teaching each other what feels good along the way? One way to avoid being a *Teen* type of lover

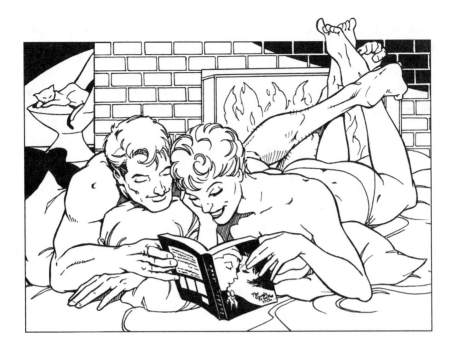

is by learning to talk to your partner about sex, about what feels good and what doesn't, and by exploring beyond what's familiar. But it's not always easy to do, which is why it sometimes helps to use props.

What to Call It Besides "Down There"?

When talking to your partner about sex, it may help if you have a comfortable name or term for your genitals. For instance, a husband and wife who had a seriously contentious relationship were in sex therapy, and the wife was asked to give her vagina a special name. She called it "jewel box." This gave the couple a basic but important building block for having conversations about what does and doesn't feel good. It was a first step in their attempt to rebuild their sex life.

Learning to Speak

By discussing sex on a regular basis, you may be helping your partner feel more receptive when you suggest that he or she try something new. Fortunately, there are "props" that can make discussions easier and more fun.

For instance, you might say to your partner, "Let's get a new book on sex every month, or check out a new Tumblr on sex every week." These don't need to be typical porn with vaginas splayed wide and penises the size of tree trunks, unless you are both into that. Consider anthologies of erotic literature (smut with a college degree!) or sites that post interesting images of sex. Browse through the erotica section of Amazon, or enter "best erotica" in your browser. And don't forget to visit *The Erotica Readers & Writers Association* at Erotica-Readers.com.

You can always highlight parts of books you find meaningful and would like your partner to know about, including this one. Or you can read sections of it to each other. Always do what you can to find humor. It helps any discussion that might otherwise be filled with anxiety.

Besides books and magazines, there are some really good videos that range from informative to hot. When searching for erotic videos, you'll find some winners and plenty of yawners.

Some couples find it fun to play board games that promote discussion about sex or physical exploration. The nice thing about these games is that none of the players are losers.

And based on the worldwide blockbuster success of the "Fifty Shades" books—horribly written as they may have been—it seems a lot of couples might enjoy reading erotica together that has themes of domination and submission. (You don't need to look far! This book's Chapter 42: *Between Vanilla and Kink* is made up of responses to our sex survey question "Are there types of non-vanilla sex that you enjoy having?" You'll be surprised at the answers. Or maybe not.)

Prevention

You might say, "Our sex life is fine right now. We don't need anything like that." Hopefully, your luck will hold, but therapists often see couples who had great sex lives two to ten years earlier. Things break down when we take them for granted, and the process of fixing them once they have fallen apart is not always pretty or fun.

It takes more to keep your sex life exciting than most couples realize.

35

Better Mating Through Internet Dating?

Internet dating can make good sense for some people. It provides access to others who are hopefully like-minded without requiring you to ever visit a singles' bar or speed date. It can also give you a much needed assist if you are painfully shy or having trouble walking up to someone and starting a conversation.

Is Internet dating a better way to meet people than at work or through friends? No. It's no better and no worse. Contrary to what the ads on TV say, there is absolutely no magic to Internet-dating services. Researchers have tried and tried to come up with ways of matching singles. Their results have been dismal failures. Internet dating services cannot match you any better than you can match yourself. They simply allow you to sort through a large pool of single people—some of whom may be telling the truth about themselves. Those with better writing skills will appear to be a better match, until they get into an actual relationship.

WARNING: Internet dating sites have become a haven for people who are trying to scam other people. So be sure you read up on how to prevent this!

What You Want and Where You Want It

You will be amazed at how many different types of Internet-dating services there are. You will probably want to join a couple. Before you decide which ones to join, you'll need to decide what it is you are looking for. Are you looking for a buddy to have fun with on the occasional weekend date, or are you looking for someone to settle down with? Are you in a "screw the ring, I just want sex" mode (aka "NSA" which means "no strings attached"). Find out what people use the online dating services in your area.

After you decide the type of relationship you want, check out the Internet-dating services that fit the bill. There are services that match people based on religion; others try to match people who are into similar kinds of kink. See how many members they have in your age group and in your geographic area. Just because a service says it has more members than the population of China doesn't mean there are any members this side of Beijing.

You will also want to compare and contrast the features that the different services offer. It's not uncommon for someone who successfully hitches up to forget to remove his or her profile. So a feature you might want is one that lists the last time the person visited the site. That way you won't waste your time responding to a potential partner who has moved across the country or a death-row inmate whose final appeal was denied months ago.

Your Profile

Most services will ask you to fill out a profile that shoppers—uh, members—get to read. It's how you present who you are. A lot of people don't take profile-writing seriously enough. If the males who have taken our online sex survey are typical of how the average straight guy writes, some of you should consider having a more expressive friend help you with your profile.

For How Long and How Much?

Some services say they are for free. You usually get what you pay for. Many of the better services charge between $20 and $30 a month, but they offer discounted three-month and six-month plans. Consider going for a longer plan. Give yourself time for the process to work. If you find the partner of your dreams in the first week, consider the extra money a tip for a service that was well provided.

Time For a Reality Check

Internet dating isn't going to make the competition disappear. Internet dating isn't going to keep you from feeling bad when someone says no. It's not going to make you seem any more appealing if you are short on social graces or high on the kind of behaviors that result in a psychiatric diagnosis.

What will be different is that the process is going to be more private and it may help you have a more focused approach. It might give you more choices. If you don't do well with romantic cold calling, being able to e-mail back and forth and then talk on the phone might be a great help. But just because you find someone whose profile looks good doesn't mean they will answer back, and it doesn't mean you would want to go out with them if they did. Assume that you will need several months of solid effort to make the process work for you. Things might start clicking right away, but that would make you the exception rather than the rule.

From Email to Sexts to Pressing Flesh

Let's say you find someone with an interesting profile and he or she thinks the same about yours. Where to go from there? While it might be more desirable to e-mail each other several times and then spend a few weeks trying each other out on the phone, someone might come along who moves quickly and next thing you know, the person you've been having the conversations with is taken. When it comes to timing, making the move from online to in-person is a subjective call, with risks each way.

The Possibility of Being Overwhelmed

It doesn't matter if you are 20 or 50, hopefully you will write a great profile and be overwhelmed with responses. But don't feel like you have to respond in detail to everyone. As you start to see the type of people who are responding, you might want to establish criteria that helps you make a quick first cut. This way you can form a short list of who you'll want to spend more time responding to. Even then, you might not have the time to respond to everyone individually. Don't be afraid to tell people when you've been overwhelmed. Say that you won't be getting back to them for awhile.

Honesty and Courtesy

It's only the Internet. What's wrong with stretching the truth a little, like when you say you've got a D-cup or seven inches when it's a B or six? What's wrong with saying you are well-read and sensitive when the only thing you've read this year is the handout at your anger-management class?

Why should honesty be any less important online than face to face? Think seriously about telling the truth, even if it's the Internet.

Next to telling lies about yourself, another form of dishonesty in Internet dating is to leave people hanging. If you aren't interested in going further with someone, have the decency to say so. Don't just disappear, and don't keep something going because you feel too guilty to say "no more." Have the courtesy to say "so long" or "it's been swell."

And Then What?

Internet dating is like arranging your own blind date. It is an attempt to meld technology with Cupid's bow. It changes the dating process, but it doesn't change the feelings that are involved in that process.

Whether we want to admit it or not, dating is a significant part of a single person's life. When a date truly clicks it can make you feel on top of the world, and when a date misfires it can make you feel deflated. Internet dating won't change any of that.

Grindr, Tinder, Whatever

You are unlikely to see some guy's dick pic on eHarmony or Christian Singles.com. But you never know on some of the hook-up apps, of which there are too many to review.

The founders of each app will trumpet its wonderfulness. Some are designed to connect with Facebook, some try to make you feel safer from trolls and stalkers, others are all about *the big fucking event*—literally, about you getting laid tonight. Nothing more and nothing less.

Your best bet is to do plenty of research, with an emphasis on the word "plenty." There was an article in The Atlantic where the author nearly soaked her panties with praise for Tinder. She kept saying how it's the one app that women use as well as men. She quoted a woman who had written a review about Tinder for HerCampus.com. So we clicked through and read that review. Here's how the HerCampus review ended, "I deleted my account after a few days because the same people kept coming up." Ooops

So be smart, do your homework, ask your friends, and have fun.

The new dating apps don't change the many mysteries of sex and dating, they just seem to help them unfold sooner. And they allow straight people to have the same kind of instant anonymous sex that gay men have had for decades on the trails and at the baths.

Thanks to Evan Marc Katz, at EvanMarcKatz.com.

36

I Knew the Bride
Long Term Relationships

This chapter is about marriage and long-term relationships. It doesn't pretend to be comprehensive, but it does speak about weddings, tradition, sex in marriage, fights, make-up sex, kids and divorce.

I Knew the Bride

One of the fun things about weddings is watching the white-laced bride taking her vows of marital bliss and wondering if she has ever handcuffed the groom and done some of the outrageous things to him that she once did to you or liked you doing to her. The memory puts a smile on your face and maybe even makes you blush. But it's not the kind of question you ask as you are working your way through the reception line—not with parents standing there, and an array of cold, clammy hands hanging out of pastel gowns and rented tuxedos waiting to shake yours.

Weddings — What's Love Got to Do with Them?

You don't have to go much farther than the average magazine rack to realize that weddings are big business. Plump, glossy zines with names like *Modern Bride* nearly bite your arm off as you walk by. The ads in these magazines reflect the many segments of our society that thrive on marriage-related businesses — bridal-wear shops, tuxedo rental centers, wedding gift registries, boutiques, kitchen appliance stores, caterers, florists, bakers, wedding coordinators, ministers, priests, rabbis, justices of the peace, churches, synagogues, reception halls, hotels, resorts, diet plans, etc.

Traditions like marriage have become an economic spectacle. Today's marriages are so choreographed you seldom get a feeling that two people are making a promise to be there for each other no matter what, and to be inseparable partners on the great climb through life. Instead, what you often get is the familiar bride-to-be psychosis, where the future bride and her mother become so savagely obsessed about things like table centerpieces and bridal gowns that any sense of love is pretty much out the window.

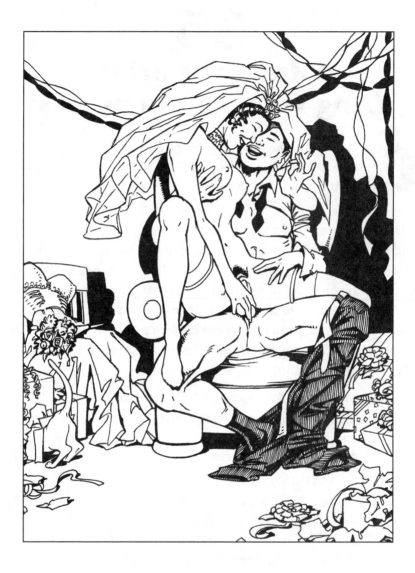

What if couples put as much effort into improving the level of intimacy and fun in their relationship as they do selecting wedding invitations? And what about those bizarre, adolescent feeding frenzies known as bachelor parties? If guys need to see high-priced women getting naked or want to lick whipping cream off silicone-filled breasts, why not just do it? Why use weddings as the excuse?

Marriage is a big step, an important step. Hopefully you won't get caught up in our culture's expectation of marriage as a generator of crippling debt, and will instead work to make your union a safe haven in a world that is sometimes anything but.

And what if couples took the money they spent on weddings and set it aside for one long weekend each and every month, just to be with each other and have fun? No phones, no texts, no Facebook, no Snaps, no work, just a three-day weekend where it's only the two of you each and every month?

Styles of Problem-Solving

Besides feeling love and friendship, an important ingredient in keeping a relationship happy is a couple's ability to solve conflicts. Couples with a knack for problem-solving tend to have happier marriages. (Duh!)

Researchers tell us that successful couples approach conflicts with a willingness to talk things over and work them out, and we are sure such couples exist somewhere. The rest of us occasionally resort to sarcasm, name-calling, stubbornness, making threats, automatically giving in, taking blame needlessly, becoming silent or pretending that there is no conflict when all hell is about to break loose.

Contrary to what you may have heard about the value of releasing anger, trying to resolve a conflict when you are still fuming at each other is not always productive. Sometimes it is best to wait until cooler heads prevail. Of course, some people will use this as an excuse to avoid confronting a partner altogether. Then nothing ever gets worked out.

The Good, Bad & Ugly

When you enter into a marriage or long-term relationship, the chances are good you will discover hidden but wonderful aspects of your partner's character. Cherish, respect and admire these. To deal with the less fortunate parts of your sweetheart's character, consider the following:

Learn how to fight constructively. This means no matter how nasty or unpleasant your fights might be, try to keep them issue-oriented so you can work your way toward a solution or compromise. This is different from fights that revert to name-calling or rehashing past hurts. These accomplish little, except to degrade whatever dignity you once may have had.

Fighting is preferable to indifference, unless you are getting violent.

Every once in a while, when you feel like wringing your partner's neck, do something really nice for him or her. This could end up being far more satisfying than fighting, and it might even get you laid.

Instead of blaming your partner for things that are going wrong or wishing he or she would somehow change, try to eliminate ways you might be setting your partner up to be the bad guy. This doesn't mean you should stay in a relationship that's no longer working, it just means that the things you control most in a relationship are those that you put into it. If your efforts to change yourself don't inspire changes in your partner, then there's not much more you can do.

Birds of a Feather Get Bored with Each Other

Long-term relationships can sometimes be a challenge to keep fresh and vital unless both partners make an effort to enjoy each other.

Think about all the extra things you did to impress each other when you first met; you probably even cut your toenails or trimmed your bikini line. Why would there be any less need for romance and wooing after you've known each other for what seems like forever? Mature relationships require more rather than less effort at romance and improvement—from cards, flowers and special dates to extra attempts at tenderness.

Single vs. Hitched

Being single makes it easier to maintain the illusion that you are a perfect human being. Long-term relationships force you to confront parts of yourself that many of us would rather not. For instance, in a long-term relationship, your husband or wife will probably get fed up with your worst faults and remind you of them at least six times a day. If you are the rigid type who is incapable of change and compromise, then you might not be well-suited for marriage. On the other hand, a reader from San Francisco comments, "It could be just what you need."

Sex after a Fight, aka "Make-Up Sex"

Fights leave most couples worn out or sad. However, some couples enjoy sex after a good fight, given how their neurotransmitters are already fired up and ready for action. On a biological level, the body might confuse a fight with sexual excitement, thus eliminating the need for tender preliminaries. Hopefully, the reasons for the fight have been resolved and the make-up sex isn't simply being used as a cover-up.

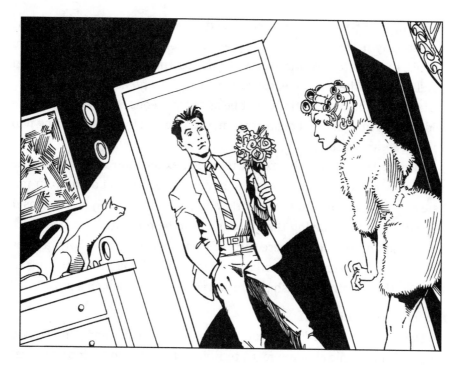

Your Partner's Bad Moods

Like colds and flu, occasional bad moods are part of the human condition. In better-functioning relationships, the partner who is in the good mood is sometimes able to maintain a healthy perspective when confronted with a partner's bad mood. He or she might even take steps that will help the other's bad mood to go away. But in difficult relationships, all bets are off.

In a difficult relationship, the partner who is in a good mood experiences the other's bad mood as a personal attack, even if it has nothing to do with him or her. Attempts to help are often filled with so much anxiety that they only make matters worse, and the partner in the bad mood might lash out at the other just for the heck of it. (Why not be nasty to the person who loves you? After all, no one else would put up with you.) Such couples usually do better if one spouse has a job that keeps him or her on the road for long periods of time.

Sex after the Baby Arrives

Our society doesn't provide many role models for caring parents who are also sexual beings. We sometimes separate the two roles entirely, as though being a good mom or dad precludes your giving great head or loving the feel of your partner's naked body next to your own. Just identifying as a parent may make you feel less sexual than you really are. Hopefully you will take the time to talk this over with your partner before having children, as well as after. There is no reason why you can't be great parents and have great sex—although the latter won't be as spontaneous as it was before the children arrived. A married reader comments: "We had lots of sex during nap time and Sesame Street."

Also, never discount the extent to which exhaustion might erode the desire to have sex, and don't expect to have sex if you aren't doing your fair share of the child care and housework. While you've probably never considered vacuuming and taking the garbage out to be romantic acts, good luck getting laid without doing these sorts of things once the new baby arrives. One reader who is a sex worker adds, "And for heaven's sake, hire someone to help with the cleaning or wash before you spend the money on a prostitute."

Divorce & Your Children

Don't assume that kids automatically do better if their parents stay together. While some children feel a terrible sadness when their parents get divorced, others feel relief. It usually depends on how bad the marriage was, how bad the divorce is, and whether the kid gets to live with his or her favorite parent, if there is one. The absolute worst arrangement for some children is spending half of a week or a month at one parent's house, and half at the other. This can be the psychological equivalent of cutting the baby in two. On the other hand, it can work if it's being done in the child's best interest as opposed to simply placating two warring parents.

What often destroys kids more than the actual divorce is the parental lunacy for years before and years after. In an emotional sense, children of divorce often end up having no parents at all because their parents are sad, joyless, hateful or frightening to be with. If you are getting a divorce, do what you can to reach through your own pain, remembering that children need to see at least some form of hope reflected in their parents' eyes. And remember that your child's psychological health will in large part be determined by how amicably you and your former spouse are able to co-parent when divorced. It is not possible to emphasize this point too much.

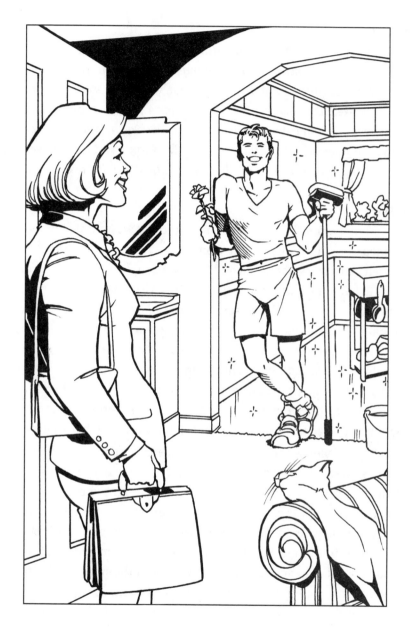

Men who help around the house get laid more often than guys who don't, causing speculation that Windex and Lysol are better aphrodisiacs than oysters and fast cars.

Dear Paul,

Friends set me up with a wonderful woman and we've hit it off really well. We've had sex four times and are building a relationship. Then I went to her place for the first time last night. (Before that, we'd always gone to mine.) Her bathroom looked like it hadn't been cleaned for a year, and some kind of alien life form was growing from the tile in her shower. She appears clean and neat, but this is another side of her that's scary. Just so you'll know, I've never been a neat freak, and don't even buy antibacterial soap. What do I do?

Tyler in Jackson Hole

Dear Tyler,

Your letter would have gone straight into the wastebasket if you hadn't mentioned the slimy ooze growing from the grout in your girlfriend's shower. Let me tell you a story about Bill and Nancy, a couple whom I feel proud and honored to have known for more than twenty years. Their house has always been immaculate—I'm talking serious sparkle. Even the litter box is clean. One night a few years ago, we'd been having too much wine and I mentioned how impressed I was with Bill and Nancy's ability to keep such a clean house. That's when Bill started hyperventilating and nearly bled from the ears. He told me about the first time he went into Nancy's bathroom when they were grad students at the University of Chicago. It took him hours of scrubbing and gallons of bleach before he could reach terra firma on her shower floor.

My point, Tyler, is the way your lover keeps her bathroom doesn't need to be a deal breaker. What's more important is the way you and she handle the situation. If you say nothing and continue to ignore her wanton disregard for disinfectants, then I'd say your relationship is in trouble. And if she is unable to handle your spending next Sunday scrubbing her bathroom, your relationship is in trouble. But if you clean her bathroom and don't make her feel bad about it, and she returns the favor with the finest blowjob you've ever received in your entire life, then I think you're onto something good.

37
Sex in the Military

66 Things the military could do to help sex be better?
Make the damn uniforms easier to get out of!"
female, age 19

It's not like soldiers leave their sex drives in their home towns. But providing helpful information about sexuality for new recruits is not always a priority of the military. Since the military does not publish reports on the sexual practices of its members, we have put this information together based on clandestine reports from the field. Hopefully, our intelligence is better than that of some governmental agencies.

The Uniform Code of Military Justice prohibits displays of physical affection while you are in uniform. The defense that you were naked and not in uniform while having sex is probably not going to wash. The UCMJ prohibits sex in barracks and sex between people of different ranks. It also prohibits sodomy, which is defined to include oral sex. If that isn't a recipe for "boring," it's hard to know what is. It also could be a bit delusional on the part of the UCMJ.

While there are some fascinating aspects to sex in the military, it is really just a cross-section of sex any place where Americans are gathered. So if you are looking for a bizarre expose, you're in for disappointment. But there are some interesting dimensions to sex in the military, especially if you are a female G.I. who likes her men well armed and ready to engage.

The "Guide To Getting It On" Recruiting for the Military?

Before we start on the cultural and sociological aspects of sexuality in the Armed Forces, consider the following observations from two khaki-wearing philosophers:

"Believe me, its the women in the military that are sex mad, but nobody complains or calls them sluts, because we would all do the same in their situation." *male age 25*

"I mean it's usually five females living in a building with 100 horny males. The girls pretty much pick who they want to sleep with that night." *male age 23*

If you are a woman who really likes sex and you decide on college, there will be somewhere around 60 women for every 40 males. For women in the military, there are 85 males for every 15 women. Plus, if you want to have sex with Uncle Sam's finest, you don't have to worry about getting a reputation, as long as you make efforts to be discrete about it. It's not like it's going to follow you 500 soldiers later, when you settle down in civilian life and marry the minister from the First Church of Christ. What happens in the military usually stays in the military.

Before those of you who are upstanding military women launch a drone strike on the offices of Goofy Foot Press, everyone knows that at least half of the women in the military are monogamous and not interested in sleeping around—which ups the odds for the rest of you to 7.5 women for every 100 men. Consider the following words of advice from a reader who knows:

"For new females—have fun! I was so eager to be the good airman, obey all the rules, etc., that for my first few years I didn't have a lot of fun with the unique situations we can get into. Most of the people you will know will be young men in good physical shape. Take advantage!!!"
female age 25

As for a man's chances of having sex in the military, these sentiments from two experienced soldiers echo what we heard time and again:

"I thought being in the military would be like taking a vow of celibacy. However, it turned out there were good opportunities." *male 25*

"Coming from a smaller town in Iowa I was a little shocked how others showed no concern that someone was married." *male age 37*

Some of the opportunities include young civilian women who have historically found the words "base adjacent" and "available men" to be music to their ears. There is seldom a scarcity of men near military bases and available civilian women. Opportunities also abound in ports of call in Europe and Asia, although in Muslim countries, the sex is mostly on base between members of the military, with some prostitution being available if you look hard enough.

As for the willingness of some military wives to offer the comforts of a warm bosom to needy soldiers while their husbands are deployed, some do and some don't. We have heard from some military wives that it's not unusual for them to share tender moments with each other rather than with other men while their husbands are away. However, the wives of officers may be held to a different standard than the wives of enlisted men.

The Culture

Sex in the military is a mirror of sex any place else where Americans live and work. However, there are a few complexities that help define sex in the military as different.

There is the never knowing when you will be put in harm's way—but always expecting it and always training for it. This can contribute to a sense of fatalism or cynicism within the culture of the military, or a *devil may care* attitude when it comes to what you do in your free time.

There's also the emphasis on the body and its abilities, the impact of group living, and constantly being moved from one base to another. This can make for a climate where the sex is catch as catch can. And soldiers are frequently immersed in cultures where sex is perceived differently than it is here. In foreign lands, sexual economies often thrive around military bases. Even here in the states, different bases have different sexual cultures.

These are just some of the factors that help give sex in the military its very own and sometimes unique perspective.

Short Tour vs. Long Tour

"My sister, who is also in the service is married to a serviceman. She recently returned from a TDY (temporary duty) assignment, and while there, engaged in an extramarital affair with another married serviceman. These things happen a lot." *female age 25*

Deployments in the military are often categorized as "short tour" or "long tour." If you are married and you are on a long tour, they will often move your family with you. If it's a short tour (under a year), your family usually stays behind. There are plenty of exceptions, especially if you are going into combat.

The Impact of Your Status

"The base where I received the bulk of my training after basic, Sheppard, is where most of the people are young, first time away from home, and have just undergone an enormous life-changing experience. There's a sudden freedom after basic training. Everyone's hormones are raging. One piece of common wisdom is, 'Don't get married at tech school!' I guess that's because lots of people jump the gun. There are lots of random hookups, some racy stuff going on at the dance clubs, and lots of alcohol. Another base I spent some time at recently, in Florida, has a greater population of 'adult' service members, so there's less of a panicky, gotta-have-it-now attitude." *female age 25*

Members of the armed forces usually fall into two groups: first termers, and lifers:

First termers are often younger and unmarried. They usually have high sex drives, and they are eager to be accepted into the military's macho culture.

Lifers are a different story. The have made the military a career, and they have often sampled many different customs and cultures. Lifers tend to be married and have families, but it is also not unusual for them to spend a good deal time away from home.

Social & Economic Class Distinctions – The Dangers of Sex between Ranks

Since there is currently no draft, there is little equity in the military. Enlisted people are almost all from the middle class and below, while commissioned officers tend to be from the middle class and above.

In addition to the political and economic divisions within the armed forces, there are strictly-enforced prohibitions regarding fraternization among the ranks. People in the military who marry other military people are expected to be in the same or a similar rank. It is a violation of the *Uniform Code of Military Justice* to even socialize with someone not in or close to your own rank. Good luck trying to explain away that little affair between a lieutenant and a private, or a colonel and junior commissioned officer.

No matter how hot that first-class private is, a commissioned officer can get him- or herself into big trouble for fraternizing when their uniforms are on the floor.

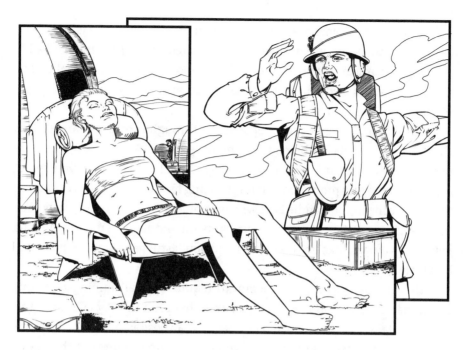

Catching some rays at the FOB—and on patrol the next day.

Women in the Military

"A female private and myself were going through an abandoned building and on the middle floor she just went crazy and started sucking me off like there was no tomorrow. She even answered her radio in the middle of it then carried on." *male age 26*

"With my coworkers, sex is not an issue—I'm a woman working a job which is, even now, pretty much a 'man's job.' I have a very non-sexual relationship with the boys in my shop. I think it surprises them when I wear civilian clothes and they remember that I'm a real girl. However, I do feel like the females are a bit of a commodity. I know several women who take advantage of the situation and live it up with all the partners they want, and others who are from conservative families/areas who wouldn't dream of it." *female age 25*

Like working women in the civilian world, women in the military often change personas between home and when on duty. Some have said that their military persona is more masculine and aggressive, while their civilian persona can be more relaxed or feminine.

In the past, sexual harassment has been prominent. It still is. But it was even worse then because a woman who wanted to report someone had to report to the officer in charge. She couldn't report to an independent person. The officer would seldom want to lose a good man, and would often ignore the charges.

In the last couple of years, reporting is through separate channels, and women's complaints are being taken more seriously. As for the reality of reporting harassment, one female soldier says it will no longer get you demoted, but forget being promoted and forget being treated decently ever again. A female Marine in the Middle East who is quoted in Newsmax.com says, "You have two choices. You can keep your pants on and be miserable and be harassed, or you can take your pants off and you'll still get harassed, but you'll be a little less miserable."

The military has recently begun to require special training regarding sexual harassment and coercion. Accounts that are SHARPly critical of this program claim it is ineffective. They say it's purpose is to placate senators and congresswomen, as opposed to genuinely trying to prevent the sexual coercion of female soldiers.

Quid Pro Quo — Where Sexual Coercion Thrives in the Military

Perhaps the biggest area of sexual coercion of women and some men in the military is referred to as *Quid Pro Quo*. *Quid Pro Quo* invites sexual assault and coercion because a solider who does not obey the wishes of a solider in command or of higher rank will not be able to advance in the military. As for the fate of a woman in the military who reports a commanding officer for *Quid Pro Quo*-related sexual coercion? We'll get back to you on that one.

Sex in Different Bases & Ports of Call

"Seemed to be a lot of screwing around going on overseas. Hell, when you are out to sea for 65+ days and come into port and see women offering sex for next to nothing, its hard not to. The Philippines was approximately $5 bar fine for a gal all night. Treat her with respect and she's yours the whole time you're there. Singapore was easy to get laid. Any cab driver knew were the brothels were located. Be careful of street walkers as many of them were benny boys (transvestites). Hong Kong–ask cabbies. Perth, Australia. OHhhhh YES! Blonde hair blue eyed beauties whose parents encouraged the relationships (short or long term)." *male age 44*

"In Greenland it was an isolated base with only a hundred or so military people and some civilians. There was probably a higher amount of cheating there than most places because it was so remote. Not much to do but drink and screw." *male age 48*

"For nearly a year in Iraq, I was under constant threat of death with my work, and I was rarely alone. I didn't have sex at all when I was there." *male age 37*

"In Washington, sex seemed more about starting a family, although I did more easily find sexually-deprived women there willing to forgo a relationship." *male age 24*

"In ports of call, the official 'off limits' list was usually a liberty battle plan because the bars had the best booze and the whore houses had the best broads. Drinking on liberty was expected, getting drunk was a badge of honor, getting wasted to the point that you can't remember where you were, what you did, who you did it to, nor how much it cost. There was honor in being a drunken whore monger." *male 58*

Saigon Vs. Baghdad

While members of the military did have sex in Iraq and Afghanistan, it was often between male and female soldiers or interpreters, and not in the best of circumstances. This was different from Vietnam, where sex was often available in bars, hotels, and at "skivvy huts" which were often close to bases. "Skivvy huts" might have three or four beds next to each other in a 12-by-12 room. Local women would be having sex with soldiers who had their pants pulled down around their ankles. There was not much privacy.

Cultures: There was more neon in Saigon than Baghdad and Kabul. In the Middle East, sex outside of marriage is strictly forbidden for women and for a woman to sell herself for sex is unthinkable. It's unusual when a soldier sees the hair of a local woman let alone makes serious eye contact, and maybe only while on a "knock and talk" and if none of the men are home.

The Military: During the war in Viet Nam, there was a draft. So the average soldier was single and somewhere between 18- and 22-years of age. In Iraq and Afghanistan, the make up of the troops was very different. Many had wives and children stateside. Many of the troops were National Guard or Reserves who tended to be older and married when compared to active duty Army or Marine Corps. Plus, today's military has a much higher percentage of females than was the case in Vietnam. There is more room for intra-armed forces fooling around.

Considering the age of the troops and the Muslim culture's attitude toward sex versus that of the Vietnamese, the respective conflicts were in different centuries in more ways than just figuratively.

Korea vs. Europe

Soldiers in Korea often move off base and set up housekeeping in a one room "hooch" with a "Moose." A Moose is a Korean woman who cooks, cleans and provides companionship, including sex. They are quite good at keeping their solider smiling. It was not unusual for a soldier to marry his moose and bring her home to the US as his wife. Most bases in the Pacific and Asia have their own form of a "moose culture." There might be some bases where the men in a military dorm pool their money and hire a group of mooses to take care of the men's needs, including their sexual needs.

In Europe, prostitutes are plentiful and legal. Contacts can be made through night clubs, bars and online.

Sex in Home Bases with Spouses of Others

"There is one extreme or the other in the military. You either have sex on the casual or you really fall in love with them. Those I knew that wanted to stay together were completely faithful to each other and some even left the military together." *male age 25*

"I had a lady friend during a remote assignment who was married to another AF member stationed elsewhere, and they seemed to have an understanding that going without sex for a long time apart wasn't a reasonable expectation. Although she and I were never intimate, she made it plain that she was willing if I was. My only sexual encounters while apart from my wife were casual, with no expectations of a lasting relationship." *male age 54*

"Most couples that I know usually ended in divorce or breaking up. I'm not sure that it was because of infidelity or not. But a lot of the women I slept with were married." *male age 23*

"Couples were fooling around a lot on both ends. There were places you could go if you wanted to pick up someone's wife." *male age 24*

While we have heard from plenty of military people who say they remained true blue to their spouse or lover, we have heard from plenty who didn't. It's not unheard of for married couples to have understandings that all is fair in love and war, or when deployed or on tour. Whether these understandings are spoken or merely understood varies with the people involved.

Masturbation

"Most guys after a while would pretty much talk about it openly. From what I gathered everyone was doing it in their bed (rack). It's enclosed on all sides and pretty much offers the most privacy. The only other place I would masturbate is in the shower. Some masturbated in the places they worked at day to day (shops). Although it is tempting because of the access to a computer, I only did this once. A few people I've know over the years were really open about it. So open as to not stop if accidentally walked in on them. They would simply ask you to come back later." *male age 24*

"I would masturbate late at night when the rest of the hooch was asleep, or in the showers. I don't recall being aware of anyone else doing it, but the general attitude was everybody did it sometime."

male age 44

"My roommates and myself were usually pretty good friends and we knew each other rather well. If one of us had to beat off we would usually just ask the other person to leave for awhile or to take their time at the store or wherever they were at the time. Or you just take a walk to the bathroom and stroke it in the stall." *male age 23*

"I did it very quietly. We had curtains on our bunks but you could usually tell when someone was solo pleasuring. You didn't say anything as everyone did it and you wouldn't like it if things were said about you." *male age 44*

E.M.H.O.s or Early Morning Hard Ons

"I don't recall any incidents where a morning erection became an issue. We joked about it a lot when coming to the end of midnight shifts. Morning erections aren't just for people waking up, there's something about dawn that seems to bring them on!" *male age 54*

Not a single man in our surveys said that early morning erections were a concern. Some said everyone had them, it was a normal part of being a guy, and no big deal. Another said he suspected the military was putting something in the food to decrease early morning erections during basic training, because he doesn't remember getting one after the first week. He does remember getting many of them after basic training. Who knows the impact of exhaustion and fear on the spontaneous erection?

Swingers & Nudists in the Military

Swinging and nudism is a fairly prominent activity in the military. This is especially true in bases in Europe or parts of Asia where the social prohibitions against swinging and nudism are not as great as they are in the US.

"Where to find sex?"

"You really don't have to go anywhere. It usually finds you." *male age 29*

"Local clubs known to be meat markets." *male age 37*

"Probably the bars on post. They are usually full of married women looking for someone to play with while their husbands are away."
male age 23

Unlike males, women in the military seldom needed any help in finding partners. For men, the Internet is now being used for finding sex. This echoes its use in civilian life. Where soldiers go online depends on what kind of sex they are looking for. USMilitarySingles.com and MilitarySinglesConnection.com appear to be legitimate dating services. They also hook up soldiers with interested civilians who live in the surrounding communities. And Match.com is said to have more military singles than all of the military dating sites combined. Just beware of the many scams aimed at military singles. Do a browser search to learn what they are so you can try to avoid them.

Between Gay and Bisexual

"There were very few homos onboard ship. It was never a concern."
male age 43

"While on ship, I had sex with as many guys as I wanted and as often as I wanted it. I had sex with men and women—in deep corners and heck, even in the barbershop once!" *male age 31*

"It's somewhat expected that everyone will date; if you don't date, coworkers will assume you're a homosexual. While this is very seldom true, it is a stigma." *male age 47*

"A lot of military in Washington use Craigslist. You would see men on the site advertise for women at first and then as the day went on you would see the same men advertising for any sex. Some of them wanting their first homosexual experience. These were guys in their early 20s, in their sexual prime."

male age 24

Contrary to what you might hear about the military, not a single one of our survey takers said he or she felt gays and lesbians were a concern for them. None reported feeling stared at while in the showers, and none listed homosexuality in others as a problem.

How you define "homosexual" in the military is interesting. There is the navy term, "It ain't queer unless it's tied to the pier," which implies a different standard for what happens on land where women are plentiful, and what happens on board ship. In years past, there was also a military joke that defined a "buddy" as a guy who would go off base while you are restricted to base, get himself two blow jobs, and come back and give you one.

There is a well established if not well hidden gay and bisexual culture in the military. The men and women who are part of this culture take extreme measures to keep it hidden. It's nothing for them to drive hours from a base to a private gay venue where there is little likelihood they will be found out. Even with the repeal of DADT, the military is not yet ready for gay pride.

Also, it can be precarious for a man or women in the military to not date a member of the other sex, as they risk being perceived as gay. Gay officers have to be particularly careful, as other officers' wives are constantly trying to set them up. A "stunt babe" is a woman who poses as a gay soldier's girlfriend at military events and whose picture he keeps on his desk. She is the military equivalent of a "beard."

Gay Females in the Military

Contrary to what you might think, lesbians can have a rough time in the military, especially those who are tomboyish as opposed to fem-looking. Everyone is expecting women in the military to be gay. Straight women in uniform can be especially sensitive to this. They consider their gay sisters as a bad mark on the family name, and often display a lack of tolerance. Lesbians in the military quickly learn this. The constant scrutiny can become nightmarish. While straight girls in the military can have a sexual heyday, lesbians in the military say they won't even risk kissing another woman in "the privacy" of a base apartment, let alone muff-diving when on government-owned real estate.

In her piece *No Ass, No Tail,* Myriam Gurba says that real military dykes aren't getting laid. She quotes one lesbian who said she believed herself to be the only dyke among 60 girls in her basic training outfit. Given the rampant homophobia, she said, "I think living in close quarters with 60 women was actually one of the most dreadful experiences I've had to endure."

While there can be opportunities for homosexual exploration, it would seem to be among women who no one suspects as being gay. Otherwise, they are too well watched for it to be comfortable.

A Talk with an Active Duty Solider

The author of *The Guide* recently had an unexpected talk about sex in the military with a young soldier who was on leave from Afghanistan. This soldier had already served two tours in Iraq. The following is a partial reconstruction of the conversation from notes scrawled on the back of an envelope.

Some soldiers say they are too exhausted or traumatized to want very much sex when they're in combat. What's it been like for you?

I enjoy sex and have it whenever I can. I have a much higher sex drive now than when I was in high school. My body is on hyper alert when I'm out on patrol and I can't shut it off just because I'm back at base. After what I see and do out there, the sex helps me reconnect with a sense of humanity.

Where do you find sex in Afghanistan?

There's a lot of sex on base!!!

What about prostitution?

I've been with prostitutes in Iraq and in Afghanistan. They're not out in the open, but you can find them if you ask around. Some that I've been with speak English. I've spent entire nights just talking with them. The women are exotic, and I find that very appealing. It's different than being with a woman here at home. The sex is incredible, but so is being with a woman from such a different culture. I know a lot of the guys just want to have sex and get off, but I want to talk for hours first.

What about the female soldiers on base? Are they up for sex?

This isn't going to sound so good, but there's a lot of people having a lot of sex on base and I don't see relationships back home being a detriment.

If you work hard to please a woman on base sexually, and you do a good job, the women will talk about you to other women. Word gets around if you're good and who you are, so it's not at all unusual for a woman to come around in the afternoon or night and ask if you're available to have sex. It's real straightforward, nobody gets embarrassed, none of the games like when you're back home. If you're available and she's someone you'd like to have sex with, then you say yes. Or maybe you'll say "I'm really sorry, but there's already someone I'll be with tonight."

And yes, the women have sex with each other. Most of the women aren't gay, it just happens. And maybe it's nice having sex with other women when you're surrounded by so many guys.

Is there much relationship drama on base?

Good God yes. Guys aren't used to women being trained soldiers, and some of these women won't hesitate to hurt you physically, and I mean hit you, pull a knife on you, and even shoot you. Everything is turned up on a base in a war zone, including the drama.

How are women treated on the bases?

Terribly. A woman who is in the military needs to have seriously thick skin. Guys are going to be talking trash to her from morning to night, "Bend over and let's see what you've got..." kind of stuff. A woman needs to be tough and able to ignore it. Guys will behave when a commanding officer is around, but the minute he or she is gone...

If the women have sex with the women, do male soldiers have sex with other male soldiers?

Before I went on leave, a friend who I've been in combat with was beating himself up because he'd had sex with another male soldier. But I don't think it's that uncommon. You suit up every morning expecting to get shot at and to lay down your life for the guy next to you. And you expect him to do the same for you. You share emotions together that a lot of husbands and wives don't share. You're in a foreign and hostile environment, and there are five or ten men to every woman.

And people are surprised that male soldiers have sex with male soldiers? They should get over it. No one has problems if two female soldiers get it on. Keep it to yourself, and that's that. What you do with your body when the enemy isn't trying to vaporize it is up to you.

What about threesomes?

I'd say there's a lot of that. Two guys and a girl. And there are times the guys will be getting each other off in addition to her. But with so many men, any woman who wants two guys at once gets two guys at once.

Sex after Combat

Thanks to better armor and more immediate medical attention, fewer soldiers are being killed in battle, but more are returning home with injuries. Some of the most common problems include traumatic brain injury (TBI), post-traumatic stress disorder (PTSD), combat related sleep disorders, burns, amputations and trauma to different parts of the body including the crotch. Many of these injuries are caused by blasts from IEDs.

Unfortunately, the VA does not want to hear about combat-related sex and relationship problems, especially those that can't be treated with pills like Viagra or Prozac.

More than 10% of combat vets are returning with PTSD, which tends to keep the body in a hyper state of alertness. This can seriously disrupt your sex life, given how the adrenaline that's surging through your system can make it difficult to kick back and feel like getting it on. Your body is in a permanent "fight or flight" mode, with sex taking a back seat to worries that bad things might happen. Just letting your guard down enough to talk about your feelings can be frightening. Plus, the sounds and sensations that happen during sex can become flashback triggers. Even the way we describe what sex feels like often includes combat imagery, "I started coming so hard it felt like an explosion..." or "There was this blast of light and energy..." Also, the sounds people make at the height of sexual passion often sound like cries of pain.

Fortunately, there are cutting-edge treatments for PTSD. Hopefully you will seek them out.

Just under 20% of returning combat vets are showing signs of traumatic brain injury. TBI can impact your ability to connect the dots in every-day life. Things you used to take for granted can become head-scratchers, especially

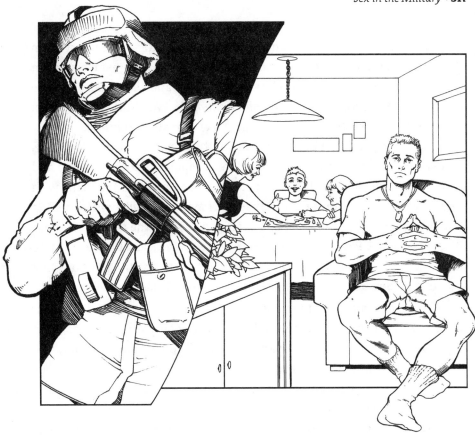

Some soldiers who return from combat appear to be totally normal, but they aren't able to feel close to loved ones and friends. It can be a real struggle to jump back into the relationship and the family life they had before.

relationships. While it's highly unlikely that TBI is making you more horny, it could be making it difficult to know the appropriate time and place to masturbate, or who to have sex with and when or where.

Even though you seem perfectly normal on the outside, a brain injury could be impacting your judgement. It might be causing to have problems expressing emotions and processing feelings.

TBI can be confusing for everyone, especially the people around you who expect you to be the person you were before combat concussed your cabeza. Like any of us, you might be trying to fake it or cover things up. You probably wouldn't know how to put what's going on into words anyway.

When possible, it's important to sort out traumatic brain injury from PTSD, as TBI symptoms can often look like those of PTSD. A great resource for learning more about TBI is a book written by Bob and Lee Woodruff: *In an Instant: A Family's Journey of Love and Healing.* Mr. Woodruff is a journalist who suffered an extensive TBI as a result of a war-related explosion.

As for burns and other tissue trauma, these can result in skin that is numb or painfully sensitive. Combat-related amputations are common and require huge adjustments to life in general, not to mention problems with keeping your balance during intercourse and having difficulty with thrusting. It's not like *Good Morning America* is going to have on the author of a book titled "Intercourse Positions for the Returning Vet Who Has a Double Amputation." The good news is, you might actually be able to get into positions that your able-bodied self could never fathom, but there will be a learning curve.

Always lurking behind any disfiguring injuries is how you feel about your body, aka "body image" and "self-esteem." How is your partner going to respond? And if you don't have a partner, how will you find one? Not only will you need to heal physically, but you'll need to become comfortable with yourself. While you will probably want and need some alone time, isolation can be a devil of its own making.

To compound all of these problems, the medications used to treat depression and pain can bring their own sexual side effects.

We are just beginning to understand some of the unique problems that today's vets are bringing home with them. You'll need to be vigilant in your search for helpful information. Do regular Internet searches, and stay connected to veteran and military related blogs.

Be sure to know the benefits you are entitled to! This can vary from state to state.

Advice from People Who Have Been There

"Military people enjoy sex pretty much the same as everybody else. The dangers of military service, and the travel and deployments, make an active sex life a little more challenging. I always appreciated a sexy welcome home, even though I realized that my being away increased my wife's burdens a great deal. Popular culture paints military members as macho types who enjoy rough sex and even rape. The truth is military people are the same as everybody else in the sex department, and what works for civilians works for GIs equally as well."

male age 54

"If it's going to be casual sex, make sure you both agree and understand this. Don't talk about any sexual partner with coworkers, ever." *male 47*

"In Iraq, it was really hard... I felt too dirty and stinky to talk to girls there, and a lot of times coming back to the fob, we'd seen contact with the enemy and were maybe upset, or are not into talking to girls because we'd just seen the edge of humanity, like a dead body or dead friend, and the last thing on your mind was having sex. Also exhaustion was a factor." *male age 23*

"After what I see and do out there, the sex helps me reconnect with a sense of humanity." *male interviewed on pages 514-516*

"I wish that I was told about the sexual reputations of all branches and how much people in military towns resented you before they even met you." *male age 24*

A Special Salute to MSgt. Glenn B. Knight, USAF Retired for advice & research. Glenn proved just how thoughtful, intelligent and perceptive soldiers can be. And a special thanks also to the active military who participated our surveys!

The Guide is also available in
a spectacular color eBook version for
your iPad, Kindle and Nook.
For more information:

wwww.GuideToGettingItOn.com

38

MRIs of Sexual Arousal
Is the Brain Half Empty or Half Full?

While researchers were looking for the parts of the brain that light up during sexual arousal, they discovered parts of the brain that were shutting down. You would think it would be the opposite, with sexual arousal causing sparks of activity arcing from ear to ear. However, it appears that in order to get into the sexual moment we need to shut down parts of our brains as well as fire up others. This would validate what women often say who take our sex survey. When asked to describe what intercourse feels like when it's really good, they often say the rest of the world disappears, for example:

> "When it's really good, I feel like the world just stops and my mind goes blank and all I want to do is feel every single move, and enjoy each breath. But when its bad, I can't stop thinking about everything other than what is really going on. My mind will be racing."
>
> *female age 22*

MRI or neuroimaging studies of the brain and crotch are the future of sex research. However, there currently exist serious limitations of brain-imaging technology and human behavior. This chapter will give you an idea of the challenges that researchers have to deal with as they are exploring this virgin territory. Understanding the limitations of current technology is especially important given the media's penchant for making way too much of findings that are tentative and have yet to be replicated and validated.

Problems with the Old (and Still Currently Used) Technology

Before sex researchers started using MRI technology to study our brains and crotches, research about sexual arousal and sexual feelings has often included tying strings around men's penises that were attached to gauges, and sticking plastic tampons containing infrared sensors up women's vaginas. We would then try to make educated guesses about what it meant when the strings got stretched and the sensors sensed. This was fraught with peril when you consider that a third or more of the research subjects would routinely be disqualified because their strings didn't stretch convincingly. There were also questions about how representative a person might be who volunteers to watch porn movies in a lab with a probe stuck up her vagina.

Worse yet, when it came to women's arousal, we've mostly been limited to measuring the changes in the blood flow in her vagina. Yet women have a clitoris that's involved in their sexual arousal. We haven't had a very good way of measuring what was going on inside of the clitoris other than slapping a glob of goo on the end of an ultrasound probe and pushing it up against the clitoris. So researchers have had to leave the clitoris out of the equation when measuring female sexual arousal.

With the newer imaging technology, researchers suddenly have the capacity to not only measure what's going on inside the entire pelvis when it's sexually aroused, but inside the brain as well. All of this while allowing the subject to remain in relative privacy—if you assume having your genitals stimulated while attempting to lie totally still in a large metal cylinder at a university lab is private.

The Current Limitations of Neuroimaging

As exciting as the new wave will be, for now we need to be mindful that brain imaging in sexual research is still in its infancy.

A research subject's head needs to be kept perfectly still for several minutes while the images are taken. The slightest movement results in signal changes that threaten to muck everything up. Worse yet, the part of the brain where some of our sexual sensations are processed is located next to a sinus cavity that the brain uses for air conditioning. Due to being located next to the brain's air-conditioning shaft, even the slightest of head movements is magnified and creates even more unwanted artifacts than if it were located closer to our foreheads.

Fortunately, researchers can use higher-resolution scans with smaller voxels or volume pixels to get reliable data. Still, try to imagine a research subject having an orgasm while needing to keep his or her head perfectly still for minutes on end. Head movements during MRI studies of orgasm are one of the reasons why these studies must be reproduced in another lab before they should be considered valid, yet few studies have been replicated elsewhere.

Also, the subjects are often shown porn clips to make them feel sexually aroused while the MRIs are being done. But how do the researchers know what the subject's brain is really processing. Is it processing sexual arousal, or the way the porn actors' bodies are moving (kinesthetics), or the changing frames in the video porn clips or some random thought that popped into the subject's mind?

There's also the question of what happens to the information when it gets inside the brain—is the information being compared to similar information that was stored in the subject's mind years ago, or is it being treated as novel information? Is the subject's brain processing the porn clip based on how the subject feels when he has had sex in the past, or is the turn-on strictly in the here and now, with no prior referencing?

Today's neuroimaging technology is still crude compared to what it will be in another twenty to thirty years. Right now, the equipment doesn't focus on the actual neurons that are firing, but on the blood that drains from that part of the brain. So let's say researchers are focusing on what's happening inside small parts of the brain called the amygdala, hypothalamus, and nucleus accumbens. Small as they might be, they contain oceans of neurons. Using the current generation of MRI equipment to nail down the exact neurons that are involved would be like trying to go to Mars using an iPod as your sole onboard computer.

There's also debate about how long to measure what it is you hope you are measuring, and whether you are actually measuring what you think you are measuring. This depends on a researcher's hypothesis about what areas of the brain are going to be activated. Because researchers use different measurements, it makes it a challenge to compare studies with each other.

The next time the media runs a big story saying that men's brains process sexual arousal differently than women's brains, you might wonder what the study was actually measuring. Was it measuring how our brains process sexual arousal in general, or was it measuring how the brains were processing the specific the porn clips the researchers were showing them to get them aroused.

Think of how you feel when you are looking forward to having sex as a partner first arrives, and the sounds, smells and actual feel of your partner's skin against yours. Is this the same way you feel when you are watching porn?[1] That's what much of the current brain research assumes—not all, but a good deal of it.

While the current MRI findings are exciting, thought provoking and will be unlocking many of the body and mind's sexual secrets—all things in good time. For now, researchers are just starting to break a sweat.

_____

[1]While reviewing this chapter, a researcher on the forefront of neuroimaging commented: "For many researchers, it's not clear that they have specific research questions when they enter the scanner. Some of the discussion sections seem like exercises in reading tea-leaves."

A Very Special Thanks to Adam Safron of Northwestern University, to Serge Stoleru of the Université Pierre et Marie Curie, and to Claire Yang and Kenneth Maravilla of the University of Washington for their helpful article "Magnetic Resonance Imaging and the Female Sexual Response: Overview of Techniques, Results, and Future Directions" in the *Journal of Sexual Medicine.*

39
What's Normal
10,000 People Talk About Sex

Twenty-five years ago, we sent out the first sex surveys for a new book that was being written called the *Guide To Getting It On*. We stapled the pages by hand and stuffed them into packets with self-addressed stamped envelopes. The responses that began arriving a few weeks later were handwritten and the pages often had coffee or tea stains on them, or that's what we hoped they were.

Deciphering the handwriting was sometimes a slow and painful process, but people's responses were so intimate and thoughtful that it felt wrong to not make every possible effort. Now, nearly 10,000 surveys later, the forms are filled out electronically by visitors to the website of *The Guide*. The coffee stains are gone, but the thoughtfulness and honesty remains.

As you will soon see, these surveys are different from typical sex surveys which are designed to collect data that can be scored by computers. Surveys that are designed to please a computer will never tell a person's story. They will never leave you feeling like you have had a conversation.

These surveys were intentionally left open-ended to encourage thoughtful responses. That's because the *Guide To Getting It On* was always meant to reflect the lives of real people.

These surveys have been a constant reminder that sex that is not simple, especially sex in relationships. They have been a reminder that "normal" incorporates a vast horizon. They have made us smile, feel awe, and occasionally turn our heads in sadness.

No generalizations can be made from the surveys we collect. These surveys speak for no one other than the individuals who answered them. In fact, when we tried to find a "representative" survey to lead off with, we couldn't. There is no single survey that represents "the women's surveys."

This chapter is a mere drop in the bucket of the surveys we have collected. We have presented each person's answers to our questions as a narrative that's made up of their own words.

FEMALE 32

I'm straight and I'm not currently in a relationship. I've had 2 serious relationships in my life. One lasted for 3 years and one for 8 years. I've had about 15 sexual partners where there wasn't much of an emotional connection.

As an adult I struggle with the timing of when to have sex in a new relationship. I'm not comfortable having sex on the first date. Now, it is assumed that everyone is comfortable with sex almost upon meeting. I never know how early to jump in. I typically want to have sex soon but not before the exchange of names! I also don't want to sleep with a jerk and can't figure out how to manage the timing.

I have used pills and the ring for birth control. I loved the pill and didn't feel like it impacted my desire or my mood at all. The ring on the other hand, put a serious damper on my mood and desire.

I find intercourse very satisfying. I have orgasms 95 percent of the time.

I am pretty good at saying what I like sexually but maybe less good at saying what I don't like, especially when I first start having sex with someone.

The worst part of giving a guy oral sex is feeling like I'm not doing a good job. The best part is just being comfortable in bed and enjoying the moment.

I have had two one-night stands. The sex wasn't that good. We were constantly moving around which wasn't interesting or good. One guy was a terrible kisser so I wanted to wipe all the saliva from my face which was distracting.

I have no problem with condoms but I don't like lubricant because it makes it too slippery and cuts down on the sensation.

My fantasy is to have sex in a public place, maybe like a rest room but I have never done that. I feel that with a long term partner we go for more intimate, less exciting sex. With a new partner I am afraid of looking like a slut so I don't ever ask for stuff I like.

While I'm female, when it comes to intercourse, I am the one who can't last very long at all which makes me feel very insecure. My partners have all told me that's a great thing and I shouldn't feel bad. With the most satisfying partners, I usually orgasm multiple times. With the less satisfying partners, I orgasm only once. I orgasm 95 percent or maybe 99 percent. I rarely don't orgasm.

I have hooked up for just a night. It is okay even though I was nervous. I played it off like it was fine and ultimately it was fine. I want them to desire me and it hurts my ego to feel that they don't, even if I don't want them.

I'm uncomfortable with the amount of fluid I produce around ovulation. The milky substance can be a little embarrassing.

I had one partner with a curved penis. I had a hard time climaxing. I couldn't find a position that was best. He just wasn't that good in bed and wasn't confident, which was a total turn off.

When I first became single after years and years of being in a relationship, I was masturbating nearly every day but then it lost its appeal. Now I pretty much only masturbate once a month. When I masturbate, I use a vibrating dildo.

FEMALE 24

I'm single and consider myself mostly straight.

I have way less sex than my peers. I voluntarily withdrew from partaking in sexcapades. I've had one serious relationship and probably about 5 hook up/friends with benefits relationships.

I find intercourse...um...pretty satisfying, I guess. I'm still waiting on the mindblowing sex. The last time, I was completely disappointed in his ability to not last. It lasted less than 5 minutes. With the one before him, sometimes I felt like he lasted too long. I mean, I'm not complaining, but by the end, my knees were on fire. I also noticed that he had a book on Tantric sex in his room and had said he was studying something about controlling his orgasms.

I rarely orgasm during intercourse. Maybe 20% of the time. Orgasms during intercourse only happen with other stimulation in addition to thrusting. Grinding worked sometimes, but the tried and true "O" button is most definitely the clitoris.

I was in eighth grade when I first fingered myself. Quite honestly I didn't feel much. I didn't know what I was supposed to feel. For the most part, it was pretty uncomfortable and after a week or so of trying I became disillusioned with the whole thing. I do remember thinking that it wasn't very big and that in no way could a living child fit through that opening, but then again, I was in eighth grade.

I first discovered my clitoris in college. My friends bought me a vibrator and it probably took me months before I mustered up the courage to use it. Before then, I hadn't even thought about touching or pleasuring myself. I didn't know enough about my body then to know what I was doing or that it could feel excruciatingly pleasurable.

After the first time using my vibrator, I felt like a whole new world had been opened to me. Quite frankly, it was one of the best sensations I'd ever felt, but at the same time I had amassed so much guilt over it. I was raised in church and, although no one explicitly said so, was taught that masturbation was sinful. To this day, I'm still not 100% comfortable with masturbation, but I've come leaps and bounds farther than where I used to be. Whether or not my behavior will ultimately damn me for eternity is to be determined, but for the time being, my clitoris and I are great, great friends.

When I do masturbate, it's when I wake up. My dreams are usually more vivid at this time and it's ample material for a good fantasy.

My best sexual experience was with a partner whose confidence was second to none. He had an insatiable, carnal need to be inside me. More importantly, I trusted him to be a good lover. I can't say I've had that trust with any other partner.

Sometimes I need to make a conscious effort to get excited about the sex. One time, I was horny and wanted sex so badly...at least I thought I did. Mentally, I thought I was feeling the whole situation, but physically, my body just did not want to take part. No matter what I thought of, or what I said, or was said to me, my body was just not in the mood for sex. I took that as a sign that my body is heaps more intelligent than I give it credit for.

I love giving oral sex. I love it! It's possibly one of the few times that I know for sure I have complete control over him. I can take my time with him; I can feel him pulsating in my mouth and knowing that he's about to come makes me that much more excited. His pleasure is pleasurable. The only down side is when I get lock jaw.

In most instances my hook ups have involved alcohol. In two instances, I have no memory of the hook up sex, but from what I've been told they were pretty spectacular. From the ones I do remember, the sex wasn't really all that great. One guy's penis was so small I couldn't feel him (wish I'd blacked out then). The others were average on the whole. Routine thrusting and no big "O" for moi. Waste of time, basically.

Hook ups are usually not an awkward experience. If something embarrassing happened the previous night (impotence due to alcohol, premature ejaculation, etc.), then there's some awkward tension. Most of my one night stands happened while I was studying abroad, so the fact that I would never see these guys again helped ease whatever awkwardness there may have been.

FEMALE 28

I'm totally straight and I have been in a new relationship for about 7 weeks. I've had 2 serious relationships and 4 hookup/ no emotional connection partners.

For birth control, I have used Alesse - a low-dose pill. I felt like it made me less horny and wet. It also made me feel less sexy because I was a little fatter and bloated. I went off it a year ago, and I do not want to go back on the pill.

I'm very comfortable talking to my partners about sex. I find intercourse very satisfying. I love it! I'd say I orgasm during sex about 85% of the time. Orgasms from intercourse require fingers on my clit or grinding against his pubic bone. My one complaint is my partners last a little too long. After a while, I don't want them to stop banging away at me.

Intercourse feels better when I know and love the person I'm with. I slept with someone a few times who was just an acquaintance, and while he was very skillful, I just wasn't that into it after the initial excitement. With someone I know and care about, it feels more intimate. Also, I'm more comfortable asking for what I like with someone I know well.

My thoughts don't usually stray during sex. I feel like I don't think at all during sex. Sometimes I do get tired of it after a while, though.

The best part of giving my guy oral is feeling his smooth skin in my mouth, and knowing that I'm giving him pleasure. Worst part is when my jaw gets tired and starts hurting. Also, it's annoying when a guy tries to last a long time during oral. Just come already!

I remember when I first started touching my clitoris, it just felt ticklish and sensitive, not really pleasurable. Once I combined it with internal stimulation, then I realized how great it can be! I still don't come from clitoral stimulation alone.

I was in high school, probably 15 or so when I first put my finger inside while taking a shower, just as an experiment. I wanted to see how many fingers I could get inside—I was a little concerned that I wouldn't be able to fit a whole penis in there. After a couple of experiments, I wanted to put my fingers inside because it felt so good.

Condoms feel less intimate. I love the way the smooth, hard penis skin feels against my skin. I can't feel that with a condom. We use them anyway, though, because I don't like the pill, and the intercourse still feels good.

There is absolutely a big gap between my sexual fantasies and the sex I have in real life. I tend to fantasize about threesomes, even though I would not want to have one in reality. Sometimes it's two men and a woman, sometimes three gay men. In the gay threesome, there is usually an age or status difference, and some bondage. Like, there will be a teenaged college student, a Teaching Assistant and a college professor. If it's two men and a woman, they are always double-penetrating her. The fantasy sex is often quite rough. In reality, I have no interest in rough sex, bondage or threesomes! I just want to have loving, vanilla sex with one partner.

I think I have ejaculated twice. The first time, my college boyfriend was going down on me, and suddenly there was liquid everywhere. I was afraid I had peed, and I was like, "Oh my God, did I just pee in your mouth?!" The second time was much later, during intercourse. It made a wet spot on the bed, but I didn't mind.

I like to masturbate at night, before I go to bed. I almost always use my fingers. I don't like things that feel unnatural - I prefer human touch. Every once in a while, I use a dildo, just to have something bigger inside. How often I masturbate depends on the week—in the middle of my cycle, I masturbate several times a week. I'm usually not as horny near my period. It's the same whether I'm single or in a relationship, unless I'm having sex every day. Then I don't need to masturbate at all.

FEMALE 33

I'm totally straight and I've been in a relationship for 12 years. I've had 3 serious relationships in my life.

I use a birth control pill. I think I'm gaining weight on it which I'm not happy about but can't afford to get pregnant. I don't like condoms. They feel like rubber, not flesh, and the friction can get painful without enough lubrication.

I don't find intercourse very satisfying. I'm sure not comfortable talking about sex. Intercourse has definitely felt better with certain partners, because of chemistry, partner's skill, and level of emotional intimacy. When intercourse is good, lasting a long time is nice, but for the past several years, the faster it's over the happier I am.

When he used to care enough to try, I would have an orgasm most of the time during intercourse. Now he can't be bothered, so I never have them. For me to orgasm during intercourse, I need thrusting and grinding. Direct contact with the clitoris usually irritates me or hurts.

With my current partner, I have to make an effort to try and stay sexually excited. Most of the time I'd rather not be having sex. Sometimes I try to get my mind in the mood. Sometimes I can't be bothered and just try to get it over with.

As for giving a male partner oral sex – it makes my jaw hurt and I loathe getting ejaculate in my mouth. Best part is it gets him hard and wet so sex is less uncomfortable and over faster.

There's a huge gap between sex in my real life and sex in my fantasies. My fantasies involve BDSM and a partner who can satisfy me easily. In reality, I'm married to a guy who couldn't care less about satisfying me, and I'm nowhere near comfortable enough with him to mention my fantasies to him, much less explore them.

I'm trying hard not to masturbate, but when I do it, it's usually first thing in the morning when I'm alone. I'm trying never to masturbate, but in reality - maybe once every couple months.

I cheated on my boyfriend once. I felt mildly guilty, ended up with neither boyfriend nor the guy I cheated with. Neither was anything special.

FEMALE 35

I'm totally straight and I'm not currently in a relationship. I've had 2 serious relations and countless "no strong emotional attachment" relationships.

Intercourse is extremely satisfying for me. I orgasm 100% of the time. However, orgasms during intercourse require direct clitoral stimulation.

In my younger days, I wasn't so choosy, now I only sleep with men that I "click" with. Sex has gotten much better since I threw chemistry into the equation.

Sometimes when I'm having sex, I feel myself sort of disengaging, letting my mind wander. When that happens, I will ask or tell my lover to do something to bring us back together. Words and sex are great together.

How comfortable I am talking about sex varies. On a scale from 1 to 10, I'm between 5 to 10 when it comes to saying what feels good and 1 when it comes to talking about what doesn't feel good.

I enjoy every bit of giving oral sex from teasing to swallowing every drop. Some favorites are: feeling his hand(s) on the back of my head, feeling him grow harder as he becomes more aroused, and feeling him throb as he comes.

When I was 18, I met a 33 year old man who showed me how my clitoris works. So even though I had been playing with myself since I was 5, I learned how to really masturbate when I was 18. Self-pleasure became much more intimate and sexy.

I've had some great one-nighters and some awful ones. Never have I wished it was more than one night, though.

From my experience, if a guy is on the smaller side, or if he can't get a full rock-hard erection, then condoms definitely impact the sensation. It often won't even go in, and if it does, it won't stay in... I'm not sure I can blame it on the condom. Condoms on a huge, rock-hard cock have very little impact. Maybe not as slippery, but nothing worth complaining about.

Sex with a partner is very different in real life from sex in my fantasies. In my fantasies, I'm very submissive. It's hard to bring that up as you're getting to know someone.

I produce a lot of fluids during sex and I'm totally comfortable with that. I love my fluids and I have never met a man who doesn't love them too.

I think I masturbate more when I'm in a relationship. Either way, it's at least several times per week. I always use my fingers, but sometime I use a butt plug for anal stimulation.

I had sex with a woman when I was much younger. I had been sleeping with her boyfriend and he set a threesome up without her finding out how he and I knew each other. The circumstances were creepy. Aside from that, I thoroughly enjoyed being with her. When she and I were together, it was like he wasn't even there... Pretty hot, really.

FEMALE 24

I consider myself mostly straight and I've been in a relationship for three years. I've had 2 serious relationships and Ohhh shit! at least 40 relationships with no strong emotional attachment.

I think intercourse is pretty satisfying. It really depends on the partner's enthusiasm, curiosity, and willingness to know MY body instead of just using "what works". Also, how much I dig the person, and circumstances like where we are doing it, and what kind of emotional place we are, how are bodies fit together can affect how good it is too. Sometimes I wonder if the sex is better when I don't have any emotional attachment or expectation! Sometimes, I have problem producing sufficient fluids. It can make sex painful. Thank goodness for lube.

For birth control, I use Fertility Awareness (rhythm method), and it definitely increased my desire. It felt good to know when it was safe to have sex. Often times I will even refrain from having ANY sex at all when I'm fertile, even with a condom.

I orgasm during intercourse about 60% of the time. It doesn't happen from thrusting alone. Fingers are a necessity! Being high allows for some of the most intense orgasms!

My one partner is just so big that when he's wearing a condom, I feel like I'm being speared... because the condom just squeezes his penis (and yes we're using the biggest condoms available) but when we have unprotected sex, it's a lot softer and more enjoyable!

When I've been emotionally involved with a partner for a long time, sometimes I have to try to keep myself present. Sex for me has always been a physical pleasure only until this relationship. Now it's like, uh, what? We do this together as well as talk about the hard shit? I have a hard time just letting go of where we are out of bed, so it's hard to just be in bed with this partner.

I LOVE, LOVE, LOVE, LOVE GIVING HEAD! I LOVE IT ALL! I have a bit of an oral fixation, and I just love how his member feels in my mouth, across my lips. If I'm having a hard time getting aroused, I'll often go down on my partner just so I can get wet! Worst parts? Sometimes his member is just too big to deep throat!

I discovered my clit when I was like four! I would put my finger in my vagina until my mom discovered what I was doing and kept interfering and telling me that it was wrong and to stop. Needless to say I have a shit ton of guilt and shame associated with masturbating, though I still do it. I remember still living at home, masturbating, being paranoid my mom was going to know, and beating myself up inside my head. I'd tell myself, "I'm addicted, I should stop", but it felt soooo goooooooooooood!

Hook ups can be good, very good. Exactly what I needed at the time! Not awkward at all. To tell the truth, with my most recent partner, we hooked up one night and never really talked about what it would mean... and then later seeing him where we hang out together was SORT of awkward, because I wasn't sure if he wanted to do it again, because I definitely did!

I masturbate 2-4 times a week whether I'm in a relationship or not. Usually at night before I fall asleep. Oh man, this is kind of embarrassing. I recently had to stop using my electric toothbrush for this purpose! I am afraid of breaking it, so I need a proper toy. I was using the toothbrush almost exclusively!

Yes, I can proudly say I've had sex with women. I really enjoyed them all! Some were at a party, others were something my ex-partner and I contrived with a mutual friend... another was a friend who said she never had an orgasm, so I decided I would try. It worked! Another was with a girl I thought I liked but she ended up being WAY, WAY, WAY too rough and she smelled/tasted horrible!

I've also had a threesome. Now I want to try two guys and me... I've had many two girls and a guy threesomes... time for something new!

I have touched a male partner's prostate. I wish more men were willing to let me stick my finger up their ass!

FEMALE 19

I totally straight and, sadly, I'm not in a relationship.

I've never had "amazing" or "mind-blowing" sex, I'm still waiting for that! On average sex can be around a 7 out of 10 for me. Foreplay and a bit of role playing work wonders though! I've had 1 relationship and about 11 hook up/fuck buddy encounters. Pretty depressing really. I definitely need to up my standards!

I've had a long-term "fuck buddy" who I saw every day at school for 2 years. We just acted like friends do, nobody ever suspected a thing! The best was when you made eye contact across the room and you gave each other a cheeky wink or smile!

Of the 12 partners, each one is different. For me, some of the best sex I've had has been with someone I connect with on an emotional level as well as a physical level. I find that the best sex is when the guy is willing to adapt and learn how I like to be touched, kissed, etc. It makes me feel like I'm the only girl on their mind at the time. Not all girls like it hard and fast. If guys take the time to ask a couple of questions, sex can be fabulous.

My mind is racing the whole time when I'm having intercourse with someone. Whether it's "should I try a new position" or "should I put on a cheeky costume"?

I'm very comfortable talking to my partners about sex. I learned years ago that if I didn't speak up and tell the guy what I liked or show him exactly how to do it, I would be left greatly disappointed. If I miss the chance to let the guy know how I like it done beforehand, I get right in there myself and show him the way if he isn't doing it for me! So far, I've had nothing but admiration for taking charge and telling a man how to do it the way I like it. After all, in the end we're all pleased!

When it comes to oral sex, men love my tongue ring! It is sexy and works wonders. When I can hear them groaning for more, it's encouraging and a huge turn on! Bit, I hate when a man pushes your head down onto his dick and thrusts into your mouth, I'm not a blow-up doll buddy!

I remember being 9 and watching the movie "Rocky" with my friend. I sat on the arm of the couch and found that if I rocked back and forth it created an amazing feeling. After that, I started experimenting with my friend. I enjoyed her weekly visits to my house because of all the new things we tried.

I remember thinking it was good fun. It's amazing the feelings you can experience at 9 years old!

I've had a few good experiences with hook up sex, but mostly I felt dirty afterwards. My experience with one nighters is that the guy doesn't really want to explore your body, doesn't ask about what you like and how you like it. It seems so desperate to me. I understand that most people don't look at one night stands that way but to me, I felt dirty.

I have an Implanon inserted into my arm. It lasts 3 years and is amazing! I don't have to worry about taking the pill everyday etc. In fact, I haven't had my period for 3 years because of it which is a bonus. It hasn't affected my sex life at all.

I believe condoms impact the sensation in certain positions. Missionary will never feel as good with a condom on. But when the girl is on top, we are dominating everything; I don't feel a difference.

For a few years there was a huge difference in my fantasies versus real life sex, but not so much now. Most of my fantasies involve putting on a show, stripping, being roughed up - most of which involves wearing very little, having confidence and just being sexy! I've had weight loss surgery and it's amazing how I now feel about myself! My fantasies are becoming more and more real situations, I feel comfortable enough to wear skimpy things and parade around in very little outfits! Nothing is holding me back now!

My previous partner couldn't keep an erection and it drove me crazy. He couldn't stay up for more than 10 minutes at a time! Any mention of "condom" and BOOM! I'd spend the next 20 minutes trying to get it back up! In the end it became so frustrating I avoided sex as often as I could! However, my most recent partner was absolutely amazing. He can keep going time and time again but I'm also aware not everyone has stamina like him!

I'd say I have an orgasm around 80% of the time. I'm a "grinder"; I have the best most intense orgasms that way. I never need clitoral stimulation. However, I'm beginning to include it when I'm masturbating!

I masturbate at night. Whether I masturbate depends on whether I've just seen an intense sex scene in a movie, or my partner is suggesting dirty things to me! On average, I masturbate twice a week when I don't have a partner compared to 4-5 times a week when I'm in a relationship. I don't ever use my fingers to masturbate—it doesn't get me off. I use a vibrator at all times. I have a couple to choose from so I never get bored!!!

I've had sex with girls, but I don't look at girls and see them in a sexual way always. I've only ever allowed one person to go down on me and that was a girl. Girls tend to know girls better, so I find it to be more intimate and naughty. It was a great experience and if the opportunity arose again, I would certainly take it up! I've never had a threesome, but I'm extremely keen!

FEMALE 26

I'm straight and I've been in a relationship for 5 years. I've only had one partner and I've never had an orgasm during sex.

I have vulvodynia so I find intercourse painful, but I still like it. I don't produce a lot of vaginal fluid because I'm always worried about the pain.

I use something like Seasonique for birth control, where you take it for 3 months straight. I've been on some form of birth control since well before I started having sex so I have no idea if it impacts my sex drive or not. I have more of a sex drive than my partner so I think I'm ok. I've used condoms but they really hurt!

It's difficult for me to stay sexually excited and in the moment because I'm always trying to block out the pain. My partner has a low sex drive and I have found basically one position that isn't painful (me on top and leaning forward). I daydream about having sex several times per week in all kinds of different positions, but it's probably never going to happen. I don't really have sexual fantasies.

As for giving my partner oral sex, my mouth is really small and he is pretty big so it really hurts my jaw.

I actually discovered my clitoris while reading an earlier version of this book when I was about 20. It was difficult and took a long time, but it turned out ok in the end.

When I was growing up, I never put a finger in my vagina because it hurt. It's hurt as long as I can remember so I never touched it until I was trying to become sexually active. I still don't touch it much and I never stick my fingers up there if I don't have to.

My partner has a curved penis. It's really curved and it curves up against his tummy so it doesn't put any pressure on the back of my vagina if I'm on top where my vulvodynia is worst (like between my vagina and my bottom). I don't think we could have sex if it wasn't for his curved penis.

I've been in a relationship almost as long as I've been masturbating. I use my fingers because most other things hurt. Sometimes, I'll use a vibrator.

Male 33

We've only included one of the men's surveys. While we've received some wonderful individual answers from men over the years, it's been unusual to get men's surveys that are as verbal from start to finish as the women's. The following highly verbal survey from a former marine truly stands out.

I am totally straight.

I left home and became a Marine. I served my country and still wish I was. I was in a Special Incident Response Team that put me at ground zero on 9/11 for a week. Did a lot of traveling up and down the east coast. I have two kids and an ex-wife. I just got done hitting rock bottom and am now remembering who I was so I can be that person again. My goal is to better myself every day. I am valuable, confident and curious.

I've had approximately 20 sexual partners. 7 of them were casual sex relationships or one night stands. I am not currently in a relationship. Since my divorce I've had two"friends with benefits" relationships. I welcomed the relationships and I was able to be very open and free with the last woman. Both instances were hot and some of the best sex I have had. The first ended because I misread the cues and I tried to take it too far emotionally. This second was different, but I still got hung up on my emotions. I trying to learn how adapt and enjoy the freedom of "this is not going to last and it is physical only".

I love to use my mouth on a woman and I love to give her oral sex. It's one of my favorite things to do. I typically will be there long enough to give her multiple orgasms. Sometimes my neck gets sore from giving oral sex. The best position I have found for me is when the woman sits on my face. Or have her sit in a chair. Slide your legs under the chair and you are right there. Advantage for her is that now she is in a really good position to watch and some woman love to watch. The key to doing oral sex right is to make her as comfortable as possible and be able to sense her reaction to what you are doing. Also, the more comfortable you are the more relaxed and the longer you will spend pleasing her.

The least amount of time I give a woman oral sex is about 30 to 45 min. But I have had my mouth between a woman's legs for a couple of hours before. From my experience, women don't start to relax until about 10 to 15 min into it. Then they go to a stage of comfort. Once they are comfortable – let the magic begin. It also depends on the amount of build-up and foreplay and the existing relationship you have. The more foreplay and better the relationship, the quicker the comfort level is reached.

One of the best sexual experiences I have had was the first time I was comfortable with pulling a girl's hair during sex. This woman put me at ease and challenged me all in one moment. She said to be as rough as you want, but just be a man. The way she said it and her look melted the paint off the walls for me. I didn't think about a thing except her hair wrapped around my hand like a lasso. She went crazy and loved it

One of my worst experiences was when I was in my late teens and a girlfriend went down on me. She was ambitious and wanted to please so she tried to put all of me into her throat. She gagged and her natural reaction was to bite down. It was horrific. Do to all of the commotion and my yelling, it wasn't long before her Dad knocked on the door to investigate. Needless to say, the most uncomfortable dinner ever.

My dad was very important in my life. He didn't do all the traditional dad stuff like show up to every one of my games or take me out for ice cream. He was a department director at a big company and it demanded a lot of attention. From him I learned how to manage people and business very well and I learned to have a strong work ethic. I want to have the same fundamentals as him and appreciate everything he has taught me. But I think it would be unfair to him and myself to be just like him. He made mistakes he does not want me to make.

I grew up with older sisters. One of the first big influences I had was when I turned 14 and my sister became involved with a man who treated me like a brother. He had a huge Influence in my life.

I do watch porn. I prefer man and woman porn. Sometimes multiple women and one guy, and girl on girl. In my younger less experienced times

I related what happened in porn to what women like and the positions that were best to perform. I soon learned that they were male generated fantasies and there is a lot more involved. It's a much more satisfying experience when you talk to each other about what works and what doesn't.

One of the worst things about porn is it gives guys a complex about their penis size. I have an adequate size and I try not to compare my dick to porn dicks. Porn is an industry that thrives on exaggeration. I am not tiny and I am not giant.

40
Bye Bye V-Card
Losing Your Virginity

There is more information in this chapter than you probably need if it's your first time. The trouble in leaving out parts is while they may not apply to you, they might be important for someone else.

Also keep in mind that couples can become VERY pregnant from their first time, even if they are doing it when a woman is having her period. And for a brief legal reminder: If you are under 18, you may be breaking some of your state's laws if you have sex. Regardless of your age, please read Chapter 13: *Consent*.

Now, for the fun part.

The Importance of Having a Good First Time

When couples have a lousy first time, it tends to negatively color the sex they will be having for the next few years. It's as if the bar gets set so low they don't expect sex to be any better. So taking charge of your first time and trying to make it a really good experience is in your best interest for now and for the years to come.

The Realities of a Girl's First Time vs A Boy's First Time

Here are some things people usually don't mention that would be good to discuss with your partner before the two of you have intercourse.

By the time most boys lose their virginity, they have had a few years of masturbating under their belt. Most will know what an orgasm feels like. And a lot of them will have tried to jerk off while using lube, so they'll at least have a remote sense of what intercourse might feel like.

Girls, on the other hand, aren't encouraged to explore their bodies. Few girls will have masturbated before their first time, so not many will know what an orgasm is. Nor will their bodies have experienced anything like a penis inside of it. A tampon, maybe, but the chances are good a boyfriend's penis will feel different than a tampon; and hopefully it won't have a string attached.

What this means is that unless a girl has a favorite dildo, her vagina will undergo more changes during her first time than her partner's penis will. This doesn't need to be a negative, it's just different.

Another thing to consider is that for most guys, the only love-making education they've had is from watching porn. Porn actors will be the first to tell you that porn was never meant to be used for sex education or as a model for having sex, whether it's your first time or your thousandth. Porn never shows couples talking about what they want to do. It never shows them discussing what feels good and what doesn't. It's all magic in porn and everyone pretends to have great sex all of the time.

Couples in real life usually spend way more time kissing and caressing each other before they have intercourse than porn actors do. Real-life couples get to enjoy each other's bodies from head to toe instead of focusing on each other's genitals. And the last thing a first-time couple should ever attempt is a hard pounding fuck like they do in porn. Easy does it is the way to go. You've got plenty of years ahead to have sex like a porn star, assuming you would want to. For now: tender and loving, yes; porn-star wannabe, no.

Preparing Ahead for a Most-Excellent Journey

"It was very hard to do, but I waited until I was 18 to have intercourse. It was with a guy who cared deeply about me, which made my first experience very fun and comfortable." *female age 36*

Most people's first time is awkward and unplanned. It doesn't need to be that way. Hopefully, it's a time you will remember with fondness—the beginning of a most excellent journey.

In Addition to This Chapter

If you'd like more information about intercourse, check out Chapter 23: *Intercourse—Horizontal Jogging.* But for your first time, you'll want to keep it simple because there are different priorities and different challenges. Just reading this Guide's chapters on kissing, handjobs, finger fucking, and oral sex will put you years ahead of the game.

Who To Do It With Your First Time

Not many of us are still with the person who we lost our virginity to. While we might have been in love with them at the time, our perspectives and romantic interests often change.

"I would have waited until I was in college. I would have saved myself years of painful, uncomfortable, inexperienced, or hurried sex. And while it just felt good to be close to the guy, I realize that I haven't thought of him in years. Girls, you ain't missing nothing!"

female age 32

Think about the difference between a crush and a friend. A friend usually has to earn your trust and respect, while a crush automatically gets it because of the way he or she looks or acts. The chances are good you will still have your friends in a year's time, but you will probably have blown through your current crush and you might even gag at the mere thought of the person.

This isn't to say you should ruin a good friendship by having sex with a friend instead of with a romantic interest. But worse things have happened. At least try to make sure your first lovemaking partner is someone who has the qualities of a friend, and he or she is not someone who pressured you to have intercourse.

Doing It Sober

Please, don't do it your first time drunk or stoned. While this is often how it happens. Every survey on first-time intercourse is chuck full of horror stories from virgins who did it drunk. Couples who do it sober will often have a better and more satisfying time.

Advice for Girls

This part of the chapter is written mostly for women. Hopefully, guys will read it as well. One of the keys to having good sex is knowing your body well enough to be able to say "That feels good" or "Let's try something else" in a way that a lover can understand. This is a skill that can take years to perfect. Even women who have had sex countless times still keep discovering new things about their bodies. So consider yourself at the start of an exciting journey that will last for much of your life.

Girls who masturbate might have a bit of an advantage their first time, but if you haven't masturbated before, not to worry. It can help a great deal if you're able to feel inside your vagina before you have intercourse for your first time. So wash your hands and get some water-based sex lube or use your own spit. Saliva is water-based and can work well if you don't have sex lube.

When you've got at least a half-hour to yourself (good luck!), or when you are tucked under the covers in bed, start exploring up and down your body with your fingertips. Spend some extra time on your neck and chest and on the area from your navel to your knees, except for your vulva and vagina. If it makes it more fun, pretend it's a partner's fingers instead of your own.

Once your fingers have explored up and down your body for at least ten or fifteen minutes, you might start to focus on the area between your legs. Let your fingertips glide up and down and around your vulva, which is the outside part of what's between your legs. For illustrations, see Chapter 7: *What's Inside a Girl*.

While one hand is exploring between your legs, there's nothing written in stone that says your other hand has to be tied to your side. At the very least, see what it's like resting it on one of your breasts.

When you think it's time to venture inside, get a finger good and wet. Slowly inch it inside your vagina, which is an opening that's buried toward the bottom of your vulva. It's where tampons and penises go. The emphasis should be on "slowly." You want to feel what your finger is feeling, as well as what your vagina is feeling.

At this point, some girls will want to put their finger in farther; others might be feeling a little overwhelmed, especially if they've been raised in a household that was not safe or supportive of their sexual growth. If you are in the "go for it!" group, let your finger keep going. And remember to keep asking yourself what your vagina is feeling. If you are so inclined, you might try adding a second finger. Given how a penis is most likely wider than your finger, two fingers is a nice goal.

If you are in the group of girls who might be starting to feel like enough is enough, then this is a good place to stop. Just letting yourself go this far is a really important step. If you can, try to go just a tiny bit farther next time, but don't be discouraged if you hit a personal wall. Maybe it would be easier to have your partner read this and ask him to explore you with his fingers, but only if you feel comfortable with that and he has good enough judgment to know the difference between a finger and a penis!

If and when you feel ready, you might practice guiding a tampon or small, tube-like vibrator into your vagina when you are lying on your back. Also practice doing this when you are squatting, as if you were in a girl-on-top position. Don't assume your partner is going to have a clue where the opening of your vagina is. Be ready to help him guide his penis in, unless you don't mind if it ends up in your belly button or up your rear end.

If all of this seems too overwhelming, maybe it's not the right time in your life to be having intercourse. There are lots of other ways you and a partner can enjoy yourselves sexually without a penis going in your vagina.

The Importance of Feeling Sexually Aroused

A lot of guys would be happy if a partner grabbed their penis and started playing with it. But women don't always do as well with surprise dives for their crotch. Women's genitals do way better if they are highly aroused before a partner touches them.

When a woman is aroused, her genitals expand as much as a penis does. This includes blood flowing into the area around the vagina so it straightens out and puffs up more. This will help make it ready for an incoming penis and it will help intercourse feel better.

Being aroused changes how contact with the clitoris will feel. Touching or kissing a clitoris might be painful if a woman isn't aroused, but it can feel exquisite after she becomes highly aroused. So it can take twenty minutes or more of kissing and caressing before her partner should reach between a woman's legs. That's way more time than they show in porn, and it's usually way more time than it takes a guy to get hard.

Hymens Don't Pop

The majority of women who have taken our sex survey did not experience bleeding during their first intercourse. Nor did their hymens (or cherry) pop. That's because it's a myth that hymens are supposed to pop or tear their first time. To understand more about your hymen, please read Chapter 8: *The Hymen*.

During their first intercourse, some women don't feel a thing hymenwise, others feel a stretching or a sting, and some feel a level of pain that you might when you get your ears pierced, or worse. But if you do the exercises with your fingers ahead of time, the chances are good you won't feel discomfort. If you do feel pain, ask your partner to stop.

If you are getting a gynecological exam before your first intercourse, it can be a really good idea to ask your gynecologist if your hymen has become stretchy enough for intercourse. If not, your gynecologist can give you some estrogen cream that you can rub on it which will help it become more elastic. *Now, for advice for members of both sexes...*

Pillows and Lube

Two accessories that might really help with your first time are lube and pillows. You have no idea how much a carefully placed pillow under a woman's rear can help with the angle of penetration and with her ability to spread her legs. This can allow her to better relax her legs and her vaginal muscles.

As for lube, put a few drops on the penis and a few drops in the opening of the vagina and you are good to go. If you don't have lube, spit can help. Just make sure things aren't dry before you try to have intercourse.

Go Slow and Ask!!!

After you've made out for a long time and are ready for intercourse, do not ram the penis in! Start with the head gently pushing against the bottom of the woman's labia. (It can be very helpful if she separates her labia and guides the penis to her vaginal opening.) If she's okay with the head pushing slightly into the opening of her vagina, ease it in a bit more, and ask again.

Once the penis is all the way inside of the vagina, just keep it there— don't start thrusting. This is the first time the woman has ever had a penis in her vagina. She should spend as much time as she needs adjusting to it being inside before there's any thrusting. This can be the most important moment of your first intercourse. It will be the only "first stroke" that either of you will have in your entire lives. Stop and savor it.

Also keep in mind that a nice sensation can result if the guy pushes his pelvic bone against the woman's while his penis is all the way in and does a slow circular motion with his hips. This may help stimulate her clitoris. She can hopefully guide him with her hands on the sides of his butt.

Orgasms, Anyone?

"Be choosy. Take your time. Touch and explore everything."

female age 36

About 80% of guys have an orgasm their first time, where it's usually less than 20% for girls. One of the things we've learned after reading thousands of women's sex surveys is they usually don't orgasm from thrusting alone during intercourse. They usually need to stimulate their clitoris with their fingers or by grinding it into their lover's pubic bone.

If you are a guy, your orgasm during intercourse might not feel as intense as when you are jerking off. After all, how many times has your penis been in your hand, and how many times has it been in a vagina? When you masturbate, your fingers put pressure on the part of your penis that helps get you off. Vaginas don't have fingers. Also the sole point of contact when you are masturbating is your hand gripping your penis; with partner-sex, your whole body is feeling her whole body.

Or how often have you had an orgasm while supporting your body's weight on your arms or elbows? And if you wank to porn, there can be a big difference between staring into a partner's eyes and staring up the crotches of porn actors. It often takes time and experience to put lovemaking together in a way that beats beating off. Give yourself time. The chances are, you're not the only nervous one between the two of you.

If He Comes Really Fast

Some of us guys can come pretty quickly the first couple of times we have intercourse. Some of us don't even get a penis inside before blowing a wad. Anxiety can do that, and there's nothing wrong with being anxious.

Coming soon might not be such a bad thing your first time. When a woman hasn't had a penis in her vagina before, here might be some rearranging or familiarizing that needs to go on inside of her pelvis. So less thrusting might be better than more. It might even be that nature intended for first-time males to launch early.

Still, if you are worried about coming too soon, get some really thick condoms made out of recycled boots to help dull the sensation.

Afterward

The time you spend together after your first intercourse can be as important as the time during and before. So don't try to do the deed minutes before your team bus is leaving for the state finals. Spend time together afterward and be aware of each other's emotions. Maybe you'll want to hold each other, or maybe you'll want to run downstairs and raid the refrigerator. Hopefully you won't feel the need to Tweet your friends before the condom is barely off.

You can't predict how you will feel afterward. Perhaps you will be relieved, maybe happy, disappointed or sad. Perhaps you'll feel extra close to your partner, or maybe you'll feel alone and isolated. That probably depends more on the quality of your relationship than anything else. Allow for a full range of possibilities and the time to experience them in the hours and days that follow.

What if It Wasn't Mind-Blowing?

"Relax and don't expect it to be like the romance novels." *female age 32*

Who knows what makes for mind-blowing sex, but don't be disappointed if it doesn't happen. If you are thinking that your first time will change your life or transform your relationship, it probably won't unless you get knocked up or get a sexually transmitted infection.

Where to Do It

"Our favorite place was on the floor in the room over my parent's garage when they were out somewhere. When the garage-door motor clicked on and started vibrating the floor we had just enough time to finish, clean up, button up, and act natural before my parents walked in." *male age 26*

For your first time, a quiet, familiar and comfortable setting might be best. But finding a private unhassled location can be a challenge any time you have sex! Ideally, find a time and place when roommates, friends or parents won't be barging in. And please don't do it your first time in a spare room at a party. You might not care now, but maybe you will in a few years. Thinking back over that could be a big regret.

Once you have lots of experience under your belt, exotic locations are fine places to have sex. But for now, safe and familiar is best. If you try it in a bathtub or hot tub, chances are good the water will wash away your natural lubricant. If you do it on a beach, the sand will find its way inside the woman's vagina.

No Time for Sex Toys

If you are so inclined, there's plenty of time in the future to bring out your stock of dildos, cuffs, and strap-ons. When it's your first time, why not stick to the lovemaking basics?

The one exception might be a vibrator, assuming the woman already uses one and enjoys it. It might not be a bad thing for her to get herself off right before you try intercourse. This can help her relax and it might help her first intercourse feel really nice. Her partner can always hold her while she masturbates or uses the vibrator.

If You've Waited until Marriage

The average reader of *The Guide* is not necessarily the kind who waits until the first night of marriage for sex, so it's not like we have a huge database of advice to pass on. But if you think about how stressful a wedding and reception can be, the night of your wedding might not be the best time to make it your first time. Then again, all that adrenaline might be just the ticket! Talk it over ahead of time.

Advice for Guys

Look over the following advice that our female readers have for women who are doing it for the first time:

"Make him go slowly and be sure that you are aroused sufficiently before you let him enter you because it will probably be a little uncomfortable the first time. If he rushes, it will hurt and you won't enjoy it at all." *female age 35*

"Make sure you really want it and it's not about being pressured. Masturbate together first. Be comfortable together. My first time was painful and humiliating; there's got to be a better way."
female age 38

"Have him read the *Guide To Getting It On* first!" *female age 30*

Men who are virgins tend to be at a disadvantage their first time because they usually don't have the courage to admit that they haven't done it before. So instead of being honest and trying to explore together, the guy tries to fake it. Hopefully, readers of this book won't be so silly.

Your first time can be special and sweet, but not if you need to pretend that you know what you are doing when you really don't. Here are a few tips for guys who are about to make their maiden voyage:

Positions Your first time is no time to get fancy. Go with the old-fashion missionary position where she is on her back and you are on top. There's plenty of time later for her to be on top. Missionary is better for the first time.

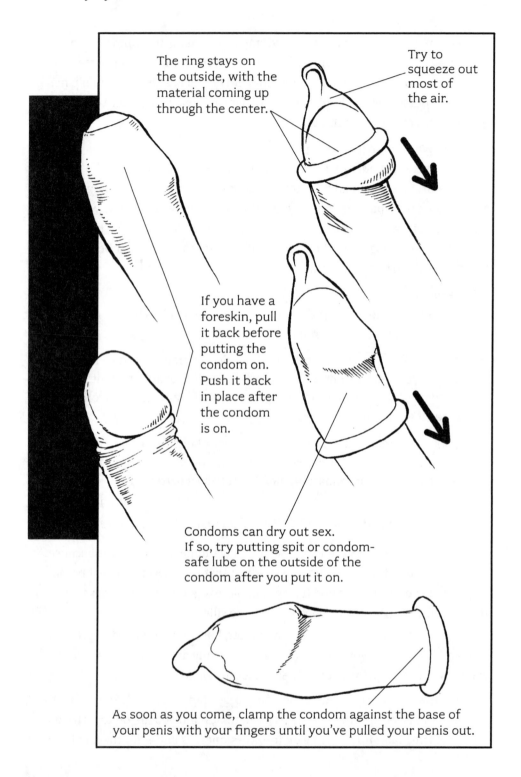

The ring stays on the outside, with the material coming up through the center.

Try to squeeze out most of the air.

If you have a foreskin, pull it back before putting the condom on. Push it back in place after the condom is on.

Condoms can dry out sex. If so, try putting spit or condom-safe lube on the outside of the condom after you put it on.

As soon as you come, clamp the condom against the base of your penis with your fingers until you've pulled your penis out.

During Intercourse If you are on top, she'll want to feel some of your weight on top of her, but not the full nine yards. So use your arms, elbows and knees to support yourself and thrust with your hips. Not to worry, you'll get the hang of it. Heck, even your dad did.

Thrusting Speed Contrary to what you might have seen in the movies, thrust slowly. Go really, really slow and enjoy each and every slip and slide. If she wants you to speed up, she will tell you.

Your Lips You will be hard-pressed to find a single woman on the planet who wouldn't enjoy it if her lover planted some tender, gentle kisses on her neck or lips as his penis is getting to know her vagina.

Porn What makes sex work in a relationship and what makes it work in porn are two very different things. In porn, the camera abhors a tender and loving touch. It comes across as being boring. In real life, tender rules. The two of you have plenty of time to explore having rougher sex after you are more experienced if that's what both of you want.

Oral Anyone? In some situations, it makes perfect sense to go down on your partner before intercourse. In other situations, this would be too over-whelming for her. The two of you need to decide together.

Erections #1 Not to worry if your erection is a bit flaky. Chances are it's never been under this kind of stress before. Keep kissing, laughing or feeling each other up instead. If you do what's described in the other how-to chapters of this book, she'll forget all about your penis.

Erections #2 First-time lovers sometimes rush because the guy might be worried he will lose his hard-on. If he does, he does. It's far more important that you take your time, with lots of kissing, touching, and more kissing. The goal of sex is to share pleasure, fun and intimacy. You don't need an erection or intercourse to do that.

Coming: It's not unusual to come quickly your first time. However, some guys aren't able to come at all. If it seems like you can't come, as her when she feels like it's been enough. Either way, too soon or really slow, don't stress it. This is about the two of you enjoying each other, not about coming.

Putting It In Your First Time

The finest GPS in the world won't help you with this one. And it doesn't matter how much porn you might have watched. Guiding your penis into a vagina can be a challenge whether it's your first time or fiftieth. If you read Chapter 23: *Horizontal Jogging,* you'll find a lot of really experienced guys still have their girlfriend or wife guide it in. You would be wise to ask your partner to guide it in as well.

Asking for a hand (or fingers) isn't a sign of being dumb or a dweeb. It means you are smart enough to know when to seek help. Otherwise, you can cause her unnecessary pain and yourself unnecessary embarrassment.

On the other hand, not all women are able to be helpful in guiding a penis into a vaginal opening. Perhaps some playful fingering will help both of you figure this one out. (See Chapter 15: *The Zen of Finger Fucking* for more ideas.)

Practicing with Condoms—Preparing For Your First Time

Unless you've really got it together and have already visited Planned Parenthood, condoms will probably be your default method of birth control.

If you are a guy, try to get a stash of condoms and water-based lube ahead of time. Condoms come in different sizes and shapes. It's a really good idea to get a sampler pack of different condoms to find which brands fit your penis best. (See Chapter 22: *Condoms—For the Ride of Your Life.*)

You'll want to practice masturbating with a condom on for at least a couple of days before your first time. Here are some suggestions:

Learn how to manipulate the condom by feel alone, as you'll often be putting it on in the dark. One of the biggest time-killers in putting on a condom is determining which way the material rolls out. Pull the tip of the condom from the center of the ring in a way that allows the ring of material to easily roll down your penis.

After you've got the condom on, run warm water over your hand so it is warm, like your partner's body will be. Then lube your hand up and start thrusting your penis into your hand. See what it's like to thrust with your hips into your lubed hand. This will give you a better sense of the condom's road-handling abilities.

Keep thrusting until you've blown a wad. Then pay close attention to what happens to your penis. If you are like most men, it will start to shrink. This is why guys need to crimp the bottom of the condom around the base of their penis as soon as they come. Otherwise, the condom will slip off, and if you keep thrusting you will push it inside your partner's vagina.

Semen will soon start running out the end of a condom after you take it off, so be sure to tie it off. Just make a knot in the middle of the condom.

If you are a girl, get extra condoms and try putting one on something penis-shaped. Learn how to open the package in the dark and how to roll it on, leaving a bit at the end with no air in it if that's what the instructions say.

Also, try to get the morning-after emergency birth control pill in advance. That way, if a condom breaks, or comes off before it's supposed to, or you forget to bring condoms with you, you'll have a better chance of preventing an unwanted pregnancy.

If you find yourself having intercourse without birth control, make sure the partner with the penis pulls out before he comes. This is called withdrawal. It's where the guy pulls his penis out of a woman's vagina before he ejaculates, and strokes himself until he comes, like when he's masturbating. This hopefully keeps his sperm outside of his partner's vagina. While withdrawal is not a particularly effective method of birth control, it's way better than doing nothing.

16 vs 26

Plenty of people don't lose their virginity until they are in their twenties. The nice thing about waiting is that you tend to be more sensible about it and you will often have a better experience. Many of the late-bloomers we have heard from say it's a much better experience. The following is from a reader who didn't lose her virginity until she was well into her twenties:

> "I was surprised at how tricky losing my virginity proved to be. The first couple of times my boyfriend and I tried, my vaginal muscles were very tight and penetration was painful. So we slowed down and tried other ways of loosening the muscles (fingers, a vibrator, etc.), I visited the ob-gyn to make sure nothing was wrong (there wasn't), and we waited for a night when I was nice and relaxed. The first couple of times we successfully had intercourse were amazing—I felt a bit of pain with initial penetration, but once my body got accustomed to him the physical sensation was wonderful, and we had a lot of fun trying different positions and experimenting with what felt good!"

A Very Special Thanks to Angela Hoffman for advice and help; to Carrie Veronica Smith, University of Mississippi, to Chris, a contented average dude from Canada; to Figleaf; and to Dayna Henry and her students at Indiana.

41
The First Time
Not What You'd Think

Researchers questioned hundreds of young women about their sexual experiences and feelings of guilt. Shock of all shocks. Girls with the most negative attitudes about their sexuality are doing it younger, with more partners and in less committed relationships than girls who feel the most positive about their bodies and their sexuality.

The girls with the most guilt are more likely to have their first intercourse with an "occasional dating partner" or with a "person just met," a pattern they continue to repeat as they get older. They tend to have their first intercourse when drinking or stoned.

The girls who feel the best about their bodies tend to masturbate more. And the girls who masturbate the most and feel the best about sex actually wait the longest before having their first intercourse and they have it with more committed partners. Most importantly, when they do have sex, it's part of a conscious decision. Not so with the girls who feel bad about sex and their bodies. More often than not, they just let sex happen to them, without thinking it through first.

So who are these high-guilt, more-promiscuous girls? High-guilt girls tend to grow up in families where the mother and father are less affectionate toward each other. They tend to regard their dads as being overly strict and they are from homes that are more religious than girls who don't sleep around as much. Their abstinence-only Purity Rings seem to hit the floor fast.

Perhaps the girls who have the least sexual acceptance at home go searching for it elsewhere. The trouble is, they go about it in such a destructive way that they end up reinforcing the bad feelings about themselves that they grew up with, and they end up with partners who are just as constricted as their dads.

Who knew that the daughters of the self-righteous would be more likely to sleep around and do it drunk than daughters of parents who have a more open, honest approach to sex and sexual feelings. It's certainly not what religious conservatives would have us believe. When are we going to learn that sex education that's based on shame doesn't work? And what about those school districts where the parents won't allow sex ed that includes discussion of pleasure? Sex education that leaves out pleasure is a lie.

Girls vs. Boys — Feelings about Sex

For a boy, puberty usually brings freedom. It also leaves a young man feeling more positive about his body, more independent and more masculine. Not so for girls. Menstruation itself often leaves a girl with a feeling that her body is out of control.

According to researcher Karin Martin, who studied teens and puberty: "The girls whom I interviewed gave only negative descriptions of their menstruating bodies. Their bodies made them feel 'yuck' or 'sick,' or as if they had 'shit their pants'.... While plenty of girls look forward to having their first period, a lot become ambivalent after the first couple of periods have come and gone."

Teenage boys may struggle with wet dreams and unwanted erections, but not many would equate these with shitting in their pants. On the contrary, a boy's growing body often makes him feel more grown-up and effective in the world, while a girl's growing body brings parental warnings about the evil intentions of men and restrictions on everything from burping out loud to learning to sit like a lady.

For a girl, her growing body represents loss as much as it represents gain. The mere fact that she suddenly has breasts causes changes in her relationship with her dad and every other man she meets. No longer will her dad be as physically affectionate, and no longer will she be as unconscious about her body. Ever hear that upbeat geezer song, *Sweet Sixteen?* It talks about a girl who was just a normal kid next door until she grows boobs and hips, and her former big-brother figure up the street suddenly has a hard-on and a hit song. Maybe the girl was happier before puberty when the universe didn't revolve around what her body looked like. Maybe she was happier when she could leave the house without having to carry tampons.

Dr. Martin tells about asking teenage girls to describe themselves:

"When I asked girls, especially working-class girls, to describe themselves or asked, 'Tell me about yourself,' they described their bodies and had a difficult time describing any other aspects of who they were. 'Can you describe an important goal you achieved?' 'I love my hair. My hair's my accomplishment…' 'What kind of things make you feel good about yourself?' 'When someone like pays me a compliment on something, you know. Like says that I look nice or have on nice clothes or something.'"

It was totally different for most of the boys. The boys felt good about themselves because of things they had done or things they felt they could do in the world. Of course, if most of these boys were more in touch with the reality of their "effectiveness" rather than their fantasies of it, they might not feel so confident. But still, when boys want to have sex, it is often with confidence and good feelings about their bodies, while girls often feel the opposite.

So how does this reflect itself in the feelings that boys and girls have about sex?

Boys thought sex would be pleasurable, and many said they looked forward to it or were curious about it. The majority of teenage girls expected sex to hurt or to be painful or scary. If this is true, why did the girls have sex?

"No matter how you look at a girl's reasons for having sex, the vast majority break down to the same simple reason: they are afraid the boy will leave, they are afraid they will lose him, or afraid he won't like them anymore."

More than half of the working-class girls and a quarter of the middle-class girls in Dr. Martin's study seemed to have an ideal or exaggerated love for the boys they were dating or wanted to date. Feelings like these will make a girl do anything to keep her man. The boys, on the other hand, did not report looking for romance or ideal love. They seemed to want a combination of friendship and sex in their relationships, although it is possible the boys kept their romantic feelings to themselves. (For a teenage boy to tell an interviewer about feelings of romantic love might be admitting to less-than-manly aspirations.)

When it comes to teenagers and sex, boys and girls often have different wants and expectations. Far more boys think that the sex will feel good, while far more girls believe it will hurt. More girls idealize their boyfriends and feel they can't live without them, or they need the boyfriend as an affirmation that they are attractive and worthwhile. For this, they are willing to have sex.

As for masturbation, many teenage girls feel it is something that boys do, and do not associate it with femininity. Nor do they seem very interested in exploring their own bodies. "Their boyfriends were allowed more access to their bodies than they allowed themselves."

Perhaps one of the most frightening findings of Dr. Martin's research is that almost all of the teenage girls felt better about shaving their legs than they did about the sex they were having with their boyfriends. It seems that being able to shave their legs provided a happy identification with their mothers or older sisters. It made the girls feel grown-up in a good way.

Few and far between are the teenage girls who feel in control of their bodies. Girls who expect sex to feel good are the exception rather than the rule.

Girls who did feel better about sex tended to have good relationships with their mothers which included lots of conversations about sex. They had good relationships with their dads, and they were also more involved in extracurricular activities like sports. They seemed to place more value on the size of their IQs than on the size of their waists. They knew their own bodies better and felt more in control of their sexuality.

Having a positive sense of your sexually is not always easy for teenage girls today. The role models we offer them are porn actresses or out of control singers who twerk across the stage. And too often, the music they listen to refers to them as bitches and hoes or as being in a clingy, bizarre relationship.

Counterpoint from a Female Reader: "Sex for me was definitely not because I was afraid of losing the guy. I don't even know if it was really about my feelings for the guy. Mostly it was my curiosity about how sex felt."

See also the prior Chapter 40: Bye Bye V-Card—Losing Your Virginity.

42

Between Vanilla & Kink

> **"** Why is it that some men just can't deal with the idea that a smart, together, professional woman like me can actually deserve their respect and still want to be thrown down on the couch and pounded like a cheap steak now and then?"   By Hanne Blank in *Clean Sheets Erotica Magazine*

In the world of sexual pleasure, "vanilla" is usually defined as masturbation, hand jobs, finger fucking, oral sex and vaginal intercourse.

And then there's kink. Kink is harder to define. So let's just call kink anything that goes on in your local BDSM dungeon.

As for defining "between vanilla and kink," it's when someone who's in the vanilla camp borrows from the kinky side to spice up his or her sex life. But definitions about sexual practices can be fickle; one person's kink can be another person's vanilla.

Rather than confusing you further, *The Guide* has turned to its readers to answer what's between vanilla and kink. What follows are your answers on our sex survey. Only about 50% of the people who have taken the survey provided an answer to our question about non-vanilla sex that they might enjoy.

So if half of you have no desire to do anything that's mentioned in this chapter, you're in good company. But if you are interested in the occasional walk on the wild side, you are in good company as well. And if you've got kinky aspirations but are afraid to tell your partner, you are in very good company!

The Question

Are there types of non-vanilla sex that you enjoy having? ("Non-vanilla sex" includes being spanked or spanking a partner, having rough sex, biting, restraining or being restrained, acting out a rape fantasy, fisting, peeing on a partner or being peed on, having her put fingers or anything else up your rear, etc.)

Your Answers

Yes or yes, yes, yes, yes or yes, no, no, no or no, no or no. *male age 18*

Love some hand spanking and rough sex. Love when he holds my wrists tight. *female age 22*

We're pretty wild. We're up for everything besides pain, peeing, or scat.
male age 27

I would really like to try out some bondage, but we haven't yet. Maybe tonight. *female age 26*

Biting is fun. Also giving orders or being fucked hard. *female age 18*

I don't do vanilla sex, haven't in years. It's one of the reasons I divorced my ex... he wasn't interested in anything but vanilla. I'm eager to try anything short of urine/fecal involvement. *female age 25*

I like rough sex occasionally (being held down and penetrated hard) and some light biting. I have done some role-playing which can be fun.
female age 28

I drool thinking about rough sex. I scratch very nicely. I love biting. I love being restraining and being spanked. I love it when he gets ready to come and gently grasps the back of my head while I blow him. I love being controlled. *female age 19*

Almost all of the above.... *male age 34*

My partner and I are in a relatively new relationship, and discussing what we might be interested in trying - I've never had anything non-vanilla before (neither has he), but we have experimented with very light restraints, biting (but more like nipping – nothing hurtful), and I am interested in forceful sex. I'm not yet sure about a full-on rape fantasy. *male age 29*

When I was having sex with my best friend, she loved it rough. I slammed her up against a door and she got so horny. She loved getting her hair pulled, and wanted me to tie her up. It was a lot of fun, but definitely needs to be with the right person and talked about beforehand. *male age 22*

Well, I like it when my partner spanks me during sex... I think I would enjoy being tied up. I would also like to add a vibrator into the mix. *female age 20*

I enjoy biting. While I've never been completely restrained, it's a huge turn-on to be held down. *female age 19*

Everything, but fisting and peeing. No poop, blood, or fire. I'm OK with everything else. Not into lots of pain but a little is rather fun sometimes. I love getting bit. Being marked means I was claimed. *female age 35*

We do anal play and both enjoy it. *female age 27*

I love getting bit. I love restraining her, spanking her and being scratched. *male age 22*

I like being restrained and blindfolded because it makes everything more intense. My boyfriend feels uncomfortable about it so there goes that... *female age 25*

I really enjoy anal play. She is happy to do it, although she would prefer to use anything other than her fingers. We are looking into toys right now. *male age 25*

Anal play and fantasize about eating cum out of her pussy or off her body. *male age 42*

I like light bondage, being tied up and blindfolded, pinned, and having the control taken away from me. Unfortunately, it hardly ever happens. *female age 35*

Being spanked, being restrained (tied down, blindfolded, etc.), rough sex, dominance play and a rape type scenario here and there. We're a rather kinky couple. *female age 19*

Rough sex, spanking or being spanked. *female age 32*

My boyfriend and I really like rough sex and sometimes he bites me. We also will sometimes have one partner give directions to the other or have one partner be "frozen" while the other does whatever the other wants to the frozen partner. *female age 21*

Being spanked, nipples bitten and rough sex. I do like it when he holds me down, but I wouldn't want it to last the entire time and I don't want to pretend that I'm feeling raped. I do really like it when I feel like he knows exactly what he wants and will take it; I guess I like it when he's very dominant, but I also like being dominant on occasion, too. *female age 23*

I love having rough sex. When my boyfriend and I are roleplaying a robbery or kidnapping, rough sex adds to the 'appeal' of the role play. It also like spanking, biting, restraining and acting out of a rape fantasy. We also have sex on every surface we can get to when we're acting out a fantasy. *female age 24*

I would enjoy being anally penetrated with toys and fingers, but my significant other isn't into that idea. *male age 38*

I like to be bitten, controlled and restrained. I love the tease. The enjoyment is the wanting to be touched somewhere and not getting it. Oh, and being marked by bites, bruises, and hickies. *female age 21*

I love everything minus rape fantasies and being peed on. I would be fine with all of that every time we had sex. *female age 21*

I like playful, gentle biting, giving and receiving hickies, back-scratching (but not necessarily to the point of bleeding), mild bondage and leather play. I have a love for piercings and tattoos and find getting them a bit of a sexual rush. *male age 31*

I enjoy being spanked while having sex with my partner, but only if we're having sex doggy style and I'm already very turned on. I enjoy rough sex some times, but not regularly or when I'm tired. I like being restrained occasionally, although my husband rarely does that to me. He has also pretended to rape me a couple times, which I enjoy, but he doesn't do it very often because of the aggression of the act. *female Age 20*

I love being "taken." I love rough sex, biting, being restrained or restraining him, and spanking. I also really like using sex toys, like dildos and vibrators. They enhance our experiences a lot. *female age 20*

I love fingers and toys up the rear. Piss play intrigues but I haven't tried it.

male age 28

Does anal and sex in public count? I enjoy anal for most sexual encounters. Sex in public took some convincing from my ex. *female age 32*

I think biting can be enjoyable and a quick smack on the ass during doggie style is nice. I like it when my husband pulls me toward his body aggressively and restrains my hands. If you saw the size of my husband's hand you would understand why I would never want to be fisted by him. Fisting seems more like a girl/girl thing with small dainty hands. *female age 30*

Having rough sex. I love that a lot. *female age 26*

I have tried the rape sex.... don't really enjoy it. It felt pretty weird. I do enjoy light spanking. I like being restrained as long as I know I can say "get off" and he will right away. No peeing or fisting though. *female age 20*

I enjoy anal play occasionally. I wish we could be more open about what we like. *male age 36*

I love being spanked, handcuffed to chairs and blindfolded. I also love schoolgirl role playing, biting, and occasionally being thrown around like a rag doll. I am a very submissive partner. *female age 19*

I love everything plus the piss. For some reason I am turned on by urine. It's not something I advertise for or roll out early in a relationship. I love light BDSM, especially getting tied up. My interest wanes as soon as the actual physical pain ramps up. *female age 28*

I love public sex, although we're usually hidden in a park. I love being spanked, rough sex, dirty talk, restraints, clitoris toys and role playing.

female age 22

Rough sex, biting, clawing, fighting a little, being restrained and hair pulling (mine and my partner's). *female age 20*

I enjoy performing anal sex on myself and being fingered while be jacked off. I like to watch women pee, I like to be peed on and pee on my partner. We enjoy public flashing and public sex and nudism. I enjoy watching others naked and having sex, and I also enjoy being watched while I have sex. *male age 25*

I guess if anal sex qualifies as "non-vanilla," that's something I enjoy, but only if I'm particularly aroused, which happens less and less often these days. *female age 27*

(Blush) I like peeing (both giving and receiving) although it's been very rare that I find a partner who is like-minded. I enjoy anal play, both giving and receiving. Frankly, if my partner enjoys it, I'm not really above doing anything. Her pleasure is the greatest aphrodisiac there is. *male age 40*

Being on the giving or receiving end of spanking, biting, scratching, wax play and bondage. There's of at least one of these every time I have sex (about once a week). *female age 29*

I love biting, but I hate being bitten. I really want to have sex with someone who won't stop every time I say "ouch." I want it rough. *female age 19*

Rough sex can be really amazing if we're both in the mood. I also enjoy women wearing plaid skirts. *male age 30*

Sometimes I like getting spanked lightly. I also prefer to be the aggressive one and not the other way around. I would rather I bite him instead of him biting me. I would rather I pin him down instead of him pinning me down. My fiance enjoys fish nets, and I swear he could almost get off just by looking at them on me or touching them. *female age 20*

I'm intrigued by hard fingering and fisting, but I have never done it. I don't think she is physically able and I don't want her to get hurt. *male age 35*

I like being spanked, and occasionally doing the spanking; having my hair pulled, pulling my partners' hair; being bitten (gently), doing the biting; I keep my nails long and it turns me on to scratch or dig my nails into my partners during sex—and most of my partners are very turned on by it. I also like group sex. *female age 25*

I enjoy strapping on a dildo and having anal sex with a man. My current boyfriend does not want to try this, but I enjoyed it immensely with a previous boyfriend. I also like the idea of restraining my partner, but I have never tried it. *female age 38*

Light bondage! Both sides, please. I love rough sex, although not to the point of pain. And anywhere that's not a bedroom is sexy, even though beds are comfortable. *male age 25*

I like being spanked, biting, being restrained and eating desserts off each other. I am open to most things. Just not peeing, pooping, screwing animals or eating flesh. Oh, or fucking dead people. That's a no-no. *female age 23*

Love being spanked and caressed and receiving love bites. I love holding my feet in the upside down straddle stretch and being pounded and adored. Being restrained by strong arms is nice. *female age 23*

My partner and I are rather kinky. We enjoy spanking, rough sex, rape fantasy, fisting, biting, restraint sex, roleplaying, and on occasion, we've even yiffed. That was a bonding experience. *female age 21*

I like to spank, and dominate my partner. I'm always switching between slow caressing and dominance. I would like to restrain her and try role playing. *male age 21*

I really enjoy being bitten and restrained. *male age 41*

I love rough sex when I'm in the mood for it. I love being restrained and restraining others! I can get a little kinky at times. I still don't think my current partner knows how to take me sometimes. *female age 23*

Whoa! Yeah, I like to spank. If I like the girl I want to be spanked. The more involved I am with a girl, the more I want from her. If she likes to bite - awesome. But if she's doing it because she saw it in a video and is trying to impress me – lame. *male age 19*

I like being spanked and spanking my partner, having rough sex, biting, restraining or being restrained, being dominated, acting out a rape fantasy, fisting, peeing on a partner or being peed on, taking dumps together and having a finger in my rear - especially hers. I love non-vanilla sex.

male age 18

Nearly every time I have sex, there's some sort of rough element, whether it's spanking, scratching or biting. I definitely enjoy being restrained or restraining my partner. But if I don't want my hands held down I'll move or try to move them. I love the idea of being dominated or overpowered. On the other hand, I hate the idea of a being a "submissive bitch", but there's something about being controlled and dominated that is erotic. Don't get me wrong, it's a give and take. I'll be restrained, but I'm going to want to give it back. *female age 21*

Yeah, I enjoy being tied up and I tie her up. I love blindfolds and anal play. We'd like to find a way to wrestle and have sex at the same time, but keeping the penis in the vagina while wrestling doesn't work very well. At least, we haven't found a way to do it. *male age 24*

With some girls it feels appropriate to be gentle. With other girls it gets rough. I guess I'm a sexual chameleon or something. *male age 25*

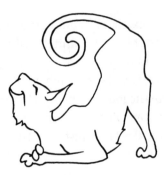

43
On Needles and Pins
Piercings, Tattoos & Sex

In the first edition of *The Guide*, piercing and tattoos didn't get a mention. In the sixth edition they rated three pages in the section on kink. Now they have a fairly substantial chapter of their own.

Tattoos, which used to be the hallmark of bikers and bandits, have become body chic and mainstream cool. Who knew that "tramp stamps" would show up on more girls' rear ends than anchors on sailors' arms or tear drops in prison-yard tattoos?

A study in the Journal of the *American Academy of Dermatology* found that 24% of people ages 18 to 50 have tattoos and 14% have body piercings. For young adults between 18 and 25, the number of body piercings increases to between 35% and 50%, and this doesn't include pierced ears.

However, according to a large study of students at Texas Tech, Baylor, Notre Dame and Purdue, less than 2% have piercings through their nipples or genitals. So while this chapter may focus on genital piercings, please don't assume that masses of people have them or that getting one is a good idea. This chapter is in response to questions about nipple and genital piercings, but is not a recommendation to get nipple or genital piercings. If nature wanted you to have extra holes through your nipples or between your legs, she would have put them there.

Warning & Disclaimer: While this chapter discusses some of the safety and health issues surrounding piercing and tattooing, it does not provide medical information and should not be viewed as a substitute for such. In two large studies, between 17% and 45% of people who had piercings experienced medical problems ranging from local tissue trauma, bleeding and bacterial infection to endocarditis and hepatitis B. Before getting a piercing, please consult the website of the Association of Piercing Professionals, and be sure to read and follow all of their safety guidelines (www.safepiercing.org). Before getting a tattoo or piercing, understand there's not much difference between an unsterile tattoo or piercing needle and the needles junkies use to shoot up with.

If you have diabetes, if you take antibiotics when you go to the dentist, or have other health-related conditions, please consult with your healthcare provider before getting a piercing or a tattoo. Also, placing metal posts through highly innervated parts of your body such as your genitals has the potential to result in permanent nerve damage, serious infection and severe bleeding.

Keep in mind that a piercing site that is healing is an open wound and needs to be treated as such. It can easily become infected, and is a source of infection to others. Follow the instructions that the piercer or tattoo artist gives you regarding your healing site, including when you can resume having sex.

Penis Piercings and Other Male-Genital Adornments

There are no scientific studies about the effectiveness of penis piercings in increasing a man's or his partner's sexual pleasure. The men often say the piercing helps to increase their own sexual pleasure as well as that of their partners. Some men particularly like the increased feeling in their urethra when they have a piercing that goes through it, although there may be a price to pay in terms of how your pee and ejaculate come out. Piercings might also make it even more fun when you masturbate.

Here are a few of the different penis piercings:

Prince Albert or PA: This is probably the most common penis piercing. It is where a ring is threaded through the urethra and out through the frenulum or part of the shaft where the foreskin attaches to the glans (see the illustration on the next page). It is said to heal sooner than most. Given that a man doesn't usually arrive for a penis piercing with an erection, it is important for the ring to have a large enough diameter so the urethra doesn't rip when the penis gets hard. The gauge should be large enough to prevent tearing, and the ball should be big enough that it doesn't drop down the urethra if it comes undone.

Reverse Prince Albert: Same as the Prince Albert, but the ring goes through the top part of the penis glans instead of the frenulum side.

Apadravya or AP: This is a vertical piercing through the head or glans of the penis. It can run through the urethra, or avoid it by sitting higher on the head of the penis. APs that go through the urethra are said to heal sooner. It seems the urine helps to clean the wound. If done correctly, the apadravya can be comfortable because it has so much flesh around it. When there are problems, they usually occur because of how it impacts the corpus cavernosum of the penis.

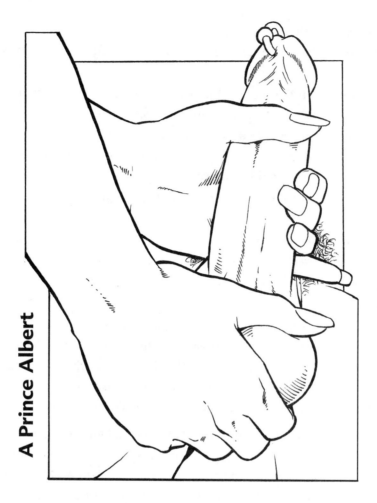

A Prince Albert

Pallang: This is a horizontal piercing where a barbell-shaped piece of jewelry runs through the head or glans of the penis. It can go through the center of the urethra, or above it.

Magic Cross: While not nearly as popular in evangelical circles as the name might imply, the magic cross consists of a pallang and apadravya through the penis head which forms a cross. If done with one stacked on top of the other, the two bars can touch or meet inside the urethra.

Dydoe: This is where small rings or barbells are placed around the edge of the head or glans of the penis. It can hurt like hell and is prone to more problems than other kinds of piercings. If the man is not circumcised, he will need a baggy foreskin for this to work.

Infibulation: Where the foreskin is pierced in a way that jewelry connects the two sides of the foreskin to prevent intercourse or the glans from being exposed.

Frenum: When the shaft of the penis is pierced along the raphe, sometimes in a series which is called a frenum ladder.

Scrotal: Any piercing that passes through the skin of the scrotum. These piercings can be difficult to heal, given that ball bags perspire, and clothes, thighs and the penis can rub and irritate the piercing site.

Scrotal ladder: A series of piercings that are aligned to make a ladder up the scrotum.

Guiche: A piercing of the perineum, or area between the balls and bum. Can run in the direction of thigh-to-thigh, or scrotum-to-bum. Perspiration and rubbing from underwear can make this kind of piercing a bear to heal.

Beading

This is where small beads are implanted under the skin on the shaft of the penis. If a sexual partner doesn't like the feeling of studded dildos or studded condoms, it is unlikely she will jump for joy when you pull out a penis with beads under the skin. It never hurts to discuss with your partner any genital alterations you might be considering well in advance.

Meatotomy, Genital Bisection, Penis Splitting and Subincision

These terms are body-mod speak for slicing a penis in two. Some of the most popular photos on the Body Modification Ezine (www.BME.com) are of this very modification. Perhaps it's due to disbelief rather than admiration ("We are so not in Kansas anymore!")—although you never know.

Penis Piercings and Your Partner's Pleasure

Aadravya (beads at 12:00 & 6:00) vs. the Pallang (beads at 3:00 & 9:00): With the AP, the beads at the ends of the little barbell are at the 12:00 and 6:00 position on the head of the penis. This means that the apadravya has the potential to stimulate a partner's G-spot area, assuming she has a G-spot area that likes being stimulated with small metal balls. As for the horizontal pallang, it's hard to see how this would add to a partner's pleasure, unless she likes extra stimulation on the walls of her vagina at 3:00 & 9:00.

Ampallang Impact on a Partner's Vagina: It can take quite the cocksman to get a penis with a steel bar through its head to slide comfortably inside a vagina. Expect a learning curve for both of you. Also expect to use a lot of lube, possibly a condom, and you'll want to make sure the bar is no longer than is absolutely necessary.

"Slowpoke" on the BME website has done a great job of reporting on the adjustments he's had to make for intercourse to work with an ampallang:

1. He uses a condom with lots of lube. The barbell does not usually tear the condom, and the condom helps his accessorized package get inside his lover's love tunnel. Experiment with whether a tight-fitting condom works better for you and your partner, or a condom with a baggy head.

2. Experiment with different kinds of jewelry to find a combination that feels best for you and your partner. A titanium barbell helps minimize the heft which can decrease cervical bruising for your partner. Also, try to decrease the length of the bar as much as possible. You don't want your penis looking like a tightrope walker carrying a balance bar.

3. Experiment with different kinds of thrusting. Slowpoke found that his girlfriend liked it best when he used shallow strokes that maximized the way the ball on the top of the barbell rubbed near her G-spot area.

4. Your partner might be nervous, which can cause the opening of her vagina to tighten. Spend as much time as she needs before you try to slide your accessorized penis into her vagina. Slowpoke tries to go in while still a bit soft. He cautions against pulling all the way out while thrusting.

5. Cleanliness afterward is important, as his AP has made him more susceptible to getting yeast infections.

Cervical Abrasion

Due to the way the cervix is innervated, the woman won't necessarily feel the surface of it being abraded by the top ball or bead of the apadravya. (There would be reasons nature made the head of the penis more like a cushion than a metal ball.) Your partner will usually know if you caused cervical abrasion by drops of blood afterward and discomfort the next day.

Showerhead Effects & Ejaculation Effects

Any piercing that intersects with the urethra can cause urine to spray out of the penis instead of come out in a stream, or in the case of a Prince Albert, the pee can cascade down the side of the jewelry. Some men are able to minimize the problem by rotating the penis 90 degrees or more when peeing. Others say a finger pushing against the lower hole can help to minimize the problem. Lord knows, you'll have plenty of opportunity to experiment and find what works best. The bottom line: If you have any kind of piercing that goes through your urethra, there is a good possibility that you'll end up needing to sit when you pee.

Your ejaculations are unlikely to paint the ceiling once a metal bar is running through your urethra. If you used to squirt, you might now ooze.

Ring Tossing

Jewelry on the end of a penis can cause a diaphragm, cervical cap, or NuvaRing to dislodge (aka "ring tossing"). Fortunately, a NuvaRing is easy to take out before intercourse and to put in after. Doing so can be a fun part of your sexplay. The NuvaRing can stay out for three hours before you need to worry. If a woman who wears a NuvaRing has a partner with a penis piercing, at the very least she or he should check after intercourse to make sure it is still in place.

Chip & Swallow

Make sure your partner's balls are firmly attached before sucking on a penis with jewelry. And while wearing a mouth guard is not called for, be mindful that teeth have been chipped by jewelry that's on a pierced penis. Back teeth are vulnerable as well as front.

Clitoris and Labia Piercings

Women often report that their genital piercings help them feel a greater sense of pride and ownership in their vulva. If done correctly and in synch with sexual preferences, piercings can also provide welcome sensations, as well as provide a fun frame of reference for vagina dialogues with a lover.

Girl piercings are dependent on each woman's particular anatomy. Decisions about what to put where need to be carefully coordinated with an experienced piercer who understands vulva landscapes. Jewelry with a larger gauge can provide more stimulation and is less likely to pinch or tear delicate tissues. You should also purchase the finest jewelry possible, as harmful bacteria can collect in any pittings that might be on the surface of the jewelry that isn't well made.

Most clitoris piercings are really clitoris-hood piercings. Here are some of the different clitoral and labia possibilities:

Vertical Clitoral Hood Piercing or VCH: This is where the piercing runs in the direction of nipples to knees and stimulates the clitoris directly. While not piercing through the clitoris, the jewelry lays on top of it and touches it directly. A woman who doesn't like her clitoris to be touched should beware, as a VCH is going to provide a lot of clitoral contact. The jewelry that goes in the piercing can be a barbell or a ring. A barbell will probably be more stimulating, as the top sits on the shaft of the clitoris while the bottom ball kisses the tip of the clitoris. **Note:** One way to see if you've got enough hood for a hood piercing is to lubricate the head of a Q-Tip and see how easily it can fit between the hood and your clitoris. The piercer will need to insert a receiving tube under the hood in order to keep the needle from skewering your clitoris. If there's not enough room or if the ring is too tight against your clitoris, consider other kinds of piercings.

Christina: This is a surface piercing that is mostly for decoration. It goes where the mons pubis joins the outer labia. It is easily rejected, does not provide sexual stimulation and can be a nightmare if you are wearing tight jeans. There needs to be some thick tissue here for this one to work, as this part of a woman's crotch often flattens out or moves with her normal range of motion. It carries with it a greater risk of infection.

Nefertiti: This piercing runs vertically under the clitoral hood from the top of the vulva where the large lips meet and exits where the clitoral hood hangs over the tip of the clitoris. Given how long the piercing is, a flexible bar made of tygon or nylon is often used, and it can take a long time to heal.

Isabella and Princess Albertina: These are dangerous piercings. Avoid them at all costs. You do not want a piercing to invade the female urethra, nor do you want to risk severing the dorsal nerve or puncturing the artery of the clitoris. Nuff said?

Horizontal Hood Piercing: A woman's clitoris and hood tend to retract when she stands, and the placement of horizontal piercings needs to take this into account. Otherwise, discomfort can occur. Placement is said to be optimal when the bead rests on the tip of the clitoris. Larger beads tend to be more stimulating. Jewelry with a thicker gauge might be preferable when a woman enjoys more pressure during intercourse. Women with a narrow pubic area or large labia or thighs that rub might not do as well with a horizontal hood piercing.

Triangle Piercing: This is where a ring is passed under the nerve bundle of the clitoris at the base of the hood. It requires an extremely experienced piercer who can locate the nerve bundle and negotiate the jewelry behind it. It can look like a sexy door knocker, assuming your clit is hung well enough to handle it. This is the only piercing that stimulates the clitoral tip from behind, and it can seriously ratchet up the sensations during intercourse. Not that many women have a clitoris that sits out far enough for a ring to be safely passed under it. A narrow crotch or big outer labia can cause the ring to twist. If that's the case, a teardrop-shaped ring might work better than a circular ring. **Note:** Piercing people refer to the clitoris in the usual "what you see is what you get" way that most of us do. However, as you can see in Chapter 7: *What's Inside a Girl,* this is only referring to the clitoral tip. The rest of the clitoris wraps around the vagina and occupies much more space.

Inner Labia Piercing: The success of an inner-labia piercing will depend a good deal on the thickness of the labia. Anything less than an 1/8" wide is likely to fail. Also, the piercings need to be placed far enough from the edge of the outer labia so they don't pull against the outer labia as a woman walks, runs and bends over. As with most genital jewelry, a thicker gauge will usually feel better and is less likely to tear these tender tissues. If a labial piercing is placed closer to the vagina, a woman's partner will be more likely to feel the sensation during intercourse. If it is placed closer to her clitoris, she might feel more sensation during intercourse.

Outer Labia Piercing: Given how outer labia have sweat glands, perspiration can be a problem as these piercings try to heal. To keep these piercings from getting irritated, let your outer lips flap free. The jewelry can also rub unpleasantly against tight panties and even your other labia.

Fourchette: This is a piercing on the bum side of the vagina that goes from the bottom wall of the vagina into the perineum. We're not talking much room to work with. This can be uncomfortable for women who enjoy intercourse, as the ring can get pulled into the vagina with incoming thrusts.

Pierced Clit: Some women have a clitoris that's beefy enough for piercing (minimum of 1/4" wide and the hood can't constrict the jewelry). Piercing an actual clit seems worrisome when you consider that the part of the clitoris that would be pierced has small chambers that become engorged with blood during arousal. Putting a post through the clitoris itself seems like it's playing Russian roulette with some pretty important neural pathways.

Female Genital Jewelry and Pregnancy

Most women with genital piercings have no problem getting pregnant. The problem can be with what happens during delivery. Talk it over with your obstetrician or midwife. The time to NOT get a new piercing is if you are pregnant or trying to get pregnant. Your body will be changing a great deal, and what was a well placed piercing during your first trimester might not be so during your third.

Beware the Navel Piercing

You would think that of any piercings, the navel would be a piece of cake. But if there is one place where you truly want an experienced piercer, your belly button is it. Wrong angle, wrong jewelry, and you are staring at six to eighteen months of healing. **Hint:** While you might have been dreaming of getting cool little ring in your navel, consider a curved barbell instead. And keep in mind that not all navels are made for piercing. An outie navel most likely contains a herniated umbilicus, and there are some asymmetrical parts of innies that do as well. The problem is if your site becomes infected, the infection might go straight to your liver via one of these blood vessels. If that happens, you may be getting your next piercing in the afterlife.

Nipple Piercing

As with genital piercings, nipple jewelry can bring its owner a sense of pride as well as being a great distraction for a partner to play with. But nipple piercings also come with a serious "ouch factor," and unless they are done right, they can migrate faster than a wildebeest across the Savannah.

The jewelry that's best for nipple piercings will depend on the size of your nipples and breasts. Also, men and women alike need to let the piercer know if their nipples are soft or erect at the time of the piercing. Jewelry that is placed in an erect nipple that later goes flat can be uncomfortable. (Jewelry that's more flexible like tygon or nylon might work better with flat nipples.)

In case you haven't noticed, female nipples tend to have a bit more going for them than male nipples when it comes to being pierced. So unless a woman has flat nipples, the piercing should go through the base of the nipple where it meets the areola, but not through the areola. (You don't want to court a case of mastitis.) It's different for boys. Unless a guy lives to be Super Sized, his nipples usually aren't as robust as a woman's. The piercing will often need to go through his areola to avoid being rejected. He also doesn't have a mammary-gland situation to contend with.

Other Nipple Piercing Considerations

Males usually don't need to worry about menstrual soreness, but a woman should weigh that before getting her nipples pierced.

Women who are planning to have their nipples pierced should inquire about the kinds of fabrics they will be able to wear. How will your nipple rings look under a conservative business suit? Lacy bras will probably be out, since the ring will constantly catch in the lacy material. Ditto for the kind of shirts you will be able to wear to work.

Wearing a bra during the healing process can put pressure on the piercing site and prolong healing, and a woman who thinks she might have an infection at her nipple site should seek medical care immediately. As stated earlier, mastitis can be a bitch.

Nursing and nipple piercings is a topic you should research if you are planning on having a baby. The advice is often contradictory—perhaps because different women have had different experiences. So look up several sources and be prepared for a number of different scenarios. (What if your normally stoic nipples become terribly tender during your third trimester? Should you remove your nipple jewelry for the duration while nursing? What if the scar sites on your nipples becomes extra sensitive?)

Tongues, Lips and Labret

A tongue piercing is something you should enjoy the feeling of in your mouth. A lot of people have tongue piercings, so be sure to ask around and get their advice. You'll want to have a sense of how far forward or back you want your piercing. Street wisdom has it that if you enjoy going down on women, you'll want your tongue piercing more forward, and if you like to give blow jobs, get it farther back–but this depends on your technique. Other considerations with placement include how much you want the outside world to know it's there. Some women change their tongue jewelry to match certain outfits. And you can get small silicone caps that fit over the bead of a barbell. These are soft and are used for decoration and for giving oral sex.

Also research the angle you want the piercing to be. The straighter it is, the more the ball will rub against the top of your mouth. Be aware that the post will angle just a bit to the side in order to avoid the web on the bottom of your tongue. The piercer might initially put in a post that's longer than what you'll need. This is to help accommodate the swelling during healing.

Tongue piercings don't usually hurt a whole lot, but expect your tongue to swell up like a weather balloon soon after. Don't expect to be talking right for the first week, and remember that eating can be a challenge with a sore and swollen tongue. The healing period will normally take a week to two weeks. The piercer might want you to avoid certain foods during the healing period, including sugars. The folks at BME caution that tongue piercings are susceptible to genital warts, and a tongue piercing might increase your chances of giving and getting sexually transmitted infections. **Note:** If a woman who gets frequent vaginal infections has a partner with a tongue piercing, bacteria in her partner's piercing might be causing the infections.

A labret is a type of lip piercing, of which there are many variations. The inside of the lip can sometimes grow over the jewelry, and gum recession and chipping of tooth enamel can be problems. Be sure ask if there's a special kind of backing you can use that might help prevent these complications.

Piercings to Avoid

Surface piercings can easily reject and can leave a scar. Hand webs are piercings in the skin between the thumb and forefinger. Not a great idea. And under no circumstances should you ever attempt a uvula (throat) piercing, unless you have no gag reflex or aren't concerned about choking.

Abandoning a Piercing

Always check with an experienced piercer about protocol for pulling out a piercing and letting the skin grow back together. And if the piercing is on your face, seriously consider getting the advice of a plastic surgeon before pulling out the post for good.

Airport Security

Airport security is unlikely to discover your piercing jewelry. One of the reasons is because it's usually made of high-quality metal that isn't magnetized. As one woman remarked, airport security didn't catch her rather stout nipple rings, but they did find a penny in her pocket. Nonetheless, the government recommends that you take out your body jewelry before going through airport security. However, you should probably try to put it back in as soon as you clear security, as holes can start to close almost immediately.

Some people who are screened frequently, such as pilots with Prince Alberts, elect to replace metal jewelry with acrylic jewelry. Other options include jewelry made of glass or medical-grade plastic.

X-Rays and Medical Procedures

You will usually need to remove all metal rings and body jewelry before having an MRI and certain medical procedures. Think metal in your microwave. You can always put in a nylon post to keep the site from closing.

Tattoo, Tattoo!

Studies done at Texas Tech found that both male and female students with tattoos were "substantively and significantly more likely to be sexually active" than nontattooed college students.

Tattoos can be very sexy, so if that's what you want to do, why not put some serious thought and effort into it and get the best you possibly can? Learn about the different styles, the different inks, and healing times and sterilization. Don't just rush out and do it, especially if you have been partying and are still trailing tequila vapor. Save your money for the absolute best tattoo artist you can possibly find. Research, research, research. Spend a few hours reading every line on the tattoo FAQ from the rec.arts.bodyart newsgroup. This incredibly well-organized, helpful, gold mine of information is lovingly maintained by Stan Schwarz. Don't be put off by the wicked URL:

http://faqs.cs.uu.nl/na-dir/bodyart/tattoo-faq/part1.html

Tattoo Logic

The first thing to consider about getting a tattoo is that it is forever. It's highly unlikely it's ever going to go away. If the reason you are getting a tattoo is because your lover's nickname is Cyclops and you think it would be cute to have a cyclops tattooed on your chest with your nipple as his eye, keep in mind that Cyclops might someday get an eye for someone else, and what do you do then? Even if he doesn't, boobs sag. Maybe not today, maybe not tomorrow, but one day you will blink and gravity will have suddenly done a number on your perky breasts. Your cyclops tattoo will start looking like things do in curvy carnival fun house mirrors. (The same is true for the skin on every other part of your body, not just breasts.)

Or what if you are bonded to your lily-white bros in your white-supremacist street gang, and you get a racist tattoo across your entire back, and in two years' time you fall head over heels in love with a wonderful girl who is Jewish or black?

Hopefully, your reasons for wanting to get a tattoo are well thought out, and you are going to spend some time and money getting the best and most interesting tattoo you possibly can.

Tramp Stamps and Ass Antlers

A tramp stamp is a lower-back tattoo that rides on the pants line. It peeks out at you when the owner—usually a woman—wears low-rise jeans or a cropped T-shirt that shows her midriff, or she bends over and her pants go low and her shirt goes high. The tattoo is often V-shaped and points down in a way that signifies the anatomy below. Tramp stamps are the kind of tattoo you can hide when you're at work if you need to. Designs range from flowers, butterflies, dolphins and tribal art to unusual symbols, geometric shapes and even sentences, although this is probably not the spot for biblical quotations.

The closer to the bones a tattoo is, the more painful it can be to get. Tramp stamps are close to the tailbone, although some women have more padding there than others. Also, tramp stamps on people over forty are known as "gramp stamps."

Some women are offended by the term "tramp stamp" because they feel the expression is derogatory and suggests that women who get this kind of tattoo like sex more than most. One can only hope. When you consider other possible terms such as "fart art" or "lower lumbar tattoo," the term "tramp stamp" starts to sound endearing.

There was a brief blogging frenzy a few years ago when a conservative blogger discovered that rub-on tramp-stamp tattoos were being sold in the vending machines at Toys'R'Us, next to the Hannah Montana stickers. In retrospect, this seems like it was perfect product placement.

Removing a Tattoo

A study of people who have tattoos removed showed that while twice as many women as men wanted their tattoos removed, at least a third of these women wanted to get new tattoos on another part of their body.

Tattoo removal will cost you dearly, and is unlikely to be totally successful. It can be painful, and you may need to opt for a cover-up instead of removal. Do lots of research and ask tattoo experts as well as a dermatologist or two their opinion before deciding on a removal process. A botched removal can leave an unsightly scar. If you go for a cover-up instead of removal, find a cover-up specialist who comes highly recommended. There are some cover-up specialists who do it often and do it well. Others will only make it worse.

Reader Suggestions

Here is advice for men from female readers on using their body jewelry to sexual advantage:

Kissing: Unless you are careful, you can bang and perhaps chip your partner's teeth. So go easy and be aware that your tongue needs more tooth clearance than one that is less accessorized. Also, women don't seem to enjoy being kissed by guys who slobber. But having a post through your tongue may keep you from sucking the saliva from it as well as you did pre-op. And some women aren't crazy about having foreign objects in the back of their throat. So when you French kiss, don't stick your tongue in very far, and remember to swallow.

Nipple Play: One woman says that dragging a steel ball across her nipples can be "a bit gnarly." Assuming your partner likes to have her nipples licked or sucked, make sure that you've coated her nipples with a heavy layer of saliva. Extra saliva on her nipples may help your ball glide rather than drag. Use the tip of your tongue when playing with her breasts and nipples. This will help keep the steel ball at bay. The best solution is to talk to your lover about this, with her giving you plenty of feedback.

Oral Sex: It is possible to give wonderful oral sex, but only as long as you know where your ball is and what it's up to. Try flicking your tongue across the palm or back of your hand. This will help you learn to steer your ball better. The last thing you want to do is bang a steel object against a woman's tender nerve endings. You will need to flick your tongue more delicately than a guy who doesn't have a steel ball attached to the end of his. To paraphrase a woman who has dated a couple of different guys with pierced tongues, flicking a pierced tongue across a woman's vulva can feel really cool, but only if the man is extremely gentle and acutely aware of the impact that a pierced tongue has. She also cautions against probing inside a woman's vagina with a tongue that's pierced.

Special Thanks to Dr. Jerry Koch at Texas Tech, to the people who maintain and contribute to BME (Body Modification Ezine) at www.bmezine.com, to Anne Greenblatt, manager of the rec.arts.bodyart Piercing FAQ, to Stan Schwarz, manager of the rec. arts.bodyart Tatto FAQ, and to Dr. Myrna Armstrong & The Body Art Team.

44
Threesomes

*D*ear Paul,
　　I was originally writing for advice about having a three-some. But my husband and I have recently met up with a third person for sex, and the experience was great!
									Bonnie from Bonneville

Dear Bonnie,

Back when I was doing my psychoanalytic training, threesomes were thought to be a very bad thing.

A few years later, a female patient told me that she and her boyfriend had decided they were going to try out threesomes, an *MMF* and an *FFM*. Having been a Freudian black sheep, I didn't sound any warnings, but I did make sure that we explored the fantasies and unconscious motivations.

As far as I could tell, the *FFM* went off without a hitch. But there was a problem with the *MMF* that threw my patient's poor boyfriend into an unexpected funk. Seems my patient ended up making the exact same noises when she was having sex with the new man as when she and her boyfriend made love. Her boyfriend was horribly depressed, realizing that "his" special magic could easily be supplied by another man.

So the first advice that I have for any couple thinking about inviting a third for play, besides talking it over for a couple of weeks and doing lots of research, is how you would handle it if you discovered that the new person gave your partner as much or more pleasure than you usually do. How would you feel if your partner was lavishing more attention on the third person than on you, although for some people, watching their partner doing it with someone else is one of life's little pleasures.

Consider a threesome only if it's something both of you are interested in, as opposed to when one partner does it just to please the other. Also, it's a bad idea to try a threesome if your purpose is to help repair a relationship that is struggling. Your relationship needs to have a foundation of trust and love for threesomes to work. Plenty of you are thinking, "How could there be love and trust if the love of my life wants us to get naked with someone else?" To that I would say, love and trust are best defined by the beholders.

One of the first couples I ever interviewed about sex were in their early 70s and had been married for more than 35 years. They were church-going pillars of the community. The most important thing in their lives were their kids and grandkids. When I sat down in their tastefully-decorated living room, the woman said, "Why don't you look through the photo album of our last vacation that we took with some good friends?"

Within minutes, my grad-student mouth nearly fell off its hinges. Not a single person in the pictures had a stitch of clothes on. Their vacation had been on board a special cruise for swingers. Then they said that just last weekend six couples had been going at it in this very living room. And then the man looked lovingly at his wife and said to me from the depth of his heart, "Mama here is the best little cocksucker of any woman in the group!" His wife beamed with pride and gratitude.

The second couple I interviewed wasn't into swinging. They were soon to be married. They were madly in love and very pleased with each other sexually. They even invited me to their wedding, which was held in a fine church. They had a traditional relationship and there's no way they would have ever had a threesome. We stayed in touch for the next two years, when their marriage suddenly split up. Divorce. I never heard from either again.

A few years later, I was having a conversation with a young woman about computer software. She eventually asked me what I did. After I told her, the volume on her voice suddenly dropped. She told me she lived with two men and was having sex with both of them. One was her husband, and the other was their roommate. This had been going on for a couple of years, and she said they were all very happy together.

So I gave up long ago on trying to predict what makes a relationship work or fail, and whether having a threesome was a good idea or bad. I figured it is a good idea for some couples, and a bad idea for others. I also gave up on any notions that swinging was for liberals and monogamy was for conservatives. One of the complaints I've heard from people in the swinging lifestyle is how conservative other swingers often are politically.

How Many Wives Can Fit on the Head of a What?

Having a threesome is not an unusual fantasy. But what about those adventurous souls who actually want to try it? It's not like you can walk up to the reference desk at your local library and say, "My wife's birthday is coming up and she's always wanted to do a guy with a bigger dick than me—do you have any books on that?" or "The three of us live together and share the same bed; do you have any books that can help our parents understand?"

Threesomes can evolve in many different ways. They can be a once-in-a-lifetime event when your husband's old college roommate visited for the weekend, or it might be something you do a couple of times a month.

Adding a third person in sex isn't like adding another cherry to your banana split. Threesomes are a declaration of war on two-thousand years of marital tradition—namely, that if you want to include another person in your sexual mix, you are supposed to lie to your partner and cheat on the side. So caution is in order. A threesome revolves around the emotions of three people instead of the usual two. The potential for everything goes up—from the level of sexual excitement to the degree of hurt and anguish.

The Definitions

There are many ways that people have sex in numbers. So before visiting the land of three, let's consider the following:

Threesome—This usually means two guys and a girl, or two girls and a guy. One of the *Ms* and one of the *Fs* are frequently in a committed relationship, with the third *M* or *F* being a free agent.

Open Marriage—This is when a primary couple agrees that each other can hook up with outsiders for sex. The past few decades have seen an increase in couples who agree on the open-marriage option from the start. However, they usually don't announce this addendum at their wedding.

Swinging or *Being in the Lifestyle*—This is when an established couple gets together with a larger group to have sex. It has many variations, from when two couples enjoy getting it on in tandem, to sex in large party rooms where almost anything goes. While the swinging couples often form friendships, it is the recreational part of sex that initially draws them together. (The term *swinging*, which replaced *wife swapping*, is now being replaced by *lifestyle*.)

Polyamory—A fluid state of friendship, love and sexual intimacy. Poly-people don't just get horny and have sex with anything that moves. There is romance, friendship and intimacy, but with more people than a husband or wife. (For more info, please see the resources at the end of this chapter.)

Wife Swapping—Wife swapping is a very dated term for anything couples did sexually that involves others. It also implied that the decisions were made unilaterally by men. As the authors of *Considering Swinging* point out, "It's the women who usually run the swinging show."

Let There Be Three

Why do people have threesomes? For starters—alcohol. Plenty of threesomes occur when three friends have been drinking enough to lose their inhibitions, but not enough to lose their erections. Threesomes created on the vapors of ethanol are seldom planned and seldom repeated. Threesomes that endure usually take forethought and planning.

Threesomes are often structured like a triangle or pyramid. At the base of the pyramid or threesome triangle is a male-female couple involved in an ongoing love relationship. The third person is the extra at the top.

The possibilities for what three people can do when they are together could fill a book. Why they decide on an *MMF* or FFM could fill volume two, although there's no reason why a threesome can't include three males or three females. If you don't know what you'd like to do and need a menu of possibilities, then maybe it's not the right time to be trying a threesome. While some successful threesomes just fall out of the sky, most take a great deal of planning and thought. Here are some things to consider:

In *MMF* threesomes, the chemistry between the men can range from "I'm fine with you doing her, but touch me with your dick and you're dead!" to "Oops, it just kinda slipped into my mouth!" The following chapter on double penetration discusses how if the two guys who are having sex with a woman are seriously homophobic, things can get a little strange. At the other end of the spectrum, guy-doing-guy play can work out well if the men are willing and the woman is turned on by everybody doing everybody. It won't work so well if she's thinking, "My idea of fun is not sitting here watching my husband with a man's cock in his mouth!"

In *FFM* threesomes, the over-riding dynamic is often the desire of the women to experience more than the usual girl-hug and kiss. This kind of threesome is often about letting the women explore, with the man providing a safe, solid, masculine backstop.

There are many ways the male in an FFM can help same-sex exploration feel safer. The women might want him to be lying on his back, with one of them sitting on his penis while the other is sitting on his face. Both women are facing each other and they can kiss and caress while being connected to a man sexually. (This combination might be more comfortable when all three are on their sides.) Or maybe the women will be happier if he just watches and strokes himself, or if he joins one in doing the other.

Unless both women are totally into it, it's usually not a good idea for an *FFM* to focus around pleasing the man. *FFM* threesomes usually work better if the man takes a background role and allows the ladies' to lead. He should never try to script the threesome or try to set the tempo, unless it's a BDSM scene with a master and his two naughty slaves.

In a threesome, the women's orgasms are seldom the end of anything. They're more like the "fasten your safety belt" sign. However, the men's orgasms in a threesome can put a definite dent in the sexual build up. This may be one of the reasons why members in an *FFM* threesome often spend the night together, nestled in each other's arms, while in *MMF* threesomes the third-wheel guy usually goes home after the final wads are fired.

The Plan

Spontaneous sex is a special gift of the gods that is bestowed upon couples who have undemanding jobs with predictable hours, no children, and friends and relatives who live on other planets. For everyone else, planning and compromise are as important to a good sex life as the twinkle in your eye and bulge in his pants. Triple that for sex with three.

The next part of this chapter is about some of the planning and logistics that are involved in having a threesome. It is divided into four sections:

1. More Than a Fantasy, But Not Yet a Plan—things to consider when considering a threesome. *2. The Pre-Penetration Plan*—from how to find a third wheel to pre-penetration negotiations. *3. Let the Party Begin*—possible positions and positions on what's possible. *4. The Morning After*—don't let the dawn get you down.

More Than a Fantasy, But Not Yet a Plan

This chapter assumes that your threesome is made up of an established couple and a third wheel. That isn't how it needs to be. There are debates about whether threesomes are best when they are made up of three individuals versus a primary couple and a third wheel. There are also debates about whether the third wheel should be a friend, an acquaintance, or a stranger. There are no studies on these options, only opinions, and good luck finding any two that fully agree. These next sections are written as if the primary couple is the main audience. A separate section for "the third wheel" follows.

A number of these suggestions are from Suzy Bauer's e-book, *Step By Step Threesomes, Nina Hartley's How-To Threesome* series of videotapes, and from Violet Blue's chapter on threesomes in her book, *The Ultimate Guide To Sexual Fantasy—How to Turn Your Fantasies into Reality.*

When you are first discussing the possibility of a threesome with your partner, avoid blurting out a list of potential lovers, such as "Your friend Ally would be sensational!" or "I'm sure Jason would add a great deal!" What your partner will hear is that you can't wait to screw someone else. If your partner is receptive to the idea of a threesome, you might ask who he or she thinks would make a good third.

Anticipate that the threesome could sour your relationship. And what if one of you fell for the third wheel? Be sure to discuss these possibilities and strategies to deal with them ahead of time.

Try to imagine the sight of someone attractive and alluring having sex with your partner. Your partner is laughing, flirting, sighing, and enjoying intense pleasure with this person. How will you deal with it when it happens during your threesome? Are there ways you can signal your partner if jealousy is getting the better of you, so she or he can help reassure you?

In a threesome, an erotic connection can sometimes build between two of the participants, with the third person being left out. This is fine as long as the third person enjoys watching, but can result in a major pout if he or she feels excluded. How will you deal with this when it happens?

What if your threesome is an *MMF*, and when the third-wheel guy drops his drawers, you and your partner drop your jaws? What if nature blessed the boy with a package of penile perfection? Ditto if you are a woman, and the second female has the kind of body that a woman only gets when she's cut a deal with the devil? Are you prepared for this kind of situation?

💡Before trying a threesome, why look at some threesome porn that shows the different positions and possibilities?

💡If you are considering an *MFF* threesome, you can simulate it by going to a upper-end strip bar where you can pay one of the girls to do a lap dance for you. It might give you a sense of the buttons that are pushed. However, think three times before taking a nude dancer or prostitute home for a threesome. She might be so experienced that it gets strange. It's better to stick with someone whose sexual perspective and experience level is closer to your own.

💡If you are considering an *MMF*, both of you might see what it's like to be in a strip bar where male dancers are the ones who get naked. Since they usually don't allow other males in the audience during male stripper shows for women, you might need to visit a bar or club where there are gay dancers who get naked. Even if your guy isn't into the same-sex aspect of an *MMF*, it will give both of you a sense of what it might be like to have another naked male in your presence. Besides, it could be worth a chuckle to see other guys trying to pick up your husband.

Whether the dancers at a strip club are male or female, it is unlikely that the third wheel in your threesome will be quite so uninhibited or look like he or she spends hours each day at the gym.

Creating a Pre-Penetration Plan

💡To prepare for your first *MMF*, the woman might consider getting a dildo and butt plug for practice. She can simulate different penetration scenarios with her partner and the toys, which can help the actual threesome to be more manageable rather than overwhelming. (Most *MMF*s don't do double penetration. But just having a penis in your mouth at the same time that you've got one in your pelvis will provide a lot more man than most women are used to.)

💡Having a threesome with a friend can deepen your friendship, or it can seriously mess it up. And while it might be good to have a threesome with someone you know and trust, it's not such a good idea if he or she has a secret crush on you or your partner. Likewise, an ex boy- or girlfriend could make a good third, or a horrible third.

☀️To find a third wheel who is not a friend or an acquaintance, swingers have clothes-on get-togethers which you might check out. Other possibilities include the Internet, certain apps, and ads in magazines or papers, although print media should be a last resort. The ads need to be carefully worded and carefully placed. Also, keep your eye out for single moms. After doing threesomes for a number of years, Suzy Bauer and her husband were thinking back over the numerous women who had joined them, and it suddenly hit them that the majority were single moms.

☀️If the prospective third wheel is an unknown entity, protect your identity. Only provide a cell-phone number or an e-mail address. If they then contact you, set up a face-to-face meeting at a neutral location where you can meet with your clothes on. Discuss things like setting up personal boundaries, safe-sex precautions, and what you hope to get from your threesome. If the pre-penetration meeting doesn't increase your desire, or the chemistry doesn't feel right, consider it a message from the heavens above that you don't have the right combination. If you do want to go through with it, you might try having your threesome in a hotel room instead of your home until you get to know the person better.

☀️Before your clothes-on pre-sex meeting, decide what is and isn't off-limits. For instance, one woman might be fine with a third wheel giving her husband a blowjob, but will morph into a psychotic puddle if the third wheel and her spouse French kiss. So make a list of the things that you'd like to encourage and discourage. Discuss them during your pre-sex meeting.

☀️If a man is being invited into a threesome with an established couple, he needs to have a thumbs-up from the primary-couple's male partner, as in "Don't worry, I won't kill you if you fuck my wife." One way to do this is for the male of the primary couple to bring up the subject of a possible *MMF* threesome to third-wheel male candidates. Likewise, for an *FFM*, the alpha female needs to invite the other woman to join. There are exceptions to these rules of the threesome jungle, but respecting them will serve you well.

☀️As with any situation where a new partner is involved, you need to protect yourself against sexually transmitted infections. Do not take a stranger's word that he or she is disease-free. Be sure to use condoms, plenty of lube, and any other safe-sex precautions that the situation warrants. Also be sure to protect against unwanted pregnancy. And if you are having an *FFM*, and the

M is going to be double-dipping into the FFs' vaginas or rectums, he'll need to change condoms when going from one girl to the next, and from one orifice to the next. So have a bunch of condoms and lube handy.

Let the Party Begin

First and foremost, consider the following advice by Nina Hartley from her *Nina Hartley's Guide to Threesomes* videos:

> "Start slow, with lots of teasing and foreplay, kissing, petting, massage. It's likely two of you will be part of an existing couple where you know each other's sexuality better than the newcomer, so don't rush. Take your time bringing the newcomer into the situation. Unlike us [porn stars], you aren't making a movie. You don't have to be so goal-oriented. Let things unfold naturally instead of pushing for the kind of acrobatics you see in porn. It may take more than one get-together to make it all work, so don't be discouraged if the first threesome ends up with a double blowjob or handjob. It may take time for the three of you to get comfortable enough for actual intercourse. It is not necessary for all three partners to be equally engaged at the same times. Kicking back and watching can be exciting, too. Don't assume that dicks in every hole at all times is a measure of a successful threesome. Do the easiest things first, and see what develops. Don't forget to talk about your feelings after-ward. You'll want to learn as much as possible from each experience."

💡Be sensitive that you are inviting a perfect stranger into your love-making lair. Don't assume that he or she has a clue of what to do or how to be. This is the moment of truth when what used to be 100 percent fantasy becomes 100 percent reality, which is not always the prettiest of transitions. Be gracious, kind, and offer the level of reassurance that you would want someone to offer you. The third wheel is not a fuck-bot who is there at your convenience, unless you are paying by the hour.

💡Just being naked together, feeling relaxed, and opening up sexually is a major accomplishment. Pay attention to the chemistry of the threesome rather than to your own need to get off. Don't try to script your threesome. It may take a couple of times together before the three of you find your groove.

☀️Your primary concern in any relationship should be that your partner feels loved and valued by you. This may mean paying more attention to your partner than to the third wheel—unless you agree that one of you mostly wants to watch. This doesn't mean you should be anything less than welcoming, but the chances are good that you didn't have children with the third wheel, and you don't share a mortgage and car payments.

☀️Be sober enough to legally drive. If you are too anxious to proceed without getting stoned or plowed, consider it a sign that this isn't something you should be doing.

☀️Don't be afraid to stop half way through the lovemaking to talk about what's going well and what could be going better. With three, you need to huddle often.

☀️There could be a time during an *MMF* when the woman is on all fours and is doing oral on the guy who's in front of her while the other guy is behind her and thrusting, aka "spit roasting." The male who is thrusting into her vagina or rectum needs to check in with her about rhythm and depth, since his thrusting might be causing her to gag on the penis of the guy who's in front. Likewise, the guy in the front needs to establish with her a comfortable pelvis-to-face distance. Both males need to be aware that the woman is between a rock and a hard place. You will probably need to work out a nonverbal signaling system, given what's in her mouth and all. Likewise, during an *FFM*, if the man has his penis inside one of the women who is giving the other woman oral sex, he needs to check in with her about the best speed and depth for thrusting. Otherwise, his thrusting might be making it difficult for her to keep her lips around whatever it is they are around.

☀️Make sure your phones are turned off and the kids are safely away at their grandparents'. Use a hotel or another location if there's any chance that teenagers might show up, and don't even think about doing this when you are on-call.

The Morning After

No matter how enjoyable your threesome may have been, expect that you will wake up the next morning with worries and bad feelings. After all, you've just violated the expectations of mostly monogamous society. If some people in this day and age still feel shame after they masturbate, imagine what you might feel after having two penises in you at the same time or your first same-sex experience while your spouse was watching.

No one should leave the morning after with self-doubt. Take the time to express your thanks and gratitude to one another—to both your primary partner and to the third wheel. If you enjoyed the experience, it's important to send the third wheel flowers if she's a woman, or something manly if he's a guy. Be sure the card has both of your names on it, and maybe even a separate line from each of you if you are an established couple.

While you have each other to talk over any morning-after doubts with, the third wheel has only him- or herself. The flowers or gift will help with that process. Do not slip up on this one. Talking it over with your partner the next day and doing something nice for the third wheel are as important as all the planning that went into making the threesome click, especially if you had a good time.

When You Are the Third Wheel

There is a certain freedom in being the third wheel in a threesome. If things don't go well, you can avoid seeing the others again. They probably live together and won't have the option of avoiding each other. On the other hand, they still have each other and can comfort each other.

🔅If you are a woman, it's likely that a big part of an *FFM* threesome is for you to explore sexually with the other woman. If it ends up being all about pleasing the man, consider bailing early, unless he's the chair of your dissertation committee. Be sure to discuss it with the couple ahead of time.

🔅Always meet with the couple ahead of time to get a sense of your chemistry together. Talk about the things the three of you might like to try. Whether you are male or female, it's an important time to discuss the kinds of things you will and won't do. Come up with safe words that will either slow or stop the action if you find yourself feeling overwhelmed. Discuss everything from sexually transmitted infections to birth control. Don't assume that because they are a couple they have their act together.

🔅You will most likely be joining an established couple with lots of history together. As a third wheel, you will need to deal with the reality that you won't be coming first, or not metaphorically, anyway.

☀You will be having an experience with three separate entities as opposed to two. You will be dealing with each of the others as individuals, as well as with them as a couple. The couple may have its own dynamics that are different from those of the individuals who make it up. This is not a problem in some threesomes, but in others, the mind-fucking can outpace the body-fucking. You didn't sign on to do couples therapy. If you find yourself being placed into that role, BAIL!

☀Things might go spinningly well, or they might get very weird. If the threesome starts to get weird, don't hesitate to suddenly remember an important meeting or a sprinkler in the yard that you are sure you left on. Do not be afraid to call it a day, no matter what stage the threesome is in. Do not for a moment be intimidated because it's them against you. If you suddenly start feeling that this is the wrong time and place, don't hesitate to grab your pants or purse and make yourself history. Be sure to drive to the location separately, or have an escape route that doesn't depend on them.

☀The three of you will have a much better time if you don't feel the need to prove what a sexual all-star you are. This is a time to blend, rather than stand out, unless they have specifically asked you to have your way with one member of the couple while the other watches.

☀If you are a third-wheel guy in an *MMF*, seek the other M's approval before trying something with his partner, even if she's inviting you to do it. It's not like you need to check with his attorney, a simple moment of eye contact and confirming nod are all that's needed. Likewise, if you are a woman, you're not there to upstage the other woman. Be respectful, and the chances are good you will get pleasure back in spades.

☀Ah, the single-dude dilemma. It is going to be significantly more difficult for a single man to find a willing couple for a threesome than it is for a single woman. It's the same problem with almost every species on the planet, be it a single bull elk, sea lion or homo sapien.

☀This is probably just a bunch of psychobabble nonsense, and even if it isn't, it's no reason not to have a great time. But try to think about any less-than-conscious reasons that might be propelling you, as a single person, to have sex with an established couple. Freud might wonder if it has something to do with unconsciously wanting to outdo one of your parents. Some

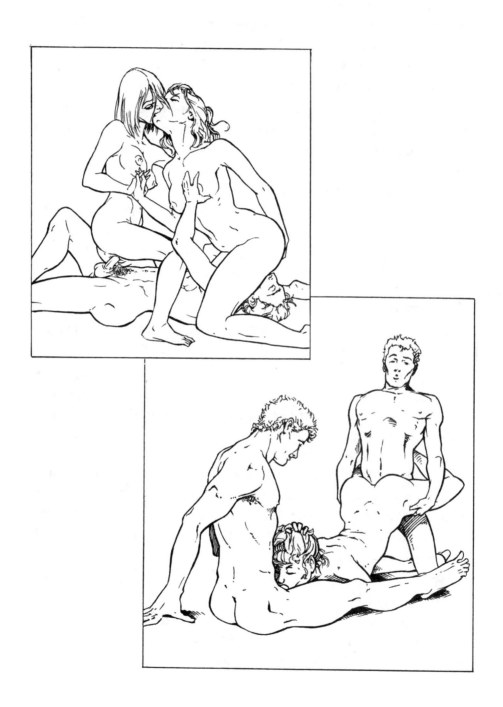

of Freud's followers might wonder if it has to do with wanting to be loved and taken care of by an idealized mommy and daddy. Again, we all do sexual things with motives that could fill anyone's psych book. That's no reason not to enjoy them. But being more aware of it can sometimes help us from getting stuck in situations that aren't always the best.

Make sure that someone knows where you are going, including the address and phone number. You don't have to tell them the truth about what you are doing, but leaving a trail and an expected return time is never a bad idea. This is just as true for males as for females. The only exception would be if you already know the people. While joining an unknown couple for sex is probably no more dangerous than joining an unknown single for sex, taking precautions is in order.

Just because they are married and say they are disease free, don't believe it. Be sure to bring your own condoms and lube.

Threesome Resources:

Diana Cage's book is definitely worth getting if you are exploring threesomes: *Threesomes, Fulfill Your Ultimate Fantasy*, Alyson Books.

Suzy Bauer's *Step By Step Threesome* e-book is very helpful. However, huge blocks of text from Lori Gammon's *Threesome* mysteriously appear in Bauer's e-book. Hmmmm. The focus of *Step By Step Threesome* is mostly on MFF threesomes. Again, while it is very helpful, Bauer's e-book, should have been less than 100 pages instead of 236. Do people really need quotes from Mark Twain and Dr. Seuss when they are trying to learn about threesomes? Many of the book's generalizations should be ignored. Still, it is money well spent if you are thinking about threesomes. Be aware that Bauer uses the Internet marketing hard-sell approach, and you might be hammered with ads if you sign up on her website at www.StepByStepThreesome.com.

While Lori Gammon has plenty of things to say in her book *Threesome*, she has a need to quote studies from *Cosmo* like it was *Scientific American*, and her enchantment with the so-called superiority of women in all matters of sex is a bit much. If women's brains and sexual nature is so darned wonderful when compared to men's, why include men at all in a threesome?

The *Nina Hartley's Guide to Threesomes—Two Girls & a Guy* and *Nina Hartley's Guide To Threesomes—Two Guys & a Girl* videos show many of the possible combinations, as long as you realize these are porn.

Violet Blue has a helpful chapter on threesomes in her book, *The Ultimate Guide to Sexual Fantasy—How to Turn Your Fantasies into Reality* from Cleis Press.

While Luna Grey's *The Kinky Girl's Guide to Dating* from Greenery Press, isn't about threesomes, it is a fine read for anyone who is thinking about stepping outside of our culture's traditional parameters for sex.

Resources for Open Marriage and Polyamory:

This is a complex subject and deserves a great deal of research if you are interested in exploring and pursuing it. The following resources are among the best that are currently available.

Tristan Taormino's *Opening Up–A Guide to Creating and Sustaining Open Relationships*, Cleis Press. This is one of the best books available on the subject of open marriage and open relationships.

Redefining Our Relationships by Wendy-O Matik from Defiant Times Press is a book on non-monogamy or love-based anarchy that a lot of people find to be very helpful. It packs a lot in its 93 pages.

The Ethical Slut by Easton and Hardy is considered by many to be the Poly Bible. The 2nd edition is available from Celestial Arts.

Loving More. The Loving More website is an online portal for all things polyamory. The information is helpful and the site is highly regarded by people who practice polyamory: www.LoveMore.com.

For an introduction to the swinging lifestyle, you can't do better than Dana and Ed Allen's *Considering Swinging* from Momentpoint Media. Don't let the low price confuse you, this book is recommended by many.

Double your knowledge about sex at

www.GuideToGettingItOn.com

45

Double Penetration[1]

Some women will tell you one penis is trouble enough. But if you've got two in your crosshairs or shorthairs, this might be the chapter for you. Double penetration is for the woman who wants a pelvis full of penises. It requires two guys and a girl. One penis is in her top bunk (vaginal intercourse) while the second is in her bottom (anal intercourse).

Is Double Penetration (DP) Safe?

There have been no studies done on DP and there is little in the medical literature about the safety or danger of it. The tissue between the vagina and rectum isn't exactly made of Kevlar and could possibly tear. It's thin enough that if you put a finger in a vagina when you are having anal sex, you can clearly feel the penis. The same is true with a finger in your bum when a penis is in your vagina. (If you enjoy this kind of exploration, remember to scrupulously clean anything that's been in the bum before it touches a vagina. This includes changing condoms. These are two different caverns with two different sets of microbes. Brown should never see pink.)

As for the advisability of whether to try DP, that's between you and your healthcare advisor. There's little in the literature about DP being dangerous, but there's little about it being safe.

Oh Nina, Oh Nina!.

After watching and rewatching porn star Nina Hartley's *Guide to Double Penetration* video, a couple of universal truths began to appear. Ms. Hartley gives the other actors verbal cues about what feels good and what doesn't. Think about that. Here's a highly-intelligent, experienced porn pro like Nina Hartley. She has hand-picked her co-stars. You would think she wouldn't have to say a word to them about what feels good. Shouldn't veteran porn stars

---

[1]It was only with the greatest of restraint that this chapter was not named after the gonzo DP porn series, *One in the Pink, One in the Stink!*

automatically know? But as you watch Ms. Hartley go at it, the opposite is true. Nina Hartley doesn't expect anyone else to know what's going on inside of her body. She makes her suggestions with humor and respect, but she lets her partners know what feels good to her and what doesn't.

So here is some very helpful and basic sex advice for any couple, whether they want to experiment with double penetration, or their sexual tastes are missionary-position that only involves the two of them:

1. When it comes to sharing sexual pleasure, only beginners think that others should automatically know how to please them. (Perhaps Nina Hartley hand-picks her porn partners not so much for their raw physical skills, but for their ability to listen.)

2. It could be that some women need couple of years of having sex before they are able to tell their partners what works. Being able to instantly convert physical sensation into words takes time, experience, and a partner who can appreciate the challenge.

Hopefully you won't think this book is encouraging you to try double penetration—even Nina Hartley avoided it until she was more than forty years old and her financial backers "encouraged" her to do a *Nina Hartley Guide to DP*. But if it is something you are interested in, the most important thing is for a woman to know her body and to be able to communicate what is going on with it. If she can't do that and do it effectively, there's no way she should be hosting a double penetration.

One That Worked and One That Didn't

Consider the experience of a woman who has tried Double Penetration with two different sets of guys. She hated it with the first set, but liked it so much with the other men that they've repeated it a couple of times.

The first pair of men were homophobic, so it became all about their need to avoid touching each other rather than being three partners in sync. They had a macho "slam-her-hard" thing going on as well. She thinks these boys had watched way too much porn.

One of the things that worked so well with the second set of men is that they weren't afraid to make physical contact with each other, so they could work as a team instead of as two men who were trying to out-straight each other. This allowed them to focus on what was and wasn't working for her.

If you are a man who would have a meltdown if another guy's arms, legs and testicles were touching your own, DP is not for you. If you would be uncomfortable feeling another guy's penis through the thin wall between a woman's vagina and rectum, forget the Robin-Batman thing.

The position this woman liked best was for the man who was doing the anal insertion to be lying on his back. She gave the example of where she faced his feet and sat on top of him while sliding his penis in. She then lay all the way back. That way, she had the full weight of her body pressing down on his, and she didn't have to worry about him getting too aggressive with his butt thrusting. The other man stood at the edge of the bed or knelt in front of them and entered her vagina that way. This is different from the DP position that's often shown in porn movies. But in porn it's all about the camera angle rather than what's comfortable. You don't see any of the preparation and planning that was done ahead of time.

Maybe the position that works best is for the three of you to be on your sides, or maybe with her on all fours, straddling the guy who's in her vagina while the buttman kneels or stands at her rear. You'll need to try different positions and rhythms.

Also, if you have been watching porn movies, keep in mind that most porn pros have rectums that can handle big rigs. Your bum might not be that practiced.

Then there's the matter of thrusting. Maybe the woman will want one man to be thrusting while the other is inside but still. Or maybe she'll want one to thrust slowly and stay shallow while the other thrusts hard and deep. She won't know what works until the show has begun.

A woman might be so overwhelmed by getting twice the bang from her bucks that her ability to speak becomes less than optimal. So before zippers get unzipped, work out a simple signaling system. If she doesn't know her body's cues for when it is getting overwhelmed, she shouldn't be trying double penetration. This is no time for passivity when all of that male energy is coming at her from both sides.

This is also no time to be drinking or getting stoned. It will keep you from being aware of important body signals and sensations. The same is true for using lubes that are desensitizing.

All three of you need to agree that your goal is your mutual fun and pleasure, and not double penetration. If the chemistry is right but DP feels like a stretch, you can always try to make it work during your second or third time together. If the time or chemistry isn't right, why force it?

A woman might start preparing a couple of weeks in advance by popping a butt plug into her rear while having vaginal sex with a real live partner. Doing it the other way around sometimes results in the dildo turning into a missile and shooting across the room once her vaginal muscles start contracting. She should also be comfortable receiving anal.

Things to assemble ahead of time include towels, condoms and lube. Be sure to banish your phones and arrange plenty of uninterrupted time. Since a double penetration involves three people, you might find the previous chapter on threesomes to be helpful. It has information about everything from hooking up with a third to the dynamics of three people having sex together.

Resources:

Nina Hartley's Guide To Double Penetration from Adam & Eve (thanks to Sinclair Intimacy Institute for sending this DVD). More porn than how-to, so it's not as helpful as it could be. However, the face-to-face interview with Nina Hartley is interesting.

Michael Ninn's *Double Penetration, Double Penetration 2*, and *Double Penetration 3*; not yet available at Target.

46
Kinky Corner

This chapter offers a brief overview of spanking, BDSM, fetishes, crossdressing, fisting, erotic asphyxiation and phone sex. None of these necessarily have much to do with each other, other than people often refer to them as kink.

One form of BDSM includes having your arms or feet tied while being kissed, tickled, caressed or otherwise made love to. For many couples, this type of activity isn't considered bondage, but merely good bedroom technique.

Men vs. Women

On the surface, it seems that men in our society are more into kink than women. Maybe that's because we define kink differently for men than for women. A woman who wears her boyfriend's boxers or briefs is at the height of fashion, but if he wears her underwear we consider him to be weird. Our society relishes her kink, but gets uncomfortable with his.

In our culture, women touch each other at will. However, if men were to touch each other with half the frequency that women do, they would be called gay. Once again, we label men for something that women do all the time.

A woman who routinely undresses in front of an open window is thought to be a neighborhood resource. Double that for a woman who plays with herself with the window shades up. But a man who does these things is called a pervert and may be locked up. There is also the biological fact that women can masturbate without being noticed. Guys can't masturbate with that kind of subtlety. The male who gets himself off in a public place is at much greater risk of being caught and labeled a sex offender than the occasional female who does the same thing.

Bondage or BDSM

The United States was originally settled by religious outcasts, malcontents, criminals and slaves. The fact that we are not all into some form of bondage is a little amazing.

BDSM often involves fantasy, role playing and an exchange of power. It can include the application of pain, humiliation or restraint. It frequently includes one person taking power and the other giving it up. BDSM can involve physical or psychological surrender, helplessness and trust. For people who are into BDSM, it's an endorphin rush that's like a runner's high. It can bring far more comfort than pain if done in the proper context.

An out-of-date perception about BDSM is that the person who takes the dominant role makes all of the decisions. This no longer works in the modern world of BDSM. Deciding on the scenarios and what's done should be shared equally between both partners and all parties. Then their fun begins.

People who are drawn to BDSM often enjoy being rendered passive. They have no choice but to enjoy what a partner is doing to them. They don't have to worry about being a "good" partner who provides pleasure in return. Performance anxiety is virtually eliminated. This can be especially appealing to people whose jobs require them to be in charge and in control.

Restraint Note Scarves and ties form tight knots that are hard to undo; wrists and ankles can be permanently damaged. Professionally made cuffs may seem expensive to couples who simply like to tickle and spank, but they are much safer than the restraints that people improvise at home.

$$\longrightarrow$$

Look at how her wrists are bound. This can cause wrist damage and is NOT the way you want to do it. Splurge and get some fake-sheepskin cuffs or look online for the latest in restraints and bedroom bondage accessories.

Painful Pleasures—Spanking

In our extensive sex survey, we asked people about things they enjoy doing or having done to them that are not vanilla. Spanking was mentioned often. (Chapter 42: *Between Vanilla and Kink.*)

There's a lot more to spanking a lover erotically than throwing him or her over your knee and having at it. An excellent book on the subject is *The Compleat Spanker* by Lady Green (Janet Hardy), Greenery Press. And the women at PleasureMechanics.com have done a video on erotic spanking that you might check out if spanking is a turn-on for you or your partner.

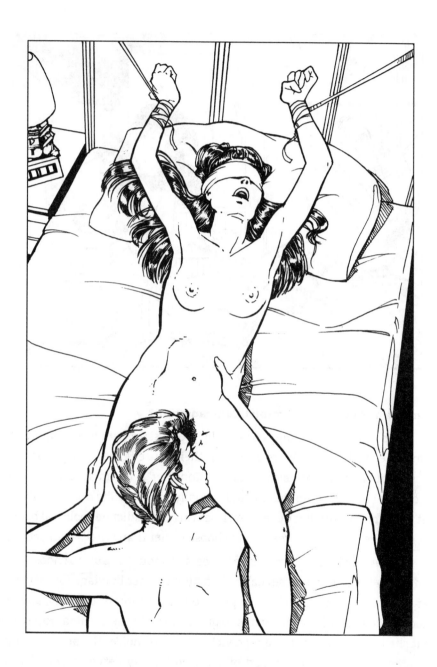

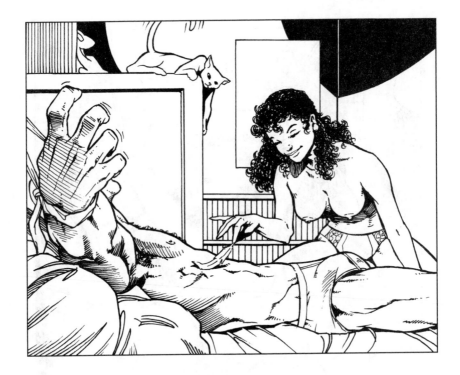

Bondage by Choice—A Feminist Contradiction?

People who are feminists or socially progressive (whatever that means) sometimes feel that they are deserting their cause if they enjoy being submissive or have masochistic fantasies. Consider a feminist lawyer whose favorite fantasy is being tied up and sexually violated. She occasionally acts out this fantasy with her male lover. Does this contradict her political beliefs? No, since the issue is the freedom to choose rather than what's being chosen.

The lady lawyer believes that each person should be able to choose what to do with his or her own sexuality. In acting out her bondage fantasy with her lover, this woman chooses to give up her position of equality, and she chooses the man whom she wants to give it up to. In the criminal-rape cases that she handles in court, the rape victim had no choice. The act was forced upon her, rather than being part of a shared fantasy between two consenting adults.

Heavy Bondage — A Little Like Life?

"Maddie's path to discovery was a gradual process. She'd been kinky for pretty much as long as she could remember. She remembered the teacher finding her tied up to the swing set at the end of recess. She didn't just play 'doctor' as a young child, she played mad scientist. Her vision was pretty dark, involving elaborate punishment scenes in a neighbor's basement. Not surprisingly, she was usually the one who got punished. She has a half-formed memory of having a bucket of coal poured over her crotch while she moaned and writhed in semi-protest. She can still remember the absolute feeling of erotic surrender, the feeling of loss of control. That memory has a sexual charge for her even today. These dirty little games continued until the inevitable discovery by a parent, at which point they abruptly ceased. She doesn't remember seeing those kids much after that... During the teenage years, her sexual awakening seemed to always involve some sort of power exchange dynamic. She chose older boys, the dangerous ones, who would use her. And she submitted to this, sometimes with great drama, but some weird little part of her loved it... The pain of losing her virginity was one of the hottest moments of her life. Unhealthy? Hell, yeah. Self-destructive? Absolutely." —From *The Kinky Girl's Guide to Dating* by Luna Grey, Greenery Press.

The more robust forms of BDSM can be a world of whips, chains, ropes, melting candle wax and devices that might put a chill up the spine of just about anyone. In BDSM, the following acronyms apply: B&D = bondage and discipline; S&M = sado masochism; D&S = dominance and submission; BDSM is a blanket term for pretty much all of it.

In BDSM, having an orgasm isn't nearly as important as the scene itself, with its undercurrent of domination, submission and sometimes humiliation. People into bondage process pain differently than people who aren't. Bondage lovers find doses of sexual pain to be invigorating and intimate, assuming it's done in a context they find arousing.

If you'd like to get into BDSM, please consider the following advice: don't pick up a stranger who enjoys beating the crap out of people and confuse that with bondage. In BDSM, there are established rules and etiquette that keep the participants from getting seriously hurt. Mind you, the definition of seriously hurt is a personal matter. If bondage is what turns you on, learn the rules and make sure that your partner know and respect them.

In almost every large city in the United States, you will be able to find an established bondage club. These clubs often have extensive calendars of events, including talks, demonstrations and social gatherings. You will often be safer in joining one of these established clubs than by experimenting on your own. You might also be amazed at how many educated, kind and helpful people you will meet at the established clubs.

Even if you aren't into bondage, don't get roped into thinking that mild-mannered people prefer being bottoms (slave or submissive role) and that aggressive types prefer being tops (master/dominator/dominatrix). There are plenty of business executives, lawyers, doctors, politicians and policemen who prefer being on the bottom. In fact, it's a problem in the bondage community that a good top is hard to find. It's also true that a number of people into BDSM enjoy alternating roles between top and bottom.

BDSM — Safety Considerations

No matter if you only use bondage once a year or are a dungeon regular, the highly regarded S&M book by author Jay Wiseman titled *SM-101*, Greenery Press, makes the following suggestions:

💡Anytime a body part that is tied up feels numb or goes to sleep, untie it immediately. And never tie anything around a partner's neck.

💡In anticipation of catastrophes like fires, earthquakes or an unexpected visit from your mom and dad, be sure to have a flashlight and a pair of heavy scissors handy. *SM-101* recommends paramedic scissors, which can be found at medical-supply stores. They cut through almost anything except handcuffs. Keep the scissors and flashlights in a place you can readily find in the dark. Ditto for the handcuff key if that's what you are using. Better yet, tie the key to the handcuffs with a string.

💡Never leave the person for long, and check them often. If any injuries were to occur, you would be legally and morally responsible.

💡Always establish a safe word or gesture which means to stop. Some people use "red" for stop and "yellow" for easing up a little. No one who is seriously into dominance and submission uses "stop," "don't," or "no more" for safe words, since any good bottom says them often seldom means it.

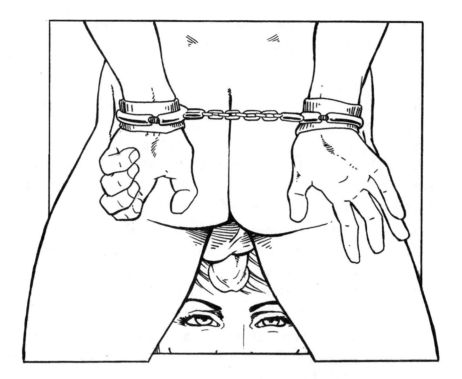

Breath Play or Erotic Asphyxiation—Do Not Do This

A reader reported that he puts his hands around his partner's neck and squeezes tightly when they are having sex—at her request. She says it makes the experience feel more intense. He is now concerned because she wants him to use a leather belt from one of her coats to get a better grip.

This kind of sex is called *breath play* or *erotic asphyxiation*. It's also referred to as *scarfing* or *terminal sex*. The side effects can include death and brain damage. There are two groups of people who enjoy their sex this way. One group is made up of boys and young men who put plastic bags over their heads or tight ropes around their necks while they masturbate. They are known as *baggers* or *gaspers*.

Baggers are often white, straight and middle-class. They fit in well socially. They keep their sexual secrets well hidden. Up to a quarter of them wear women's underwear while they masturbate on death's doorstep.

It is thought that several boy baggers die each year in this country. Their deaths are often reported as suicides. But people who are trying to kill themselves don't hang from door knobs and they don't design safety releases into their death devices. Boy baggers fully intend to free themselves after squeezing out their blurry-eyed orgasms.

Horrified parents will often spruce up the death scene before the ambulance arrives. Instead of being reported as masturbation gone awry, the coroner thinks it's a suicide and none of Nathan's friends can understand why a kid who seemed so well-adjusted would want to off himself.

The other group of people who are into breath play are normal-appearing couples. They have no fear of the boy-bagger's fate. They assume that the person who is applying the pressure is like a designated driver who can put the brakes on before it's too late. "Not so!" says Jay Wiseman, author of *S/M 101*:

> "As a person with years of medical education and experience, I know of no way whatsoever that either suffocation or strangulation can be done in a way that does not put the recipient at risk of cardiac arrest.... If the recipient does arrest, the probability of resuscitating them, even with optimal CPR, is distinctly small."

You could be hooked up to state-of-the-art heart monitors and have a partner who is a board-certified cardiologist, breath play would still be Russian roulette in your birthday suit.

Another thing that has healthcare providers concerned is the risk of brain damage. Those like Charles Moser, a physician who is highly respected in the world of kink, worry about the long-term consequences of breath play.

Fetishes: An Overview

There once was a popular song where a man was imploring his lover to take off all her clothes, except for her hat. If a man can't enjoy sex unless his partner has a hat on, we might say he has a hat fetish:

> FETISH—1. Reliance on a prop, body part, scene or scenario in order to get off sexually. 2. The prop can either be fantasized or exist in actuality. 3. One philosopher has described "fetish" as being similar to when a hungry person sits down at a dinner table and feels full from fondling the napkin.

If both people in a relationship enjoy the same fetish, then its presence is a welcome event. But if only one partner is into the fetish, the other person might feel that she or he is not nearly as important as the fetish itself. For instance, the woman in the song might start to feel like a human hat rack.

Fetishes come in many different forms; some include objects, others include actions that need to be repeated over and over.

Normal Sexual Turn-on vs. a Fetish

Let's say your boyfriend loves to feel your legs when you have pantyhose on. He's a really sweet guy and you enjoy the extra attention, but your mother says it's a fetish.

As long as it feels like he is more turned-on by you than the pantyhose, they are probably just a fun prop for him. He won't go into sexual mourning if you swear off pantyhose for no-show socks. But what if he can't become aroused unless you are wearing pantyhose, or he gets off more and more by your pantyhose and you feel like a mannequin? Rather than being an erotic accessory that helps to spice things up, the pantyhose would be way too important. That's when you're talking a fetish.

Some people have fetishes for objects or materials like leather, rubber, latex, underwear, shoes, socks, boots, smelly feet, hair, breasts and even diapers. There are websites with adults wearing diapers, and not because they need to. Other people with fetishes have scenarios or fantasies that get them off, e.g., the guy who likes his partner to urinate or defecate on him. Or the fetish might be as hidden and subtle as the kind of haircut his partner has. He suddenly goes bonkers if she changes it. (Ever notice how some guys date or marry only women who are the spitting image of each other? Is it the woman he loves, or a certain look that she has?)

People with fetishes sometimes get comfort from the fetish that they can't get from human beings. The fetish becomes the missing piece that completes their sexual circuit. The fetish evolves into a sexual partner who isn't demanding or humiliating. (It's far easier to control a pair of pantyhose than to control the woman who is wearing them!) The fetish provides an exciting sense of relief.

One problem with having a serious fetish is the loneliness that can sometimes be a part of it. No matter how many times you fondle them, a pair of rubber panties or a woman's feet can go only so far in providing the closeness or friendship that many of us value in a sexual partner. In fact, some people refer to the fetish as a compromise between the fear of human closeness and the need for it.

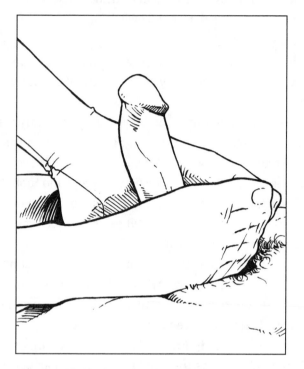

Is this activity:

a. fun
b. a fetish
c. both
d. who cares?

This wouldn't be considered a fetish if it is something you enjoy doing but can also do without. Psychologists would call it a fetish if the man couldn't become aroused without seeing or touching the woman's feet, or if her pantyhose were so important to him that he needed them rather than her to become sexually excited. How do psychologists know? Because they are as kinky as anyone else.

Crossdressing

Some women occasionally dress up like men, to the point of wearing a fake penis. This is a form of accessorizing known as "packing." One woman reports that if she's been packing for an extended amount of time she even stops having her period—without taking a single male hormone. Once she is through packing and the fingernail polish goes back on, her periods become regular again. However, crossdressers are mostly men. Crossdressing is the way that men who have an inner woman or an inner vagina allow her out to play.

Crossdressing could have been included in the chapter on gender-bending or transsexuals, but transsexuals often don't consider crossdressers to be part of their tribe. It could have been placed in the same-sex chapter, but most men who crossdress identify as straight. As for whether crossdressing is a matter of gender identification, a form of kink, or something else, it varies depending on the man. But for a lot of crossdressors, gender identification is more the issue than fetish or kink.

The only reason crosdressing was placed in this chapter is because none of the other chapters of this book felt it belonged, which is the dilemma that most crossdressers face. Their dilemma is described by Amy Bloom in her book, *Normal–Transsexual CEOs, Crossdressing Cops, and Hermaphrodites with Attitude:*

> "Heterosexual crossdressers bother almost everyone. Gay people regard them with disdain or affectionate incomprehension, something warmer than tolerance, but not much. Transsexuals regard them as men 'settling' for crossdressing because they don't have the courage to act on their transsexual longing, or else as closeted gay men so homophobic that they prefer wearing a dress to facing their desire for another man. Other straight men tend to find them funny or sad, and some find them enraging....."

There are hundreds of thousands of transvestites or male crossdressers in the United States alone. Many are quite masculine when they aren't wearing a bra and panties. Many appear quite masculine when they are wearing a bra and panties. They are often married. A lot of crossdressers value their sports-page loving side as much as their inner girlfriend, but struggle with finding ways to enjoy both at the same time.

Contrary to what you might imagine, male crossdressers aren't necessarily drawn to professions that welcome a guy's feminine side. The average crossdresser is as likely to be a baseball player, fireman, policeman, auto mechanic or business executive as a hairdresser or florist.

A lot of crossdressers have a perpetual crush on their female persona. She often calls to them, imploring them to give her life by dressing as a woman. The bra becomes her breasts, the panties her female genitals that he so loves. So there he stands, in front of the mirror, admiring his "breasts and vagina." This will allow some crossdressers to have the erection they need in order to masturbate, others don't want to be reminded of the male genitals behind their frilly lingerie.

Therapy will not change a crossdresser's need to crossdress. However, if a man is compulsive about crossdressing, therapy can help him with that aspect. Many crossdressers hope that marriage will cure them of their desire to dress like a woman. But the envy and allure of their wife's underwear drawer will soon rear its head and so much for good intentions.

Men who are reading this book while wearing their favorite DKNY dress might be concerned about being found out. This is a fear shared by many crossdressers who are not out of the closet.

If you are a wife or girlfriend who suddenly discovers that your man has a secret cache of frilly garb, try to give yourself a three-month chilling-off period before doing anything drastic. Talk to your partner about what he does and why. He must love you a great deal if he's worked so hard to hide something that's so darned big. If you can, check out the site of the Society for the Second Self or Tri-Ess at www.tri-ess.org. This national organization is for crossdressers, their wives and their families. Search out anything written by Francis Fairfax, particularly the *Wives' Bill of Rights*. Some women also find the books by Helen Boyd to be helpful.

Given how this is not the sort of thing you can necessarily call your mom or sister about, see if there is a support group in your area for wives of crossdressers. The folks at Tri-Ess can help you find them. Talk to these wives about what they will and won't put up with. There are plenty of things you don't need to agree to, like meeting your man for lunch when he's dressed like Britney Spears. And if for some reason he thinks he can dress up in front of the kids or gets so deep into the crossdressing scene that he stops being a good husband or dad, crossdressers' wives will offer all the support you need to confront him. In other words, you don't have to condone what he's doing but you don't need to divorce him either.

For a lot of women, it would be easier to accept their husband if he said he were gay. But to see him dressed up like Little Bo Peep and hear him say he's straight.... Wives tend to fear they will lose the manly part of their crossdressing man. Hopefully, he'll be the same man he was in bed before you found out about the heels and gown. Part of a wife's fear may have to do with humiliation that someone else will find out.

After chilling off, a wife or girlfriend might see that there are worse things a man could do than wear women's clothes, fashion crime that it might be. She might also realize that he has the same good characteristics that he had before she found out about his hidden side.

There's no shortage of publications on crossdressing. Some people value the books by Peggy Rudd, a therapist and the wife of a crossdresser. Others aren't so comfortable with her crossdresser-as-visionary point of view. Your public library may have them, but perhaps you'll want to try Amazon.

HIGHLY RECOMMENDED: The book "Alice in Genderland" should be at the top of any crossdresser's reading list. It's by Alice Novic, a crossdressing psychiatrist. And need a gift for a man who cross-dresses? www.wayout-publishing.com.

Phone Sex—When 911 Isn't Enough to Put Out Your Fire

Ever wonder what goes on in phone sex, when a man pays several dollars a minute to get a good talking to? A young woman who worked as a phone-sex operator after graduating from an expensive private college was kind enough to offer the following description:

"The fantasies ranged from men who wanted me to physically beat myself on the phone with a hairbrush, to those who wanted me to force them to have oral sex with other men and those who just wanted to hear me have an orgasm. What struck me is that men have more gay fantasies than I would have expected. There seems to be a correlation between men who have powerful jobs and their sexual fantasies. One client, who I later found out was a senior partner in a financial firm always wanted me to 'force' him to do things, mostly to other men and sometimes to me. Others wanted to escape from their life, shed their responsibility and their maleness—they explored their imagination with me and pretended I was their dominatrix, their she-male, their whore. I gave them permission and encouraged them to be who they wanted to be and that's what they needed.

"I always wondered about clients. I was madly curious. I wanted to know who they were, how much money they made, if they were married, if they were straight and if they were the kinds of guys I knew. And often, I'd 'interview' them and I'll admit that I looked up what I could find on Google. I couldn't help myself. I wanted to know why they were calling me, how it played into their real sex life and what I was to them. In some instances, I was the woman on the phone who was their mistress, but in the most controlled way and they would call on a regular basis. Some got attached to me and I was fired and then rehired and in my absence, I was missed (as I learned later)."

Vaginal Fisting (Handballing)

Vaginal fisting is finger fucking times five, and then some. This Guide first became aware of the concept when reviewing lesbian tapes produced by and for women. Some women enjoy having a partner's fist inside their vagina.

But that kind of fisting is being done by women to women. Most women have significantly smaller fists than men. A fist the size of a man's could take a potentially pleasurable experience and turn it into something akin to childbirth. On the other hand, a leading sex therapist believes a number of straight couples are getting a fist up.

If vaginal fisting is something you want to try, please plan far enough ahead to read a book or two that covers the subject. Greenery Press publishes *A Hand in the Bush: The Fine Art of Vaginal Fisting* by Deborah Addington. This subject is also discussed in the *Good Vibrations Guide to Sex* by Anne Semans and Cathy Winks, Cleis Press and in the *On Our Backs Guide to Lesbian Sex*, edited by Diana Cage, Alyson Press.

Please check with a health-care professional before attempting any kind of fisting, and in no instance should you proceed if you experience anything but the slightest amount of pain. Perhaps you can find the name of a physician or nurse practitioner who is familiar with fisting through a gay and lesbian health center, since your local HMO might not be particularly well versed in the practice. You should never attempt fisting if either of you has been drinking or doing drugs, and you certainly shouldn't try it before reading the advice of women who do it.

Anal Fisting

Some couples, straight as well as gay, are into anal fisting. You shouldn't even think about trying this unless you really, really, really know what you are doing. Technically, this act is possible without causing physical damage, since surgeons occasionally stick an entire hand up a person's rectum. On the other hand, receiving a fist up the bum requires the kind of relaxation that is beyond the capacity of the average anus.

Couples into anal fisting often recommend a book on the subject by Bert Herrman, *Trust—The Hand Book*, Alamo Square Press. Tristan Taormino's *The Ultimate Guide to Anal Sex for Women, 2nd edition*, Cleis Press is an excellent resource. There may also be organized groups of fisters in the nearest large city who give talks and demonstrations. Please check with a health-care professional before attempting any kind of fisting, and in no instance should you proceed if you are not completely sober or experience anything but the slightest amount of pain.

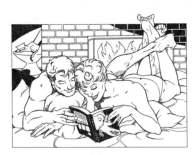

Dear Paul,

Do you have any advice about going to a dominatrix?

Policeman by Day, Schoolboy by Night

Dear Officer,

To help answer your question, I called my friend Lorrett, who runs a house devoted to BDSM and fantasy play. She offers the following advice:

1. BDSM is about creating a fantasy scene, and then acting it out. In creating the scene, you need to talk to the person you are hiring about things like boundaries, safe words, and how you want the scene to play out. You should feel comfortable with the person, and feel that they are comfortable with you in negotiating the scene. If they come off as being abrupt or domineering when setting up the scene, then what follows isn't going to be play. Instead, you are going to be acting out their agenda, and what follows will be anything but consensual.

2. Trust your instincts. It's fine to be nervous or anxious, but if you feel frightened or uncomfortable, go elsewhere.

In domination and fantasy games, the dominatrix doesn't actually get you off. You are free to get yourself off in her presence, but she won't actually give you an orgasm the way a prostitute will. That's why it's not illegal for you to hire a dominatrix.

RESOURCES

The New Bottoming Book—2nd edition by Janet Hardy and Dossie Easton, Greenery Press, 2015.

The Ultimate Guide to Kink: BDSM, Role Play and the Erotic Edge by Tristan Taormino, Cleis Press, 2012.

The New Topping Book by Janet Hardy and Dossie Easton, Greenery Press, 2011.

SM 101: A Realistic Introduction—2nd edition by Jay Wiseman, Greenery Press.

The Compleat Spanker by Lady Green, Greenery Press.

Special Thanks to Lorrett at Fantasy Makers in Berkeley and Janet at Greenery Press—two of the nicest people around.

47

Vulva Care
Keeping Your Kitty Happy

Male readers have indicated that some of the women they've gone down on didn't seem to be paying attention to general crotch care. When it comes to shaving, waxing, or trimming—the women were on top of it. It's the hygiene basics they were wondering about. When we asked our gynecology consultant about this, she went on a rant:

> "It fascinates me how many women come to the gynecologist with a smelly puss. For heaven's sake, give the kitty a little wipe-down before you spread your legs."

Healthcare providers have been telling us for years about young women who won't use the Nuva-Ring because they say it's gross to stick their fingers in their own vagina. Ditto for OB tampons. And a lot of young women today feel it's nasty for women to masturbate. They will let some guy whose first name they hardly know stick his fingers and penis between their legs, but when it comes to taking pride and ownership of their own genitals, it seems to stop at their bikini line.

If women are uptight about their genitals, they might have a tendency to over clean them in a scrubbing-douching frenzy, or they might ignore that part of their body altogether and spend the time doing their nails. So here's a chapter on kitty care.

Crotch Care Basics—From Wiping to Giving Your Puss a Bath[1]

Cleanliness is next to godliness—but only in moderation

Do not overclean. It only needs soap once a day at the most, and that should be a bland bar of soap like Basis, Pears, Dove Sensitive Skin or better yet, the ultra-mild SebaMed Cleansing Bar which has a low pH and nothing in it that will irritate a vulva. (Just because Ivory says it's pure doesn't mean it's not harsh. Besides, why would you want something *pure* between your

---

[1] For women who have vulvar pain, infections, concerns about their vaginal health or any medical condition: please seek out the advice of a gynecologist.

legs? The women at Goofy Foot Press want anything that's going between their legs to be bad to the bone!)

Wiping. "Always wipe front to back for pee as well as poop" (our gynecology consultant's words). If we guys had vaginas and had to wipe from front to back, our vaginas would be infected running sores. That's why we've got penises: there's no way you could ever train us to wipe from front to rear.

Do not use liquid body gels or cheap washes. Our gynecology experts go nuclear at the thought of using body gels and cheap washes, including the bubble bath soaps:

> "I always tell women not to use bubble baths/bath beads. This is basically douching with those chemicals. These products are mainstream and are often in gift baskets—it's like, 'Here my friend, have this lovely yeast infection and happy birthday to you!'"

Lower pH Can Be a Good Thing: Let's say your kitty is a persnickety puss who doesn't like soap every day. Unless your gynecologist says something to the contrary, you should still clean her with water. One reason for her not doing well with soap might be the kind you are using. Your vulva and vagina are a bit acidic, with a pH of around 5.2. However, most bar soaps are alkaline, with a pH of 10 or higher. Consider trying a high-quality, low-pH soap like SebaMed between your legs. Some women who have struggled with vaginal infections swear by the lower-pH soaps like SebaMed. These soaps don't have a lot of alkali in them like cheaper soaps, and they are a bit acidic just like your vagina. They also make a SebaMed Feminine Intimate Wash that's just for the vulva. It has an even lower pH and is especially gentle and mild. You can find it at www.sebamedusa.com. (Some women readers have reported feeling "way fresher for much longer" after switching to a low-pH soap.)

Your Vulva Is Not a Pot: Never scrub between your legs. Using your fingers instead of a wash cloth is best. It's fine if you have a hand held shower head and know how to hit your sweet spot with it.

Smegma? Isn't that Just a Penis Thing? To help prevent clitoral-hood adhesions or smegma—yes, smegma—from forming where a man likes to lick, pull back your clitoral hood and separate your inner and outer lips while rinsing with water. Again, use your fingers, not a washcloth.

Avoid Shampoo Run-Off from Your Head: Shampoos tend to be harsh and perfumy. Make sure your shampoo and conditioner don't stream between your legs and through the lips of your vulva when you are rinsing your hair. This can be avoided by bending over when you are rinsing out the shampoo and conditioner.

Pat, Don't Rub! There's a perfectly good time to rub between your legs, but not when drying yourself after a shower or bath. While some experts advise drying your vulva with a hair dryer on cool, others warn against it. They all agree that gentle patting is good.

Wipes, Lotions, Feminine Sprays, Douches & Perfume: Do not use baby wipes after peeing or pooping, and never use powders, lotions or perfume. They tend to be irritating. If nature intended your crotch to be perfumed, she would have planted roses between your legs. Also, avoid feminine-hygiene sprays, douches and talcum powder. (Talcum powder has a possible link to ovarian cancer). According to our gynecology experts,

> "The puss is a natural cleansing area and douching makes it smell. Douching is acceptable only if it's right after your period and hot sex is coming that night."

Normal Smells

Your vulva is an orifice. It has sweat glands and it's covered with hair. As one of our gynecology experts says, "This can lead to all sorts of interesting smells, most of them completely normal." (Of course, our guy crotches never smell anything but wonderful!) It's normal for a vulva and vagina to smell musky, and it's normal for the odor to change throughout your cycle.

Also be aware that female vulvas and male scrotums have apocrine glands embedded in them. These glands respond to stress situations and are the olfactory version of land mines. There's not a thing you can do about it, except maybe move to a tropical island paradise where you can lounge by the beach all day and forget stress altogether.

So there's musky, and there's bad. If your vagina smells bad as opposed to musky, it probably needs a visit to the crotch doc. You might also be more prone to an infection early in a relationship, which is pretty common. This might happen "as his stuff gets used to your stuff." If your vagina smells really fishy after your partner ejaculates inside of you, consider the possibility that you have a vaginal infection. (Semen is alkaline, which creates an odor-releasing chemical reaction with the secretions in your vagina. The odor can be way worse when you have a vaginal infection.) Or your partner might have chronic prostatitis, which a urologist can check for. But most likely, neither of you have issues that require medical attention.

Thongs & Pads vs. Going Commando

While our gyno expert agrees that thongs can look hot, thongs abrade and tear up the vulva. She sees lots of redness, rubbing and irritation due to thongs. She recommends going commando (wearing no undies) instead. She also says that wearing pads or pantiliners to "feel fresh" simply trap moisture and are irritating to the vulva. If leakage is a problem, try using a cotton handkerchief to line your panties with, or a 100% cotton pad.

It's also possible the part of your thong or G-string that sits on top of your anus can act like a zip line for bacteria from your butt to hop into your vagina.

Our other gynecology expert gets her panties in a wad over women sleeping in their panties. She says that vulvas need to breathe, and there's no way that's going to happen if you sleep while wearing your underwear, even the kind with a cotton crotch.

Both of our gyno experts are proponents of going commando as often as possible. That's because your vulva needs air to breathe. As for the occasional Britney Spears moment, if anyone notices, tell them you are doing your bit to help beautify the homeland.

Peeing, Shaving, and Popping Hair Bumps

Shaving can be really irritating, and so can hair-removal products. If you want your hair short, try a bikini trimmer. It won't be porn-star bare, but who needs that?.

Our gynecology expert thinks that a lot of women would have happier crotches if they had less pubic hair, because it would allow more air to circulate around their lips. She just doesn't want you to abrade your skin in the process. So consider trimming your pubic hair short instead of shaving it away with a razor.

If you shave and get little bumps around the hair follicles, NO POPPING. There is a high risk for *staph* infections from doing this. Try warm, moist compresses and antibacterial ointment, and see your healthcare provider if you are concerned or irritation continues.

The opening of the urethra (peehole) is above the opening for the vagina. So if you dribble urine while sitting on a toilet, the urine will drip into the opening of your vagina.

If you have labial adhesions or you dribble after peeing, pull your pants all the way down and urinate with your knees apart. This will help prevent urine from pooling into your vagina. (Throughout most of human existence, women would squat to pee with their knees far apart. Sitting on a toilet with knees together is a very recent development, and the vulva has not had time to evolve around it.) If the problems persist, it might help for you to pull the labia apart with your fingers when you pee, so the urine can exit freely. Ask your healthcare provider.

Chronic Crotch Irritation?

Almost all toilet paper has formaldehyde and chlorine residues, especially the nicer feeling premium toilet papers. If you are having chronic crotch irritation, you might try not using toilet paper, or not the premium, soft, fluffy and really white kind. Also pat your vulva instead of wiping it.

What to Wear Down There If You Can't Go Commando

Wear 100% cotton underwear. Do not wear underwear that is nylon on the outside but has a cotton liner, as the nylon shell will keep the cotton crotch from breathing. For workout gear, fabrics that wick away moisture are good, but take off your work out gear as soon as you are done. Thigh highs (nylons) are better than pantyhose for your crotch, and you don't need to take them off if you are having a quickie. Also consider cutting the crotches out of your panty hose.

How to Wash What You Wear Down There

When washing your underwear, use a mild, unscented laundry soap such as Tide Free, All Free and Clear, Dreft, Ivory and Kirkland Free and Clear. Detergents like these have earned the *Good Crotchkeeping Seal*. Also:

💡Use less detergent rather than more; if your washer has an extra rinse option, use it.

💡Do not use fabric softening or antistatic sheets in the dryer when drying your underwear as these leave residues in the fabric that can easily rub off on your skin. If you have static between your legs, masturbate.

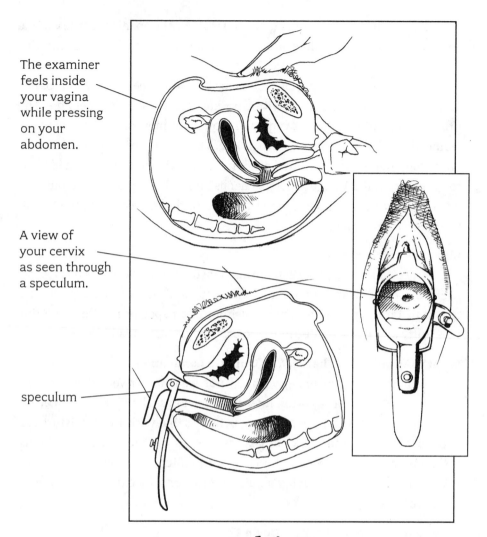

The examiner feels inside your vagina while pressing on your abdomen.

A view of your cervix as seen through a speculum.

speculum

Pelvic Exam

No intercourse the night before!

Dear Paul,

My friends have gone recently to their first gynecologist exam, and the stories they told me really scared me. One girl said it was really uncomfortable, and the other said it was downright painful; she was actually crying. Both mentioned something about the doctor sticking their whole hand inside them; is this true? I am starting to worry because I can't even get a tampon in there: last time I tried it was too painful and I gave up. Do some girls have unusually narrow vaginas?

About to Have My First Pelvic Exam

Dear About to Have,

For the exam itself, you will go into a room and trade your shirt and blue jeans for a paper gown—sometimes purple, sometimes blue, whatever the latest is in disposable gyno fashion. Usually a nurse and doctor will come in for the exam. They will ask you to lay down on an examination table. You will put your heels in metal stirrups and scoot your bum all the way to the end of the table. They will then shine a light on your genitals. The doctor will put a speculum in your vagina to help expand it and insert a little stick-like device to scrape some cells from your cervix. This shouldn't hurt, but you still might feel something. The cells will be put on a slide and sent to the lab for testing. Then they remove the speculum, and the doctor will insert one or two fingers inside your vagina to feel your cervix, ovaries and whatever else Mother Nature put up there. She will also feel the outside of your abdomen with her other hand. Most doctors will examine the lips of your vulva and some doctors will do a brief rectal exam. The doctor or nurse will also do a breast exam. It's best to abstain from intercourse the night before, but if you must, use a condom. Here is advice for you from our women readers:

> "I remember how scared I was before my first exam. The best thing to do is to tell the doctor that you are anxious and ask him or her to explain what is going to happen before the exam begins. A good doctor will explain things in as much detail as it takes to help calm your nerves. The worst part for me was the feeling of embarrassment that someone was looking at me. A pelvic exam should not hurt, and if it does for some reason you should tell the doctor immediately so that he or she can stop. As far as tampons are concerned, I have the same problem, and you might want to check out the tampons that are marketed as "slim fit" or even the ones that don't use an applicator. I find that these work best for me. Also try to relax. The more nervous you are the tighter your pelvic muscles will be." *female age 22*

> "It's not that bad, and no MD has EVER put his or her whole hand in me for a regular exam. Your friends are probably being overly dramatic." *female age 18*

> "He doesn't put his whole hand in there, darlin, it just seems like you are very full because of the speculum. It is pressing you open from top and bottom and it is what you mostly feel. Also not all

girls are a straight shot in. I had some discomfort on a regular basis until a male doctor pointed out that my cervix was tilted to the right-hand-side of my body. I now know to tell the doctor about this before going in so I don't get banged in the wrong direction. Unless the doctor is using one of the new disposable speculums, they do come in different sizes as well. I am very petite and know that a smaller size will be more comfortable. Some of this comes from experience, but it is your part to speak out on these issues with your doctor." *female age 33*

"I am a very small woman. My first pap was done with the instruments they use to test small children for molestation, if that tells you anything. I have since had many pelvic exams, all of which have been done with standard equipment. Breathe deeply, and try to think of other things, and let the doctor do her job. And don't let them give you an exam while you're on your period. It's uncomfortable for you, take my word for it." *female age 22*

Last but not least, for a report on getting a pelvic exam from half way around the world (count your lucky stars, girls in America!):

"Each examination room is shared by two doctors. So when I entered, there was another patient splayed out on the table, having a pelvic exam, right next to the door. She appeared to be accompanied by half a dozen people, both males and females; the preceding patient and her entourage were also there, in addition to my coworker and myself, and the two doctors. The door to the lobby was wide open. The first question the doctor asked me was translated as, 'Do you have the sexy life?' (As in, 'Are you sexually active?') Naturally, all eyes turned to me–foreigners are something of a novelty here–and of course, I'd just started dating a guy after six months of celibacy, so I said yes. After several more questions, I was led to a table in the corner of the room and instructed to disrobe. No paper gown, no curtain, no closed door. So, my legs spread for what felt like the world to see, up the speculum went." *female age 24*

A Very Special Thanks to Maureen Whelihan, MD, the gyno-goddess of greater Florida, and to Rachel Pauls, MD, FACOG, Urogynecologist and Director, Center for Female Sexual Health at Good Sam in Cincinnati.

48

Male Genital Care

Wash your package daily. If you've got a foreskin, pull it back and wash there, as well. That's it. Dick maintenance is a breeze when compared to what a woman goes through. No periods, no pads, no tampons, no pregnancy, no vaginal infections, no gynecologist, few bladder infections and no shaving or waxing between your legs. *Be thankful.*

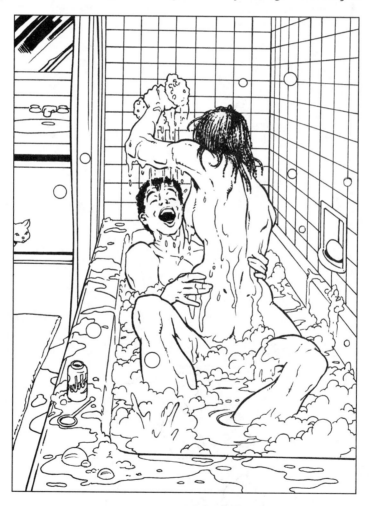

A fine way to clean male genitals.

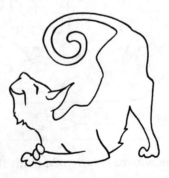

49
A Trip Inside Amber's Vagina

There are plenty of reasons to take a trip inside Amber's vagina. Let's say you want to know what causes yeast infections in a woman's vagina. Or your boyfriend's finger starts to sting when he's had it in your vagina for a while and you want to know why. Or maybe you want to know why it is unwise to assume that over-the-counter drugs will automatically make a vaginal infection go away.

Amber's vagina will be our gynecological version of *The Discovery Channel*. So let's look at what makes Amber's vagina hum, besides sweet texts and kisses from her boyfriend.

For this to work, we will need to shrink until we are very small. So small that we can take a trip up Amber's vagina. Given how a healthy vagina is fairly acidic, some of you might think of this as an acid trip. If Amber's boyfriend gets his prayers for sex answered before we are done, it will probably feel like an acid trip.

Amber's Vagina vs. The Vagina of a Rabbit, Hamster or Macaque

The vaginas of almost all mammals have a pH of around 7 which stands for neutral. They are neither acidic nor alkaline. This is very different from the pH in the human vagina. From puberty to menopause, the human vagina is acidic.

Before Amber went through puberty, the pH in her vagina was the same as the pH in her blood, which is about the same as the pH in water. But once puberty struck, Amber's vagina became acidic. (The average pH for adult women who haven't reached menopause is between 3.5 and 4.7.) After Amber goes through menopause, her vagina's pH will go back up to around 7 and will almost become neutral again.

There are times when the pH in Amber's vagina will briefly rise. During her periods, the pH will go up to around 6 or close to neutral. It will also go up for a few hours after she's had sex. That's because her boyfriend's semen is not acidic, so it causes the pH of her vagina to climb, and her sexual lubrication is not acidic either. And last but not least, the pH can rise when a woman has a vaginal infection. A high pH in a woman's vagina is one of the hallmarks of some vaginal infections.

Amber's Vagina—Home to Several Colonies of Bacteria

While we could view Amber's vagina as a warm, wet, heavenly place that lots of guys and some girls would like to visit, it's also like a rainforest that has an incredible ecosystem of bacterial flora and fauna that keep it all in balance.

One of the most important residents of Amber's vagina is a group of bacteria called Lactobacilli. When things are in balance, families of Lactobacilli produce hydrogen peroxide and lactic acid in just the right amounts. The hydrogen peroxide helps kill undesirable bacteria and the lactic acid helps to maintain an acidic environment that's so essential for healthy functioning. It also makes the fingers of Amber's boyfriend sting when they are inside of her vagina. This is a property of all healthy vaginas. Their acidic nature will make most people's fingers sting if they stay in there long enough.

The Lactobacilli have tiny projections that stick out from their cell bodies. These projections clasp onto the cell walls of the vagina and prevent germs from attaching at these points. You might think of it as special siding for the inside of Amber's vagina.

When Amber Takes Antibiotics and Things Go Wrong in Her Vagina

A very positive effect of the Lactobacilli is they keep the pH in Amber's vagina low. This helps keep out unfriendly bacteria that can cause infections. If something happens that disturbs the ecosystem in Amber's vagina, the stage is set for infections and uncomfortable conditions.

For instance, let's say Amber starts taking antibiotics for a lung infection. This kills off the wicked bacteria in her chest, but it also starts to kill off the Lactobacilli in her vagina. The lactic acid that's produced by the good bacteria will decrease and the alkalinity in Amber's vagina will increase. As the alkalinity or pH rises, fewer Lactobacilli will reproduce. A nasty spiral is created where the population of the good bacteria stars collapsing.

As the population of the good Lactobacilli begins to crash, another of its important by-products (hydrogen peroxide) will be in short supply. With less hydrogen peroxide, unfriendly bacteria will have an easier time taking up residence in Amber's vagina. Also, the Lactobacilli that was protecting the walls of Amber's vagina will weaken. Anaerobic bacteria will invade the cell walls in Amber's vagina and she may get bacterial vaginosis or BV. One of the most common symptoms of BV is a discharge with a fishy odor.

Why a Vagina with an Infection Will Sometimes Smell Fishy or Bad

When the levels of hydrogen peroxide go down, there is even less oxygen in the vagina than normal. As a result, anerobic bacteria that grow in low oxygen environments start to flourish. Instead of processing oxygen, they feast on sulfur and produce sulfur-like compounds. This kind of bacteria is responsible for the smell of bad breath, smelly feet, and Limburger cheese. It is one of the reasons why a vagina that has an infection will sometimes smell unpleasant. A fishy smell is also caused by the cellular death and destruction that's going on in the vagina as part of the body's efforts to make things right again.

Why Yogurt Won't Help

Lactobacilli is found in yogurt, so you would think that eating a lot of yogurt or plastering it between a woman's legs would help her infection go away. But the kind of yogurt that's in milk is very specific to cow intestines. So while yogurt might be good for a woman's calcium intake and maybe for her digestion, the yogurt we eat is unlikely to help at all with problems in the vagina. Researchers are hoping to find microorganisms (aka "probiotics") that will help treat conditions like bacterial vaginosis. This would provide a much more elegant solution than we currently have for treatment.

The Opposite Problem — Amber's Vagina Becomes a Distillery

Another kind of calamity can occur when the population of Lactobacilli suddenly rises and it produces too much lactic acid and hydrogen peroxide. Natural sugars start being fermented into carbon dioxide, alcohol, formic acid and acetic acid. This causes itching and irritation inside of Amber's vagina. When this occurs, Amber's boyfriend will need more than prayers and flowers to get between her legs.

This kind of situation shares the same symptoms as a yeast infection: including itching, burning, painful intercourse and a slight discharge. It is often misdiagnosed as a yeast infection. This is why a woman who is having problems with recurring vaginitis needs both a sharp gynecologist and a good knowledge of how her vagina works. Over-the-counter drugs for yeast infections won't touch these kinds of situations when the vagina becomes a distillery. (These conditions might be good for making beer and whiskey, but not for Amber's vagina.)

A third problem that can occur in Amber's vagina is when she really does get a yeast infection, commonly referred to as Candida. A fourth type of infection is caused by a protozoa known as Trich or Trichomonas Vaginalis. And then there's Noninfectious Vaginitis. Instead of being caused by funky organisms, the source of irritation for Noninfectious Vaginitis can be anything from feminine hygiene spray and body soap to premium toilet paper, laundry detergent, exercise bike-seat irritation, and period gear.

Researchers' Fascinating Findings about Amber's Crotch

Not long ago, physicians believed that the ecosystems in most vaginas were alike. They were wrong. Very wrong. We now know that there are five distinct communities of bacteria that can live in a human vagina. While these communities are fairly stable in some women, they can transition frequently in the vaginas of other women. (It might seem like there would be more vaginal infections in women whose vaginal communities transition more frequently, but that does not appear to be the case.)

The equilibrium in some women's vaginas can fluctuate widely when they have their periods, while the bacteria remain fairly stable when other women have their periods. There can also be fluctuations after women have sex. And black women are more likely to have a kind of bacterial community that is different from what is found in the vaginas of white women. As a result, the vaginas of black women might have a different pH than the vaginas of white women. Researchers are just beginning to find out about the different ecosystems that are inside of women's vaginas.

Coming Down

That does it for our trip inside Amber's vagina. Hopefully, the next time you see Amber, or any other woman, you will appreciate what an incredibly wonderful and complex ecosystem exists between her legs.

Special Thanks To Jacques Revel, University of Maryland School of Medicine, Greg Gloor, the University of Western Ontario, and Jeanne Marrazzo of the University of Washington.

50

Surfing the Crimson Wave
From Period Gear to Period Sex

If guys had periods, you could tell when by looking at the color under our fingernails or the stains on the top of our socks. That's because we'd either be checking out our vaginas like they were the Stargate, or because no one's going to stop a game of Halo or basketball just because he started bleeding or his flow was a tampon's worst nightmare.

So it's the strangest thing that so many men act awkward when dealing with their partner's periods, or why everyone gets quiet and pretends to ignore it when an ad for tampons or pads is on TV.

Part of the strangeness has to do with privacy. Many women prefer to keep periods private, which is not a bad thing. But there are ways of respecting a woman's privacy without acting distant or like you've just encountered an alien with a slime disease. And there are ways of dealing with tampons and pads without behaving like a dork.

Hopefully you'll find this chapter to be a squirm-free alternative to what you might have been told about periods in a health or biology class—where talk of eggs and Fallopian tubes ruled the day instead of information that might actually be useful in your life and relationships.

This chapter talks about bleeding, leaking, cramps, period gear, stain removal, menstrual cups, period panties, and more than you'll find anywhere else about period sex, including why a lot of couples say it feels so good.

Nearly 20% of the Women You Know Are Having a Period Right Now

At this very moment, nearly 20% of all non-pregnant women between the ages of 15 and 50 are having their periods. That's nearly one-in-five of the women who are skiing, running, swimming and playing baseball, basketball or soccer—women who are students, office workers, doctors, lawyers, accountants, teachers, mothers, dancers, actresses, waitresses.

When you put it in that perspective, it's hard to understand why people think there's anything unusual or embarrassing about periods.

More to the point, there is no evidence that a woman's intellectual or job performance is affected by her menstrual cycle. Plenty of women have won Olympic medals and recorded platinum songs while having periods.

The Pad and Tampon Wars

Two young boys walk into a pharmacy one day, pick out a box of tampons, and proceed to the checkout counter.

The man at the counter asks the older boy, "Son, how old are you?"

"Eight," the boy replies.

The man continues, "Do you know what these are used for?"

"Not exactly," the boy says. "But they aren't for me. They're for him. He's my brother. He's four. We saw on TV that if you use these you would be able to swim and ride a bike. Right now he can't do either one."

Not too long ago, people believed that women needed to rest during their periods. (Today's women would love the luxury!) The wisdom of the day had it that females of the better classes shouldn't exert themselves with strenuous activities or sports during that time of the month. Not so for the maid or cook who was expected to work a full day regardless.

The experts who championed these theories in the late 1800s believed that women were the more delicate sex and their bodies were more frail than men's. They were sure that women didn't think about sex, and that the female brain was too small for the demands of college and higher education. Then came the convenience of pads and tampons, and the "frail woman" nonsense started to get tossed out as fast as a used tampon.

Today's academic feminists have been cramping in disgust at the way women's periods have been portrayed in advertising for pads and tampons. But they miss a salient concept that a number of these ads have championed: while a woman's period might be annoying and distracting, it isn't debilitating. More importantly, copy from the ads like those that follow reminded people that the modern woman had social and economic opportunities that her mother didn't:

"The Girl of Today demands perfect freedom and comfort. She wants the best and will not tolerate the drudgeries that held her mother in bondage." *Modess 1929*

"Old-Fashioned ways cannot withstand the merry onslaught of the modern girl..." *Modess, 1929*

"Every Day of the Month Is a Day of Freedom." *Tampax, 1936*

"Don't Give Up Athletics Any Day of the Month." *Tampax, 1939*

"You're the Fun in His Furlough... Why let trying days of the month rule your life? You don't need time-out... that is, if you choose Kotex sanitary napkins." *Kotex, 1942*

And what about this over-the-top text from the 1929 Modess pad campaign that championed self-reliance and rejection of old-fashioned ideas:

"Life is so much more fun when one is not afraid. It is her happy courage—the zest with which she welcomes every new delightful freedom—which is the charm of the modern girl... In a gloomier age, women were resigned to drudgery. Today, young womanhood does not permit drudgery to cloud her joy of living."

These ads refuted ideas from the 1800s that women's bodies and brains were inferior. They took the onus off of the body and put it on the pad—a woman wasn't the slave of her period as long as she bought "the right" period gear. Long before the feminism of the 1960s and 1970s, these ads were telling women that they could do anything that men could, with smaller strings attached.

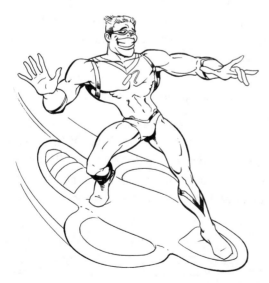

Captain Menstruation's Extreme Makeover: Before the 8th edition of *The Guide*, Captain Menstruation was a guy. He was a parody about the ridiculousness of period gear ads showing pads with wings flying through the air. But women kept telling us it would be more empowering if Capt. Menstruation were a girl. So Daerick gave him a sex change. *Turn the page for the new Captain Menstruation!*

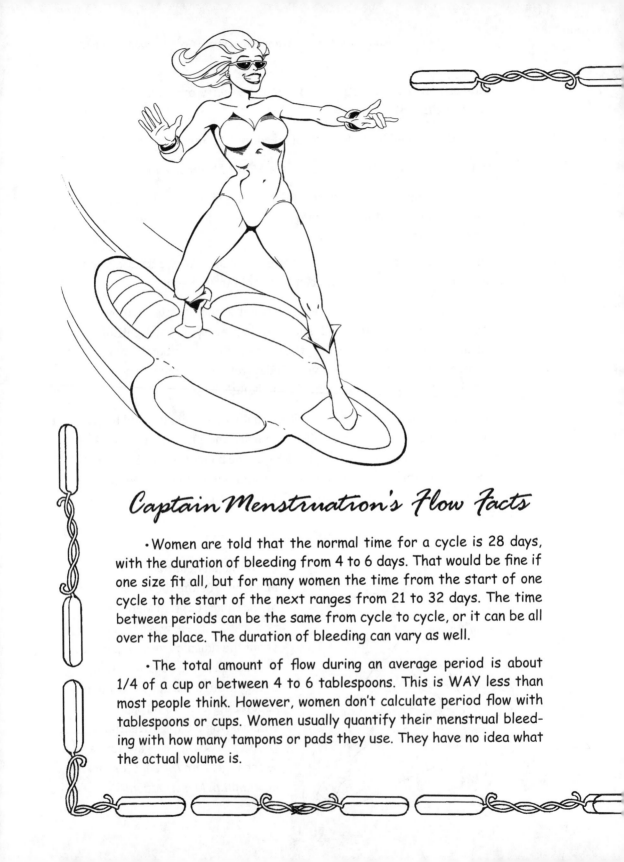

Captain Menstruation's Flow Facts

• Women are told that the normal time for a cycle is 28 days, with the duration of bleeding from 4 to 6 days. That would be fine if one size fit all, but for many women the time from the start of one cycle to the start of the next ranges from 21 to 32 days. The time between periods can be the same from cycle to cycle, or it can be all over the place. The duration of bleeding can vary as well.

• The total amount of flow during an average period is about 1/4 of a cup or between 4 to 6 tablespoons. This is WAY less than most people think. However, women don't calculate period flow with tablespoons or cups. Women usually quantify their menstrual bleeding with how many tampons or pads they use. They have no idea what the actual volume is.

• Oh joy! Period cramps are related to labor pains. Both are mediated by prostaglandins. This is why prostaglandin inhibitors like Midol, ibuprofen, ponstel and celebrex can help if you have cramps. The trick is in taking ibuprofen a day or two **BEFORE** you think your cramps will begin. Birth-control pills can also help decrease cramping because the progesterone in them can quiet the roar in your uterus and might help even you out hormonally.

• For pain relief once your period starts, orgasms can help. Orgasms pump powerful pain relievers into the body and the contractions can help push accumulated fluids out of your uterus. In spite of the benefits, can you imagine a mother telling her daughter, "Honey, if you're having cramps, why not masturbate?"

• The faster period blood drips out, the more red it's going to be. The slower it drips out, the darker it might be. That's because when it flows more slowly, it spends a longer time in the upper part of your vagina and becomes oxidized, which can result in its turning brownish. The reason why period blood often looks brown on pads is because it has mixed with oxygen and has oxidized. If period blood comes out really slowly, it might look like a dark, tar-like paste.

• The clumps in your period flow are from your body's clotting mechanisms. Our gyno consultant said that when there's heavy flow, she likes to see clotting, because it means the body is working to decrease the amount of bleeding. It concerns her when there's a lot of bright red blood that is thin like Koolaid and has no clots in it. She also said that as a woman gets older, "she'll start to shed tissue from the lining that looks like 'strings' of tissue."

• After a woman turns 40 or so, the volume of blood flow might seriously increase, but for only 1 to 3 days rather than the whole time. There might be more clumps, as well.

• If you are concerned about any of this beyond the basic annoyance that it has to happen to you, please ask your physician!

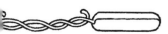

Why Guys Freak Out

There are two things about women's bodies and their periods that have freaked men out (and women) over the ages. The first is how a woman's vagina, ovaries and uterus are on the inside. Ergonomically, this isn't nearly as bad as having your testicles and penis hanging on the outside where they are in harm's way, but we still tend to fear what we can't see.

The second issue: blood. We humans have a one-tracked mind when it comes to bleeding. We see it as a sign of injury or disease.

So if you combine monthly bleeding with where the blood drips from— you start seeing cultures throughout the ages that have come up with rituals regarding menstruation to help deal with their fear of the unknown. Some of the rituals were sadly isolating and punitive, while others appear to have been empowering for women.

Women, too, must have wondered about the strange spirits that took over their bodies and made them bleed every month. Some still do.

From Evil Spirits to Eggs & Fallopian Tubes

Unless she is seriously late or is trying to get pregnant, the last thing a woman thinks about when she's having her period is that an egg had dropped down her Fallopian tubes but didn't implant. Yet that's pretty much what periods have been reduced to in the way we teach about menstruation in school.

The story of how monthly bleeding relates to reproduction has become the new mythology to help allay our fears about menstruation. It's a scientific narrative that helps reassure us that periods are really OK. But given the silence in the room when a tampon commercial comes on TV, you can't help but wonder. Is the silence because the ad is a reminder that a woman has a vagina? That blood come out of it? Are people as uncomfortable when an ad comes on for Viagra?

While modern science has better answers about menstruation than philosophers like Aristotle and St. Augustine did in centuries past, we still don't know why women menstruate every month and whether it's a good thing or a bad thing. There is currently a huge debate over the long- term safety of using birth control pills to stop a woman's periods altogether, and we still don't know why some women's breasts get tender at different times in their monthly cycle.

What Girls Really Want to Know, and What Guys Should Know

Are eggs and Fallopian tubes what girls want to know about periods? Of course not. Girls in their teens want to know how to control the mess, how to control the cramps and backaches, how to get stains out of their panties and pajamas, how to better predict when their period will arrive and how heavy the flow will be. They want to know how to carry period gear inconspicuously, and how to deal with the embarrassment when boys find out they are having their period and try to tease them about it.

When girls get older and become sexually active, they also want to know about period sex, and no matter how young or old they are, girls who are having their periods want to know "Why me? Why does this happens to women and not guys?"

As for men, once you get into a long-term relationship, menstruation is something that happens to both of you. That's why guys who live with girls will do better in life if they try to understand more about periods. Males tend to relate periods to a possible decrease in sex, while for women periods are about blood, tampons, pads, and for some, cramps, tender breasts and lower back pain. And until a guy becomes a dad who has to pay for tampons and pads, he is usually not aware of how much period gear costs every month.

Period Gear

Period gear has come a long way since the days when women wore funky belts to hold thick pads that were just shy of being mattress-sized between their legs. Here's a story from back, when pads had tails instead of wings:

My mother taught me to read when I was four years old (her first mistake)...

One day, I was in the bathroom and noticed one of the cabinet doors was open. I read the box in the cabinet. I then asked my mother why she was keeping 'napkins' in the bathroom. Didn't they belong in the kitchen? Not wanting to burden me with unnecessary facts, she told me that those were for "special occasions" (her second mistake).

Now, fast forward a few months.... It's Thanksgiving Day, and my folks are leaving to pick up my uncle and his wife for dinner. Mom had assignments for all of us while they were gone. Mine was to set the table.

When they returned, my uncle came in first and immediately burst into laughter. Next, in came my father, who roared with laughter. Then in came Mom, who almost died of embarrassment when she saw each place setting on the table with a "special occasion" napkin at each plate, with the fork carefully arranged on top. I had even tucked the little tail in so they didn't hang off the edge! My mother asked me why I used these and, of course, my response sent the other adults into further fits of laughter. "But, Mom, you said they were for special occasions!!!"

Quick Change Artists & Talking the Talk

While teenage guys need to have certain strategies to deal with unwanted hard-ons, not too many have to worry about a friend tapping them on the shoulder and whispering that a BIG blotch of blood leaked through the back of their pants.

Periods can arrive with little rhyme or reason, especially during the first couple of years, so a young women has to cope with everything from blood leaking out to how she's going to change a pad or tampon during a five-minute break between classes—all while acting like nothing's up because she's worried guys will make fun of her if they know she's having her period.

On the other hand, periods give girls an excuse to talk with each other about their own reproductive anatomy. Sharing experiences and information about periods can be a source of bonding, not to mention an outlet for sharing personal horror stories, like when the cutest guy on the planet got behind you in the checkout line at the supermarket after you just put a super gigantic sized package of Kotex on the conveyer belt.

Being able to talk with their friends about periods might also help girls share information about their bodies in a time when parents still refer to female genitals collectively as "your vagina" or "down there," and a lot of teenage girls don't even know what their clit is.

When a Woman Drops a Tampon

Researchers designed a study where a woman "accidentally" dropped either a tampon that was still in its wrapper or a hair clip on the ground. They then asked people who viewed the woman dropping the objects what they thought about her. When she dropped a tampon, the woman was considered to be less competent and less likeable than when she dropped the hair clip.

(What do you think the response would have been if she had dropped a condom? Would we rate a male who dropped a condom more favorably than a woman?)

A Sweater or Shirt to Tie Around Your Waist and Period Panties

While some young women wear sweaters or shirts tied around their waists to hide their butts, it never hurts for them to keep an extra shirt or sweater in their locker or car in case they end up with a blood stain on the back of their pants or skirt. Unfortunately, this is not an option for women who have to wear uniforms. Keeping an extra pair of pants or jeans and undies in their car or locker is also a good idea. (Are these things that guys ever have to worry about?)

The cool way to store a stash of tampons is to keep them in a Vinnie's Tampon Case.

A lot of women have what they call *period panties,* which in some cases were panties they really liked but have ended up with stains in the crotch that refuse to come out. They only wear them when they are bleeding. Others will wear dark underwear that won't show stains, and some get inexpensive Walmart specials to wear when they are having their periods.

Making Your Own Custom Pads

It's fairly easy and fun to sew custom period pads. They look great and help save landfill space. You can also make them from 100% cotton. There are a number of websites that have patterns and show how to make pads. Enter "period gear" in the search box at www.GuideToGettingItOn.com.

Cycle-Related Breast Tenderness

Some women's breasts get really sore when they are having their period. Other women experience breast soreness at a different time, like when they are ovulating. And instead of being painful, some women's breasts become sensitive in a way that welcomes kisses and caresses during certain times of the month. So if you are in a relationship, breast tenderness is important to talk about.

Period-related breast soreness can be slight, or it can be so extreme that just driving over speed bumps can really hurt. Some women say their breasts will feel like they are bruised. Both breasts can become tender, or just one. Breast tenderness can be helped by taking birth-control pills, or it can be caused by taking birth-control pills. Go figure.

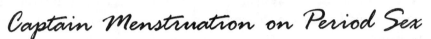

Captain Menstruation on Period Sex

Some couples are afraid of having intercourse when Aunt Flo comes to town. Fear not! Period sex causes no harm to either partner. Better yet, it can bring buckets of smiles. Here are some reasons why:

- Period flow can make a vagina feel super-lubed. Some couples say the flow feels better than store-bought lube. Other couples need to add store-bought lube for period sex. That's because a woman's estrogen level tanks during her period, which can result in less natural lubrication.

- Menstrual swelling can help a woman have a really nice orgasm. Who knows if it makes intercourse feel better, but a woman's cervix drops when she's having her period. As a result, some couples might prefer certain period positions. Explore and see what feels best for you.

- Some women get extra-horny during their periods. This might have to do with a change in hormones, or perhaps they feel more relaxed since it's harder to get pregnant.

Some couples feel all primal and cool being drenched in period sex blood; others act like they've just arrived at a crime scene. You can vary your flow exposure with the following tips:

- Put a towel down to catch the flow, or have sex in the shower.

- Use a male condom or the female condom.

- Wear a diaphragm or use Instead menstrual cups. These are little domes that cradle the cervix and catch most of the flow.

- For period-sex-fantasy fun, have sex while one of the vampire shows is on the TV!

- If period sex proper isn't for you, you can always get each other off by hand, with a vibrator or dildo. Orgasms can help ease period pain.

- Anal sex can be an option if both of you enjoy it, but it's hard to think that a woman who enjoys anal sex would have a problem with vaginal sex while she's on her period.

- DO NOT wear a tampon during intercourse!

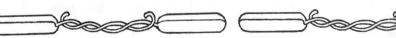

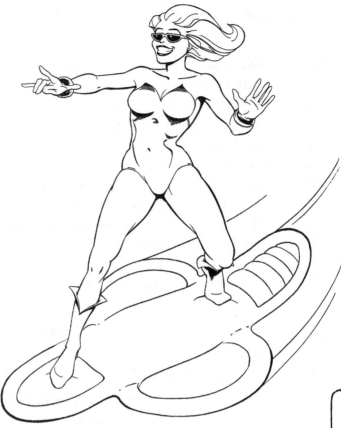

Tips for receiving oral sex while on your period:

• Splash some water into your vagina, then insert a tampon before a partner goes down on you. The tampon will catch most of the flow. If intercourse follows, be sure to take the tampon out first.

• Do it in the shower.

• Wear a diaphragm, Instead or a menstrual cup: Some women get a diaphragm for the sole purpose of having period sex. Some couples start with it in for oral sex, but take it out for intercourse.

• Wrap it! Cover your vulva with a barrier or plastic wrap. A little lube between the vulva and plastic wrap might help.

• Some guys like going down as is, flow and all.

• **Important Health Note:** You CAN get pregnant from having period sex. You can get dangerous STIs like hepatitis or HIV from period blood, even if the woman shows no symptoms.

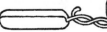

Getting The Red Out—Removing Period Blood

It's difficult to have periods and not stain things. If you've been having periods for a while and haven't stained a whole bunch of things, consider getting treatment for an obsessive-compulsive disorder.

It's always best to treat blood stains as soon as possible, but who's got a laundry room handy when most stains occur? For triage while on the run, try hitting a new stain with a wad of saliva and blotting it up, or better yet, if there's some contact-lens saline solution handy, try that. The reason for using saline or spit, which is saline with some enzymes and food particles added, is that saline will help the blood cells float out instead of smearing them on the fabric like cream cheese on a bagel.

Also, the percent of blood in period flow can be high or low, depending on the day. So what might work for stains one day might not work the next.

 Soak the item in cold water, overnight if necessary.

 Try applying Clorox 2 Stain Fighter and Color Booster directly to the stain. It can occasionally work miracles.

 Use unpreserved saline solution on the stain, the kind people use for contact lenses. Or mix one cup of salt in 2 quarts of cold water. Soak for half an hour. Then blot, don't rub. (Blotting is the operative word as rubbing bursts the red blood cells and will stain the fabric even more.)

 If Big Red is still there, add a bit of mild bar soap. Rinse with cold water.

If the stain refuses to surrender, consider this: blood stains can become really nasty when the hemoglobin in the blood mixes with oxygen in the air. This binds the stain to the fabric. Since hemoglobin is made up of iron, what you might be dealing with in a blood stain is a rust stain. Even the folks at Tide mention using rust remover if the usual removal techniques fail:

1) Carefully apply Whink Rust Remover or other liquid rust remover following the instructions on the package. Apply over a plastic or glass dishpan, as the rust remover can be gnarly on certain surfaces. 2) Rinse in 1 quart of water to which 3 tablespoons of baking soda have been added. 3) Air dry and repeat the procedure if necessary.

Hydrogen peroxide is often used to get out blood stains. However, hydrogen peroxide can make the fabric weaker. That's why hydrogen peroxide is not a product of first choice, unless you were hoping for crotchless panties.

Period Parties & "You Are Becoming a Woman"

This Kotex ad from 1942 shows how period education used to be:

> ~ Mothers ~
>
> Why get all involved trying to explain the facts of menstruation to your little girls when there's a simple, easy way to do this dreaded task?
>
> Let the new booklet "As One Girl To Another" do this job for you! It will spare you a session that may only end in confusion, and embarrassment.

Fortunately, things are changing. A lot of mothers today are framing a girl's first period as an important milestone in a girl's life. Some moms take their daughters out to a special lunch or dinner, and some even have parties—which might be a bit much as far as some daughters are concerned. But if parents feel the need to mortify their kid with a cake and party to celebrate their daughter's first period, at least it's a step in the right direction.

How to decorate a cake to celebrate your first period is another matter. We at Goofy Foot Press would most likely edge it with pads and tampons made of marzipan, and a confetti of Midols made from sugar. As for the cake's interior, do you stay with a classic white cake with alternating layers of strawberry and raspberry, or do you make a bold statement and go with a red velvet cake?

As for saying that a girl has "become a woman" after her first period, that seems to be stretching it a bit when you consider how early girls are having their periods. The concept of womanhood is more social than biological, and to think that a 11- or 12-year-old girl in Western culture has reached womanhood begs a reality check. A girl's first period marks an important biological passage, but it's more reasonable to think of her high-school graduation as a transition into womanhood.

Perhaps the most significant passage a first period marks is it allows a girl to enter into the same "club" that her mom, friends and older sisters are in. This can be empowering and socially important. Some girls who have their first period later than their friends feel left out of this "club" and can't wait to join it—until they have their first cramps.

Hygienic Hysteria and What about Odor?

Toward the end of the 1800s, germs started to become a big deal, not that they hadn't killed billions of people in the years prior. But with Lister's discovery about germs there was no turning back, and menstruation seemed like a perfect target for people who were concerned about contagion.

Some of the greatest perpetrators of menstruation as a hygienic catastrophe were women themselves. Their advice columns for much of the 1900s had the signature of self-loathing and obsessive cleanliness. Yet when it comes to female genitals, cleanliness is next to Godliness only if it is done in moderation. Also, when it comes to germs, your vagina will never be as gross as your mouth or your partner's mouth.

With so much hygienic hysteria, it was only natural that the companies that made sanitary napkins would play the odor card. However, if there is period-related odor, sanitary napkins may actually be a source of it. Period flow contains blood cells and dead tissue. All dead tissue contains organic compounds like putrescine and cadaverine. No one will ever confuse putrescine or cadaverine with perfume.

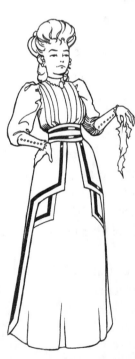

However, a bigger problem occurs when period flow mixes with butt bacteria (e coli). And the place where that's most likely to happen is in a pad or sanitary napkin that is trapping period flow from your vagina and moisture from your rear end. Sanitary napkins are the perfect delivery system for one to meet the other. If a pad is what you need, consider using a natural cotton pad that breathes.

A lot of women use pads like the Luna pad that are washable and can be reused. This is one of the reasons why a woman should change her pad as often as the manufacturer suggests, only it's unlikely that makers of sanitary napkins will tell you about the problem with butt bacteria mixing with period flow. (Our gynecology consultant doesn't feel that thongs and g-strings are too far behind the sanitary napkin when it comes to possible ways of transporting butt bacteria into your vagina.)

For First-Time Tampon Users

"I didn't realize the cardboard was supposed to come out (while the cotton wad stays in). It was a rather uncomfortable first hour, 'til I finally asked a girlfriend, 'What the hell?'" *female age 28*

"I mostly use pads, but they used to get stuck in my pubic hair. OUCH! Tampons are only useful for pools and hot tubs, otherwise it feels really weird walking around feeling like you have a soft dick stuck in you all day." *female age 21 [Editor's note: this could be happening because she isn't pushing the tampon in far enough.]*

"Pads were so horrid, even though I used them for many years. They were just so gross, it felt like wearing a diaper, but I could never get the hang of applicator tampons, so I just used pads. When I got to college we got a free trial pack of OB applicatorless tampons and I fell in love instantly and have never looked back!" *female age 20*

"I hated pads because I felt gooey and gross when I wore them. The blood never absorbs like the commercials say it does. I hurt the first couple of times I put a tampon in, and had to force it, but eventually that stopped and I didn't have a problem anymore." *female age 21*

"I never had a problem using tampons, and I hate it when my pubic hair gets stuck to the bloody pad. YUCK. So I'm a tampon girl—though I have to use the slim kind, as the larger ones hurt." *female age 20*

A number of our female readers have reported strange or painful experiences when they first tried using a tampon, including trying to pull out the tampon while it was still dry. This probably resulted from wearing a higher absorbency tampon than was needed and the tampon ended up sticking to the sides of their vagina. Ouch! Tampons come in a couple of absorbencies. It's best not to use one that is more absorbent than you need.

As for common tampon questions, a tampon can't get pushed in "too far." That's because your vagina ends in a cul-de-sac. Tampons won't ever float away inside your body, so you don't need to worry about doctors having to fish one out from behind your lung. Tampons are not like penises—you shouldn't be able to feel them. If you can, it's probably because you didn't push it far enough inside.

Here are some tips on tampon insertion from our female readers. However, always read and follow the instructions that come with the tampons.

The companies that make these products don't want to get sued, and so the information in their instructions is usually the latest and greatest. Do not leave the tampons in longer than the manufacturer says. If you are concerned about tampon-related sickness, see the section in this chapter on TSS.

Most tampons come with applicators or plungers. Some tampons, like O.B.s, use the inserting device that Mother Nature provided: your finger.

Putting tampons where they need to go requires three steps: pushing in the applicator, pushing in the plunger, and pulling out the applicator, unless you are using O.B.s, where there aren't any messy plungers to throw away that eventually wash up on our beaches.

It might help to coat the end of the tampon with a lubricant like KY Jelly. If you can't score the jelly, try dabbing a little saliva on it.

Buy or borrow the skinniest tampon you can find. You might try Tampax Lites or Playtex SlimFit regulars for your first time.

Find your vaginal opening. It's down there somewhere, at the bottom part of your vulva. Spread the lips of your vulva and put your finger in a little way. This is where the tampon will go.

Some women put tampons in while standing with a little squat action or with one leg higher and out to the side. Other women put them in while sitting on the toilet.

Spread your lips with the fingers of one hand, and insert the applicator into your vagina with the other. *Aim it toward your tailbone and not up toward your stomach!*

Insert the applicator so that the wider part of the barrel is almost all of the way in—with just enough sticking out to hold on to. If you don't insert the tampon far enough inside, the ring of muscles in the first part of your vagina can clamp it, making it feel uncomfortable.

Once you've got the applicator in, hold the barrel firmly with your fingers. Push the plunger in. Bingo!

As you pull out the applicator, try not to pull on the string or you'll pull the tampon out and you're back to square one. If this happens, push the tampon back in with your finger.

☼ Make sure the string of the tampon is hanging out of your vagina. If it isn't, don't worry. Squat and push down as if you are trying to take the mother of all dumps. Reach a finger inside your vagina to see if you can feel the critter. You can always use your thumb and finger to pull the string out. If you have no luck, ask your mom, aunt, grandmother older sister, best friend or boyfriend for help, or call your healthcare provider and speak with a nurse. Again, it's not like the end of the world, but you will need to get the tampon out in the next couple of hours. Pulling out a lost tampon is not much different from pulling out a lost condom.

♥ Your vagina might be dry on the last day or two of your period. Don't hesitate to dab some lube on the tampon before putting it in.

☀ Sorry to be repetitive, but do not have intercourse with a tampon inside. While it's not going to end up in the next county, it's best not to have tampon getting smooshed behind your cervix by the head of a guy's penis.

Tampons, Sponges & Toxic-Shock Syndrome

Toxic-Shock Syndrome (TSS) is a rare but sometimes fatal disease caused by the toxins of bacteria that grow in the bodies of both men and women. TSS is now mainly associated with surgery and severe burn cases, but during the early 1980s some women died from TSS following the introduction of a new superabsorbent tampon called Rely.

Contrary to what scientists first believed, the killer tampons were not a breeding site for TSS bacteria. Rely contained two synthetic fibers (carboxymethyl cellulose and polyester foam) that are thought to have irritated the vaginal lining in ways that triggered the TSS bacteria to produce a dangerous toxin. Tampons are now made from only cotton and rayon. As a result, the occurrence of TSS among tampon users is rare. Your chances of getting killed in a car wreck are 500 to 1,000 times greater than the risk of death by tampon.

It was originally thought that wearing the same tampon for several hours increased your chances of getting TSS. Not so. But the risk does go up when you use nothing but tampons throughout your entire period, even if you change them every three hours. If you are a tampon user who wants to greatly reduce her chances of getting TSS, don't wear tampons throughout your entire period. For instance, alternate using tampons and pads, or ditch the traditional period gear for a more environmentally sound menstrual cup.

Also, some people are naturally more susceptible to TSS. If you have ever had TSS or appear susceptible to it, you are better off not using tampons.

Warning signs of TSS: sudden high fever (usually 102 degrees or more) that includes vomiting and/or diarrhea, fainting or near-fainting when you stand up and dizziness or a sunburn-like rash. Symptoms usually appear very quickly and are often severe. Symptoms can vary, and might include aching of muscles and joints, redness of the eyes, sore throat, and weakness.

If you are on your period, have a sudden high fever and one or more of these TSS symptoms, ditch your tampon at once and make tracks to an emergency room. This would not be a time for modesty—claw your way to the front of the line and let the clerk know you are on your period and have been wearing a tampon.

There are rumors that tampons contain dioxins that cause TSS. That might be possible if anyone could actually find dioxins in tampons, but the amount of dioxins in tampons is virtually nil. We are exposed to much higher levels of dioxins in the environment than from anything that comes in a box and has a string on the end.

Turning Your Crotch Green

The average woman uses 10,000 or more pads or tampons in her lifetime. If your choice is between pads and tampons, it would seem as though a tampon without an applicator, such as O.B., or a pad made of washable cotton, would be the more environmentally friendly choice. Disposable pads contain layers of engineered petroleum products. Tampons are mostly cotton. And the gynecologists who have consulted on this book aren't exactly big fans of disposable pads (sanitary napkins), especially if a woman is experiencing crotch irritation. A pad made of cotton cloth is much preferred for vulva health, but the final decision should be between you and your healthcare provider.

If you do use tampons, you might try to use O.B.s or tampons without applicators. Nature gave you your own applicators—your fingers. If they haven't met your vagina, what are you waiting for?

Also, it wouldn't hurt to investigate using menstrual cups rather than tampons or pads. Women who use menstrual cups often rave about them. While the learning curve is high, it is possible you will have a better user experience.

Menstrual Cups—A Cross between a Diaphragm and A Shot Glass

A menstrual cup is a soft, flexible container made of soft silicone rubber or latex that is inserted into the vagina to collect period flow. It looks a bit like a small, upside-down funnel, although the stem is not hollow and the body of the cup is more rounded than a funnel. There are a number of different brands of menstrual cups, such as the Lunette, Diva, Moon Cup, Lady Cup, Femmecup, Miacup Keeper and Pink Cup. Most are made of medical grade silicone, with each having a slightly different length, softness, rim, stem and color.

Once it's in place, a menstrual cup forms a seal that allows it to collect the blood as it flows from the cervix. Unlike a tampon, which absorbs the natural healthy secretions of the vagina in addition to period flow, a menstrual cup collects only period flow. As a result, it won't dry out a vagina.

A lot of women who are devoted users say they originally thought the concept of a menstrual cup was gross or disgusting. But they experienced so many advantages in using menstrual cups that they wouldn't think of going back to pads or tampons.

Menstrual cups hold enough flow for most women to handle a light day without emptying it until evening, although you might need to empty it a couple of times a day when the flow is like the Mississippi. Menstrual cups last for nearly ten years. They are a little spendy to begin with, but quickly amortize with each new period, as you won't have to buy pads or tampons.

Some women worry that a menstrual cup isn't sterile, as if a tongue, penis, fingers or a tampon are. Depending on the manufacturer's instructions, some women clean the cups with soap, soak them in hydrogen peroxide, or use other solutions before storing them until their next period. Unlike tampons, they have never been linked to Toxic Shock Syndrome.

In order to insert a menstrual cup, it needs to be folded and then pushed into the vagina until it's just below the cervix. There are different ways to fold menstrual cups, including the c-fold, origami, "7" fold, and punch-down fold. A virgin can wear a menstrual cup, as well as a woman whose vagina is on the smaller side.

Some women get the hang of using a menstrual cup the very first time, others require a few efforts. Since menstrual cups don't dry out your vagina, you can practice inserting them before you have your period. According to users, here are some of the advantages of using a menstrual cup:

Tampons can seriously dry out your vagina. Menstrual cups don't. They are soft, flexible and don't absorb your natural moisture.

Once they learn how to make the cup sit right, a lot of users say they don't get the kind of leaking that they did with tampons. With less leaking, the chances are lower that a woman's favorite underwear will be stained and have to become period panties.

Some cup users say they experience less cramping than when they used tampons.

No more late-night runs to the store to buy tampons or pads.

During the years that a woman has periods, those who use menstrual cups will put approximately 10,000 fewer pads, tampons, and their wrappers into our landfills, sewers, and beaches.

At the time of publication, there were two excellent websites for women who are thinking about trying menstrual cups:

http://community.livejournal.com/menstrual_cups/tag/faq

www.ecomenses.com

Period Suppression

Period suppression refers to a woman preventing her period from happening by doing things like ditching the placebo week of birth-control pills or keeping her NuvaRing in for all four weeks instead of for just three. (You should never attempt this without first discussing it with your gynecologist. It will work with only certain pills or other hormonal methods and there might be health concerns that could make it a bad idea.)

There is still a lot of debate about the safety of period suppression. On the one hand, there are theories that nature never intended women to constantly have monthly periods because women were pregnant so often. The reasoning goes that having as many periods as women do today is not good for you. Other theories claim that a monthly fluctuation in hormones that happens with periods is good for a woman's body and is one of the reasons why women outlive men by five years or so.

While menstrual suppression appears to be quite safe, we don't have the kind of long-term studies yet.

The Female Athlete Triad

It is not uncommon for women athletes to stop menstruating or have irregular periods. This is because the woman does not eat enough food to make up for the energy she is burning. Far from being benign, this can result in brittle bones and severe injuries. It is part of what is now called The Female Athlete Triad. It tends to be worse in sports where being thin is an advantage. It can also be a problem for cheerleaders and dancers.

Some gynecologists mistakenly believe that giving an athlete hormonal birth control will even out her periods, and that the estrogen in the pills will make up for the estrogen that is missing due to insufficient diet. Research does not currently support this idea. Putting an athlete on the pill simply removes the important symptom of irregular or missed periods.

(It is with restraint that your author tells about the time during his freshman year of college when he lifted weights with the women members of the Soviet National Shot-Put Team. He never thought to ask Olga, Svetlana, and Georgia if they menstruated regularly.)

Tipped Uterus Considerations

Some women with a tipped uterus experience period pain more as a back ache than a pain in their abdomen and they may have diarrhea during their periods as well. Some women with a tipped uterus know when their period is coming because they start having loose stools that might be caused by a release of prostaglandins.

PMS

PMS is short for pre-menstrual syndrome. It refers to period-related mood fluctuations. To this day, PMS remains such a loosely defined concept that in addition to women, most men qualify as having it.

During World War II, when the bulk of American males went to war, millions of American women manned the nation's industrial-war machine. Our female-dominated workforce turned out an armada of planes, tanks, ships, and guns that was unprecedented in history. It wasn't until the men returned from war and needed their jobs back that the myth of women's so-called hormonal instability began to rear its head. It fit well with our society's need to get women out of the workplace and back into the home.

An entire PMS industry sprung up during the 1990s that attempted to turn hormonal mood fluctuations into a disease. This helped fuel the notion that women as a group are flakier than men. Just as flaky, absolutely; flakier, no. While period-related mood fluctuations can definitely result in mood swings, this usually doesn't make a woman emotionally unstable unless

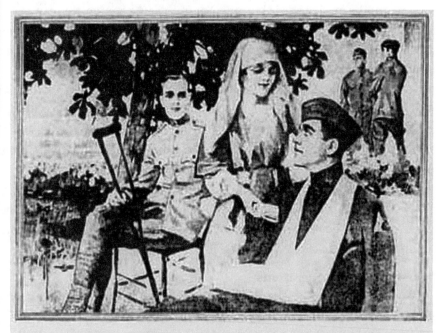

To Save Men's Lives Science Discovered

KOTEX

Wisconsin Historical Society

*This 1920 ad was rejected for magazine placement because it contained
too many men in a product that was for women.*

she's emotionally fragile to begin with. Studies show that men have as many
monthly mood swings as women, but there's no psychiatric diagnosis for that.
Something that might help women with severe period related mood swings
is birth-control pills. However, some women find that the pill creates mood
swings or makes them worse. Depends on the pill and the woman.

Brief History of the Napkin and Tampon

Kotex was the first widely marketed sanitary napkin. It was invented
shortly after World War I. Before then, women used rags that they wadded up
and pinned to the inside of their underwear. The modern tampon was born
in the late 1920s or early 1930s. It was called an "internal sanitary napkin."

⇐ *The ad on the left was created in 1920. It is a prototype of the very first Kotex ad ever done.*

Kotex had its origins during World War I. Since cotton was in short supply, companies started to make bandages from cellulose. Army nurses found that the cellulose bandaging made an excellent substitute for the menstrual rags that they usually wore. It was cheap, absorbent, and they could throw it away.

As soon as the war was over, Kimberly-Clark, the company that made the bandages, looked opportunity in the crotch and created Kotex, which stood for KOtten-Like-TEXture. They hoped that by using a cryptic name such as "Kotex," women would be able to buy the product without the embarrassment of male clerks knowing what it was. Sure.

Another challenge for the Kotex people was to create an ad for their new product that magazines in the early 1920s would run. This was advertising for a product that went between a woman's legs at a time when this kind of item was still new and possibly scandalous.

Look at the headlines that went with this ad. Can you see a similarity with the way we sell products today by claiming that they were "Developed by NASA for our astronauts." Also, whatever the nurse is handing to the wounded officer is about the size of a Kotex, and it is placed in the illustration in front of her crotch. (Thanks to the Museum of Menstruation: www.mum.org, and the Wisconsin Historical Society for permission to use the Kotex ad.)

It did not have an applicator or a string. It was wrapped in gauze, which formed a tail that a woman pulled on in order to remove the tampon.

Another early tampon was called Paz. In 1936, the Tambrands company bought the Paz company and started selling Tampax, which was the first tampon with an applicator. It's interesting that they changed the name of the Paz tampon to Tampax, when Tampaz (TAMbrands + PAZ) would have made more sense. Perhaps it was because the very first tampon was made by another company and was called FAX. "Tampax" includes Tam+Paz+Fax.

One early problem with using tampons is they required women to touch their genitals. There were widespread fears that this would lead to wanton immorality. There were also fears that tampons would devirginize teenage girls. As late as the early 1990s, Tampax ran ads to help dispel this fear. After then, even the people at Tampax gave up the virginity ghost.

As for newer technology, a few years ago we heard about a new menstrual product called the "inSync Miniform." It was about the size of a tampon but fit between the labia. It was supposed to be used on light days, but who reads the instructions? Our research assistant volunteered to try it out. This nearly resulted in a worker's compensation claim against Goofy Foot Press.

  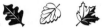

NOTE: According to Publisher's Weekly, the classic period book "Are You There God? It's Me, Margaret" by Judy Bloom has sold roughly 7 million copies since it was first published in 1972. It continues to sell more than 100,000 copies each year. This makes it one of the best-selling books of all time.

Highly Recommended—Be sure to check out the amazing *Museum of Menstruation* website: www.mum.org, which rates *Two Tampons Way Up!* or would that be 5 *Panty Liners out of* 5? It includes anything you would ever want or need to know about menstruation. Also, if you are doing research on menstrual products patented in the United States from 1854 to 1921, get a copy of a paper of the same name by Laura K. Kidd and Jane Farrel-Beck, published in *Dress*, 1997 Vol. 24 pp. 27-41.

While the following book title is a tad on the academic side, it could be the most spot-on period book to date. This chapter owes much to it and it should be in the library of any women's studies major:

"Girls in Power: Gender, Body, and Menstruation in Adolescence" by Laura Fingerson, Albany, New York, State University of New York Press.

Special thanks to Maureen Whelihan, MD, gynecological goddess, and to Rear Admiral Anne Schuchat, MD, from the Center for Disease Control and Nina Bender at Whitehall Laboratories for their help on TSS. Also, thanks to Harry Finley at the *Museum of Menstruation* for consultation on the history of sanitary napkins and tampons, and to Jane Farrel-Beck for being so generous with photocopies of her articles! The original negative of the 1920 Kotex ad belongs to the Wisconsin Historical Society.

51

Shaving Down Below

We have managed to put golf carts on Mars and we are engineering cows with genes that nature never intended. But we have yet to find a particularly good way to remove unwanted body hair. In this chapter, we look at temporary methods for removing unwanted body hair, then at permanent methods.

IMPORTANT: *Both of our gynecology consultants have encouraged our women readers who shave to use a bikini trimmer instead. They are not opposed to getting rid of pubic hair, but they are concerned about the extensive amounts of vulvar skin irritation they see due to shaving.*

Body Hair Removal

"I'm more aware of myself and my sexuality when I'm shaved. It feels sensual, like the first time you wear silk underwear. It's too much trouble to keep up, though. If there was an easy way, I think I'd do it more often." *female age 36*

"Shaving is painful and I look about 12 years old, it grosses me out. Trimming works! Borrow a beard trimmer and go for it! One crew cut coming up!" *female age 29*

"My husband really likes to trim my pubic area for me. He gets turned on by this. I think it's highly arousing, too." *female age 45*

Women have shaved or plucked their body hair for thousands of years. However, here in the U.S., the current trend of shaving the female frame got its start in the year 1915, when the Wilkinson Sword Razor company began an ad campaign to convince women their arm-pit hair was unfeminine and unclean. This coincided nicely with the introduction of the first sleeveless evening gowns. Razor sales started to soar.

Now, almost a hundred years later, even men are getting into below-the-neck pruning, although not to the extent of women. It used to be a man who did this was considered limp-of-wrist. Now he's liable to be a member of the football team.

As for sex differences between men and women, a hair follicle is pretty much a hair follicle, there aren't boy ones and girl ones. Some follicles might be more androgen-sensitive and grow a thicker hair, but the underlying mechanism is the same. What is different among the sexes is the timing and predictability of hair growth.

By the time a male is 25, he's got a pretty good idea of how much body hair he is going to have, and where. Not so for women. Nature has reserved the right to play wicked hair tricks on a woman's body at any point during her lifespan. A female reader sums it up quite aptly:

> "I used to have this lovely, neat, wonderfully behaved triangle of pubic hair. And then I turned thirty, and the thing started to spread..."
>
> *female age 32*

Trimming vs. Shaving the Male Crotch?

When we first started asking our sex survey takers whether men trim or shave between their legs, we expected to see a 10% to 20% "yes" rate. We didn't expect to get blown away with 50% and more. Nor did we expect to see nearly total agreement between the men's numbers and the women's assessment of their partner's pubic-hair status. (Men and women can't agree on how much sex they've had with each other, but when it comes to crotch trimming, detente abounds!)

However, while a lot of guys say they trim their pubic hair, most only do it once a month and very few men shave their pubic hair. So there's not even close to equality between men and women when it comes to removing pubic hair.

When men did shave their pubic area, it was usually the scrotum. They report their wives and girlfriends prefer a kinder and gentler scrotum for giving oral sex to. And that's exactly what we heard from female survey takers: they went on and on about how annoying it is to get a pubic hair stuck in the back of their throat. Many of them commented on how much nicer it is to lick and suck on a well-trimmed or shaved scrotum, but they thought it a bit weird if a guy shaved off all of his pubic hair, saying it was like sleeping with a Cub Scout. The women appreciated maintenance as opposed to scorched earth, and they rewarded it by giving more oral sex.

Men with hairy backs and shoulders are likely to shave, wax or laser that part of their body, but we haven't done any surveys on that.

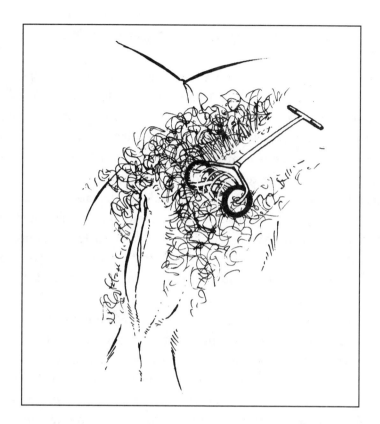

Not Everyone Wants Their Partner Bare

Some people prefer their partners with pubic hair, or at least some of it. One guy says he thinks it's sexy when a woman has more than a tiny landing strip, and a woman tells us she's fed up with her boyfriend's bare scrotum that feels like the fruit on a cactus. So before you go to the pain of waxing or plucking your privates, why not ask your partner what he or she thinks?

Shaving & The Big Myth

Contrary to what you often hear, there is no truth to the myth that shaving results in a thicker hair follicle or increased hair growth. The reason hair might look thicker after you shave or trim it is because you are cutting the hair off at the thickest part, around the base. A normal, full length hair is thickest at the base and tapers toward the tip. So instead of a soft, well-worn tip like that on a fully grown hair, a newly shaven hair will look like a tree stump and have a nasty, sharp edge. En masse, they create the 5 o'clock shadow.

Shaving is by far the safest method of temporary hair removal because it does no damage to the follicle. There are two different kinds of razors to consider, depending on whether you are shaving a large flat area, like your legs, back or chest, or something more rounded, like your face or pubic area.

For chest, back and leg hair, try a woman's razor for leg hair. It doesn't matter if you are male or female, women's razors are often made for large, flat areas. If you are shaving your crotch, you'll want a razor with a head that swivels, like many of the razors that are for men's faces. A razor designed to navigate the chin will make small-time of the scrotum. Experiment and find what is best for your hair and skin type. No matter what parts you are shaving, it may take weeks before your hair and skin settle into an obliging routine.

If you are shaving between your legs, it is often easier to do it in the shower or bath. Or, you can warm the area for several minutes first with a wash cloth. Getting it warm and wet can help make shaving easier. You might try using shaving cream that's for sensitive skin or the "bikini area," although there's little difference between shaving cream that's marketed to women as opposed to men, except for the fragrance. Keep extra cream in the hand that's not holding the razor, so you can reapply it each time you are going over an area that you've already done. You don't want to pull a razor across skin that doesn't have shaving cream on it.

For the first month, you might try shaving in the direction the hair seems to grow in and not against it, although this can be a challenge in the pubic area because the hair often grows in swirls. Be satisfied with an okay job instead of a great job. An okay job means shaving with one stroke or two, and not against the grain.

If you've been at it for a couple of weeks and want to experiment with going against the grain, give it a try. But wait until you get a good sense of the different directions that the hair can grow in, and the price your skin might pay for a perfect shave. Doing an obsessively neat job often results in shaving off some of the skin, especially the little bumps in the skin that frequently populate the labia and scrotum. These are called Fordyce spots.

The skin on your genitals is not as resilient to shaving as the skin on other parts of your body. For that reason, the latest and greatest five-blade razor that works great on your face or legs might behave more like a meat-slicer on your labia or scrotum. It may also be necessary to pull the skin in your pubic area tight in order to get a good shave. Throw a pair of gonads under the surface, and good luck. Assume there will be a learning curve.

A lot of people experience itchiness and discomfort for the first month of shaving. If you have concerns, a dermatologist or a licensed hair-removal professional is good to consult. And if you are using an electric shaver, beware those with rotary heads. They may not be the best choice for pubic hair.

The "pimples" that can form after shaving or plucking aren't pimples at all and should never be popped. (They can take up to five days to form after waxing.) While these are often caused by pockets of pus resulting from bacteria that have gotten into the follicle, they do not have the structure of a pimple. If you are concerned about them, check with your healthcare provider. Antibiotics might be necessary.

To help prevent ingrown hairs *(pseudofolliculitis barbae)*, a number of shaving experts suggest that you exfoliate often. Try using a loofah or skin-scrubbing product, or a liquid exfoliant like Tend Skin. Some people say to do it right before you shave, and others say to do it right after. If ingrown hairs remain a problem, try using an electric razor and shave only every other day. Also check with a dermatologist to come up with the best strategy for your skin type. For one of the best discussions you will ever find about ingrown hairs, click on the "razor bumps" section at www.hairtell.com.

Loofah Note: There is some concern that natural loofahs can harbor bacteria. Some people suggest using synthetic loofah-like materials instead, although there's no science to guide us either way.

Hair on Women's Nipples and Assorted Hair Facts

Number of Hair Follicles: All of the hair follicles anyone will ever have are formed while we are in the womb. The average newborn (and adult) has 2 million hair follicles and sweat glands. Hair follicle density is similar in women and men.

Nipple Hair: It is very common for women to have nipple hair. The hairs around the nipples tend to grow out in pairs and crisscross over each other due to the placement of follicles.

Hormonal Birth Control: Hormonal birth control can impact the growth of body hair. For some women, it can result in less body hair, and for others it can cause more. Pregnancy can cause a hormonally-related increase in body hair. Things usually go back to normal in six to twelve months after delivery.

Inner Lips: The inner labia of some women end up sticking unpleasantly to the sides of their legs when all of their pubic hair is removed. When this is the case, it might be better to use corn starch for a possible remedy as opposed to talc, since partners can't taste corn starch when performing oral sex and talc use in the genitals may cause an increase in cancer. (Check with a gynecologist before putting any kind of powder on your vulva.)

Hair on the Shaft of the Penis: It is not unusual for males to have hair that grows up the shaft of the penis. This might best be taken care of with electrolysis, but few guys will do that. So if you shave your shaft, shave carefully.

Will It Grow in More Thickly?

Shaving hair does not cause it to grow in more thickly. What causes hair to grow more thickly is an increase in hormones related to puberty, pregnancy, menopause and certain metabolic disorders such as PCOS. Medications such as certain inhalers, corticosteroids, some antidepressants, and some hormonal methods of birth control can cause an increase in hair growth, as can an increase in blood circulation.

Other Ways to Get Hair Off

Depilatory: This is a form of chemical warfare that dissolves the hair at the surface of the skin. You've probably heard of Nair. Depilatories don't do any better job than shaving, but some people like them. Others find they irritate the skin. Be sure to follow the instructions. Make sure they are safe to be used on the genitals and never use a depilatory on the scrotum. (There are some hysterical parody reviews on Amazon from men who have supposedly used a depilatory on their scrotum.)

Vaniqa: This is a prescription cream that started life as an anti-cancer drug. The reason it sometimes works on reducing hair growth is because tumor cells and hair follicles have much in common. Vaniqa also helps cure African Sleeping Sickness. So people coming out of near-death comas from sleeping sickness who were treated with Vaniqa might find their unwanted body hair gone as well. Vaniqa only removes body hair on 58% of the women who use it, and only temporarily. What's truly bizarre is that in clinical tests for Vaniqa, more than a third of the women using a placebo cream also had "improved" or "markedly improved" results with their unwanted body hair. Vaniqa hasn't been tested on men, but its safety and effectiveness hasn't been tested when it is applied to pubic hair. Plus, you need to get a prescription and it is expensive.

Tweezing: Contrary to what you might think, tweezing can do nasty damage to the hair follicle. This can be a cosmetic bummer if you radically tweeze your eyebrows and find you are stuck with the bald eyebrow look for life. The most common body parts that get tweezed are eyebrows and nipples. Warm the area with a wash cloth to trick the follicles into relaxing their grip on the hairs. *To prevent over-plucking of eyebrows, www.hairfacts.com recommends you draw the line you would like with a concealer first, then pluck the little villains that reside on the other side.*

Waxing and Sugaring: If you are waxing for the first time, be sure to have it done professionally or by a friend who is highly experienced. Infections and broken hairs can result. If you are a woman, the pubic area seems to be more tender when you are having a period, so wait until later for waxing. If you are a man, be aware there are scrotum-horror stories about the wax pulling off more than pubic hair. If you are going to wax a scrotum, get special wax that is meant for that, and only work in small areas at a time. For either sex, there is no evidence that waxing decreases hair growth, unless it creates scar tissue over the follicles. While some people can go for a month or two between waxings, others have visible hair growth after only a week. Wait at least two hours after showering before waxing, and try not get sweaty for 24-hours after waxing. Facial hair needs to be at least one-eighth of an inch before waxing, while pubic hair needs to be at least one-quarter of an inch. The pain of waxing is often worse the first few times; the pain receptors in the skin don't seem to revolt nearly as much by the third or fourth time if you wax on a consistent basis.

Rotary Epilators: These are electronic torture devices with rows of tweezers that yank hairs out by the root. Some people swear by them, others swear at them. The Braun model comes highly recommended, as does the Cleancut Personal Shaver (formerly called the Seiko Cleancut). People who use the Cleancut recommend getting the companion trimmer. You need to pull the skin tight when using an epilator on your genitals, and the hair has to be long enough for the mechanical tweezers to yank them, but not too long. The most pain occurs the first time you use a rotary epilator. Some of the epilators have a special attachment for the first time which reduces the number of hairs pulled out during each pass.

Threading: This is plucking with a thread. It's a traditional form of removing hair from the faces of Indian and Muslim women.

Bleaching: This isn't a way of removing hair, but trying to make it look less obvious. *Warning: bleaching can make hair look thicker because the bleach gets absorbed inside the shaft and puffs it up. Plus, it can make the hair stick out more from the skin.*

Head Trips? If you are a fan of the naked noggin, you'll find all kinds of head-shaving tips at www.baldrus.com.

Permanent Hair Removal—Electrolysis

With electrolysis, a technician sticks a thin electrified needle into the hair follicle. He or she then zaps it electrically. Think of it as being like sending your hair follicles to the electric chair.

There are three different kinds of electrolysis: galvanic, thermolysis or Flash, and blended. The blend method is a combination of thermolysis and galvanic. It is said to be the best method for removing pubic hair.

An average male might have 25,000 or more hair follicles running from his navel to behind his scrotum. A woman will hopefully have fewer hair follicles, and no scrotum. One of the reasons why it is difficult to estimate how many hours of electrolysis it will take to clear your crotch is the density of hair follicles. Jacob might have only 20 active hair follicles in an area that's the size of a quarter, while his girlfriend might have 200.

When trying to conceptualize hair follicles, think of a cave with a sleeping bear inside. That's because a large number of hair follicles on our bodies are resting at any time. One of the keys to successful electrolysis is being able to start with a full initial clearance. Then follow up with several electrolysis sessions over a course of twelve to eighteen months to zap new hairs that have come out of hibernation since your last appointment.

A knowledgeable electrolysis expert offers the following perspective:

"In the pubic area, there are well over 20,000 hairs packed into that small area, so one would need to remove at least 2,000 hairs just to effect a 10% removal. Proper treatment requires longer and more frequent appointments in the beginning, and tapers off to minutes every 3 to 6 months at the end. If the aggressive schedule is not followed, one could go once a month for an hour for the rest of one's life and only get a minor reduction."

This means that you and an experienced electrolysist need to make a treatment plan and follow it. You'll want to be sure to get total clearance during the initial phase, which will require more and longer sessions at the start. Don't just go in for an hour or two and think it's going to work. Figure on at least ten or twelve hours to tame the wild beaver.

As for the pain, it can vary from almost none to excruciating, depending on the person who is doing the electrolysis, the person who is having the electrolysis done, and the particular part of your body that's being zapped. For instance, logic might tell you it's far more painful to have your scrotum done than the hair at the base of your penis, but the opposite is usually true. You will definitely want to talk to the technician about pain-relief options.

With all of the special handling that goes on during hair removal of the male genitals, it's not unusual for guys to get an erection. Most attendants know about this, and the erection actually helps the process because it stretches the skin more tightly. Even if you don't have an erection, you will find the electrologist will probably ask you to stretch the skin with your fingers to help the process go faster. The problem for guys who want electrolysis on their penis or scrotum is that most electrolysists are women, and not many will work on a guy's crotch.

To find a competent electrolysist who will do crotch hair—especially on a male—here are two possible options: visit the forums at www.HairTell.com, although you'll want to ask for references and be sure the person is licensed and legitimate. (There's never any harm in checking with the state licensing board and the Better Business Bureau to see if there are any complaints on the person.) Also, you might search online for suggestions posted on the subject by M2F transsexuals. They need a lot of electrolysis before they can have bottom surgery, and they usually know who will do it and who is good.

Between Waxing and Electrolysis—Laser Hair Removal

Laser hair removal works best if you have very light skin with dark hair growing out of it. That's because lasers work by targeting the melanin in the hair follicle. This is the compound that gives hair its color. The laser emits a very narrow bandwidth of light that can be absorbed by the melanin in the follicle. The heat that gathers in the melanin then radiates to the rest of the follicle and hopefully fries it. If your skin is olive or dark, or the hair is blond or gray, or the laser isn't well-matched for your skin type or isn't working correctly, the destructive energy can be absorbed by your skin instead of the hair follicle and nasty things can happen. (Forget using lasers for removing nipple hair. You'll end up with a nipple fry, as the dark skin will absorb all of the energy.)

This is why you should always have a test patch done first and not schedule any appointments for at least a week or more to make sure your skin doesn't become pigmented. Then be sure the same attendant does all of your treatments using the same machine.

Also, be aware that no fertility studies have been done to demonstrate the safety of using lasers on a guy's scrotum. (The lack of smooth skin on the scrotum can create its own problems with laser hair removal.) No studies have been done on whether laser hair removal impacts the sensitivity of the clitoris.

The people at HairTell.com have a laser hair removal consultation form you can print out. Take it with you if you are visiting a laser hair-removal center. Please read their suggestions on how to select an electrologist and what to ask.

As for the home hair removal kits, there is not enough science-based information yet to say much about them. Be sure to read the consumer reviews—which tend to be mixed and you never know how many were written by PR people from the manufacturers. Calculate the added costs of replacement cartridges, and don't expect the home units to do as good of a job on pubic hair as professional equipment that costs thousands of dollars. Also, do not expect these to work if you have dark skin or light hair.

Permanent Hair Removal Precaution

This chapter has barely touched the surface of permanent hair removal. If you are considering it, please spend a few hours doing research.

Permanent hair removal can be safe, effective, and satisfying, or it can permanently damage your skin. It can also be painful, and it is almost always time-consuming and very costly. Make the experience work for you by knowing as much as you can before you take off your shirt or drop your pants and plunk down your hard-earned money.

Hormonal Problems that Cause Plentiful Hair Growth

Some hormonal conditions can cause women to have hair so thick on their faces that they need to shave twice a day. Some of these women live in dire fear that they will get into an accident and have to be hospitalized and won't be able to shave their faces. At the same time, there are men who find hairy women to be a sexual turn on.

According to Sarah Rosenthal, author of *Women and Unwanted Hair*, the causes of excessive hair growth in women can include too much androgen secretion (polycystic ovarian syndrome), overactive adrenal glands (such as with Cushing's disease), hair follicles that are too sensitive to androgens, certain drugs (including some oral contraceptives, steroids, and dilantin), insulin resistance, hyperthyroidism, endocrine disorders, genetics, obesity and stress.

If you are bothered by the amount of hair you have, or if you suddenly start growing gobs of new hair, try to find an endocrinologist who specializes in hirsutism. Just because the physician is an endocrinologist doesn't mean he or she is either sympathetic or knowledgeable about hormone imbalances and excessive hair growth.

A Big Thanks to Andrea James for an eye-opening education about getting rid of body hair.

For frequent updates, visit the book's website at

www.GuideToGettingItOn.com

52

Gnarly Sex Germs

The most common reason for reading this chapter is when you are worried about having an infection that you'd rather not have, or when someone you had sex with a few weeks ago just sent you a text that starts with "BTW..."

This chapter provides an interesting look at the STI landscape. STI stands for "sexually transmitted infection." The old term used to be VD or venereal disease, which referred to Venus the goddess of love. But that term fell out of favor and STD took its place. STD stands for "sexually transmitted disease." But the word "disease" isn't totally correct. The more accurate term is infection. However, it's unlikely your crotch will care. Call it whatever you like, just understand that a little prevention can go a long way in keeping you from having to consult this chapter again.

In the pages that follow, you'll see why condoms are effective in preventing some STIs but not others. You'll hear that getting an STI like herpes is not the end of the world. You'll learn why STIs that have no symptoms still need to be treated. And hopefully, you'll remember that HIV remains the mother of all STIs. It's just as easy to get HIV as ever. You want to avoid it at all costs. On the other hand, a new strain of antibiotic resistant gonorrhea has recently surfaced. This is not good. Fortunately, condoms work well in preventing the spread of both HIV and gonorrhea.

Unfortunately, nothing you read in a book can take the place of a seasoned observer armed with fresh lab test results. So if you are concerned about having an STI, be sure to visit a healthcare provider or STI clinic. They'll probably ask you to drop trou. They might take blood, and they'll most likely have you pee in a cup. That's a small inconvenience for the benefits you'll be getting. (See more on this in the section on STI testing.)

Also keep in mind that the information on the pages that follow is just that: information. It is not meant to take the place of diagnosis or treatment by a trained healthcare provider and it is only up-to-date as of press time.

Sometimes, It's a Numbers Game

There would be a big drop in the number of sexually transmitted infections if people dated for a few weeks or months before getting naked together. By then, you would know more about a potential partner than how they fill out their jeans. You might decide "Looked hot, still looks hot, but not someone I'd like to sleep with." Or maybe it would be the opposite, with the erotic tension that's been building paying off in extra pleasure once your pants hit the floor.

Epidemiologically speaking, draining a few cappuccinos together and seeing a movie or two before you round third makes really good sense.

Defining an Acceptable Level of Risk

Each year 32,000 Americans die in car accidents. Thousands more are seriously injured. Yet most of us consider driving to be an acceptable risk. However, if 32,000 people started dying each year from a new sex disease, that was killing straight people, there would be an outcry against sex.

Perhaps we believe there is something inherently good about driving and something inherently bad about sex. Or maybe we get more satisfaction from driving. Whatever the case, you can greatly decrease your chances of being killed in a car accident by not drinking when you drive, by wearing a seat belt, and by driving sensibly. The same is true for sex, except for the seat belt, unless you are into BDSM.

Besides using condoms and being picky about new sex partners, getting checked for STIs is an important way to stay sexually healthy.

Getting Tested for STIs—How, Where and When

Just because a partner looks totally hot and hygienically perfect doesn't mean he or she is STI free. Unless you are in a true-blue never-fool-around relationship, it's smart to get tested every year, even if you have no symptoms.

Two websites that will give you the addresses and phone numbers of nearby testing locations are www.hivtest.org (the Center for Disease Control's site for STIs) and www.plannedparenthood.org. Click on sexually transmitted disease link and enter your zip code. If you're a college student, be sure to call your student health service and ask where you can get tested.

The cost of STI testing can vary, so if finances are an issue, be sure to look for low or no cost testing centers. Along with needing to visually look you over, it's likely they'll have you do a urine test for chlamydia and gonorrhea. If you are pee shy, ask them if you can fill the cup at home, or get an STD test kit from Walmart. Follow the instructions and include a check for $99. If the people at the post office inquire whether the package contains hazardous materials, you don't need to answer yes. They ask everyone that.

If you're a woman, don't assume you're getting an STI test when you get an annual gynecological exam. You need to tell them you want an STI test.

The STIs That Condoms Help You Avoid and Why

Some STIs are spread when the genital secretions from someone who is infected make contact with the mucosal membranes of someone who isn't infected. Other STIs are transmitted mostly by skin-to-skin contact.

Since condoms capture genital secretions, they will help prevent the spread of STIs such as HIV, gonorrhea, chlamydia, and trichomoniasis. They aren't as effective in stopping STIs such as herpes, syphilis and HPV which can be spread by skin-to-skin contact.

STIs and Your Mucosal Membranes

Moist mucosal surfaces are the passageways in and out of the body, such as the urethra (peehole), vagina, mouth and butt. We utilize them when we eat, use the rest room, and have oral sex or intercourse.

If you can keep an infected partner's genital fluids from making contact with your moist mucosal surfaces, you can do a lot to prevent catching some of the worst STIs. Condoms are your best bet for achieving this.

Skin To Skin

Some sexually transmitted infections such as genital herpes and syphilis are known as genital ulcer diseases. They can use the skin for entry into the body, in addition to moist mucosal membranes.

You would think you could tell from looking at a person if they have something as gross-sounding as a "genital ulcer disease." But the ulcers can be so small that it's nearly impossible to see them. At the very least, you might need a bright light and a magnifying glass. Good luck getting a potential partner to take their clothes off and let you do an inspection like that.

Condoms aren't as effective in preventing the spread of genital ulcer diseases because there's lots of skin where the ulcers can be hiding. You'd have to wear a wet-suit version of a condom to get really good protection.

While HPV or human papilloma virus isn't a genital ulcer disease, it's a tough one to prevent the spread of when you are having sex. Condoms can help, but miracle workers they aren't.

Condoms Work Differently for Men and Women

If a male partner is already infected with an STI, the condom works by collecting and isolating the fluids that might drip, seep, or shoot out of his penis. That way, the infected fluids don't make contact with your moist mucus membranes.

If it's the woman who is infected, the condom will keep the STI-infected fluids in her vagina from getting inside the urethra or peehole of the penis.

Good News: Prescriptions for Partners

As of press time, healthcare providers in 32 states were allowed to write prescriptions to treat partners of STI patients without having to examine the partners. With many STIs, treating your partner is as important as getting treatment yourself. Otherwise, you'll just end up with an STI ping-pong effect, where the untreated partner keeps reinfecting the partner who has been treated. Some states will only allow this option for heterosexual partners, due to higher prevalence of HIV and syphilis infections in male-male relationships.

STI Reduction Odds and Ends

Before presenting you with a blow-by-blow summary of each and almost every sex germ, here are some practical issues to consider about keeping yourself safe from sexually transmitted infections:

Monogamy Only Works for Some It would be one thing if people who say they are going to stay monogamous would actually stay monogamous. But that's not how it always works. Don't try to fit yourself into a monogamous square if you belong in a round hole. If there is a chance you or your partner might have sex outside of the relationship, keep using condoms.

When Symptoms Go Away If you have STI symptoms and they suddenly go away, do not assume the disease has gone away. The most common symptom of a sexually transmitted infection is no symptom at all. It is very common to have an STI and not be aware of it.

25 and Under You won't believe how many people who are twenty-five and under get sexually transmitted infections. If you are young and frisky, be sure to get tested for STIs every year.

Pregnancy and STIs? You also won't believe how many women who are single and pregnant get new STIs while they are pregnant or during the first six months after giving birth. One reason is because they figure they can only get pregnant once at a time, so they stop using condoms. If you are pregnant, please remember about STIs and your baby.

Blow Jobs Using a condom while blowing a guy makes sense if you are not in a long-term relationship. Find a brand of flavored condoms that doesn't taste too hideous. (Of all the different condom flavors, no one makes one called "Semen Flavor." Hmmm. Wonder why?) Do not use the same condom for oral sex as for intercourse, because it's easy for your canine choppers to leave little rips in the condom.

Muff Diving Using latex dental dams when going down on a woman is someone's idea of a really bad joke. Using Saran wrap isn't nearly as bad, although you are unlikely to find "Cunnilingus Directions" on the side of the box. And don't use cling wrap version. This is not a family picnic and you aren't trying to keep your partner's pussy freshly sealed for refrigerating and microwaving later. The pluses of using Saran Wrap are you can see through it, your tongue doesn't drag across it, and it has no taste. Have the woman lather some of her own spit on the side of the plastic wrap that you are laying over her vulva, then lay it in place. You will automatically lubricate your side of the wrap with your mouth. Then make her casserole sing.

Cold Sores If you have a cold sore on or in your mouth, you could give herpes to the person you are having oral sex with. So it's best to try finger fucking after you've washed your hands or give a hand job until the cold sore heals up, assuming intercourse is not an option.

Precum When it comes to sexually transmitted infections, precum is just as high-octane as semen. If the penis has an STI, pre-cum will definitely transmit it.

Rimming or Booty Licking Rimming is when you use your tongue on a partner's anus. If you are in a long-term monogamous relationship, you share many of the same intestinal flora, fauna, and bugs, so there's probably not an increased risk associated with rimming that you haven't already incurred. But in more casual relationships, you should be concerned about getting things like hepatitis, E. coli, salmonella, shigella, amoeba, giardia, and cryptosporidiosis.

If you enjoy rimming but aren't in a true-blue relationship, at the very least get a hepatitis vaccination. Straight or gay, you are being a fool if you don't get vaccinated for hepatitis when you enjoy rimming. Using plastic wrap could be an effective preventative for rimming-associated germs, but tongues that like to rim usually prefer to feel the real thing. Another strategy is to hop into the shower first and soap up. A post-doc fellow at UCLA did a study on germs and hand-washing. She discovered that if you soap-up, rinse, and soap-up a second time there will be a substantial decrease in the amount of germs as opposed to soaping up and rinsing only once. The first soaping helps remove the dead layer of skin cells, but it takes the second soaping to get germs that are hiding underneath. This sounds like particularly good advice for when you're licking someone's butt. However, it's far from fool proof, given there's a germ-shedding rectum behind the butt you are licking.

Handjobs The chances of catching an STI from giving your partner a hand job are about the same as breaking your neck from falling out of bed, although you never know about HPV. What you want to avoid is taking a hand that has a partner's sex fluids on it and rubbing it on your genitals, unless neither of you has an STI. You also want to avoid getting a partner's sex fluids into an open cut if you have one.

Intercourse Concerns (Penis into Vagina) It is highly unlikely that the cute fraternity guy you are about to have sex with is going to say, "I'm totally low-risk except for that little butt-fucking incident last month with the captain of the wrestling team." Nor will the former high-school cheerleader you're about to bang admit to having spiked heroin "during my rebellious phase last summer." Great looks and a clean exterior mean nothing when it comes to a partner's ability to give you a sexually transmitted infection.

Pulling Out While pulling a penis out and squirting off to the side may win you the *Birth Control from the Middle Ages Award*, it won't keep you from getting an STI.

When to Bag It? Put a condom on a penis as soon as a guy gets wood. A hard penis starts dripping long before it gets to where it's going.

Intercourse (Anal) The only time you should consider having anal sex without a condom is if you are in a long-term, true-blue relationship and you have no concerns about sexually transmitted infections. In that case, one of the main concerns about barebacking (anal sex without a condom) is even if you wash the penis, tiny bits of fecal matter might still have lodged in the peehole and can end up shooting into the vagina. Barebacking can also be a risk factor for bacterial vaginosis. It is possibly a risk for a male to get a prostate infection, but it's not very likely.

Adding Trust to the Thrust in Anal Sex Sex educators are now adding the word "trust" to discussions about anal sex. That's because people tend to relax their rear ends when they are with a partner they trust. (Can you imagine writing a grant application for a study about that?) If you are on the receiving end of anal sex and you are not relaxed enough, your anal sphincters can clamp a penis so tightly as to rip the condom. That's why they say trust is important. (Why you would let someone you don't trust stick their penis up your rear end is a another story for another time.)

Urine Play If you are not in a monogamous relationship, don't shoot urine into people's body cavities. Using a partner as a urinal is something that should wait for marriage or a long-term relationship.

You Can't Scrub Them Away Washing your crotch or douching will not keep you from getting STIs, although you'll sparkle all the way to the VD clinic. Douching can also lead to bacterial vaginosis and candida.

Increase Your Chances of Getting HIV Being infected with other venereal diseases will greatly increase your chances of getting HIV if you are with a partner who has HIV.

Non-Essential Drugs A healthy immune system can fight certain STIs and keep them from being persistent. But non-essential drugs can tax an immune system. So try to eliminate all non-essential drugs from your body, whether prescribed or recreational. This includes recreational drugs such as meth and cocaine to prescription drugs such as antibiotics and antifungals. If you don't need them, don't take them.

— Sexually Transmitted Infections —
Those That Condoms Help Prevent

Please visit the website of the Centers for Disease Control and Prevention or your local healthcare provider for the most recent information about sexually transmitted infections.

Chlamydia

Chlamydia is caused by a bacteria. You can get chlamydia in your vagina, penis, anus or mouth. It is one of the most common sexually transmitted infections, with almost 3 million new cases in the United States each year.

Chlamydia is called a silent STD because most people who have it don't have any symptoms. If you suddenly start having symptoms, you'll probably assume you just got chlamydia. But you may have had it for some time and your current partner is not necessarily the one who gave it to you.

If most people don't have symptoms, why get treated? Because chlamydia that's left untreated can cause pelvic inflammatory disease, chronic pelvic pain, permanent damage to the uterus and fallopian tubes, ectopic pregnancy and infertility. It can also cause pain during intercourse which can become difficult to resolve. What's startling is how chlamydia can do so much harm without causing the kind of symptoms that would normally send someone to the doctor. This is why if you are sexually active, you should be tested for chlamydia at least once a year.

Chlamydia can be easily diagnosed and treated as long as you and your partner both get treatment. Otherwise, you risk reinfecting each other.

Men who are sexually active need to get tested for chlamydia, even if they have no symptoms. This is especially true if their partner has chlamydia. Otherwise, they'll keep giving it back to each other. The good news is, the test for chlamydia is a simple urine test!

What are the symptoms? If you have symptoms, the most common ones are an unusual discharge, burning and itching. Four out of five women who have chlamydia don't know they have it until they get serious complications such as Pelvic Inflammatory Disease. In more advanced cases, symptoms can include pain in the lower abdomen, nausea, fever and bleeding between periods. For men who do have symptoms, there can be a liquid discharge, painful peeing, or nongonococcal urethritis or NGU. (NGU is an infection or inflammation of the urethra that is caused by something other than gonorrhea, such as chlamydia.)

As long as you are sexually active, you should talk to your healthcare provider or gynecologist about having a yearly urine test for chlamydia.

Using condoms can help decrease your chances of getting and transmitting chlamydia.

Gonorrhea

Gonorrhea is a common STI. It used to be called "the clap." It is caused by a bacteria and grows easily in the warm moist parts of the reproductive tract. In men, that would be the urethra (peehole). In women, gonorrhea can grow in the urethra, cervix, uterus, and fallopian tubes. It can also grow in the mouth, throat, eyes, and anus of either sex. If not treated, gonorrhea can spread into the blood and joints.

Gonorrhea can cause pelvic inflammatory disease in women. This can lead to chronic pain, pus-filled abscesses in the pelvis and sterility. Gonorrhea can increase the risk of having an ectopic pregnancy, and it can increase your chances of getting HIV. Gonorrhea can cause sterility in men.

Men are more likely to have symptoms of gonorrhea than women. These include a burning sensation when they pee, or a white, yellow, or green discharge from the penis. Some men with gonorrhea will find that their testicles become painful or swollen. This is most likely due to epididymitis which is a painful swelling in the tubes leading from the testicles. If you get symptoms from gonorrhea, they will usually show up within one day to two weeks after being infected.

Women usually don't get symptoms from gonorrhea. If they do, they are generally mild and are sometimes mistaken for an infection of the vagina or bladder. Symptoms can include burning or pain when peeing, extra vaginal discharge, and bleeding between periods. Whether a woman has symptoms or not, gonorrhea that is not treated can lead to serious complications including pelvic inflammatory disease, tubal pregnancy and sterility.

Symptoms of rectal gonorrhea can range from no symptoms at all to a sore or itchy butt, discharge, bleeding, or pain when pooping. Infections in the throat usually don't cause symptoms, other than a possible sore throat.

Gonorrhea is becoming drug resistant. There is now only one class of antibiotics that can treat it. It is called Cephalosporin. However, Cephalosporin does not work against the new strain of antibiotic-resistant gonorrhea. This may herald an unfortunate return to the days of old when gonorrhea could land a person in the hospital. The prospects for a good outcome are by no means guaranteed. Fortunately, gonorrhea is one of the STIs that condoms can help prevent, so please use them.

Trichomoniasis: A Vaginal Infection

Trichomoniasis is caused by a parasite. It is the most common curable sexually transmitted infection. There are almost 4 million new cases each year in the United States. More women get trichomoniasis than men. Only 50% of women and 10% of men with trichomoniasis have symptoms. However, people who don't have symptoms can still give trichomoniasis to others.

Trichomoniasis moves from genitals to genitals during sexual activity. It can also be a sneaky opportunist, using an infected person's towel or bathing suit as a medium for entering a new person's crotch. So be careful what you borrow.

Women will tend to get trichomoniasis in their vulva, vagina or urethra. Men will most likely get it in the penis (urethra). When men get symptoms, they might include itching, penile discomfort, burning after urination or ejaculation, and occasional discharge from the penis. When women have symptoms, they often include irritation of the vulva and a discharge that is yellow-green and can have a strange smell. Trichomoniasis can also make sex feel unpleasant.

No one knows why some people have symptoms and others don't. Trichomoniasis can also impact the hands, mouth and anus, but not nearly as often as the genitals.

Trichomoniasis can increase your chances of getting HIV. It can also increases a woman's chances of having a low-birth weight or pre-term birth by approximately 60%.

There's no one sure test for trichomoniasis. Visual inspection is important. Then, if necessary, swabs can be taken, cultures grown, microscopic investigations done, as well as other tests depending on the symptoms.

Trichomoniasis can be eliminated by taking a single dose of metronidazole or tinidazole. As is the case with most STIs, it is easy to get reinfected if your partner isn't treated at the same time. Avoid having sex during treatment, and keep in mind that the reinfection rate is 17% in only three months. Without treatment, the infection can last for months or even years.

Using condoms can help prevent, but not eliminate, the spread of trich.

HIV/AIDS

The human immunodeficiency virus (HIV) attacks the body's T-helper that allow you to fend off infections. AIDS is one of the diseases that you get after HIV shuts down your immune system.

If you get either HIV or AIDS, you will need to take HIV/AIDS drugs for the rest of your life. These drugs are so expensive that a month before press time, the director of the American Public Health Association informed a senate subcommittee that we may at some point need to ration the drugs for HIV/AIDS because the government cannot afford to pay for them. It is not unusual for someone with HIV or AIDS without insurance coverage to pay more than $25,000 a year for HIV/AIDS drugs in North America.

Equally disconcerting are recent reports in the medical journal Lancet that drug-resistant cases of HIV/AIDS are starting to show up. This is not unexpected when more than 8 million people are taking HIV/AIDS drugs.

Is there a single partner on the planet who is sexually hot enough to risk getting such a terrible disease? What remains so mind-blowing is that HIV is usually preventable by using condoms.

HIV is spread through the exchange of body fluids, including blood, semen, pre-cum, vaginal fluids, breast milk and anal mucus. A common way to get HIV is by having vaginal or anal sex with someone who is infected. Infected fluids can get into your bloodstream through microscopic rips or tears in the moist mucous membranes that line the vagina, vulva, penis and rectum. Almost everyone has tiny tears in their moist mucous membranes.

Another common way of getting HIV is through intravenous drug use. Babies can get HIV from their mothers, healthcare workers can get it through accidental needle sticks and cuts. Before better screening tests were available, people could get it by receiving a blood transfusion.

You cannot get HIV from hugging someone who is infected or by shaking an infected person's hand. You can't get it by using the same toilet seat, towel or by sharing the same cups and eating utensils. That's because HIV doesn't survive well when outside of the body.

It is possible but unlikely to get HIV through having oral sex or kissing. It is next to impossible to get HIV through giving a hand job unless you've got a cut on your hand. You can't get HIV from an infected person's saliva. However, if you are kissing them and they have a sore in their mouth that is shedding infected blood-related products and you have a sore that their saliva makes contact with, there is a slight chance that you can get HIV that way. Likewise, you can't get HIV from poop, snot, sweat, tears, urine, or vomit unless there's infected blood in those fluids and it somehow gets into your blood stream.

You can't get HIV from insect or mosquito bites. When an insect or mosquito bites a person, it doesn't inject its own blood or the blood of someone else it has bitten. Instead, it injects its saliva, which does not carry HIV. (No such luck with malaria and yellow fever.)

There are no known cases of getting HIV while playing sports. However, playing around after playing sports is a different story.

Having a sexually transmitted infection such as syphilis, gonorrhea, chlamydia or herpes can greatly increase your chances of getting HIV because they can cause irritation of the mucous membrane. They can also cause sores that HIV can use to get into your blood stream.

As for AIDS, there is still much that we do not know about it. AIDS is one of the most complex and deadly diseases of our time. You are STRONGLY encouraged to do all you can to avoid getting HIV, which is an effective gateway to getting AIDS. The best way to avoid getting HIV is by using condoms unless you are in a relationship with a partner who is not infected and not at risk for becoming infected.

The FDA recently approved a drug called Truvada for the prevention of HIV in people who are at high risk. This would include those whose partners have HIV, those who don't trust the judgment of a partner, and those who don't trust their own judgment. Unfortunately, the protection that Truvada offers is much lower than 100% and you still need to use condoms. Truvada currently costs $1,200 a month, and the side effects can be considerable. So there is the good with the bad. If you feel this drug might be helpful for you or a partner, please speak to a healthcare provider about it.

— Sexually Transmitted Infections —
Those That Condoms Aren't
As Effective In Preventing

Human Papilloma Virus (HPV): The Strains That Cause Genital Warts

Human papilloma or HPV is one of the sexually transmitted infections that condoms might help prevent but not with any degree of certainty. HPV is a virus that lives in the flat cells on the surface of the skin and on the moist mucosal membranes in the body. These include the urethra (peehole), vagina, cervix, penis, anus and throat.

There are at least 120 types or strains of human papilloma virus. While many of the HPV strains cause no symptoms, others can cause warts, like the warts people get on their hands and feet, or on their genitals, anus and thighs. Some of the HPV strains can cause cancer. The cancer-causing strains of HPV are discussed in separate sections that follow.

Approximately forty of the HPV strains are passed through sexual contact. These can infect the genital areas, including the skin around the vulva, cervix, penis or anus. They can also infect the mouth and throat. Most sexually active people will get HPV at some point in their life. It's nearly impossible to avoid. It's also nearly impossible to know who you got HPV from because it usually doesn't have symptoms. Most people never know they have it. You might have only had sex once ten years ago and still not know you have HPV.

One of the fascinating things about HPV is that 90% of people who have it get rid of it on their own within one or two years. It doesn't matter if it is one of the strains that causes warts or cancer. Most people's immune system clears it.

Genital Warts: About 1% of men and women have genital warts at any given time. Most genital warts are caused by HPV types 6 and 11. Genital warts are usually harmless but potentially gross looking. They are small growths that can sprout up on your genitals or anus.

Genital warts seldom hurt, except maybe your pride. Genital warts can be single or in groups. Some are flat, some are raised, some big, some small. Genital warts pose no health risk to you or your partner unless you have HIV. They won't turn into cervical cancer.

It is possible to get genital warts from someone who has no warts and no symptoms. HPV is like that. It can take weeks or months for genital warts to show up after you had sex with an infected partner. Women can get genital warts on their vulva, vagina, cervix, anus or thighs. Men can get them on the penis, scrotum, anus or thighs.

Be sure to have a healthcare provider diagnose whether you have genital warts and discuss the treatment options. Unfortunately, treating the warts won't necessarily make them less contagious.

Treatments to remove genital warts include surgery, medicines and freezing the warts off. One of the treatments is made from an extract of green tea. It is the first botanical to be approved as a prescription drug in the US. None of the treatments for genital warts work better than the others, although one type of treatment might be better suited to your particular situation. Another treatment strategy is to not have the warts treated and see if they go away on their own. Sometimes they do, sometimes they don't.

If you want your warts removed, you can have a healthcare provider do it or you can use a home treatment. Current over-the-counter products for genital wart removal include podofilox and salicylic acid. There may also be homeopathic remedies. A pharmacist should be able to help you find whatever over-the-counter products are available if that's what you decide.

Whether you or your healthcare provider remove the genital warts, the chances are good they will return and you will need to do more treatments.

If you currently have genital warts, you should tell a partner about them and avoid having sex until the warts are gone or removed. However, it's not yet known how long a person can pass on genital warts after the warts are gone. So once the warts have come and gone away, no one knows if you should tell a future partner that you formerly had them. Talk to your healthcare provider about this.

Note: Some healthcare providers will apply a 3% to 5% solution of acetic acid to the skin of your genitals to see if you are HPV-infected. This is not a specific test for HPV and is not recommended.

Human Papilloma Virus (HPV): Strains That Cause Cancer

Cervical Cancer: While the vast majority of HPV strains do not cause cancer, there are a couple of stinker strains that do. Cervical cancer is caused by HPV—mostly strain 16 and 18. What's fascinating is that a lot of women will be infected with these strains of HPV, but their immune systems will clear the infections in an overwhelming majority of women. So there are other factors or cofactors that cause the infection to remain or be persistent in a small minority of women. And even then, less than 20% of women under the age of 55 who have a persistent infection with a carcinogenic strain of HPV will go on to develop cervical cancer.

So an important question is "What causes an infection to go from persistent to cancerous?" Smoking is a significant factor, but women who have never smoked can also get cervical cancer. So there must be something that causes the cancer switch to be thrown: perhaps there's a genetic tendency in your family toward one type of cancer or another, perhaps it's environmental or anything else that impacts a woman's immune system. There is still much that we don't know about cervical cancer.

Fortunately, women can protect themselves from getting cervical cancer by having routine pap smears and getting treatment if necessary. That's because it can take a long time for cervical cancer to develop and the cells on the cervix usually show warning signs. This is why it's so important to get pap smears. If a pap smear is unclear or irregular, a woman needs to follow up as recommended. If abnormal or precancerous cells are found, those areas can be cleared with cryotherapy or freezing. This will prevent the cancer from forming.

Anal Cancer, Vulvar Cancer, Vaginal Cancer, Penile Cancer These are rare cancers that are also caused by certain strains of HPV, particularly #16 and #18. One of the problems with these cancers is there are no methods to detect them early. Once they get bad enough to send the person to the doctor, they are often far along and can be difficult to treat.

Certain Oral Cancers: Cancer of the Tonsils and Cancer of the Back of the Tongue: Please see the section that follows on the next page.

HPV Vaccines: There are currently two HPV vaccines. One was designed to protect against the two strains of HPV that cause cervical cancer, HPV # 16 and HPV #18. The second vaccine was designed to protect against the HPV strains that cause genital warts in addition to cancer. Unfortunately, we don't yet know for sure if the vaccines will fulfill their promise of eliminating cervical cancer. We won't know that for another decade or two. However, it's now been almost ten years since the first group of human test subjects were vaccinated, and the vaccines appear to be performing as expected, which is encouraging. On the other hand, women will still need to get Pap smears, and whether a woman is vaccinated or not, most cervical cancers can be prevented with routine gynecological care. If you are under the age 26 and are interested in taking the HPV vaccines, speak with your healthcare provider.

Oral Sex and HPV-Positive Oral Cancer?

Years ago, researchers discovered that strains 16 and 18 of the human papillomavirus caused most cervical cancers. They also found that women who had a greater number of sexual partners had a higher risk for getting cervical cancer. So when researchers recently discovered that cancer of the tonsils and cancer of the back of the tongue could be caused by HPV as well as by smoking and drinking, they started asking questions about sexual behavior. As it turned out, some of the studies showed that people who had the oral cancers that were associated with HPV had a higher number of oral sex partners than people who didn't get these cancers. So it seemed reasonable to claim that oral sex was the cause of HPV-positive oral cancers. Researchers also noticed that the HPV-positive oral cancers, although uncommon, were on the rise. This matched nicely with the idea that oral sex must be the cause, because oral sex has become increasingly popular during the last fifty years.

A headline-grabbing oral-sex panic was in the making. Captions such as the following from CBS News in 2011 were becoming common: "Oral sex now main cause of oral cancer" followed by "What's the leading cause of oral cancer? Smoking? Heavy drinking? Actually, it's oral sex." It wouldn't be long before an exuberant HPV-oral cancer researcher would be releasing advisories to the media that parents should warn their children about the dangers of oral sex.

What the media forgot to mention is the average age of people who are diagnosed with HPV-related oral cancer is sixty-one years. This means it will be thirty-five to forty-five years before today's teenagers start getting oral cancer—if they get oral cancer, which very few will. The chances of a teenager being killed in a car wreck during the next thirty years are almost a million times greater than the chances he or she will die from oral cancer during that time.

The media also forgot to report that billions of people have had oral sex with multiple partners, yet only a tiny percent have gone on to have an

HPV-positive oral cancer. Clearly, something else is involved besides just oral sex. Otherwise, oral cancer would be the most common cancer on the planet instead of being one of the most uncommon.

Contrary to the reader-grabbing headlines, we don't yet understand what leads to persistent HPV infection in the throat and mouth, and we don't understand why a very small group of people who do get persistent oral HPV infections will go on to develop oral cancers. We also don't know why men get HPV-related oral cancers at a much higher rate than women. Fortunately, oral cancer is an uncommon cancer, being number 14 on the list of cancers that women get and number 8 on the list of cancers that men get. And a significant percent of these cancers are caused by tobacco and alcohol rather than HPV. This will continue to be the case as long as people smoke, drink, and chew tobacco. Unfortunately, oral cancers can be devastating regardless of the cause.

According to the National Institute of Health, while HPV is certainly involved with some of the oral cancers, we don't know yet how it's involved, as we do for cervical cancer. This is a different story than has been presented in the media. As for the role of oral sex, one study concludes: "...oral sexual contact in the form of both oral-oral and oral-genital contact could play a role in the transmission of oral HPV." That's the most we currently know. It will probably be years before we know the rest of the story. *If you have any concerns about HPV or any other infection, please consult with a physician.*

Genital Herpes

Herpes is a virus, not a bacteria. There is no cure for it, although antiviral drugs can help with the symptoms. Condom use can reduce the risk of transmitting herpes by half, and antibiotics are totally ineffective against herpes.

Genital herpes is transmitted through sexual contact including intercourse, oral-genital contact, and rubbing naked genitals together. Seventy percent (70%) of new herpes cases are transmitted by someone who shows no obvious symptoms. Most genital herpes symptoms are mild. They are easy to miss.

Many people who get herpes fly into a panic when they are first told, thinking it's the end of their sex lives. Before we get into the nuts and bolts of herpes, please take the following section to heart.

Herpes in Perspective — It's Not Leprosy!

Many people know that cold sores or fever blisters in the mouth are a form of herpes, but they assume that genital herpes is so much worse. Yet these two forms of herpes are very similar—and the symptoms each causes are also similar. So why do we need special dating sites for people who have herpes in the crotch, but not for people who have herpes in the mouth? Why the added stigma for genital herpes?

On the website of the American Social Health Association, it says that most of the 50 million Americans who have genital herpes do not even know they have it. According to the CDC, most individuals with genital herpes have very mild signs that they don't even notice. Yet people behave as if genital herpes is a terrible disease. Perhaps that's because it shows up below the belt as opposed to above.

This is not to minimize the impact of genital herpes. The symptoms can be severe for some people. So if you know you have it, you need to inform a potential partner before you have sex. And if you don't have herpes, try to protect yourself from getting it. But if you are searching for perspective, the same should be true for oral herpes.

Oral herpes resides in a part of the body that is much closer to the brain than genital herpes. Some researchers are starting to worry about a possible connection between oral herpes and Alzheimer's. As upset as people are about genital herpes, no one has ever suggested it could someday cause you to lose your mind.

So please, if you find out you have genital herpes, learn all you can about it, stay healthy, and try to keep it in perspective.

The Different Types of Herpes

Herpes Simplex Virus 1: Oral Herpes The most common form of herpes is Herpes Simplex Virus 1 (HSV1), which causes cold sores on the lips, nose, chin and other parts of your face. People usually get HSV1 during childhood and most symptoms go unnoticed because they are minor. About 56% of people over age 14 in the US display evidence of a previous HSV1 infection when their blood is tested.

Herpes Simplex Virus 2: Genital Herpes HSV2 is associated with genital herpes infections. About 16% of people in the US over the age of 13 show evidence of HSV2 infection when their blood is tested. Of those infected with HSV2, only about 10% know it.

Genital Herpes is classified into 3 categories:

Non-primary: This is a first-episode infection of HSV2 or genital herpes in someone who has previously been infected with HSV1 (cold sores, etc.). Symptoms are less severe and may go unnoticed. As many as 80% to 90% of first-time genital outbreaks go unrecognized.

Primary: This is an outbreak of genital herpes in someone who has never had HSV1 or HSV2. Primary symptoms are sometimes severe and can range from headaches, aching joints, tiredness, fever, pain in the legs, and flu-like symptoms. The lymph nodes in the groin can become enlarged and tender. Lesions and sores may appear in the throat or mouth. Genital symptoms may also include sores, painful urination as well as itching and discharge from the penis or vagina. The sores begin as blisters, then break open to form ulcers in the skin. Women may not notice sores on their labia. They will normally have lesions on their cervix as well. Men may have lesions inside their urethra. Frequently, a new crop of lesions will appear 5 to 7 days after the 1st batch.

Recurrent Infection or Flare Ups: Flare ups occur at the same site or near it in people who have had previous HSV infections. For genital herpes, this includes having outbreaks anywhere in the "boxer shorts" area. That's because herpes hibernates in the nerves, and a single group of nerves supplies the genitals, thighs, lower abdomen, rectum and buttocks. Herpes can move along that group of nerves and cause an outbreak anywhere on the skin where those nerves go. So while some people will have outbreaks in the same location, others might have a new outbreak on their thigh or rear end or lower abdomen. This also means you don't need to have had anal sex for an outbreak to occur around your anus. During the first year, it is not uncommon to have four or five recurrences. The average recurrence lasts 2 to 10 days. However, the recurrences can be so mild that people are hardly aware of them.

Luck of the Draw: While most people with herpes have symptoms that range from extremely mild to moderate, some people with herpes have symptoms that are severe. Talk to your healthcare provider about medications that can help reduce the severity of future flare ups.

Timing of Herpes Infection vs. Timing of Outbreak

A person could have herpes for thirty years, not know it and then have their first recognized occurrence. When they finally do have an outbreak that they can recognize, it can cause unwarranted suspicions of infidelity. Ouch!

Oral Herpes in the Genitals

Oral herpes (HSV1) now causes about one-third of the first-time genital herpes outbreaks. The way this happens is when someone with a cold sore or other kind of oral herpes gives a partner oral sex. So the partner can get a case of oral herpes in the neighborhood where genital herpes usually lives.

At the start, the partner is unlikely to notice much of a difference in how the oral herpes behaves. It will seem just like genital herpes. However, because it's not genital herpes, it won't have the same affinity for the nerves in the genitals as genital herpes would. As a result, the person whose genitals get infected with oral herpes is much less likely to have recurrences.

Other Herpes Information

Prodrome: *Prodrome* is a set of symptoms that occurs before an actual outbreak is present. Itching, tingling, a crawling under the skin feeling, pain down the leg or in the butt are some of the symptoms. About half of the people with genital herpes experience prodrome.

Triggers: Things that can trigger a herpes outbreak include menstruation, sunlight, pregnancy, birth control pills, diet, friction (prolonged intercourse, oral sex or masturbations), stress, illness, and heat.

Tests for Diagnosis: Visual inspection and viral cultures can be done to diagnose herpes if there are sores. The problem with viral cultures is that they give false negative results up to 76% of the time. This means that up to 76% of the time, when a viral culture comes back negative the person really does have herpes. All negative cultures should be followed up by a more accurate blood test 3 to 4 months after possible exposure. Blood tests can also be done when you are between outbreaks, although according to the CDC, the results are not always clear-cut.

Treatment: The following medications are available to help alleviate the symptoms of herpes: Acyclovir, Valtrex, Famvir and CS 21 Barrier Genital Gel. 80% to 90% of people who take the drugs have greatly reduced frequency of outbreaks or do not have outbreaks while taking the drug. If a woman should become pregnant while taking an antiviral medication, she should discontinue its use and inform her healthcare provider.

Transmission: The greatest concern sexually has to do with transmitting the virus to another person. Intercourse should be avoided completely during outbreaks for maximum safety when one partner is infected and the other is not. Even though someone who has herpes has never had severe symptoms, a person they give it to could have severe symptoms.

Pregnancy: According to the CDC, the infection of a baby with herpes from a pregnant mom is very rare. However, if a woman has active genital herpes at the time of delivery, a C-section will often be performed as a precaution. Pregnant women who are considering having sex with a new partner should be aware that contacting herpes late in the pregnancy can substantially increase the chance of transmitting herpes to the baby. The baby's chances of dying or being developmentally disabled from neonatal herpes are much greater when the mom is first infected with herpes when she is in the third trimester of pregnancy. If the mom was infected with herpes before she got pregnant or before the third trimester of pregnancy, the chances are good her immune system will help protect the infant."

Herpes and HIV: Like most sexually transmitted infections, herpes can increase your chances of getting HIV and it can make people who have HIV more infectious.

Disclosure to a New Partner

It is essential to disclose your herpes status to a new sexual partner prior to having sex. Give them the chance to make an informed decision about the future of their own health. Let them know that even if you don't have active symptoms, you can still give them herpes. If you don't tell your partner until after sex, they have good reason to question your integrity and your ability to be trusted. If you are having casual sex, keep in mind that people who have herpes seldom inform casual-sex partners about it.

Herpes Resources

By far, the best online resource for herpes is the Westover Heights Clinic: www.westoverheights.com/herpes/the-updated-herpes-handbook/. You can download the *Updated Herpes Handbook* for free. It is updated frequently by its authors, Terri and Ricks Warren. You can also phone the National Herpes Hotline at (919) 361-8488 or the National STD Hotline at (800)227-8922.

Hepatitis A, B, or C

Hepatitis refers to a chronic inflammation of the liver. While you can have hepatitis without ever knowing it, hepatitis can also lead to liver failure and to cancer of the liver. So hepatitis has many forms, from a silent infection that your body clears without needing treatment, to a disease that can easily kill you.

Hepatitis is usually caused by one of six viruses that are not related to each other. Hepatitis can also be caused by heavy alcohol use as well as medications, toxic chemicals, and certain illnesses.

The word "hepatitis" simply refers to a liver that is damaged, as opposed to what is causing the damage. This is different from STIs like herpes, HPV, and HIV, which are named after the specific microorganism that causes them. Also keep in mind that while alcohol abuse can cause hepatitis all on its own, a hepatitis virus can damage your liver without you ever having had a drink.

The reason why hepatitis can be so devastating is because we rely on the liver to filter out toxins in the body and to produce bile to help break down fat. There is no living without a liver.

The six viruses that cause hepatitis are often lumped together in discussions like this one because they all impact the liver. But they are by no means the same. This is why reading about hepatitis can be confusing. Just trying to understand the different ways the viruses are spread can cause your liver to ache. One of the hepatitis viruses is spread by fecal contamination and by oral-anal contact. One is spread by regular sex and kissing or sharing a toothbrush. Another is only spread by contact with infected blood. Three of the viruses are common in North America (hepatitis A, B, and C) while the others are more common in other parts of the world. There are vaccines that help prevent two of the viruses, but not for the other four.

Hepatitis A is primarily spread through fecal contamination, so beware rimming or having anal-oral contact with strangers or casual sex partners. You can also get hepatitis A by eating food and drinking water that is contaminated with microscopic pieces of poop.

Hepatitis B is found in infected blood, semen, saliva and vaginal secretions. So it is spread through sexual contact including kissing, and it can be spread by contact with the blood of an infected person. This would include intravenous drug use, sharing needles, sharing razors for shaving and even through sharing a toothbrush.

Hepatitis C is the most common blood borne infection there is. It is primarily transmitted through injection of blood (blood transfusions, drug use and accidental needle sticks in healthcare settings). It is possible that hepatitis C can be spread through sex and through sharing razors or a toothbrush, but these are not very efficient ways of transmitting hepatitis C.

A lot of people who have hepatitis don't experience symptoms, but others do. These are the same kinds of symptoms that people have when their liver is failing or not functioning correctly. They can include abdominal pain, dark urine and clay-colored poop, jaundice or yellowing of the skin and whites of the eyes, fever, fatigue, loss of appetite, nausea, vomiting and joint pain.

Symptoms can last from weeks to months or longer. Some kinds of hepatitis infections will clear up on their own, others won't. People who have no symptoms can still be carriers of one of the viruses.

Getting vaccinated for hepatitis A and B viruses is a really good thing to do even if you are a total virgin. It can be even more important if your sexual boundaries are a bit porous or you enjoy barebacking and rimming. Condom use might help decrease the spread of hepatitis B, but condoms are of only limited help in preventing other hepatitis viruses.

Syphilis

Syphilis is caused by a bacteria. It is transmitted when you make contact with a syphilis sore that is on a partner's genitals, vagina, anus, rectum, mouth or lips. A lot of people with syphilis don't have symptoms but are at risk for serious harm if the syphilis is left untreated. Syphilis can also increase the chances of getting HIV by two to five times.

Syphilis is one of the most famous sexually transmitted diseases in history. At one time, when there was no treatment for syphilis, half of the hospital beds in the world were filled with patients who had syphilis. (See the history of syphilis at the end of this chapter.)

Syphilis infections occur in stages. The first stage is a painless open sore or sores on the genitals, rectum or mouth. These are called chancres. They disappear in a few weeks. The second stage starts as the chancres are disappearing or have disappeared. During this stage, people often develop a rash, especially on the hands and feet. However, the symptoms can mimic those of so many other diseases that syphilis is sometimes called the great imitator.

If left untreated, syphilis goes into a hidden or latent stage for 3 to 40 years. Then, people can get *late stage* or *tertiary syphilis*. This can result in severe damage to the heart, brain, nerves, bones, eyes, organs and muscles.

Syphilis is easy to detect by blood test and sometimes with direct observation. Syphilis is also easy to treat during its early stages with penicillin. Condoms are not very effective in stopping the spread of syphilis.

While not many people get syphilis today, this disease can be so devastating in its late stages that it is important to get tested for it every year if you are sexually active and not in a monogamous relationship. Pregnant women should always get tested for syphilis, because it can be passed on to the baby with devastating results.

Bacterial Vaginosis (BV)

Bacterial vaginosis is a puzzling condition. While it is the most prevalent vaginal infection in women of reproductive age, the latest research is indicating that it may be overly diagnosed.

Researchers are not yet certain whether BV is a sexually transmitted infection, although the evidence does stack up in that direction. Symptoms for BV can range from little or no symptoms at all to a creamy discharge, a fishy smell after intercourse, itching and painful peeing.

When a woman has bacterial vaginosis, the pH of her vagina is usually higher or more alkaline than normal, although some women's vaginas are more alkaline than others and this should not be automatically associated with bacterial vaginosis. With bacterial vaginosis there may be several more types of bacteria in the vagina than is normal, however, it is normal for many women to have more types of bacteria than was originally thought.

BV increases a woman's chances of getting pelvic inflammatory disease. It can also endanger pregnancies, cause premature birth, premature rupture of membranes and inflammation of fetal membranes, pelvic inflammatory disease, and it can increase your chances of getting HIV and other STIs.

While antibiotics are the treatment of choice, they are not effective in 15% to 20% of women. Recurrence rates are as high as 75% in only a year's time.

Risk factors for getting BV include recently douching, having a new sex partner, sex with multiple partners (either male or female), having sex with another woman, sharing insertive sex toys, recently using sex lube, and not using condoms. It is important to carefully clean sex toys and not share them. Anything that's been in a woman's anus should stay far away from her vagina. It is recommended women abstain from vaginal sex during treatment for bacterial vaginosis. Using condoms during the first month after treatment will possibly help.

Currently, treatment of the male partner has not improved BV-related outcomes in women. Douching is not recommended in any way, shape or form, and various "yogurt cures" and probiotics have not proven effective. Most preparations that are intended to help acidify the vagina have not been shown to be helpful in clinical trials for the treatment of bacterial vaginosis.

There is a great deal of research being done on BV. These recommendations might have changed by the time you are reading this, so be sure to check with your healthcare provider. The hope is that with time and research, we will understand how to manage the vaginal environment in ways that promote health rather than often having to use antibiotics.

If you are interested in learning more about the normal bacterial cultures in the vagina, see Chapter 49: *A Trip Inside Amber's Vagina*.

Yeast Infections or Candida Albicans (Thrush)

Candida is a fungus that normally occurs in the body. Symptoms of candida can include itchy genitals and a heavy, whitish, clumpy discharge that can smell like yeast. The discharge almost always looks like cottage cheese.

Candida is not really a sexually transmitted infection because most healthy people have at least some of it. Also, people who have never had sex can get a candida or thrush infection. Something needs to disturb the body's natural balance for a candida or thrush infection to occur.

Up to 75% of women get candida or thrush in their genitals at least once in their life, although you can also get it in the mouth and on the skin. 40% to 50% of women have a reoccurrence of candida.

Most women have no identifiable precipitating factors that lead to candida. It would probably be easier to list the things that candida is not associated with than the things it is associated with. Recurrent candida has been associated with spermicide use, douching and using feminine hygiene products (especially panty liners). Candida can be caused by wearing anything that's tight enough to cause a camel toe, including tight jeans, leotards, swimwear and panty hose, but not the crotchless kind (thank goodness!). Candida has also been associated with vaginal intercourse and possibly receiving a healthy amount of oral sex, taking antibiotics, using birth control pills (especially those with higher amounts of estrogen), with being pregnant, having diabetes, and with yogurt consumption or a diet heavy in carbs.

Women are often misdiagnosed as having candidas when they actually have genital herpes, linchen planus, recurrent bacterial vaginosis, contact dermatitis, atrophic vaginitis or a urinary tract infection. Women who are self-treating for candidas are often treating themselves for the wrong thing.

As of press time, treating a partner was not recommended unless a woman is getting recurrent infections or a man has a form of candida called balantitis or a yeast infection of the foreskin.

— Mites, Lice and Things That Crawl —
Condoms Are of No Help in
Preventing the Spread of These!

The Louse Family (aka Lice)

There are three different kinds of louses or lice that can take residence on the human body. One is the head louse that gets onto your head. The other is the body louse that gets on your body minus your head and pubic area. The third is the pubic or crab louse, which is the perv of the group because it lurks in the bush around your genitals. While all three louses can be spread by intimate contact, the pubic louse is the one that's consider to be sexually transmitted.

Each of the louses has adapted to the part of the body where it lives, so it's unusual for a louse to be living outside of its normal hood. You generally won't find a head louse living where body or pubic lice live. It's unusual for a body louse to be living above your shoulders or below your belt. And if there's a pubic lice on your eyebrows, eyelashes or beard, you may have gotten it while you were giving head because pubic lice normally prefer to be in your pubes.

The reason lice cause a person to itch is because they inject saliva into the skin before they suck the blood out. This is to keep the blood from clotting as they draw it up. It's probably your body's reaction to the lice's saliva rather than the actual blood sucking that can make you itch to the point of near insanity.

In the next three sections, you'll discover much about the three different kinds of lice. This will give you interesting things to talk about the next time you have dinner with your partner's family.

Pubic Lice (aka Crab Lice)

Pubic lice are called crab lice because they look like crabs when under a microscope. They are broader and flatter than their cousins, the head and body lice, which look more like tiny beetles.

You will know you have pubic lice when you find yourself needing to scratch so badly that you'll even do it in front of friends or co-workers. However, you can have crab lice for two to six weeks without experiencing any symptoms or itching. That's probably because your body's immune system hasn't yet learned to pitch an itchy fit when the crab lice injects its saliva into your skin. This means you can infect others without knowing you have crab lice. Fortunately, crab lice do not transmit disease, although you can get a bacterial infection from scratching yourself too much.

Lice related discomfort might be worse at night because lice are apparently nocturnal, or at least head lice are. The day-night cycle might be less of an issue for crab lice, given they live where the sun don't shine.

Crab lice are usually transmitted through acts of sexual congress. While it's possible to get crab lice from sharing clothes, towels or bed linens, the lice don't live for long when away from the warmth and blood of their human brethren. Plus, they can't hop like fleas do, so it generally takes an actual groin grinding for crabs to move from person to person.

People with shaved pubic hair are probably less likely to get pubic lice because there's less of what pubic lice need to hold onto. However, no studies have been done on this subject, so no one really knows. In other words, don't go shaving your pubic hair for the sole purpose of avoiding crab lice.

Each of the lice's six legs have claws for feet that are especially made to grab onto hair. This makes crab lice phenomenal at holding on to pubic hair. However, lice aren't nearly as epic when it comes to staying on a glossy surface like a toilet seat. This is why you can't get crab lice from toilet seats.

Dogs, cats, birds and livestock have their own unique families of lice that don't like the taste of human flesh. So you can't blame a case of crab lice on the family dog, even if you and the dog have an especially close relationship.

Crab lice organization is somewhat like that of a fraternal order. The female lice will lay 30 eggs or nits during their lifetime, which lasts about a month. If the eggs hatch, a mini-me version of the adult crab lice will emerge which is called the 1st nymph. After the 1st nymph sucks enough blood, it molts and becomes a bigger version of itself, which is called the 2nd nymph. The 2nd nymph will suck more blood until it molts and becomes the 3rd nymph, which will suck more blood until it molts and becomes a full-fledged adult or grand master louse, which will suck even more blood until it grows old and dies. As soon as the former female nymphs become mature enough, they will have sex and start laying eggs in your pubes.

Treatment for crab lice is available over-the-counter. Follow the instructions carefully and be sure that you and anyone who you've had sex with during the past month is treated. You might be instructed to use a special nit comb or a tight flea comb to get the nits or eggs out. Wash any clothes, towels and bed linens that you've used in the last two or three days in hot water and put them in a hot dryer. If you have clothes or bedding that you've made contact with that can't be washed, you can save on dry cleaning costs by putting them in plastic bags for two weeks. The nits will hatch within 10 days, but they can't live after hatching for more than two or three days without having a human groin to grab on to.

The louse literature from the CDC says it's only "occasionally" that someone will get crab lice from clothing or linens, given how lice die in one or two days after falling off a person. Also keep in mind that a lice infection is not the end of the world. There's no need to fly into an obsessive-compulsive panic and wash everything in the house. Lice are not a sign of having a dirty house. Lice don't care if you are dirty or clean. They are much more interested that you have sex with different people so their species can keep marching on.

Be extra careful about the treatment if you have lice or nits on your eyebrows or eye lashes. The usual treatment is toxic to the eyes. You might be able to get the nits and lice with your fingernails or a nit comb. If not, you'll need to use ophthalmic-grade petrolatum ointment to the eyelids to suffocate the crabs with.

There is a fairly high association of other STIs with crab lice. So if you were with a partner who gave you the crabs, it's wise to get checked for other sexually transmitted infections.

Head Lice

Head lice are about the size of a sesame seed. They can live on your head, eyebrows and eyelashes. The females cement their eggs to the shaft of the hair follicles. It's easy to confuse head lice with dandruff or flaky scalp.

Head lice will generally make your scalp itch. They tend to be night owls, so you are more likely to feel a tickling sensation on your head at night. The only disease that head lice can spread is social annoyance, so if the school calls and says your kid has head lice, there's no reason to rush and pick him or her up. By the time a diagnosis has been made, the head lice have most likely been there for a few days or weeks. Simply pick up some head lice medication on your way home.

The little pincers of head lice are designed to hold onto the shaft of actual hair, so it's unusual for them to be on hats or clothing. The way people usually get head lice is from making head-to-head contact. Not from borrowing someone's cap, hat or helmet. So you are more likely to get head lice from sleeping together than from wearing your partner's clothes.

The traditional treatment for head lice is an over-the-counter medication that has pyrethrin in it, but there are rumors that modern head lice have become wise to pyrethrin. So do a browser search on the latest research about head lice (as of press time, the best work was being done by Dale Pearlman). Check out the reviews for products on Amazon as well as with your physician, although it's surprising how many physicians aren't up on the latest research about head lice.

If you get a reinfestation, it's probably because you didn't get all of the lice out of the person's head to begin with. So don't get all crazy about washing and fumigating every square inch of the house. Head lice don't live for long once they exit your cabasa. One or two days with no blood and heat from a human head, and the louse is history.

Focus your washing and drying efforts on the clothing and bed linens that an infested person wore or used in the last two days prior to treatment. Using hot water and high heat in the dryer will do the job, or maybe just ten minutes in the dryer. Again, check out the latest research about this.

There's no need to give the family dog or cat a bath. Lice that like human heads want nothing to do with dogs, cats and other pets. However, you do want to soak any of your family members' combs and brushes in hot soapy water for at least fifteen minutes (130 to 140 degrees) or soak them in Lysol for an hour.

If you think it will help, vacuum the carpets and furniture in the area where the infected person sat or lay. However, the CDC says the risk of getting infested by lice that are in your carpet or on your furniture is very small. That's because head lice don't hop. So they can't act like fleas and leap on you from the carpet or furniture. Your carpet and furniture will soon become a cemetery for any louse that falls on it.

Body Lice

Body lice live and lay eggs on your clothing. They only move to your skin when they are hungry and want to feed. Treatment for body lice is simple. It revolves around removing the body lice from their immediate habitat, which is usually your clothes. So all that is generally needed is good personal hygiene, washing your clothes and wearing clean clothes on a regular basis.

Scabies

Saying "scabies" is much easier than saying *Sarcoptes scabiei var. hominis,* which is the name of the parasitic mite that causes scabies. The scabies mite is a tiny arachnid that is barely visible to the human eye. The male and female scabies only mate once. That's all it takes for the female to be fertile for the rest of her life. Thank goodness it's not the same for human females.

Scabies-related nastiness begins when the female burrows under a person's skin to lay her eggs. Every day, two or three of the newly hatched mites will crawl out from under the skin and make short burrows on the surface of the skin called moulting pouches. The skin will respond by breaking out into a pimple-like rash that's made up of red pustules that can be very annoying and itchy. It's also possible that the eggs and mite poop that are in the upper layer of the skin can cause itching.

You can have scabies for four to six weeks before you start having symptoms. But if you've had scabies before, the symptoms will often appear much sooner if you are reinfected. People who are infected but don't yet have symptoms can pass on scabies to others.

Aside from the garden variety type of scabies, there are Crusted Norwegian Scabies which are highly contagious. This kind of scabies often targets people whose immune systems are compromised. These scabies form crusts which are highly infectious.

While scabies have an affinity for skin around the genitals, scabies can inhabit virtually anyplace on your body. They particularly look for skin folds, like on wrists, elbows, armpits, fingers, toes, nipples and knees.

Since scabies outbreaks can occur in preschools and nursing homes, transmission of scabies is by no means limited to sexual activity. However, rubbing a scabies-infested crotch against a partner's uninfected crotch is a way to share the scabies love. Scabies can also spread via clothing, towels and bedding, but the risk is not very high unless the person has crusted scabies. Then, all bets are off.

Scabies is treated with a cream or lotion that's called a scabicide. Unfortunately, you can only get scabicides by prescription. Follow the instructions carefully. All sexual partners and other household members should be treated, especially anyone who has had prolonged skin-to-skin contact with a person who is infected. The itching should stop in two to four weeks. If it doesn't, reapply.

Never use a treatment for scabies on humans that is intended for animals. While animals do have scabies, they have a different kind than humans. Humans can not get scabies from animals.

Scabies cannot live away from human skin for more than two to three days. So when it comes to clothes and bedding, you can either wash them in really hot water and use a hot dryer, or simply wait at least 72 hours as long as there is no human contact with the infected items. In 72 hours, the scabies on clothes and bedding will have died. So fumigation and dry cleaning are not necessary.

Other Sexually Transmitted Infections

When it comes to new diseases, we don't know what's out there. So rather than focusing on one type of disease, why not try to keep your entire body healthy? First and foremost, this means not doing recreational drugs such as crystal meth, poppers (nitrile inhalants) or shooting anything into your veins. The reason for avoiding recreational drugs is that there is a strong association between using recreational drugs and getting sick. People who party and do drugs tend not to use condoms, nor do they always exercise the best judgment.

Keeping your entire body healthy means staying fit, eating well and avoiding all non-essential drugs, including antibiotics if you don't need them. If you aren't monogamous, it means using condoms during oral and vaginal intercourse as well.

Anyone who has been in more than one sexual relationship during the past year should have a check-up for sexually transmitted infections. Talk to your healthcare provider about a throat culture if you have been performing oral sex and a rectal culture if you've been taking it up the rear. It's a good idea to get routine checkups even if you use condoms and don't have symptoms, or if you had symptoms but they went away.

Know yourself, enjoy yourself, and protect yourself.

Gnarly Sex Germs in History

Some people believe that AIDS is the most deadly sex disease that ever was. Sadly enough, the prize goes to syphilis. Even a couple of popes died from syphilis.

Before 1492, when Columbus came to America, there had been no recorded cases of syphilis in Europe. But syphilis did exist in the part of the New World where Columbus and his crew landed. Shortly after Columbus's return, a vicious strain of syphilis began to spread throughout Europe, quickly killing a sizable portion of the population. Smallpox got its name because the lesions it caused were small compared to those of syphilis, "The Great Pox." During its first fifty years in Europe, from about 1493 until 1550, syphilis was a savage killer.

In what may have been one of the first recorded instances of biological warfare, the Spanish army seems to have sent syphilitic prostitutes to infect the Italian army.

After 1550, syphilis went from being a quick killer to a slow killer, more like the syphilis we know today. Instead of finishing off its victims in short order, syphilis began to linger in the body for years after the initial infection, eventually targeting organs like the heart or brain. Syphilis remained a potent killer for four hundred more years (from 1550 to 1940).

In the 1920s, a medical doctor received the Nobel Prize for infecting syphilis patients with malaria. The high fever caused by the malaria helped burn out the stubborn syphilis infection. Unfortunately, there was no cure for the new cure. Some scientists speculate that more people died from the attempts to cure syphilis than from syphilis itself. Until the discovery of antibiotics, popular syphilis therapies included treatment with arsenic and mercury.

Syphilis is less of a problem today because it can now be treated in its early phases by antibiotics, which weren't discovered until the 1940s.

Lonely Shepherds, Scared Sheep

Folklore has it that syphilis was originally caused by lonely shepherds who prodded their sheep with something more personal than carved wooden staffs. The reason for the sheep/shepherd rumor is a simple matter of poetry. In 1530, a great physician, poet, and scholar named Fracastor wrote a poem about the disease of syphilis which hadn't been named syphilis yet. In the poem, a 16-year-old shepherd boy named Syphilis made the horrible mistake of building an altar on the wrong plot of land and praying to the wrong gods. This was the 1530s equivalent of wearing the wrong colors in a gang-controlled neighborhood. It angered the god Apollo, who struck the youth's genitals with a chancre-laden thunderbolt.

Fracastor's poem tells about the rapid spread of the "new" disease:

"I sing of that terrible disease, unknown to past centuries, which attacked all Europe in one day and spread itself over part of Africa and Asia..."

This sounds like AIDS!

In five hundred years, people will think of our modern efforts to fight disease in the same way we think of strange cures from the past. But before you are too harsh on ideas like infecting syphilitic patients with malaria to cook the infecting virus, keep in mind that our main defense today against sexually transmitted diseases is even more crude. We have the technology to send motorized vehicles to Mars, but the best we can do to protect ourselves from sexually transmitted infections is to put a plastic bag on a penis.

NUMBERS:

National STD Hotline: (800) 227-8922

National Herpes Hotline: (919) 361-8488

National AIDS Line: (800) 342-AIDS

WEBSITES:

The website for the CDC (Center for Disease Control) at www.cdc.gov/std

A VERY Special Thanks: to Angela Hoffman, birth control and sex education expert, for much help over the years; to Matthew Grober at Georgia State University and Adam Safron at Northwestern. Also to the people at the CDC for providing so much helpful information about sexually transmitted infections on their website at www.cdc.gov/std.

If you have any questions about STIs or anything else mentioned in this chapter, please consult with a healthcare provider and read all you can on the website of the CDC.

53

Dyslexia of the Penis
Improving Your Sexual Hang Time

I t's easy to understand why most men would be too embarrassed to call a healthcare provider about premature ejaculation. The reception-ist always wants to know why you want to see the doctor. *"Uh, 'cause I come in about three seconds?"*

Worse yet, most healthcare providers know more about the rings of Uranus than they do about premature ejaculation. That's why this chapter is kept as up-to-date as possible, and why some of the world's top researchers are consulted. Perhaps you and your doctor can learn together.

Terms like premature ejaculation, PE, early ejaculation, and rapid ejac-ulation are used interchangeably, but they all mean the same thing. You would think it would be easy to define premature ejaculation, but it was only recently that a diverse group of researchers and clinicians finally agreed on a working definition. Even then, their definition is more limiting than many would have wanted. You'll see why in the pages that follow. You'll also see that there are many myths and misperceptions about PE.

This chapter begins with a look at what PE is and ends with the treat-ments that are currently being used.

Partners of Men with PE

One of the biggest problems with premature ejaculation is that a man's partner is seldom part of the conversation or the solution. That's not good. This chapter is for sexual partners as well as for men with PE. Hopefully you'll both read it and discuss the sections that are meaningful for you. There's no reason why PE needs to ruin your enjoyment of sex.

ISSM on Jizzing

According to the International Society for Sexual Medicine (ISSM), pre-mature ejaculation is when a man usually comes in less than a minute, has little if any control, and feels distress as a result.

Depending on whose statistics you use, almost 98% of men are able to last for more than a minute. This leaves between 1.5% and 2.5% of men who qualify as having PE. But if you add another thirty seconds to the ISSM definition by including men who come in less than a minute and a half, up to five times as many men have premature ejaculation, as long as they feel a lack of control and it's causing them distress.

The reason why ISSM has taken such a conservative approach is that it wanted to limit its definition to what is truly known and can be validated with research. Otherwise, there is a chance PE would not be accepted as a legitimate diagnosis in the medical world. Treatment would not be reimbursable and drug companies might stop their research. Unfortunately, using only a minute as a definition of PE allows drugs that don't work very well to appear to be more effective than they are.

The Problem with "What's Average"

In a study of nearly 500 couples from five countries who timed their intercourse, half of the men lasted for less than six minutes, and half for more. The lion's share of the men lasted between two and nine minutes. Few men lasted longer than eighteen minutes. Condom use and circumcision did not have an impact one way or the other.

The men over-estimated the amount of time it took them to come by an average of 31% or almost two minutes. So guys who came in six minutes thought they lasted for close eight. Also, there is more variation in how long each individual male lasts than was previously thought.

A lot of PE researchers don't think it's relevant to list an average time for intercourse. That's because there are men who last for a minute and who satisfy their lovers with all the things they do rather than just intercourse. And there are plenty of men who can last for ten or more minutes and aren't satisfying lovers.

The researchers would want you to remember there's way more to being a good lover than how long you last. Consider this book: only one chapter out of almost ninety is on intercourse. That should tell you there is way more to satisfying sex than when a penis is in a vagina.

Parallel Parking and Premature Ejaculation

Another problem with defining premature ejaculation based on the clock alone is that it doesn't speak to the speed and intensity of the thrusting. Some of the men who were part of a huge study said they are able to last more than a minute but that they ejaculated within ten thrusts or less. That works out to about six seconds per thrust. ("One Mississippi, two Mississippi, Three Mississippi, Four Mississippi, Five Mississippi, Six Mississippi" for each in and out.) This would be like having intercourse in slow motion—and some men do that in order to last longer. Also, men might have to think about dead animals or when they dropped the winning touchdown pass in a championship game in order to last longer. This makes sex less fun for themselves and their partners.

Most men who don't have PE are able to get control by stopping for a bit or pulling out and changing positions. They don't have to slap a governor on their sexual excitement from start to finish. Doing so is one of the burdens of having PE.

Female partners will often keep their hips still and mute their excitement in an attempt to help a partner with PE to last longer. They throttle down their sexual excitement, which results in their being less satisfied.

The Grim Reaper of Sexual Fun

For most men who come in less than a minute, premature ejaculation feels like a joke their body is playing on itself. Their penis feels like it's had hundreds of thrusts before their partner barely has her panties off. As much as they would love to have intercourse, they start to dread it because they feel like losers who can't please their partners.

And some women feel that premature ejaculation is "his problem," that their partner is the one who needs to fix it. However, a man with PE can no more will his wad to wait than he can will world peace.

Erections don't fare well in an environment of dread. So a lot of guys with PE not only worry about coming too soon, they also worry about not being able to get it up or keep it up once they do. And their orgasms are not always as enjoyable as for men who have better control. There are plenty of men with PE who fear new relationships or avoid them altogether rather than having to face the embarrassment of PE.

Is Premature Ejaculation Inherited?

According to the latest research, there seems to be a genetic influence that impacts some men who have PE. So it is possible that a man with premature ejaculation may have more in common with his father and brothers than meets the eye. Or maybe not.

While genetics might be a factor in PE, there is not a specific gene for premature ejaculation. To quote a researcher, "PE is influenced by many things, most of which are not understood. The genetic influence on PE is likely to be indirect." This means the genes that effect PE probably influence other things first, such as your mood, appetite, emotions, and temperament. These may or may not have an effect on your ejaculatory control.

So it's a long and winding trail from what's happening in your genes to what's happening in your jeans. Saying that genetics can influence whether you have PE simply means the chances are greater that you will come sooner than someone without that particular gene configuration. Beyond that, we do not have enough knowledge about PE to be more specific.

If you are the partner of a man with PE, it's best to leave the genetic research to the geneticists. Do not succumb to the temptation of asking your lover's mother, "Mrs. Snappy, does your husband come as quickly as your son?" But in case you do, be sure to let us know what she says.

El Prematuro Loco

There are a number of men who are sure they have PE when they don't. The majority of the men who describe themselves as having premature ejaculation do not have anything close. When a man assumes he has PE but doesn't, we say he has a case of *El Prematuro Loco.*

Someone with a real case of premature ejaculation can hardly last a minute. But a man with *El Prematuro Loco* can go for several minutes during intercourse while thrusting at a satisfying clip for both he and his partner. He is within the range of average, sometimes at the high end of average. Being able to last that long would make a man who really does have premature ejaculation smile from ear to ear.

Fortunately, education, reassurance, and sometimes counseling is enough to help a man with *El Prematuro Loco* stop focusing on what he perceives to be his short-comings, and to work instead on finding ways to give his partner extra pleasure besides just thrusting. So if you are a man who feels he has premature ejaculation, why not start by talking to your partner about your concerns? It could be she wants something different in bed than for you to last longer.

And if she does want you to last longer, some of the retraining techniques mentioned later in this chapter might help. If you can already last for a few minutes, you've got a lot more room to teach yourself to improve your hang time than a guy who lasts for 30 seconds. You might not have to be fighting your body's genetics, neurology or psychology in order to last longer.

Also, a reality check is in order for today's porn-inspired couple who assumes that every guy can thrust like a robot.

Control Issues

Surveys have shown that 50% of men feel they can control when they ejaculate during intercourse. Being able to control when you come is beyond the comprehension of a man who has premature ejaculation. Unfortunately, research also shows that partners of men with PE often believe that a man can control it if he tries. For most men with PE, this is not possible.

While some women blame themselves when a partner has erection problems, they tend to blame their partner when he has PE. Couples would have way more fun if they learned to have sex that's based on more than what a man can do with his penis. Making it safe for your partner to act out some of her sex fantasies with you would make you a better lover than most.

Lifelong vs. Acquired — How Psychology Can Impact Biology

Most men who have PE have had it in varying degrees from the time of their first intercourse. This is known as lifelong premature ejaculation. However, there are some men who have fairly decent control until the PE Fairy waves a wand of quickness over their penis. So if you were okay to begin with and then start to ejaculate rapidly, you might have "acquired PE."

Consider the case of Bill, who is a construction worker and who scheduled an appointment with a urologist to deal with his premature ejaculation. Bill rarely had trouble with his ejaculation until recently.

If Bill's urologist had been too busy to ask about Bill's relationships, he would have missed that Bill recently started dating Jenni who is a corporate CEO. She is high-powered and white-collar, while Bill carries a hammer and is blue-collar. Bill has felt inadequate from the start with Jenni, given that she's drop-dead gorgeous and makes about ten times as much money as he does. Bill's premature ejaculation started soon after he began dating Jenni.

Bill got his PE along the way as opposed to always having struggled with it. What Bill needed were some sessions with a therapist to help him deal with his conflicted feelings about being in a relationship with Jenni. (Thanks to sex therapist Stan Althof for providing this example.)

Possible Risk Factors

If you have recently started to ejaculate rapidly and no earthshaking life changes have occurred that might explain it, such as finding your wife in bed with the teenager who mows your lawn, then it is a good idea to have a complete physical exam.

Before assuming PE has a physical cause, be aware there has been little evidence to support a medical or psychological cause of premature ejaculation. As of press time, the best that can be said is more and better studies need to be done.

To date, one study found that between 50% and 70% of men with a hyperthyroid have PE. After receiving successful treatment for their thyroid problem, the rate of PE dropped from 50% to 15%. On the other hand, there was not a single case of hyperthyroidism in a study of 620 men who have lifelong PE. So while any man with acquired PE should get his thyroid checked, it's unlikely that thyroid is the cause of PE in a man who's always had premature ejaculation.

There are some indications that prostate infections might be a cause of PE. The trouble with these studies is they aren't particularly sound from a scientific point of view. Prostate infections are something to be aware of regarding PE, especially PE that is acquired, but that's about it.

There's a high association between premature ejaculation and erectile dysfunction in men who have diabetes, and a moderate association between PE and erectile dysfunction in general. In these cases, trying one of the boner drugs like Viagra might be a consideration.

Early ejaculation has also been reported as a side effect of withdrawal from SSRI antidepressants. Some recreational drugs might also contribute to premature ejaculation.

Aside from genetic influences, one study suggests that a short frenulum could help trigger PE in men who have lifelong premature ejaculation. Theoretically, having a shorter frenulum could cause excessive tension in the area of the glans corona, which is one of the most sensitive and nerve-filled parts of the penis. However, controlled studies need to be done regarding the short-frenulum theory before any credence is given to it.

In time, it's possible that physical causes of PE will be discovered. Currently, the data is limited and sometimes contradictory.

Your First Time vs Youthful Exuberance

In a recent study in Finland, a lot of men who don't have PE reported ejaculating in under a minute the first time they had intercourse. Many of these men ejaculated before their penis got its first feel of their partner's vagina. But they've had normal ejaculation times ever since. So there's a big difference between mastering the anxiety and inexperience of your first couple of times and coming quickly for the rest of your life.

In most men with PE, ejaculation-control doesn't improve with age. And in many cases, premature ejaculation gets worse as relationships get longer. That wouldn't be the case if time and experience were the cure for premature ejaculation.

A Reality Check with Your Partner

Women often assume their male partners are not concerned about having PE when the man himself might be an anxious mess. At the same time, here is often a major disconnect between what a man *thinks* his partner wants and what she really wants.

So if either of you is concerned about PE, the first thing to do is to talk about it together. She might prefer that you spend more time kissing, caressing, or sharing oral sex. Maybe she wants you to be more of a take-charge kind of guy when it comes to sex. Or she might want you to last longer, but hasn't let you know because she's been afraid of hurting your feelings. Either way, talking it over is an important step when one or both of you is concerned about premature ejaculation.

Myths To Fry

In trying to understand more about PE, it is helpful to look at what people used to believe caused it. Some sex educators and therapists still adhere to these myths:

Goat Gonads! Premature ejaculation was first described in medical literature in the late 1800s. That's when PE, impotence, and just about everything that could possibly go wrong with a man was blamed on masturbation or "self-pollution." Even having intercourse more than once a week was a concern among the anti-ejaculation fanatics of the day. To help revitalize and rejuvenate the body, more than a thousand men were given testicular grafts from sheep, monkeys, goats, deer, and other men.

Vasectomies to Prevent the Spilling Seed: In the late 1800s and early 1900s, there was so much concern about losing semen that men would get vasectomies to keep their sperm inside their bodies. That's how vasectomies originally became popular—not for birth control, but as a way of returning a man's "masculine essence" into his own body. Even Freud got a vasectomy when he was 67, clearly not for birth control.

Being Pissed Off: In the 1920s, a psychoanalyst by the name of Karl Abraham suggested that PE resulted from a man's unconscious anger at women. Rapid ejaculation was a man's way of symbolically peeing inside of his partner's vagina. How charming. We have since discovered that men with PE aren't more angry at women than men without PE.

A Headache in Your Penis: In the early 1940s, another German psychiatrist, Bernard Schapiro, speculated that PE was a psychosomatic illness, like anxiety-related headaches. He said that PE was the result of a man's psychological conflict expressing itself bodily. This, too, has been proven false.

PE from Jerking Off Quickly: In the late 1970s, renowned sex therapists Masters and Johnson changed the premature ejaculation landscape by claiming that PE was a learned experience. They believed PE was something males taught themselves when they rushed their way through masturbation or had rushed sex in a car or did it with a prostitute. We now realize that popping out quick ones is not the cause of premature ejaculation. However, it is possible that if a man was born with a shorter fuse to begin with, the rushed experiences he had when he was a teenager could have had more of a lasting impact than if he had been born with a penis that was wired like a porn star's. In this situation, the squeeze-technique that Masters and Johnson suggested might be helpful in extending his hang time (explained in the treatment section of this chapter).

From Zero to Sixty in 2.46 Seconds: In the late 1980s, sex researcher Helen Singer Kaplan proposed that men with PE never developed the ability to experience a gradual buildup of sensation in their penis. Kaplan believed most guys have an early warning system in their penis and are able to say to themselves, "It's starting to feel like I'm getting close—I'll slow down my thrusting or change positions so I can delay coming." But for the man with PE, ejaculation arrives like a sneak attack. He gets no warning signals until it's too late to delay. Kaplan also felt that anxiety fueled PE.

Her theories held sway for many years, and they shouldn't be quickly dismissed. But when men with PE are given medications that allow them to delay their ejaculation, they can have the same range of sensory awareness in their penis as guys who don't have premature ejaculation. It is also interesting that tramadol and SSRIs, which are drugs that help with anxiety, also help decrease PE. However, it's more likely these drugs delay ejaculation by impacting the centers in the nervous system that trigger ejaculation.

Porn Causes PE: This is one of the most recent and more bizarre theories about the causes of premature ejaculation. If porn were a cause of premature ejaculation, we would have seen a huge increase in the number of men with PE during the past two decades. There has been no such increase. However, if this theory were true, it would be interesting to know if men with DSL come faster than men with dial-up used to!

Research Findings on the Man with a Pronto Penis

When researchers placed sensors on men's penises and showed them sexually exciting materials, they expected the men with PE to have a more rapid sexual response. Yet they weren't able to find any differences between men with PE and those who had good control. Time to erection was about the same.

So the researchers made the situation more like real life. They put "pleasure devices" on the men's penises so the men would feel physical stimulation while they were watching dirty movies. And that's when they found that nearly 60% of premature ejaculators would quickly blow a wad as opposed to only 5% of the men who didn't have a problem with coming too soon. This finding helped give credence to the idea that men with premature ejaculation might be wired to come sooner than men who don't have PE. But it doesn't mean they can't retrain themselves.

Semen Samples

Anxiety about sex with a partner does not appear to be the cause of premature ejaculation.

There are anecdotal reports from researchers who have had premature ejaculators and controls masturbate in the lab to give semen samples. The men who were premature ejaculators came out of the rest room with their semen in a cup faster than the men who were controls. Given that they were masturbating, anxiety about sex with a partner was not the reason why the men with PE produced their semen samples sooner than men without PE.

Research Findings—Neurology, Heart Rate, and Erections

When men who don't have PE are having intercourse, their heart rates slow down after their penises get hard, even though they are getting aerobic exercise from thrusting during intercourse. When they are about to ejaculate, their heart rates speed up again.

But when a guy with PE gets sexually aroused, his heart beat is likely to remain rapid from the moment he gets hard until he ejaculates. His nervous system doesn't shift into the intercourse version of cruise-control. He is on the verge of ejaculating from the get-go. It is possible that by doing the retraining techniques listed later in this chapter, a man with PE can learn to drop his heart rate like one who doesn't have PE.

Erection Issues

You would think that men with PE would get erect sooner than controls. However, the opposite is true for some groups of men with PE. A number of men with PE also have varying degrees of erectile dysfunction. This dovetails with why some men with PE respond well to erection drugs such as Viagra, Cialis, and Levitra. Perhaps these are men whose PE is related to erectile dysfunction. Or maybe their erectile dysfunction is due to their distress about having PE, and the erection drugs help alleviate the fear that they won't be able to get it up.

Some men who don't have PE complain that the boner drugs make their penis feel somewhat wooden. This would be a case of one man's poison being another man's cure.

Even if the erection drugs don't help them to last longer the first time, they do help most men to get an erection after ejaculation more sooner. Most men will be able to thrust longer the second time.

Emotional Reaction

Men with PE often have more negative feelings about sex than men who have control over their ejaculations. Therapists used to assume it was the negative feelings that were causing the premature ejaculation rather than being a result of it.

But the men with PE did not look forward to having intercourse because they believed they were going to disappoint their partner. Many of the negative feelings that men with PE have about sex stop once they are able to get more control over their ejaculations.

What's Often Missing: A Partner's Perception

The results of a recent FDA trial on a treatment for premature ejaculation trumpeted how it added extra minutes to the men's thrusting times. But in spite of the great results, the men's partners didn't report significant increases in their own sexual satisfaction.

So maybe the problem wasn't as bad as the guys with PE assumed. Or maybe sexual satisfaction is more complex than we think. Sexual problems don't exist in a vacuum. When it comes to sexual intimacy, mutual pleasure can't always be measured with a stopwatch.

This takes us back to a central theme throughout this chapter: men with PE are often so focused on their failure that they aren't able to enjoy ways of making sex more fun and rewarding. By the time a man with PE tries the retraining techniques or uses drugs for it, sexual excitement in the relationship might need to be rekindled.

Plenty of men learn to compensate for PE by becoming really good at pleasing a woman with oral sex or different kinds of massage. Some couples act out fun scenarios and fantasies together. Others might want to read Chapter 42: *Between Vanilla and Kink*. There's no reason why coming quickly should get in the way of having great sex.

The Other 97% of Your Body and Mind

It can be helpful for a man with PE to become more aware of the sensations in other parts of his body in addition to his penis. Not enough can be said about allowing a partner to touch you from head to toe while you let your body relax. This kind of non-pressured exploration is often the cornerstone of sex therapy.

To help become more aware of sensations, some couples enjoy using a variety of materials and fabrics to massage each other from head to toe. Good results can be had with feathers or furry mitts, as well as a silk scarf or piece of rayon. Some couples might be into leather, latex, or rubber. Others find the feel of a partner's fingertips to be exquisite.

Motivation

None of the treatments on the pages that follow are a cure. However, they can help, sometimes a great deal. But they do require motivation and a long-term commitment.

The Most Important Ingredients

In helping a man to last longer, don't forget to have a sense of humor. Humor is the sexual lubricant for the soul. The chances are, a man with PE is angry and frustrated with himself. Humor and a tolerance for frustration can go a long way.

Your Partner's Orgasms

The couple must find ways for the man's partner to get off besides having intercourse. That way she won't feel resentful, he won't feel guilty, and both partners will get to experience what it is like when she can open up and no longer needs to mute her excitement in order to help him last longer. This is one of the first things a couple should work on, as opposed to just focusing on the man's penis.

Relationship Fears & Resistances

Helen Singer Kaplan said that the men who were unable to complete her program for rapid ejaculation usually had wives or girlfriends who did not necessarily want them to last longer.

The three gentlemen mentioned below were rapid ejaculators as well as contributors to *The Guide*. They were kind enough to share their personal stories for you to read.

Zeus suspected his wife didn't want him to improve his sexual function and that she would resist helping him do something about it. He was right. His wife didn't enjoy sex, or not with him anyway, and the faster he came, the better. In addition, she didn't want him having sex with anyone else. She assumed he would be less likely to have extramarital affairs if his problems with PE remained.

Lancelot was afraid his girlfriend wouldn't want to invest the time and effort in helping him to last longer. He was mortified to even ask. As it turned out, he was wrong. She was happy (and relieved) that he wanted her help in solving the problem. They took on the problem together with historic results.

Heathcliff had a secret and didn't know if Catherine would want to help. While caring greatly for each other, their sex life had never been a central part of their relationship. After several years, he finally asked for her help with his premature ejaculation. He received an unexpected reply. She told him she often masturbated after he went to sleep, keeping her sexual needs to herself because she didn't think he was interested. They began masturbating together and started feeling sexually intimate for the first time in their lives. They found many ways to please each other sexually. By this time, Heathcliff had become such a changed man that not even his neighbors could recognize him.

Rather than bulldozing ahead with the treatments that are mentioned in this chapter, why not start by having a couple of long talks about it first? You might want to include a discussion about what it would be like if you were able to make changes in your sex life. Even if you both want changes, each of you might have your own fears and concerns about them.

Treatments

The rest of this chapter lists drugs, creams, condoms, and behavioral techniques that are being used to treat PE. Since PE isn't a disease and it doesn't have a specific cause, the best treatment will depend on your biology, psychology, and partner situation. In exploring different treatment options, you will need to be flexible and adventurous—two qualities that men are not always known for, according to the women who take our sex surveys.

A logical treatment to try first would be the retraining techniques. One version is free, and these methods have no side effects.

Teaching an Old Dog New Tricks: The Squeeze Technique

The squeeze technique for premature ejaculation has been around for almost as long as the penis itself. It has had different variations, one being called "the start stop technique." The goal is to take you to the edge of ejaculation, but not over. This will help your body learn how to be in a high state of arousal without ejaculating.

You would think there would have been dozens of studies investigating the efficacy of this technique; not so. Since the squeeze technique is free, drug companies aren't lining up to fund the research. And our government rarely chomps at the bit to fund studies on improving sexual pleasure.

Two studies that were done on the squeeze technique during the 1980s showed that a number of men had success with it initially, but most of the gains were lost over time. This is not unusual regarding sex. Sex therapists often schedule follow-up appointments for any kind of problem every six months after successful treatment. That's because sexual problems have the tenacity of the cockroach. There can also be a placebo effect with any kind of sexual intervention, which means it works at the start because you believe it will. So don't be surprised if you need to do squeeze-technique refreshers every couple of months. But this should be fun. Seriously, what's not to like about a partner stroking your penis?

Warning #1: Get a Grip—Stop Apologizing

Some of the most annoying aspects of premature ejaculation that women report are the constant apologies and self-criticism that men express after coming too soon. This puts their partners off. If you decide to work on these exercises together, the man needs to promise he will no longer apologize or berate himself for coming too soon.

Warning #2: Feel Your Sexual Excitement

Men with PE often try to think about something unsexy, which is about as productive as a race-car driver thinking about golf when he's entering a high-speed turn. All of us are occasionally distracted when having sex, but to intentionally think about something besides sex is not a good way to last longer. It could lead to erection problems, so you'll then have ED and will still come too soon. Let yourself feel totally turned on.

Squeeze-Technique Particulars

You both get naked and kiss and fool around. Then you kiss and fool around some more. At some point, which is totally up to the two of you, the female partner says, "On your back, dude!" She then starts stroking his penis handjob style. While it's usually done without lube, there's nothing that says lube can't be used. See what works best for the two of you.

The man's job is to tell his partner what he's feeling in his penis. As soon as he feels like he is reaching the point of no return, he asks her to stop stroking and that's her cue to start squeezing—right below the head for 10 to 20 seconds. Then, after a minute or so, the man's urge to ejaculate should subside, and his partner can start stroking his penis again. Repeat at least three

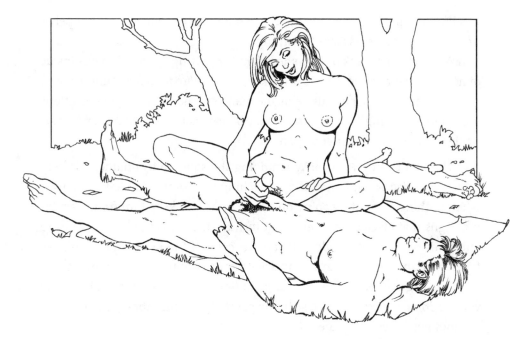

The Squeeze Technique

or four times. When the two of you decide his penis has had a good enough workout, she can stroke him to ejaculation.

After a few weeks of doing it this way, the woman might experiment with switching techniques. Rather than stopping and squeezing when her partner tells her he's about to come, she might try rubbing the head of his penis instead. So she goes from choking his chicken to polishing his helmet.

As for erections, don't worry about them. What you are interested in is trying to tolerate more sensation.

A variation on the squeeze technique is called *the stop-start technique.* Instead of squeezing when the man is close to coming, his partner removes her hand from his penis. It's totally your call as to which technique you'd prefer to use.

From Squeezing to Intercourse: When the two of you feel you are getting more control over the situation, the woman might try stimulating the penis with her lips instead of her fingers, or by sitting on top of the man and rubbing his penis with her vulva. This is called femoral intercourse. It is where the shaft of the penis glides through the lips of the vulva like a hot dog in a bun. The penis doesn't go into the vagina. The woman can lift her pelvis up when her partner is close to coming.

After another week or two, she might try putting the man's penis inside of her vagina while she is on top. Try keeping it there for a few minutes without thrusting very much. This helps the man get used to the warm sensations, and there's nothing that says she can't be caressing her clitoris or breasts while his penis is inside her vagina.

The Point of No Return: When doing the squeeze technique, it is helpful to recognize when a man is approaching the Point of No Return. This is when nothing short of stepping on a land mine will keep him from ejaculating. Signs that ejaculation is eminent include: the veins in his penis start to bulge, his penis gives a sudden throb, the color of the head darkens, his testicles suck up into his groin, his muscles start to tighten, his hips thrust, and he starts to groan or invokes the name of God or Allah. Appreciate how well you are doing if he can stay close to the point of no return for several minutes without going over the edge.

Also, it helps if the couple can cut themselves plenty of slack. There will be times when a guy reaches the point of no return before his partner can squeeze or pause. It's no big deal. Doing the squeeze technique should be fun, and occasionally funny. It's not a competition.

Prolong: A Vibrator Version of the Stop-Start Technique

One of the top PE researchers did a small study where men with PE used a new vibratory device called "Prolong." The device is a vibrator that's embedded into a half-round silicone sleeve. The man lubes up the most sensitive part of his penis and rubs it with the device until he's almost ready to ejaculate. Then he stops, and repeats this a few times.

There are currently two downsides for men in North America: as of press time, the device was not available in the US or Canada. And even in Europe, it was about $250 US dollars. Hopefully it will soon be available. If it works, this would be a far more preferable approach to treating PE than using drugs, which all have side effects, and men can use it on their own. Also, it might be helpful to use a device like Prolong in conjunction with the squeeze technique. **PE DRAMA:** It seems the Prolong website has been hacked by one of the well funded companies who makes an ejaculation delaying spray. So keep doing browser searchers to find the device.

Pelvic Floor Exercises

Researchers from the University of Rome recently (2014) published a study titled *Pelvic floor muscle rehabilitation for patients with lifelong premature ejaculation: A novel therapeutic approach.* You are encouraged to do a browser search and read the study. This study seems to demonstrate that a number of men with serious lifelong PE can be helped without drugs.

Promescent—A Delay Spray That May Be Worth Trying

Sprays and creams for PE that help numb a penis have been around for decades. All of these sprays and creams contain similar numbing agents, such as lidocaine, prilocaine and benzocaine. The problem has been with the delivery system. Most of the numbing agent molecules have remained evenly distributed throughout the creams they are mixed in and do not make contact with the skin. As a result, they are not quickly absorbed and the man has to wear a condom to keep the numbing cream from touching his partner's clitoris. The creams also have a tendency to numb out the penis.

Drug companies have spent millions of dollars trying to create a delivery system for the numbing agents that allow just enough of the molecules to get to the skin of the penis where they can be rapidly absorbed without leaving a residue that will numb a partner's genitals. The well-funded company that invented Promescent believes they have succeeded. They also believe that Promescent will not numb out a man's penis if he begins to have intercourse within five minutes of application.

Promescent is a cousin of a product called SD502 that is used for pain relief for burn victims, although not necessarily burn victims with premature ejaculation. Promescent is not a cure for premature ejaculation, but something a man can use five minutes before intercourse. Promescent is anything but cheap, but it doesn't require a prescription and there appear to be no side effects. You can order it from www.promescent.com.

NOTE: When this spray was in Phase II clinical trials, it seemed like the researchers were having to move heaven and earth to squeeze significance out of the results. However, Phase III trial results looked more promising. The proof will be in the ejaculating.

A concern we have with this cream and the company that makes it is the degree of hype and the huge amount of marketing dollars that are being spent. If you are looking for a delaying cream or spray, this is probably the one to try. But you might do just as well with the squeeze technique, or perhaps a combination of the two.

Trojan Extended Pleasure and Durex Performax Condoms

These condoms have benzocaine gel on the inside to desensitize or numb out the penis. It is fascinating to read user reviews. They tend to either be 5 stars or 1 star, with guys and their partners either loving them or hating them. The biggest complaint is that these condoms numb out the penis so much that some men lose all sensation, and their erection as well. The biggest praise is that they numb out the penis enough so a man can last longer than he normally does.

Men who have tried both brands tend to prefer one or the other. So you might try both and see if one works better for you. Do not put these condoms on too soon before intercourse. Otherwise, your penis could feel like your gums after getting novocaine at the dentist's office. Do read the instructions, and be careful not to get the gel from the inside of the condom on a woman's genitals. And as one woman with a numb mouth flamed on a user forum: *Do not give a blow job after a man takes one of these bad boys off!*

Treatments —The Drugs

Most of the drugs that are now used for PE were not designed for PE, just like Viagra was not designed for ED. The ejaculation-delaying properties of drugs like tramadol and SSRI antidepressants were first discovered as unwanted side effects. These drugs have not yet been approved for treating PE and may never be approved for it.

PLEASE consider the squeeze technique listed on the prior pages or Promescent or numbing condoms before taking drugs to help with premature ejaculation. The drugs do not necessarily work well and all have side effects.

The Ugly Side of Progress

More and more research is being done on premature ejaculation, especially since the drug companies realize they would have a pharmaceutical gold mine on their hands if they could come up with a pill that helps men last longer without putting them to sleep, zapping their sex drives, or making their penises feel like lead pipes. The problem will be in how drug companies will market the PE drugs. They'll try to convince young men that their sexual self-esteem will rise exponentially if they take the new *intimacy-*

enhancing pills. Soon enough, men who last "only" six minutes—which is close to what half of men last—will assume they have premature ejaculation and will want to take the new drug. So while there will be a definite upside to a medication that works for men who truly have PE, there may also be an ugly underbelly.

Treatments—Pills

As of press time, no pills have been approved in the US as treatments for premature ejaculation. Using them would be off-label and the wisdom of doing so is between you and your healthcare provider. The following summaries are for information only and might not reflect the latest research.

Also, all of the medications mentioned have side effects which could be negligible for some men, but truly bothersome for others. The possible side effects include dry mouth, nausea, headaches, weight gain, insomnia, erectile dysfunction, low sex drive, the occasional suicide attempt, drug addiction, fertility problems and liver damage.

Up to 90% of men who start taking drugs for PE discontinue them because they either don't work as well as promised or because of the side effects.

If the pills alone don't extend your range, some physicians suggest combining them with the squeeze technique or layering them, such as using an SSRI with a boner drug, or a boner drug with a delaying spray. There are currently only a few studies to guide us on combining medications for PE, and when studies are paid for by the manufacturers of the drugs, we have no idea if the results are truly valid.

SSRI Antidepressants (brand names include Paxil, Prozac, and Zoloft): A common side effect for SSRI antidepressants is delayed ejaculation. The delay in ejaculation can be so significant that for a man who doesn't have PE, that taking SSRI antidepressants can make him feel like he's wearing a dozen condoms. This is why some SSRIs could be just what the doctor ordered for men with premature ejaculation if it weren't for the other side effects.

There are some SSRIs that delay ejaculation more than others, but the additional side effects can be problematic. The front line SSRI that one sexual medicine expert prescribes is Zoloft (generic name is sertraline). He says there are other SSRIs that might be better for PE, but he finds Zoloft is better tolerated. He also likes the fact that Zoloft has a generic version that doesn't cost his patients as much.

Keep in mind that SSRIs can have wicked sexual side effects including ED and killing your libido. They can cause headaches, nausea, drowsiness, weight gain, and other physical and mental nastiness. There is concern that young men who are taking them are at an increased risk of suicide. Also, some men with PE who find early success with SSRIs report their PE returns after several months. *Please, do not even think of taking SSRI antidepressants for premature ejaculation if you are bipolar.*

Dapoxetine (Priligy): Some researchers assumed that a fast-acting SSRI with a short half-life would be a good on-demand solution for premature ejaculation. While one SSRI by the name of **dapoxetine (Priligy)** has been approved in other countries for on-demand treatment for PE, our own FDA was not particularly impressed. Up to 90% of men who are given this drug for PE stop using it before the end of a year. This should say volumes about the side effects vs. the lack of efficacy.

Erection Drugs (brand names are Viagra, Levitra, Cialis, and Stendra): Can boner drugs help men with PE? Yes and no. A number of men with PE have erection-related problems. So is it the erection problems that are causing premature ejaculation, or does PE cause men so much distress that they end up having ED? Research to date has not found that Viagra helps men with PE to last significantly longer. However, the men with PE who used Viagra reported increased confidence, a greater perception of control, and more overall sexual satisfaction. There might be two reasons for this: Viagra may have resulted in more reliable erections, which was a big relief. Viagra also helps men with PE to get it up more quickly after coming the first time. Most man can last longer the second time if they can get it up again and rally for another ride. (Research by the Levitra people found Levitra to be helpful for PE as well.)

If you and your healthcare provider decide to give the boner drugs a go, it's best to get samples and try each one. You might find one works better for you in terms of PE. Also, you might talk to your healthcare provider about using erection drugs with the non-prescription delaying spray Promescent or with one of the retraining techniques.

Clomipramine (brand name is Anafranil): This is a tricyclic antidepressant that has been used for a long time to help people with obsessive compulsive disorders. One of the side effects is that it delays ejaculation, which is why they started to use it for men with PE. A 25-mg dose taken 4 to 24 hours before intercourse is sometimes recommended. This can be raised to 50 mg, but with that can come increased side effects. A study was done in which a 10-30 mg dose was given on a long-term basis with satisfactory results.

As with SSRI antidepressants, be sure to understand the side effects, as there could be an increased risk for suicide among young men, although it's not known if that would be the case for young men who are taking it for PE and who are using it on demand as opposed to daily. Do not take this if you are bipolar or have erection problems.

Tramadol (brand name is Ultram): This is a centrally-acting opioid analgesic that appears to have few side effects at the low doses being used to treat PE. The doses of tramadol used in PE studies are between 25 mg and 89 mg (the drug is approved for 400 mgs a day).

There is conflicting and limited research with an on-demand dose of 50 mg of tramadol for PE. Men who could only last for 19 seconds started lasting four minutes, and a 25-mg dose had men who normally ejaculated in a minute going for more than six minutes. This drug is optimally taken two hours before intercourse.

While studies in 2007, 2008 and 2011 found tramadol to be effective for PE, a 2010 study comparing the on-demand use of tramadol for PE with daily use of the SSRI antidepressant paroxetine (Paxil) found paroxetine shredding tramadol when it came to delaying ejaculation at 12 weeks. The authors of the Paxil study also say that Tramadol had a negative effect on erections, while Paxil had a positive effect. In responding to the Paxil results, the lead researcher in one of the tramadol studies insists that tramadol humbles Paxil as a drug for PE and claims his team never saw erection problems with men in their tramadol studies. Plus, it's hard to find ED listed as a side effect for men taking 400 mg a day of tramadol, let alone only 50 mgs every couple of days. Also, if you are considering Paxil for PE, keep in mind it can have wicked side effects.

Unfortunately, little is known about the effectiveness of tramadol on PE after being used for extended periods of time. Tramadol is one of the only opioid drugs that is not a controlled substance in many parts of the world. It has been around since the late 1970s and is even sold over-the-counter in some countries. However, in 2010 the FDA listed some new side effect warnings for tramadol, and it is unlikely tramadol will ever be approved as a PE drug because it is an opioid. Mind you, it is commonly prescribed for backaches in much higher doses.

WARNING — Tramadol has become a highly abused drug worldwide. Some clinicians do not feel it is worth the risk of giving young men prescriptions for tramadol due to its potential for abuse as a recreational drug. While the dose used for PE is a fraction of that which is needed to get a pain-killing effect, this is an important warning and should be taken very seriously. Tramadol can be a bear of a drug to get off of if you become addicted.

Treatments—Penis Injections (Do Not Use These for PE!)

Penis injections can be helpful for men with erectile dysfunction who don't respond to the usual array of boner drugs. However, unscrupulous healthcare providers have been advertising the use of these injections for premature ejaculation. The *Journal of Sexual Medicine* has strongly warned against using penis injections for PE. Long-term penis damage can result.

Be sure to look up the side effects of any drug you are taking. Also be aware that if your healthcare professional prescribes these or any other drugs for PE, it would currently be an off-label use.

A Special Thanks to: Patrick Jern of the Åbo Akademi University in Finland and the Sahlgrenska Academy in Sweden; New York City psychiatrist and sex therapist Stephen Snyder; Jason Feifer, an editor at Men's Health, Donald Strassberg of the University of Utah; David Rowland of Valparaiso University; Marcel D. Waldinger of University of Utrecht; Joseph Marzucco, urology specialist; Stan Althof of the Center for Marital and Sexual Health in South Florida; and Michael Metz, co-author with Barry McCarthy of *Coping With Premature Ejaculation*. Michael Metz recently left us—may he rest each night in emerald meadows surrounded by naked women.

54
Delayed Ejaculation

Delayed ejaculation is when a guy can get a rock-hard erection and have intercourse for a really long time, but can't ejaculate or he struggles to ejaculate. It doesn't matter if he's having oral, vaginal, or anal sex, or if his partner is giving him a handjob — either he can't ejaculate or it can take him close to forever to come. Or maybe he can come by masturbating in a certain way, but not with a partner. The problem is not in getting an erection and keeping an erection; rather it's with having an orgasm and ejaculation.

For those of you who have delayed ejaculation or are dealing with it in your relationship, be aware that very little research has been done on this subject and virtually none of it is the double-blind kind that you can take to the bank. Delayed ejaculation (DE) is poorly understood. No one has been able to come up with a universal set of causes, physical or emotional.

There appear to be two different types of delayed ejaculation: the primary type, where a man has always had it, and the secondary type, where he was perfectly fine and then it starts to occur. If you have the secondary type, be sure to rule out physical causes such as diabetes, multiple sclerosis, pelvic surgery, dystonia, spinal cord injuries, or a big old tumor. Fortunately, these are rare causes of delayed ejaculation. Medication side effects are more likely to be culprits behind secondary DE. We'll discuss this in a few more pages.

Delayed Ejaculation: A Partner Speaks

A sex educator who uses *The Guide* in her college course has been married for more than thirty years to a man who has delayed ejaculation. She offered to write this section for partners of men with DE. If you've done any research on delayed ejaculation, you'll appreciate that what she has to say is far more helpful than most of what's been written on the subject to date. Here goes:

> I've been married to a man for 31 years who has never been able to ejaculate with me in the ordinary way. I married him knowing this was true, but thought that we would be able to solve the problem.

I didn't know at the time that delayed ejaculation is the most difficult of the sexual problems to solve or change, even more difficult than desire discrepancy.

Early in our relationship, I looked this up in a book on sexual problems by Masters and Johnson who were famous sex researchers. I discovered that they had only worked with a handful of men with this problem; mostly couples who were worried about whether the women could become pregnant. They used the technique of the man masturbating to the "point of no return" and then the woman would get on top and the man would ejaculate inside her. If the couple was able to do this, then this was considered a successful outcome.

We were able to do this and have two beautiful daughters who are now grown. However, that did not feel like a success to me and my husband was not really interested in doing this for recreational sex. We have explored a lot of sex therapy and psychotherapy, individually and together trying to come to terms with this problem.

As Paul describes in this chapter, my husband has a style of masturbation that is very hard to duplicate with my hand, let alone with my vagina. It is very, very fast and very hard. He has had some success changing his masturbation style, but because it is difficult for him to orgasm, even when masturbating, it is hard for him to want to change his style. Because of this, I have never been able to bring him to orgasm in any way, orally, anally, vaginally or manually.

Overall, I think my husband has come to see this as normal for him; he has never been any different with any other partner. I have had to accept that this sexual style is not something that he really wants to spend a lot more time or energy worrying about. After all these years, we still like to be sexual together, and I count my blessings. He really likes intercourse and has no problem with erections. Unfortunately, I am one of those women who don't come with vaginal stimulation only, so I don't get the benefit of having a partner with this problem that some women do.

Here are some things I've learned that might help the partner married to someone with this problem.

💡DON'T TAKE IT PERSONALLY. IT IS NOT ABOUT YOU! I am a skilled and experienced lover and have never thought that my vagina wasn't tight enough or I wasn't sexy enough to please him. Also, he had this problem with all previous lovers.

💡Don't decide it is a sickness or a pathology. In one of the articles that Paul mentions, the author talks about a bell curve of sexual responsiveness on which men and women naturally fall. Some men and women orgasm extremely easily and some orgasm with a lot of difficulty. Most are somewhere in between. Rather than thinking there is something wrong with your partner, try to think of DE as something he is born with, like dark hair or intelligence or needing glasses.

💡Don't marry him if you need him to change. It may be impossible and it's better to go into it knowing that.

💡Use your sexuality as an opportunity to develop greater intimacy. Talk to each other, use the ideas that are in this book, improve communication, have fun. Focus on loving your partner and feeling emotionally connected and physically close.

💡Don't fall into the trap of "goal-oriented" sex instead of "pleasure-oriented sex". Goal oriented sex says that all good sex ends with orgasm. Pleasure-oriented sex says that any sexual behaviors that feel good count as sex.

💡Count your blessings and enjoy the fact that you will never be able to do "cookie cutter sex". Use it as a way to rebel against the Hollywood myth of perfect sex and keep it creative and fun.

💡Don't tell too many friends about this. They will never have heard of it and will think it is really weird and will make you feel worse, most likely.

Looking Under the Hood of Delayed Ejaculation

Delayed ejaculation used to be known as retarded ejaculation, until we decided that calling a man a "retarded ejaculator" was a bit harsh. While modern medicine still calls the condition retarded ejaculation, some people refer to it as inhibited ejaculation. People who are trying to sound medical refer to it as a DED, diminished ejaculatory disorder. Honest.

How many men have delayed ejaculation? We aren't really sure. The guesses range from 1% to 3%, but even if it were only 0.5%, that's still a lot of guys whose corks won't pop.

This condition can present itself differently in different men. It can be intermittent or it can happen every time. It can be lifelong or something that crept up along the way. It can be mild, moderate, severe, or super-severe.

If you are stopwatch obsessed and hellbent on quantifying delayed ejaculation, consider that an average guy lasts somewhere between three and eight minutes during intercourse. One researcher has cooked the various standard deviations of how long an average intercourse lasts and suggests if you can't come after 25 to 30 minutes of thrusting, then you probably qualify as having delayed ejaculation. But here's a problem: for some couples, 25 minutes is just getting warmed up, while for others 25 minutes would be a nightmare of excess. So in order to declare a man has delayed ejaculation, both he and his partner need to consider it a problem. There are also situations when a man is able to come after fifteen minutes, but his partner wishes he were done after five.

Forget calling it delayed ejaculation if the problem only happens when a man is using a condom. If that's the case, a dab of water-based lube on the head of the penis before sliding the condom down the shaft might help increase sensation.

What's particularly fascinating about delayed ejaculation is that the majority of men who have it are able to ejaculate when they masturbate. It's when you put a flesh-and-blood partner between the guy's hand and his penis that he usually has the problem. It can get so bad that his intercourse partner is able to figure out the plot lines to her next three novels before he's even close to coming.

As you'll see, there can be numerous factors that contribute to how fast or slow a guy launches his load, from the biology he was born with to how he processes things like excitement and anxiety. Please keep in mind that while one man with delayed ejaculation might respond to X, Y, or Z, another man might do better with A, B and C, and a third won't respond no matter what. So we'll take a shotgun approach and mention a number of possibilities. Your job is to decide which, if any, apply to your situation.

Biologically Delayed vs. Faster Than a Speeding Bullet

Let's start with biology. A man might be pre-disposed to delayed ejaculation if he has a slow stick for a penis that's not as sensitive as most other guys, or if his body is wired in such a way that he needs to reach a higher level of excitement than others before his ejaculation button gets triggered. He can't do any more to change the way he's wired than you can blink and your Ford turns into a Maserati or your Suburban into a Prius. So what we'll focus on are some of the possible work-arounds that you might consider.

On the other hand, if you have premature ejaculation and come faster than Han Solo in a Millennium Falcon, you might be thinking, "What's the big deal—I'll trade my premature ejaculation for his delayed ejaculation in a heartbeat." But unless you've been there and done that, it's hard to understand just how cumbersome or what a burden on a relationship delayed ejaculation can be. It can make sex hard work for both partners.

Although premature ejaculation and delayed ejaculation are on opposite sides of the cum spectrum, they both result in the man's ejaculation taking center stage. Instead of his being able to have fun with his partner and sharing pleasure, sex becomes more about his equipment and its failure to ejaculate when he wishes it would.

Reverse Misogyny

Here's a caution about delayed ejaculation that you won't read elsewhere. Not many years ago we used to say that a woman who couldn't have an orgasm from intercourse was "frigid." We would give her a medical diagnosis as if she had a disease. While "frigid" is nicer than "retarded," we now consider ourselves more enlightened. We tell people today that a lot of women can't have orgasms from thrusting alone during intercourse and that it's completely fine and normal if they have their orgasms from masturbation. In other words, we've tried to make the female orgasm something a woman is allowed to have by her own hand, rather than it being an experience she needs to put on parade during intercourse.

We are neither as kind nor as generous with men. If a man can come only from masturbation but not intercourse, we call him a "retarded" or "delayed" ejaculator. He feels horrible about himself, and his partner is sure it's because he doesn't find her sexually appealing. Or she doesn't feel like she can do anything good for him in a sexual way. So sex can become a source of dread and anxiety for both partners.

If you are a man or a couple with this problem, why not at least try to remember that there are plenty of ways you can enjoy intercourse and sexual intimacy without needing an ejaculation to signal that you are crossing the lovemaking finish line. What if you agree on a sign your partner can give during intercourse for when she or he is satisfied and wants to stop? This takes the pressure off of both of you.

Women invented and have been using a special "I want to stop having intercourse" signal since the beginning of time. It's called faking an orgasm. Unfortunately, a guy can't get away with that on a regular basis. If he could, few people would know there was such a thing as delayed ejaculation.

Beyond the Basic Symptom

Let's look at some of the possible causes and treatments of delayed ejaculation with an emphasis on the word "possible." That's because much of the current information is based on anecdote, which means if it is real science, it's only real science by accident. Please keep in mind that what follows is strictly for informational purposes. This is not meant to take the place of a meeting with your healthcare provider, although few health care professionals will have a clue on how to deal with delayed ejaculation, aside from eliminating various medical causes.

It's important to be sensitive about the couple aspect of delayed ejaculation. A couple's chemistry, ability to talk it over, and willingness to deal with the matter are all important if they hope to make progress. And if a man's partner tends to be passive during sex, helping him deal with his delayed ejaculation may require that she step outside of her comfort zone.

Patience, Prudence, Drug Side Effects and More

If you're the kind who's looking for a magic pill, it's unlikely the ejaculation gods will be blowing too many sticky kisses your way. If you want it to be like TV talk shows where patients solve massive problems in the span of two commercials, forget it. And good luck if your goal is to be like porn stars—where the male actors are human thrust-and-come machines who have no emotions or need for feedback and communication with their partners. Actually, at least one sex therapist believes a lot of male porn stars suffer from delayed ejaculation; they've just managed to make a career out of it.

Speaking of magic pills, you want to rule out the possibility that the ejaculation problem is a side effect of any drug or medications you are taking. Anti-depressants are at the top of a list of possible causes that includes antipsychotic medications, methadone, heroin, opiates, other analgesics, tranquilizers, sedatives, medications to lower your blood pressure, various muscle relaxers, pregabalin, gapapentin, benzos, GHB, poppers, marijuana, cocaine, alcohol, and possibly cigarette smoking.

Don't assume that drugs will include delayed ejaculation as a possible side effect on their warning labels. There are medications that don't list heart attacks as a possible side effect when they probably should, so don't expect them to put "delayed ejaculation" on the side of the box even if they truly do cause problems with ejaculation.

If your problem with delayed ejaculation hasn't been lifelong, try to think back to when it was that your ability to come suddenly went. Were any new medications introduced around that time? Likewise, delayed ejaculation can be secondary to erection problems, or these conditions can occur in tandem. So if you aren't having good erections, see if your healthcare provider can help you with that.

You also want to be sure that delayed ejaculation isn't due to neurological problems, multiple sclerosis, spinal-cord injury, diabetes, thyroid issues, prostate-related problems, certain surgeries, or other pelvic unpleasantries. Low testosterone can also be a suspect. While most cases of delayed ejaculation don't appear to be caused by drugs or disease, it's important to rule out these possibilities.

Religion, Abuse, and Other Possible Semen Stoppers

You might explore whether there were any traumatic psycho-social events that occurred around the time when you started to come slower than a slug in Super Glue. Did you come home unexpectedly to find your wife and best friend going at it with her screaming, "I've never come like this with that loser husband of mine!"?

Religious prohibitions about sex can be a contributing factor for men with delayed ejaculation. One study found that a disproportionate number of men with delayed ejaculation were raised in conservative religious homes or had conservative religious beliefs. Even without a conservative religious upbringing, guilt and shame can keep a man's semen parked in his pelvis.

Another possible psychological semen stopper is if a man is having fears about his partner becoming pregnant. Other issues that might be getting in the way include deep-seated anger and having a withholding personality.

On the other hand, if anger, conservative religious upbringing and fears of getting your partner pregnant were sure to cause delayed ejaculation, almost all men would suffer from it at one time or another.

Is Your Penis Lying?

The erect penis of a man with delayed ejaculation sometimes lies. This can be confusing, because when a guy is sporting a seriously hard penis, you'd normally assume he's highly aroused. But that might not be the case. Even though he's really hard, he might not be allowing himself to experience as much sexual excitement as other guys with hard-ons. To use psychological terms, his erection might be out of sync with his internal state. If that's the case, he may need to work on increasing the level of sexual excitement that he allows himself to feel. Focusing on the sensations that make him feel good sexually might be helpful.

Sometimes men with delayed ejaculation appear to be so focused on giving their partner pleasure that they won't let themselves be aware of their own sexual excitement, or they don't take in enough pleasure to reach the ejaculatory point of no return.

Too Much Focus, Too Little Excitement

There are situations in which the man is trying so hard to ejaculate, often to make his partner feel better, that he's focused on his penis at the expense of the rest of his body. This makes him even more numb to his own sexual excitement.

So consider doing a lot of exploration of the man's body from head to toe—and not just trying to find some magic spot or button that makes him ejaculate. Try to discover some of the subtle things that feel good, and work on talking more easily about them. For some men, this might include long lingering kisses up and down the side of the neck or on his chest, nipples, or back, or maybe a finger up his bum. Experiment and explore. Or you can get seriously Cosmo and run silk scarves or soft make-up brushes up and down his body. You might try to stimulate his genitals at the same time that you are kissing his neck or nipples. This can help him double up on the excitement and sensation he is feeling.

Again, the goal of this approach is to focus on pleasure rather than on orgasm. You're trying to help him experience more pleasure and excitement. Technically, you're trying to storm the guard that's keeping sensation away from his orgasm trigger. You'll need to be sensitive to how much he can handle. Some men will enjoy whatever you've got to throw at them. Others will reach a point of overload, after which all you are doing is increasing their resistance.

Note: Some therapists advise that the man not attempt to have intercourse until he can actually feel that he's sexually excited as opposed to just having an erection. Hopefully, you really will focus on pleasure as opposed to ejaculation. Sex is about sharing pleasure. Even if he never ejaculates, he might learn how to feel more pleasure and joy than guys who are able to come on command.

Harsh, Draconian Masturbation Techniques!

You'll hear a lot about the possible role of masturbation in men with delayed ejaculation. There are at least two factors to consider: the physics or mechanics of how a guy strokes himself, and the fantasy he calls up to help himself get off. We'll consider the fantasy aspect in another section.

One of the few researchers who has actually studied delayed ejaculation feels that super vigorous or unusual masturbation habits can be a contributor in some cases. He thinks that changing masturbation habits is essential in situations where the guy pounds his meat like he's making chicken fried steak. This researcher often tries to get the man to stop masturbating for several weeks or months, with the hope that he will have to rely on his partner to help him come. When the man does masturbate, a goal is to masturbate in a way that is kinder and more gentle. He's encouraged to use his other hand, or perhaps to use oil in a way that makes masturbation more like intercourse.

If a forceful masturbation technique is the source of the problem, you don't want intercourse to have to compete.

Sunny Side Up

Masturbating face down is thought to contribute to delayed ejaculation. If you have trouble coming and masturbate face down, see if you can teach yourself to start stroking it when you are on your back or while standing up.

Masturbation-Gone-Wrong? Or Is This One of Those Chicken-Egg Things?

One trouble with the masturbation-gone-wrong theory is that there are plenty of men who pound their meat mercilessly and have no problem ejaculating during partner sex. There may also be guys who masturbate face down and whose partners find them to be prolific comers.

So if these are problems, maybe they are only problems for certain guys who have some of the other contributing factors that we've talked about. Perhaps the man's penis is less sensitive than most, or his threshold to reach ejaculation is higher, so he learned to masturbate the way he did because it's the only way he can have an orgasm. If that's the case, his strange way of masturbating isn't the cause of the problem, but the result of it. Still, it's hard to see a downside to at least try to change hands or ease up on the grip, or to masturbate face up rather than face down, or to turn over the reins to a significant other.

The Role of Fantasies

It's possible that some men with delayed ejaculation have specific fantasies that they need in order to get off. But the realities of having sex with a partner might get in the way of being able to call up those fantasies.

Let's say a guy has a secret fantasy where his partner is stroking his penis with her feet, or maybe she's dressed in a special corset, or she pees on him, or he or she is being gang raped by Dopey, Grumpy, Happy, Bashful, Sneezy, Sleepy and Doc. These fantasies might work great for him when he's strokin' it alone. But how does he lose himself in them when he is having intercourse with a real-live partner whose physical presence is a sad reminder that the Seven Dwarfs are nowhere to be found?

One of the challenges for him and his partner will be to allow enough of the fantasy to safely emerge to help him get off during intercourse. This means that exploring masturbation fantasies might be fruitful in some cases of delayed ejaculation. This might not be a problem if what turns a guy on is his partner wearing a certain bra or maybe a pair of pantyhose with the crotch cut out. Most women won't be offended by those kind of requests; some will even be turned on by them.

But things can get a little dicey when his fantasies are at the extreme end of good taste and propriety, or when he feels guilty about them. It can be particularly difficult to share a fantasy with a partner when he needs the same rigid scenario to get off each and every time. The partner can begin to experience sex as a mechanical ritual.

For That Rare Man Who Doesn't Abuse Himself

There are situations when a man with delayed ejaculation can't or won't masturbate. If that's the case, you might start to explore the reasons and beliefs that are behind that decision. This will require introspection, which is not necessarily the hallmark of males, let alone those with delayed ejaculation. Some men who are too embarrassed to masturbate might try doing it in stages. They can start while they are home alone, and work up to where they can do it when their partner is home but in a different room. Eventually they might try to do it when she's in the same room but without the lights on.

When Porn Might Help

It could possibly help for a man to watch porn just before or while he is making love. The rationale is that it might increase his level of stimulation or excitement. This could theoretically help him learn to ejaculate during intercourse, or at least learn to associate ejaculation with the feelings of intercourse. Think of it as the ejaculatory equivalent of using training wheels. On the other hand, there's absolutely no science to back any of this up.

Streaming your favorite porn while making love might not sit too well with your partner. On the other hand, it could be absolutely fine with her. So it's important to talk it over first.

We consider the possibility that porn might help a person with ADHD to focus better while making love in the last part of this chapter.

When Porn Might Hurt

As a result of watching so much porn, you may have conditioned yourself to need more visual stimulation than most men in order to come. It's unlikely you'll get the kind of visual hyperstimulation from real-life lovemaking that you get from porn.

If you watch a lot of porn and have delayed ejaculation, weaning yourself from porn might be a sensible thing to try. Unfortunately, there are no easy answers.

Threshold Clinging

A consultant to this book offered his own theory on delayed ejaculation. When most men feel the sensations that tell them they are about to ejaculate, they either choose between letting themselves ejaculate or slowing down or changing positions in order to delay coming. However, some men with delayed ejaculation seem to have trained themselves to automatically go the other way once they start to feel an increase in sensation. That is, they mentally decrease their sensation or level of excitement even though they are still thrusting at the same speed.

This urology specialist advises the men to stop intercourse once they have backed away from the point of no return more than three times in one session of lovemaking. He feels that to keep thrusting away simply reinforces the tendency to delay ejaculation, which only teaches men to become even better at delaying ejaculation.

Unfortunately, this is anecdote rather than science, but it might have meaning for some readers.

Old Advice vs. New

It used to be that the advice for dealing with delayed ejaculation was to try having intercourse in novel situations or in places where there might be additional excitement from the lack of familiarity, like in the kitchen or in the back seat of a car. However, this doesn't seem to be mentioned in the more recent articles on delayed ejaculation.

This novel-situation approach attempts to distract the man from his usual modus operandi where he's thought to be the master of control. The goal is to help him relinquish his need for control, assuming that's one of the things that might be causing the problem.

Another strategy has been to have the man bring himself close to ejaculating with his own hands, and then quickly put his penis in his partner's cheering vagina and begin to thrust away. Hopefully he is able to ejaculate. As a result, he can start to appreciate that he can ejaculate inside of his partner without the world coming to an end. However, this assumes that he and his partner will find this to be of value as opposed to being yet another form of torture and torment.

Sex Toys?

Sex toys, including a vibrating cock ring or vibrating butt plug, might provide the extra stimulation that some men need to help them ejaculate during intercourse.

Just Imagine

One thing that sex therapists sometimes ask couples to do is to imagine what would happen if the problem were to suddenly disappear. The point of this is to see if certain fears or concerns might emerge.

Is there something about the problem that's keeping both partners within a certain comfort zone? Would the man's partner worry he'd want sex more often if he didn't have the problem? Would he be tempted to try his newfound skills on other women? Would he be concerned that his partner might make new demands on him, or would he sense a loss of control? None of these fears need to be grounded in reality in order to be impacting sexual response.

Are There Drugs That Can Help?

In a word, none, as of press time. No drugs have been approved for delayed ejaculation. Dopamine agonists and anti-serotonergic drugs have been tried, but side effects can be significant and there doesn't appear to be anything on the immediate horizon.

ADD, Bipolar Issues and Abuse As Contributors

A very perceptive sex therapist who has treated men with delayed ejaculation believes that some of his patients with attention deficit and bipolar issues might be at risk. He feels that some men with ADHD and bipolar problems could have trouble reaching high enough levels of sexual excitement to ejaculate during sex with a partner. This is because they are tuning in to everything in the room as opposed to the sex they are having. He wonders whether some of these men watch porn while having intercourse in order to help them focus on the sex so they can eventually ejaculate.

If you have delayed ejaculation and struggle with attention issues, perhaps his observations will be meaningful for you. While no one is encouraging you to have porn blaring on a 60-inch screen during intercourse, perhaps there are things you and your partner can do to help keep you more focused on the sex you are having and on the building excitement in your body.

This same therapist has also seen men who were sexually abused as boys who he feels may have trouble ejaculating as a result.

RECOMMENDED READING:

Michael Perelman's chapter on delayed ejaculation in the *Principles and Practices of Sex Therapy 5th edition*, edited by Y.M. Binik and K.S.K. Hall, Guilford Press, 2013.

David Rowland's ten-page section on delayed ejaculation in his book *Sexual Dysfunction in Men*, Hogrefe Publishing, 2012.

Additional Resources: Marcel Waldinger's 2007 chapter on delayed ejaculation in the 4th edition of Sandy Leiblums' *Principles and Practice of Sexual Therapy*, and Perelman and Rowland's chapter on delayed ejaculation in David Rowland's 2008 *Handbook of Sexuality and Gender Identity Disorders*. Special thanks to Stephen Braveman and Joe Marzucco.

55

When Your System Crashes

While this is a chapter on sexual problems, please keep in mind that it's only a brief overview. You are encouraged to read articles and books on sex that offer a more detailed perspective, and check with a sex therapist or physician as needed.

This chapter starts with male trouble and ends with female trouble.

Deadwood—The Bummer in Your Pants

It is amusing to look at the impotence ads in the sports section of major newspapers. They are usually located next to the ads for hair removal and hair restoration, above the ads for nude female mud wrestling and sometimes on the same page as the penis-enlargement ads. Most of the men in the impotence ads are older, same as they are on TV.

Contrary to what the erection ads show, hard-on problems happen to men of all ages, from teenagers on up. It's not unusual for erection problems to occur at the start of a sexual relationship. Call it performance anxiety, call it fear—it's not unusual for a man to need a couple of weeks or months to find a comfortable groove. Giving him any less time to get it up is silly and shortsighted, as long as your relationship is solid and there is a strong sense of mutual attraction. The real danger is not with the lack of erection, but with what each of you makes of it. Short-term problems can become long-term problems if the man sees himself as a failure or the woman needs his erection to validate that she's desirable. Consider the following from a young man in his early twenties:

> "Last week we had attempted sex again. Once again I went from an erection to completely unerect in a short amount of time. It happened when she said do you want to have sex. I had a feeling of uneasiness run through my entire body. It's almost like when you blow past a cop doing 80 and you get that feeling in your chest. It's a penetrating feeling through my body, that I won't be able to get an erection and it becomes self-fulfilling and self-defeating. I don't have control over my body and that is what is so frustrating."

A combination of sex therapy and a Viagra-like drug might be the approach of choice for this young man.

Several kinds of erection failure are discussed in the pages that follow. Whatever the cause, hopefully a man will be able to utilize moments of hydraulic failure as an excuse to explore and please his partner with his fingers, mouth and imagination. At the same time, a partner's lips and caress can feel incredible on a penis that's soft, and there are plenty of sexual fantasies the two of you can act out that don't require a penis at all.

Boners Are Not an Instant Fix

There is an interesting sex problem that some men have that is called delayed ejaculation. We talk about it more in Chapter 54: *Delayed Ejaculation*. Fortunately, there are things that can be learned about what goes right by investigating problems such as delayed ejaculation.

While the "average man" ejaculates and goes soft in approximately three to nine minutes, men with delayed ejaculation can often stay hard for forty minutes or more of serious thrusting. Some keep going for longer. With the way most men think of it, if five minutes is good, forty minutes would be eight times better. Yet that's not how it is for the men with delayed ejaculation. They have sex less often than five-minute men and they don't enjoy it nearly as much. Even though they have magnificent hard-ons, there is little magic and awe when their partner is saying "enough already."

Likewise, while drugs like Viagra help many men with erection problems get hard, more than 50% of men stop taking them. What we have learned is that it's not always a good idea to give a man an erection without a few sessions of counseling for himself and his partner first. When it comes to making love, relationship issues trump penis issues. When you haven't had sexual interaction with a partner in a couple of years, suddenly introducing a hard penis into a bedroom can create as many problems as it solves. The man might be horribly anxious about performing after all these years and the woman might wonder if he's really turned on by her or if it's the drug. There can be hundreds of other issues.

So hopefully you will stop thinking that a hard-on can fix all that ails you. Erections are marvelous wonders, but a satisfying relationship they do not make. Unfortunately, when the penis doesn't get hard or when it comes too fast or too slow, it becomes it's own vortex that sucks up all of the energies that a couple could otherwise use in pleasing each other. There are plenty of

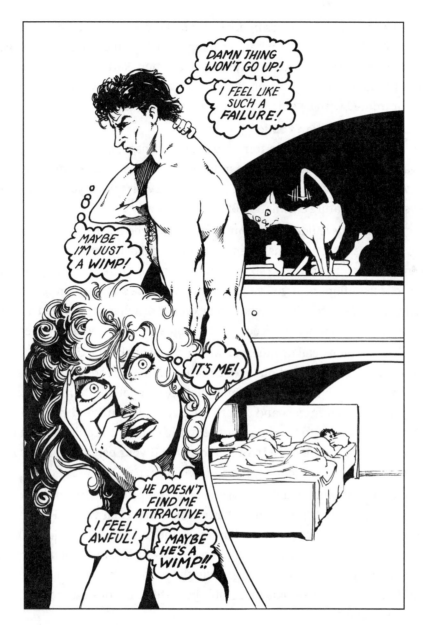

situations where a woman would be perfectly satisfied with her partner if he would focus on her instead of on what his penis is not able to do.

Suggestion If a penis stalls out, try not to give it the power to ruin your sexual intimacy. Easier said than done, but what about necking for a long time, finger fucking, oral sex, using a vibrator or dildo, tying each other up, or acting out a fantasy? That way, a potential downer might evolve into something sweet and hot. Success in life is often about what we are able to make of our shortcomings, even when it's hanging between our legs. The biggest problems with impotence isn't the lack of erection. Rather, it's a lack of playfulness and resourcefulness on the part of the man and woman when they are confronted with a penis that's being contrary.

When Your Posse Won't Ride

Books on sex often use terms such as "self-hatred," "self-loathing" and "devastating" to describe how a man feels when he is—gulp—impotent. You know, the horror when he can't get it up. (So you won't think you are all alone, guys with premature ejaculation often feel this way as well.)

Perhaps this Guide is way out of step or maybe it's just insensitive, but *devastating* is what happens when your wife or child dies or when you've just been told that you only have six months to live. *Self-hatred* is what you feel if your business flops or if you've just blown your life's savings on something really dumb. *Self-loathing* is what you experience when you've had a major stroke or accident and can't feed or bathe yourself or wipe your own rear.

Call us callous, call us rude, but we can think of about a thousand things worse than if a man's hard-on takes a hiatus, even if it's forever. Sure, it's frustrating and even humiliating at times, but so are a lot of other things in life. You still have your fingers and mouth for giving pleasure, and you still have what's in your heart to love your partner with. And if you can't count at least five things in your life to be thankful for, even if your penis never gets hard again, then your priorities are in seriously bad shape.

Contrary to what you'll read elsewhere, penis problems, regardless of the cause, are an opportunity to have better sex rather than worse. Fortunately, there are plenty of ways that modern medicine can help a recalcitrant penis to get hard, but it seems a shame to employ a quick cure without allowing yourself and your relationship to grow in the process. You won't believe how many times Viagra-like pills will result in better erections but not in better sex for either partner.

People who survive heart attacks and cancer learn to approach life differently as a result of the disease. A woman who is overcoming orgasm problems has to welcome a new way of embracing her body and her sexuality. It's a journey, a process. Impotent men, on the other hand, just want their dicks to get hard—no learning, no journey.

The Sufis have a saying that you have to let yourself die before you are truly born. Sometimes a guy has to give up his penis as a symbol of masculinity before he can get on with his life. Sometimes he has to realize that there's more to being a man than getting an erection or lasting for a prescribed number of thrusts. Then he sometimes has to convince his partner.

This is not to say that a man shouldn't inquire about the various remedies that modern medicine has for erection problems. He should also have a full physical to make sure that the erection problem is not a symptom of something else. If there are medical problems, they need to be treated.

Note: No kidding about getting a physical exam. Men who begin to experience a gradual increase in impotency might be seeing the first signs of an impending stroke, heart attack or diabetes. Impotence may be a better predictor of cardiovascular disease than the stress test. The arteries in the penis can start to gum up before those in the rest of the body. A physical exam may allow physicians to help a man before something bad happens to his most important organs—his heart and brain. Also, researchers are now finding a high correlation between obesity and impotence. Who knew that the drive-thru at McDonald's could do your dick in?

A Modern Medical Approach to the Great Groin Grinch

If your penis is impotent, it is likely you are muttering under your breath that we can take our Sufi logic and stuff it where the sun don't shine. You want a traditional Western approach. You want a magic bullet that does not require introspection or lifestyle changes. Good enough. The advice that follows is a spoof on a modern medical approach to fixing erection problems. While it conveys some wisdom, it still focuses on fixing the penis instead of helping the man behind it and the woman in front of it. It is an approach that attempts to turn the clock back to a time when the penis worked just fine. It's a regressive fix rather than a step forward, one that is oblivious to lessons that might be learned or frontiers of trust that are waiting to be crossed.

Dear Dr. Goofy Foot,
My bowling partner recently started having erection problems and is
too embarrassed to seek help. Can you offer advice?
                                                    Bob from Boston
Dear Bob,

If your bowling partner has stopped throwing strikes for more than a couple of weeks, it's a good idea for him to take his pokey pecker to a physician for a checkup. It's smart to rule out underlying medical conditions.

Modern medicine has decided that more than 99.999% of erection problems are due to physical causes, from diabetes to who-knows-what. Doctors can fix almost anything, unless your friend is a cigarette smoker. If that's the case, he might as well call a mortuary and have himself interred.

Is your friend able to get erections at all, like in the morning upon waking or when he jerks off? To explore this further, his urologist might send him home with a device he attaches to his penis when he sleeps. The device won't help to get him off, but it does tell if he has erections in his sleep and for how long. If a man can get a rigid sustained erection in his sleep or while masturbating, the plumbing below his belt probably works. Then a question to explore is if the problem resides in his psyche.

Some physicians will send your friend home with samples of Viagra—or Levitra, Cialis if they have stock in Glaxo or Lilly. If the pills don't work, then they'll do a work-up. Or they might give your friend's penis an injection that's a pecker-picker-upper. Don't worry, no one's going to pull out a syringe with a hollow nail for a needle and say, "Drop your drawers." It's an itty-bitty wisp of a shot that hurts less than getting a pubic hair stuck in your zipper. If the penis gets hard and is able to stay hard, then the underlying plumbing is intact and the problem can probably be fixed with a prescription.

If the shot does not make the penis hard, or it gets hard but doesn't stay hard, then it's likely there is a circulation problem. This can range from hardening of the arteries (strange term for when it happens in the penis!) to leaky valves. More tests would need to be done to peg the exact cause.

It is also possible that there is a neurological problem which is disabling the body's ability to begin the hard-on process. This is similar to when you turn the ignition key on your car and nothing happens. Another thing to check is if your friend is taking medications that might be cold-cocking his penis. Suspicious meds range from alcohol and heroin to prescriptions and over-the-counter drugs. Some say that Tagamet can do a dick in. (Your friend isn't one of those meth-abusing party boys, is he? Recreational drugs can be very bad for a penis.)

If they can't find anything medical, they may consider the unlikely possibility that your friend's erection problem stems from emotional causes or a combination of something emotional and physical. To explore the emotional possibilities, some questions are in order. For instance, what was going on in your friend's life around the time when his soldier stopped marching? Did his ability to get an erection decline gradually, like the fall of Rome, or did it shut down all at once, like Bear Stearns, Wachovia or Lehman Brothers? Was there a change in his job status? Did his team not go to the Superbowl because of a lousy call in the closing seconds? Was there a change in his relationship with his partner? Did his wife leave him for another man? Did she leave him for another woman? Was he pulled from an important project, or did he lose a promotion he had his heart set on? Did he receive an unkind inquiry from the IRS?

Also, it is helpful to inquire about his relationship with his spouse. If he instantly says, "Naw, it's fine," ask him to describe some of the things that are fine about it. See if he conveys a sense of love and fondness, or if he sounds like he's reading the instructions on a bottle of Kaopectate. If the relationship has fallen on–dare we say–hard times, then he and his wife need to focus on fixing that rather than on fixing his penis, which is merely the messenger.

In order to treat erection problems that are caused by relationship problems, your friend and his partner might try to forget all that they know about each other and start over again as if they'd just met. This can be difficult, especially if they have had some really lousy times together. They might try taking a month or two doing things like hugging, touching and talking, with no attempt at intercourse. They also might try sharing romantic dinners, movies and the types of things they enjoyed doing when they first met. How about racking their bowling balls and taking a trip around the country? They might discover that there really is life after bowling. On the other hand, some couples do better when they spend less time with each other. This can be especially true when they are newly retired and suddenly find themselves in each other's face 24 hours a day.

He and his wife should be reminded that the more mature the penis, the more hands-on play and wooing it needs in order to get hard. Lots and lots. Also, there's the possibility that your friend had erection problems before he and his wife met. And if none of that helps, there's this Sufi saying....

Soft Hard vs. Hard Hard

Most younger men don't realize that there are at least two separate mechanisms that make for an erection. That's because when they are sexually aroused, their penis can go so fast from the first step to the second step that it's all pretty much a blur.

The first step is when the penis starts to get bigger and becomes just hard enough for intercourse but is still kind of floppy. It requires a separate mechanism or a second step to take an erection from bigger-but-floppy to seriously hard. (In urology speak, the first step utilizes the veno-occlusive mechanism while the second step requires cavernosal artery perfusion pressure.)

While a lot of men with ED are able to achieve the first step, failure to complete the second step leaves them with a "soft erection" that's maybe hard enough to stuff into a vagina. This can result in intercourse that doesn't last as long as it used to, or intercourse that isn't as much fun as it used to be. So there are at least two issues to be aware of if you are having ED problems— whether your penis can get big enough, and then whether it can get hard enough. For many men, erection drugs help make the second step more doable. On the other hand, Viagra isn't going to transform a middle-aged or older penis into that of an 18-year old. It's an assist, not a miracle.

The Finest Viagra Quote

One of the finest quotes about Viagra is from the *Boston Globe*'s Ellen Goodman:

> "I can't help wondering why we got a pill to help men with performance instead of communication. Moreover, how is it possible that we came up with a male impotence pill before we got a male birth control pill? The Vatican, you will note, has approved Viagra while still condemning condoms."

Viagra & Friends—Be Sure to Read the Instructions

Remember how Barbie had friends like Skipper and Midge? Viagra has pill friends, with names like Levitra, Cialis and Stendra. People often prefer Cialis because you don't have to take it soon before intercourse. Another problem with Viagra is that you need to take it on an empty stomach. This is a major reason why Viagra doesn't work very well for some men: they don't take it on an empty stomach. If you are taking boner drugs, be sure to carefully read all of the instructions

Also, do not buy boner drugs from online sellers unless you know they are a licensed pharmacy. There is a lot of counterfeit Viagra on the Internet.

Viagra in the Cockpit

Pilots are not allowed to take Viagra for twelve hours before a flight. The FAA does not want the co-pilot to accidentally grab the pilot's erection instead of the landing-gear controls. Viagra also inhibits an enzyme in the penis which helps the blood vessels dilate. A similar enzyme in our eyes might possibly be impacted by Viagra. This is why there has been concern that Viagra could result in altered color perception. Pilots who are taking Viagra have apparently seen flying vaginas in the friendly skies. **Note:** Researchers are now saying that if the pilots are seeing vaginas, it's because a stewardess is dancing around the cockpit naked. Hard as they tried, they weren't able to show that Viagra was impacting vision. If you are having visual issues after taking, try switching to one of the other boner drugs that has less of an affinity to impact the enzymes in the eye.

Levitra as a Thrill Pill?

At least the Viagra people have had the decency to market their drug toward guys who might actually need it. No such claim can be made by the makers of Levitra, which is clearly going for the younger man who gets it up just fine. In one of their ads, they show a young stud trying to throw a football through a tire. It bounces off to the side. After Levitra is mentioned, the boy gets the ball through the tire several times. He is then joined by his smiling wife or girlfriend, whose tires he seems to have rotated quite nicely.

The interesting thing about boner drugs is they don't add a whole lot to the experience if you're able to get a good erection to begin with. And as is related in Chapter 5: *On The Penis,* the recreational use of boner drugs can cause psychological dependence on them.

Other Chemicals That Make You Hard

There are some compounds that cause a diehard erection when they are injected into the penis, assuming the penile plumbing can maintain an erection once the penis gets hard. A compound called Papervine was formerly used for this purpose, but now there are different combinations of ingredients used in the injections. One popular combination includes papervine, phentolamine, and prostaglandin E1.

Also, there is a kind of prostaglandin which a man shoots into his urethra (peehole) to help give himself an erection. It's like a fertilizer stick that you shove in the soil next to your droopy houseplants.

There are other orally-prescribed drugs that can help some men to get hard. One drug that is sometimes prescribed is called yohimbine. Yohimbine is native to Africa. It can often be found in health food stores. Since the cost of yohimbine isn't much more by prescription, why not get it from a urologist? That way you will be monitored for side effects and you can be sure you are getting the yohimbine in consistent doses, which is not true for the yohimbine in health food stores. The doc can also rule out other possible causes of the erection problem. Other drugs for impotence that are being tested include one that is administered in cream form. The problem is getting the cream to penetrate through the part of the penis that surrounds the vascular tissue. Another problem is stiffness in your fingers after applying the cream.

"Ejaculate Like a Porn Star," "Add an Inch in Two Weeks," "Natural Male Enhancement," "Recharge Your Libido"— Some Seriously Iffy Ideas

There is probably not a living human being who hasn't seen ads for herbal pills that promise to get you horny, big and hard. Some of these products are cleverly marketed to make them look legitimate.

Some of the companies that produce these pills are being shut down for consumer fraud. Also, if your in-laws wanted to make herbal supplements in their garage where their fourteen cats sleep, they could. And they could sell them on TV. There is no regulation on herbal supplements. They can put strychnine and cow plops in herbal pills. The only way the government will test herbal pills is if about a dozen people suddenly die.

If there really were a pill that could put a smile on Bob's face and do all of the things the scammers and spammers say their pills can do, don't you think the multi-billion dollar drug companies would be selling it?

Mechanical Devices for Getting Hard & Surgical Implants

Some men find that the vacuum pump is a useful erection aid. It is a little bulky and cumbersome, but worth a try if you are in search of a lost erection. What do you have to lose, unless there are medical reasons why you shouldn't. There are different suppliers for vacuum pumps. Be sure the pump you get includes gaskets which keep your scrotum from getting sucked up into the vacuum tube. Some of the penis pumper companies that market to gay males sell excellent units for less than half of the ones that are medicare approved. Still, expect to pay $100 for a decent rig.

There are different surgical implants, from semi-rigid shanks to implants with little pumps that will give a man an erection. Frequent improvements are being made in the technology. Please research this subject carefully before making an incision—uh, decision.

The Tour de France in Your Pants

Urologists have been saying for years that bicycle seats are causing erection problems for hard riders (or formerly hard riders). They've been seeing case after case of young riders with numbness in their crotches and erection issues. It's not so much that riders can't get it up, but that it won't stay up. Instead of wanting to study the matter further, some of the bike magazines tried to discredit the concerned physicians.

But the bicycle industry underestimated the steadfastness of the crotch docs who spend hours each day with their faces between mens' legs. The crotch docs wired bicycle seats with more sensors than the Sands Casino when it was demolished. They did studies on bicycle-riding policemen whose penis heads were connected to oxygen sensors. They found that the typical bicycle saddle robs the penis of 80% of its oxygen and causes a decrease in erections during sleep. Plus, there's a major nerve to your penis that runs between your legs. It takes a terrible thrashing when you are using a traditional saddle. You know that tingling sensation after riding a bike for awhile? It's not normal. It is from crotch compression which can damage the nerves in your penis or clitoris.

When you sit in a chair, your weight is distributed across your entire butt and thighs. Because of the wide distribution of weight, the circulation in the crotch is not compromised and the nerves aren't damaged. But when you are on a bike, the entire weight of your body is bearing down a very small part of your crotch that provides the oxygen and nerves to your genitals. As for the newer bike saddles with the cut-outs? They can actually make the problem worse, as there's even less area to distribute your weight over.

Unfortunately, women are no more immune than guys. Researchers found a measurable decrease in sexual sensation for women who ride seriously. They've also found a condition on competitive riders called "Bicyclist's Vulva" where one of the labia can grow really big due to the pounding a girl's crotch takes from the seat.

The solution? There are two. The first is to raise the handlebars above the level of the seat so you sit up instead of crouching over. This will help somewhat. The other solution is to get a saddle without a nose called a no-nose saddle. Inner-city cops who chase criminals on bikes swear by them. For a list of no-nose saddles, visit www.no-nose.com.

Peyronie's Disease (PD)

This is a condition that results in a curving or bending deformity of the penis. It can range from mild to so severe that intercourse is not possible and there can be pain with erection. PD results from plaques forming on the tunica albuginea of the penis. This results in scar tissue that prevents that side of the penis from expanding during erection. This causes curvature during erection and sometimes pain. (Think of what happens if you put a piece of tape on one side of a long balloon and then try to blow it up.)

Most PD patients are between 45 and 65 years of age, with the average onset occurring at 53 years. The causes of PD are not fully understood. There is no approved treatment for PD. Attempts to treat PD have included intralesional nicardipine injection, vacuum therapy, vitamin E, potaba, colchicine, tamoxifen, carnitine, pentoxifylline, PDE5 inhibitors and surgery. Treatment options and success often depend on the stage and severity of the PD. While there is spontaneous repair in some cases, these would be in the minority. Men with moderate to severe cases are often clinically depressed, describing themselves as "feeling like a freak." Pyronie's-related depression can take its toll on a relationship. If it's a problem for you, find a urologist who specializes in the treatment of Peyronie's Disease.

Pharmaceutical Sex Assassins That Impact Both Men and Women

You wouldn't believe how many over-the-counter or prescription medications can mess with everything from your ability to get hard or wet to your feelings of desire. For instance, just taking a common antihistamine can keep a woman from lubricating. Extending this into a worst-case scenario:

1. A woman takes an antihistamine to help with her runny nose. It dries up her nose, and her vagina.

2. Because of the dry vagina, she starts having painful intercourse.

3. Because of the pain, the muscles in her vagina tense up whenever she sees her husband's penis get hard.

4. The tensing up in her vagina becomes a learned response, and continues for long after she's stopped taking the allergy medicine.

5. Because of the constant pain, she experiences a decrease in sexual desire, which causes her insecure husband to have an affair. She finds out about it and files for divorce. All because she took a

couple of Sudafed! Or maybe she's taking an antidepressant which decreases sexual desire. How sad, a divorce due to an antidepressant.

At the top of the list of sexual suspects should be any medication that says, "May cause drowsiness. Do not drive or operate heavy equipment." Assume when they say "equipment" they are also referring to your sexual equipment or your sex drive.

Whatever your sexual problems or concerns, the absolute first thing to do is to make a list of all the medications you are taking—from simple over-the-counter drugs to prescription medications to herbal teas and vitamin concoctions to heroin, cocaine, pot, poppers, ecstasy, meth, or alcohol. Then check these over with a pharmacist. Medications may not be the cause of the sexual problem, but they're the first and most obvious thing to rule out.

The Warning that Should Be on Paxil, Prozac, Zoloft & The Other SSRIs

According to the *Journal of Sexual Medicine*, any person who has been given a prescription for an SSRI antidepressant should be given a warning such as the following:

> "There is a high probability of sexual side effects while on SSRI medications. There are indications that in an unknown number of cases, the side effects may not resolve with cessation of the medication and could be potentially irreversible."

SSRIs are antidepressants that include Prozac, Zoloft, Paxil, Lexapro, Luvox, Celexa, Effexor, Serzone and Remeron.

A Question of Desire

Some people think that "low desire" is a sickness like the flu that a woman needs to get over. They assume that she's cured of her low desire if she can happily hop on her partner's erect penis. But low desire can mean different things, some of which require a reworking of the relationship outside of the bedroom before there will be any changes between the sheets. The mind-set of trying to recreate what the woman was like in the past is not productive. None of us are the same as we were a few years ago. Our sexuality needs to reflect our current situation, and in some cases of low desire, that is exactly what it is doing.

It is also possible that low desire can result from physical causes or metabolic changes. For some women, taking birth-control pills or certain medications can cause changes in desire that last after they discontinue the pills or medications. We know that anti-depressants can do horrible things to a person's sex drive.

Drug companies are trying very hard to get products containing testosterone approved for women with low sexual desire. This might be helpful if a woman has had her ovaries removed or if she has a metabolic disorder, but women should be cautious about these preparations. Their use as an elixor for low desire is controversial.

Highly Recommended: Remember the finger that you used to masturbate with? Why not put it to use by turning the pages of books like *Wanting Sex Again: How to Rediscover Your Desire and Heal a Sexless Marriage* by Laurie Watson, Penguin, 2012, and Kathryn Hall's helpful book *Reclaiming Your Sexual Self: How You Can Bring Desire Back into Your Life*, John Wiley & Sons, (2004). These books treat low desire as a messenger rather than as a disease. Men and women both will be able to find approaches to help them better understand and give meaning to lost desire. Neither author is beholden to the drug companies. They realize the short-sightedness of automatically throwing pills or patches at whatever ails you.

When Excitement Is Too Much

Some of us can't tolerate much excitement. Somewhere along the line we got the feeling that sexual excitement is dangerous or disorganizing. As a result, we experience conflicts when becoming sexually excited. People with this problem sometimes numb themselves between the navel and the knees. That way they don't have to face the anticipated dread that sexual excitement holds in their imagination.

Those who want to work through excitement problems need to experience pleasurable feelings slowly and without goals such as having an orgasm. Pressure to feel sexual takes them out of the moment and makes them feel numb. With time and effort, sexual excitement can be tolerated in the here and now, assuming that's what you want.

Some people have trouble managing sexual excitement when they are alone. They can't masturbate or even feel sexual on their own, but do just fine when they are with a partner. Perhaps they need to experience a partner's excitement about them before they can feel their own excitement.

Orgasm Fears & Tears

Although orgasms are usually welcome events, this is not always the case. Young girls or boys who are having their first orgasms can sometimes feel that they have done something wrong or broken something inside.

Adults can have mixed feelings about their own orgasms, especially when sadness, loneliness or guilt are triggered by the orgasm. The sadness can be about a former real-life partner, or maybe the orgasm taps into a deep emotional pain that suddenly gets released. Some people cry after an intense orgasm because it touches a sadness that's deep inside.

There are also people who treat their own orgasms with cold detachment, especially when they feel a need to masturbate. Perhaps the need for sexual relief brings up feelings of weakness or self-loathing. Whatever the case, they are not particularly gentle or tender when handling their own genitals. There are also people who dislike orgasms because they experience them as a form of losing control. It's a fine testament to the power of orgasm that more people in our society don't have problems with them.

Painful Intercourse

The 2010 National Survey of Sexual Health and Behavior found that 30% of women reported some pain during their last intercourse. It is likely that the kind of pain the majority of these women are experiencing is because they were not adequately aroused during intercourse. The causes can be everything from clumsy lovemaking to relationship conflicts.

However, there's another kind of sexual pain that happens to some women regardless of how much she wants to have sex or aroused she might be. This kind of pain can happen to men as well, but more often to women. The pain is not necessarily limited to the vulva, vagina, or bladder, but can also result from problems in the floor of the pelvis.

If you are having pain during intercourse, be sure to check with a physician or physical therapist who specializes in pelvic pain. If you are a woman, try to determine whether the pain is at the opening of the vagina or is caused by deep thrusting. Deep-thrusting pain is sometimes caused by constipation or pelvic inflammatory disease. Shallow-thrusting pain has a larger range of possible causes, from adhesions under the clitoral hood or episiotomy scars to yeast infections, herpes sores, or vaginal changes associated with menopause. Other questions to explore about painful intercourse include whether it happens all the time, how long it has been happening, if it happens with all partners or just one, and if added lubrication helps.

This kind of pain is very real and it can have horrible effects on a sexual relationship. The woman (and couple) who is experiencing it needs the same kind of support as anyone who is experiencing a chronic-pain disorder.

Here are some of things that might be going on:

VULVODYNIA: this would be Latin for "a great big pain in my pussy." Symptoms include discomfort or burning pain in the vulvar area of unexplained origin, which means that no infections or neurological disorders appear to be present. Often described as a chronic burning or knife-like pain, this disorder is very complex and can be a serious challenge to treat. Most healthcare providers throw their gloved-hands up in despair, which means that the patient will need to do a lot of research and find a specialist who works with vulvodynia. Just to give you an idea of the complexity, vulvodynia can be broken down into pain that is generalized or localized, and these categories are further broken down into pain that is provoked, unprovoked or both provoked and unprovoked. While few physicians who specialize in treating vulvodynia believe it is the result of psychological problems, a lot of patients and their healthcare providers mistakenly do. This isn't to say that stress and anxiety can't make the symptoms worse, but the are unlikely the cause. We have an entire chapter on this type of sexual pain, Chapter 56: *Damn That Hurts! When Sex Is Painful.*

VULVAR VESTIBULITIS: a form of vulvodynia where the pain or discomfort is localized to the vulvar vestibule, which is the part of the vulva that's between the inner lips. In some cases, the pain has been there since their first tampon or intercourse, in others it started long after. Could be from any of a number of different causes, including the use of oral contraceptives. We have an entire chapter on this type of sexual pain, Chapter 56: *Damn That Hurts! When Sex Is Painful.*

VULVITIS: an inflammation of the vulva. There can be as many causes as there are vulvas.

INTERSTITIAL CYSTITIS: pain or discomfort in the pelvis that is related to the bladder. Symptoms often include a persistent urge to pee or the need to pee frequently, as often as a couple of times an hour. This is not called "painful bladder syndrome" without good reason, as the urge can feel quite extreme and it can be accompanied by spasms and pressure. People can have pain while urinating, pain while driving, and pain while having sex. In men, there can be painful ejaculation. The cause is not known, although a number of theories are on the table, and it could be there are different things that cause it. There are a number of different treatments, with one of the main goals being in decreasing the pain. People with this disorder are often very depressed as a result, in part due to the pain and discomfort, and in part because it causes such incredible interference in their lives.

PELVIC INFLAMMATORY DISEASE (PID): inflammation of the female reproductive organs, often the Fallopian tubes, which is usually caused by a bacterial infection.

HIGHLY RECOMMENDED: *When Sex Hurts: A Woman's Guide to Banishing Sexual Pain* by Andrew Goldstein, Caroline Pukall, and Irwin Goldstein, Da Capo Lifelong Books. This book was written by three of the top specialists in the research and treatment of women's sexual pain. If you or your partner is experiencing female sexual pain, there is no better place to start than with this book.

Women's Orgasm Problems

Plenty of women don't have orgasms with thrusting during intercourse. This doesn't mean that they have sexual problems. All it means is that both partners need to explore what gets the woman off and include it as part of their lovemaking, unless it happens to be the man's best friend, though some couples might enjoy that, too. (See Chapter 23: *Intercourse—Horizontal Jogging* for more on stimulating the clitoris during intercourse.)

One of the first things therapists look for in women who don't have orgasms is a history of sexual abuse. Yet plenty of men and women who never had a shred of sexual abuse still have sexual problems. Being raised in a highly religious household can cause sexual problems that appear similar to those of sexual abuse, including the person's feeling vacant, depersonalized, or numb when having sex. Good luck having an orgasm with all of that going on. Books on this subject that are often recommended include *The Elusive Orgasm: A Woman's Guide to Why She Can't and How She Can Orgasm* (by

Vivienne Cass), *For Yourself* (by Lonnie Barbach) and *Becoming Orgasmic* (by Julia Heiman & Leslie LoPiccolo).

Vaginismus — Gridlock in Your Groin

Vaginismus is a tightness in the vagina that causes discomfort, burning, pain, penetration problems, or complete inability to have intercourse. The muscles surrounding the vagina can close so tightly that they won't allow anything to go inside. The reaction can be so severe that a woman can't even insert a tampon.

Vaginismus is no longer considered a separate disorder, because it is often difficult to distinguish from other chronic pelvic pain disorders. An excellent source of information and help for vaginismus is Lisa and Mark Carter's website and online community at www.Vaginismus.com. Also, please see Chapter 56: *Damn That Hurts! When Sex Is Painful.*

Persistent Genital Arousal Disorder (PGAD)

This is an unusual and difficult disorder that has only recently been recognized. It is when a woman's genitals are physically aroused for hours, days, weeks or longer, but she doesn't feel any desire to have sex. Having sex provides no relief, and orgasms don't help her arousal to reside. This would be similar to if a man had an erection for weeks at time, where he desperately wanted it to go down, but the most earth-shaking orgasm and ejaculation would not bring a smile of satisfaction or a dent in the tent in his pants. Some medications can be helpful, but there is no cure.

Based on what is currently known, PGAD is a syndrome with a wide array of possible causes. Areas that have been studied the most are 1.) PGAD as experienced by women who tend to be post menopausal and who appear to have a pudendal nerve neuralgia but no pre-existing psychological illness. This kind of neuralgia would impact the dorsal clitoral nerve; 2.) PGAD has been associated with withdrawal from some SSRI antidepressants; 3.) PGAD has been linked to Tarlov cysts on the spine; 4.) Some women with PGAD have a fairly extensive history of affective disorder, obsessive-compulsive disorder, and sexual assault. This type of PGAD is considered to be a psychosomatic illness, where the women misinterpret genital sensations and experience them as negative events; and 5.) There has been an association of some cases of PGAD with restless legs syndrome and overactive bladder.

CHAPTER
56
Damn That Hurts!
When Sex is Painful

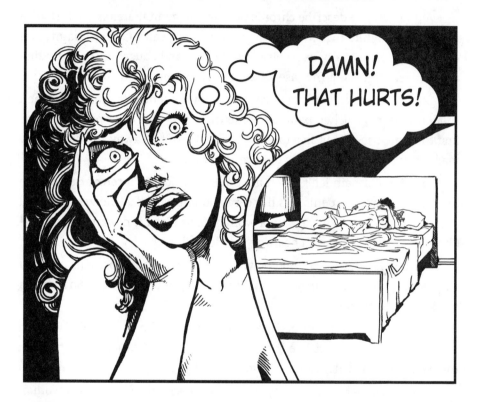

Few men understand how painful sex can be for some women. This isn't pain from the kind of rushed and rough sex that's typical in porn. Instead, think of when a Q-tip is pressed against a woman's genitals and it causes her to flinch in pain. Or when intercourse with a gentle lover creates an intense burning sensation in her vagina or makes her feel like she's being stabbed with a knife. Or when the muscles around the opening of her vagina are clamped so tight she can't insert a tampon.

Fortunately, for plenty of women with sexual pain, it's not this severe. But it still makes sex something they endure rather than enjoy.

Many of us assume there are two times in life when sex hurts for women: their first time and after menopause. We don't realize that more than 20% of women in their teens, twenties, thirties and beyond can experience pain during sex, and not just once or twice. This is chronic sexual pain that lasts for months or years.

What Chronic Pelvic Pain Isn't

A good way to describe chronic pain in the genital area is to start with what it isn't. While rushed or clumsy lovemaking can make sex painful for women, this can usually be resolved with effort and education, or by finding a new lover. That is not the case when there is chronic pain during sex.

Sometimes a woman can have great sex with a man for years, and then suddenly develop pelvic pain. Or sometimes she will have pain from the first time she tries to put in a tampon and it doesn't go away, no matter how many different lovers she tries to have sex with.

This kind of pain isn't when a woman is enjoying intercourse and the head of her partner's penis hits her cervix and it feels like she was punched in the stomach. Nor is it the pain a woman feels if she is dry and needs lube. Chronic sexual pain doesn't go away by adding lube.

A woman can't fix chronic pelvic pain by changing positions or wrapping her legs around a partner's waist instead of around his neck. So it's not a matter of lube or logistics.

A lover's penis might be three clicks bigger than huge and a woman may need to do exercises like they teach in childbirth classes to fit it in, but that is not usually what causes chronic sexual pain.

Chronic sexual pain is pretty much there each and every time a woman has intercourse, assuming she is able to have intercourse. It doesn't suddenly get better if she has sex with another guy or her partner's younger brother.

While menopause may bring it's own set of issues that can lead to pain during intercourse, the type of pelvic pain this chapter is about is not because of menopause.

What Pelvic Pain Might Be *(The Rest of This Chapter Is Addressed to Women)*

A problem with defining pelvic pain is that whatever caused it probably occurred long ago. This might have been an infection inside your vagina or it might have started from a dermatological condition in the sensitive area between your lips called the vulvar vestibule. The vulvar vestibule is like a small platform that the urethra (peehole) and the opening of the vagina are mounted on.

The pain might have developed in response to an uncomfortable gynecological exam, or a sudden surge of hormones in your body that went back to normal in a few days, weeks, or months. It could have been caused by taking oral contraceptives, or by an allergic reaction.

As long as there are no current conditions that might be causing the pain, the cause is not what's important. The problem you are probably dealing with now is the reaction (or over-reaction) of your nerves and muscles to something that happened long ago. But as far as your body is concerned, this doesn't make it any less severe or less painful than if it happened yesterday.

Creating a Strategy

There are a number of books on sexual pain, some of which are recommended in this chapter. Unfortunately, many offer an approach that doesn't take into account the complexity of the problem. Here are some of the steps that may be required to help resolve your sexual pain. Some researchers say it will require all of these steps to effectively fix the problem:

- Getting a thorough exam to rule out medical conditions that might be causing pain. This can be done by a gynecologist or a physical therapist who specializes in pelvic pain disorders—in a perfect world, you would see both.

- Learning all you can about chronic pelvic pain before you try various solutions.

- Retraining your central nervous system.

- Retraining the muscles in your pelvis.

- Involving your partner if you have one.

Eliminate the Obvious

While the original cause of your pelvic pain may be long gone, you will need thorough exam by a competent gynecologist to rule out any causes of pain that still might be ongoing.

Deep-thrusting pain is sometimes caused by constipation or pelvic inflammatory disease. Shallow-thrusting pain has a larger range of possible causes, from adhesions under the clitoral hood or episiotomy scars to yeast infections. There are a number of pain-causing conditions with names that are difficult to pronounce. Some are listed in the preceding chapter.

It would seem that most gynecologists would know how to treat chronic pelvic pain, but few specialize in this area. This is why the next step is so very important.

Knowledge—The Key to Any Strategy to Zap Pelvic Pain

To help assure a positive outcome, you need to be well informed from the very beginning.

Fortunately, pelvic pain is not as hopeless as it used to be—far from it. Research is now being done and there are helpful resources. But it will be up to you and your partner to form a strategy, or just you if you don't have a partner.

Assuming you are in good gynecological health, one of the first things to do is to read the resources that are suggested in this chapter. Please do this *before* venturing on an odyssey through the healthcare system to cure your pelvic pain. Hopefully you will find other resources as well, but a good place to begin is with the *When Sex Hurts* book and at the website of the *National Vulvodynia Association*. (See **Resources** at the end of the chapter.)

Is the Pain in Your Head? YES!

Whatever caused the pelvic pain in the first place is usually gone by the time you see one of umpteenth healthcare providers who women with pelvic pain often see. So you will soon start to hear that the pain is in your head. And for the most part, this is true! That's because all pain comes from our heads, or our brains, anyway. It doesn't matter if you step on a nail or break your arm. The pain is controlled by your brain, which decides when to turn the pain on and when to turn it off, as well as when to turn it up and down.

What probably happened is your nerves and the muscles between your legs responded to the initial provocation exactly as they should have. Your brain assessed the incoming data from the nerve receptors in your genitals, decided there was a problem, and started setting off pain alarms. And then the muscles in your pelvis probably started clamping down to help protect you from what your brain perceived was a threat.

But after the threat was gone, your brain and the muscles never got the memo. They might still be fighting a in a war that's long been over. They are still on hyper alert, as if the cause of the pain was never resolved.

Whatever happened in your vulva or vagina ended up creating the perfect storm, especially if you have a genetic predisposition to being tense or anxious.

The Pain Is Also on Your Forearm and in Your Feet

Researchers have discovered that women who have chronic pelvic pain are more sensitive to pain throughout their entire body. This is called pain amplification. It's a nice way of saying things are messed up.

When researchers put noxious substances on the forearms and feet of women who do and don't have pelvic pain, the women who have pelvic pain notice the pain much more. It's as if whatever went on in their genitals created a glitch or hypersensitivity throughout their entire body. The skin all over their body becomes more sensitive to tactile sensation. This is often the case with pain disorders. Pain in one part of the body can make us more sensitive to pain in other non-related parts.

Some women with chronic pelvic pain become so hyper alert that even thinking about sex can cause them pain. Sexual fantasies which, in the past, may have made them want to masturbate or jump their partner on the spot might now cause them to feel pain in their genitals. This pain is every bit as real as the pain when you hit your finger with a hammer.

The good news is that it's possible to retrain a nervous system that is on hyper alert. To learn more about how, you'll want to read the *Why Pelvic Pain Hurts* book that's listed at the end of the chapter.

Pelvic Floor Muscles — The Pit Bull in Your Panties

The muscles in the pelvis are usually players in chronic pelvic pain conditions. Sometime they are the key players, other times not. But by the time a woman has chronic pain during sex, her muscles are usually doing things they shouldn't.

One pelvic pain specialist who works with elite athletes says that a number of her patients who do repetitive motions on one side of their body have pain during intercourse as a result, eg, tennis players, volleyball players, golfers, shot putters, javelin throwers, etc. The muscles on that side of their pelvis become tense or tight, and can make intercourse very painful. So for these women, physical therapy involves biofeedback that helps them learn to relax the muscles on one side of their pelvis.

The sexual pain for these athletes began in their pelvic muscles. In other women with pelvic pain, the muscle problems in their pelvis began after the original cause of the pain. One or more of the pelvic muscles tightened up to help protect the women from the source of the problem. Muscle groups in the pelvis that control the opening of the vagina may have started clamping shut whenever something like a finger or penis touched a woman's genitals, and they continue to do so. The muscles might stay relaxed until there is touch, and then they go ballistic.

For other women, the muscles in their pelvis never relax. They are like a pit bull in your panties.

There can also be trigger points along various muscles in the pelvis. Touch or pressure on these trigger points can cause excruciating pain.

This is why a strategy to eliminate pelvic pain will most likely need to include teaching the muscles in your pelvis to relax. The *Sex Without Pain: A Self-Treatment Guide* listed at the end of this chapter shows some of the ways it can be done.

Your Partner: Ally for Intimacy or ???

Most approaches to pelvic pain list involvement of the woman's partner as a footnote somewhere along the way. Unless your partner is a useless tool, he or she can be your biggest ally.

Women who experience sexual pain often try to avoid sexual intimacy with their partner. This is a mistake. It almost never turns out well. The job of a couple is to figure out the types of sexual intimacy they can enjoy that don't cause a woman pelvic pain. Once a woman can be sure her partner won't reach for her crotch, there are many ways the two of them can enjoy sexual intimacy. We list some of them in a bit.

Partner Profiles

Different partners respond to a woman's sexual pain in different ways. For simplicity' sake, let's assume there are three different types of partners:

What a Dick! This is a guy who either doesn't believe your pain is real or doesn't care. He's angry that he's not getting the sex he thinks he deserves. The last thing he tries to be is reasonable, supportive, or helpful. Why you stay with him is beyond the scope of this book and probably has your friends stumped as well. The prognosis for pain-free sex with this type of partner is on the unlikely side.

Mr. "I feel your pain!" This type of partner is so solicitous and afraid of causing you pain that he becomes a pain himself. Rather than being a ray of hope, he ends up reinforcing sexual pain. Pelvic pain has compromised your intimacy and put a serious dent in your sexual satisfaction. You need an ally who will inspire you in battle, not a wimp who is going to bring you aspirin. You need someone who is strong as well as sensitive.

The Man! This is the guy who is going to help keep sexual intimacy alive in your relationship without creating more sexual pain. This is the partner we all want to be, and on some days, we are!

This is a man who wants to learn about your pelvic pain. He wants to backstop your efforts, but doesn't need to take over. He understands the shots are yours to call, but he isn't afraid to offer the point of view of a third party who might understand things about you that you don't.

He's a man who isn't afraid to say, "If that hurts, let's find something we both like to do that doesn't hurt." He's not afraid to be an unflinching advocate for sexual intimacy with you.

Reconnecting with Your Partner

While women who have sexual pain do not have anywhere near the level of sexual satisfaction as other women, their satisfaction with their relationship is often the same as women who don't have chronic sexual pain. It seems that sexual pain can bring some partners closer together.

However, there are plenty of situations where a woman will begin to avoid her partner's touch in order to avoid having sex. Maybe she'll go to bed earlier or later than he does, or when he says sexy things to her she freezes up rather than smiles. He will often assume her distance is because of something he's done, or because she would rather have sex with someone else.

A strategy to treat sexual pain will often involve reconnecting with your partner. Maybe this is something the two of you can do together, or maybe you can use the help of a couples therapist or a sex therapist. At the very minimum, it would be a good idea to ask him to read this chapter.

Sexual Intimacy With Your Partner When You Have Pelvic Pain

Only one chapter out of the eighty-seven chapters in this book is on sexual intercourse (penis into vagina). That should speak volumes for how many ways there are to share sexual intimacy without having intercourse.

Here are just a few suggestions for how a partner can be sexually intimate with you without touching your vagina:

💡 Smother your inner thighs with kisses, avoiding the part of your crotch that hurts when it's touched.

💡 Shower your abdomen with kisses, from your navel to the top of your mons pubis (landing strip area) and from one hip bone to the other.

💡 Did your partner used to be the incredible make-out king? Many of his make-out skills may have gone into the deep freeze after the two of you began having intercourse. Dust them off and give them new life!

💡 Are there fantasy scenarios that turn you on or you used to enjoy acting out together? Do you ever do role playing?

💡 Is it possible the two of you will like reading erotica together?

💡 Maybe you like breast play. Perhaps it's in the form of tender kisses from your neck to your nipples, or below your breasts. Or maybe you like a firm approach to breast play. If you have a favorite pair of nipple clamps, he should be on it.

💡 If you enjoy anal stimulation or anal sex, there shouldn't be anything stopping you.

💡 If you like being restrained or spanked, your partner can learn just you like it.

💡 Some women with pelvic pain are able to masturbate. Your partner can hold you or kiss and caress the parts of your body you enjoy the most while you masturbate. Or maybe you can masturbate together.

The purpose of this is for the two of you to share sexual intimacy. It is not—repeat—not a step on the way to having intercourse. This is your safe harbor of sexual intimacy. Making it a milestone on the way to intercourse will only ruin it.

As for what you can do for him, stop assuming there are rules that sex isn't sex unless a penis goes inside a vagina! There are dozens of ways you can give your partner sexual pleasure without your vagina being involved. If you are short on ideas, why not read together the chapters in this book on handjobs, blowjobs, the testicles, the prostate, and more. Or read the chapters separately and highlight the things that look interesting. If there are parts you both highlighted, then you are off to the races.

Just kissing your partner's neck and nipples, or letting him kiss you while he's masturbating might lead to way more sexual satisfaction than a lot of couples have.

Dissociation vs. Pleasure

One of the bigger problems in the treatment of sexual pain is when its focus is to allow intercourse instead of being about sexual pleasure. The woman will often try to dissociate or mentally leave her body in order to ignore the pain, to achieve the goal of intercourse.

While this is easy to understand and may even be admirable, it is unlikely to work. Besides, is this how you want sexual intimacy to be—where the woman mentally numbs herself so her partner can get his penis inside of her vagina? (Physical therapist and pelvic pain specialist Talli Rosenbaum has written about this. See the references at the end of the chapter.)

Hormonal Contraceptives

Contrary to popular belief, men's bodies make estrogen and women's bodies make testosterone. The skin on a woman's vulva is sensitive to testosterone. It needs a certain amount of testosterone to be healthy. The problem with hormonal methods of birth control is they decrease the amount of testosterone in a woman's body—considerably.

This can cause a thinning of the skin in a woman's genitals. It also could be the reason why women who use hormonal contraceptives are six times more likely to experience pelvic pain than women who don't use hormonal contraceptives. And it's one of the reasons why physicians who specialize in pelvic pain will often suggest you discontinue using oral contraceptives, or contraceptives that may be decreasing your body's level of testosterone.

Can Bicycle Seats Create or Contribute To Chronic Sexual Pain?

Research has found an association between bicycle seats and clitoral numbness, but there's been no research on bicycle seats and chronic sexual pain. That research is just beginning. For now, if you have chronic sexual pain and ride a bike, consider switching to a no-nose saddle. *Enter "bicycle" in the search box at www.GuideToGettingItOn.com for links and resources on no-nose saddles.*

When "The Cure" Adds to The Pain

For the past couple of decades, Kegel exercises have been suggested as a nearly universal "cure" for all things going on in the female pelvis. Yet Kegel exercises that are not done properly can contribute to pelvic floor problems, and even when Kegel exercises are done properly, they can make an already painful situation worse. This is particularly true when some of the muscles are clenching or have too much tone and you aren't aware of it. It's one of the reasons why it is so important to be examined by a physical therapist who specializes in pelvic floor problems if you are experiencing chronic pain during sex. If your personal circumstances prevent this, at the very least, read the books mentioned at the end of this chapter to learn more.

The same cautions apply for Pilates core exercises that are designed to strengthen pelvic floor muscles and certain Yoga regimens. While these exercises can be beneficial when done correctly by women who have no pelvic floor problems, they should not be used as a treatment for pelvic floor pain without an evaluation first.

The Journey Forward

If you have insurance or the financial means and are in proximity of a gynecologist or physical therapist who specializes in female pelvic pain, then a hands-on examination would be essential. Women who have pelvic pain tend to dread gynecological exams, but rest assured, if you can find a specialist who specializes in sexual pain, it would not be like your past visits to healthcare providers.

BOOKS

Whether you are able to see a specialist in pelvic pain or not, here are two of the most important books you can read at the start of your journey to eliminate sexual pain:

When Sex Hurts: A Woman's Guide to Banishing Sexual Pain by Andrew Goldstein, Caroline Pukall, and Irwin Goldstein, Da Capo Lifelong Books. This book was written by three of the top specialists in the research and treatment of women's sexual pain. You won't find a more competent resource on sexual pain anywhere.

Why Pelvic Pain Hurts—Neuroscience Education for Patients with Pelvic Pain by Adriaan Louw, Sandra Hilton and Caroly Vandyken. This little gem explains what's going on in the nervous system of people with pelvic pain. It is easy to read and incredibly helpful. It suggests ways of retraining a nervous system that is on hyper alert.

This third book is recommended but with reservations:

Sex Without Pain: A Self-Treatment Guide to the Sex Life You Deserve by Heather Jeffcoat. Active Orange Publishing.

The *Sex Without Pain* book does a good job of explaining how to examine your genitals and do the type of retraining exercises that are often used to help retrain the muscles in the pelvic area. Books like these can be especially helpful for women who do not have the resources to see a pelvic pain specialist. They also provide important knowledge about pelvic floor retraining for women with sexual pain. The reservations about this book are because it tends to promise a one-dimensional cure to pelvic pain, when treating pelvic pain can be much more complex than retraining the pelvic floor muscles. Also, the author frequently suggests readers use the resources on her website including her list of specialists as if it is a thorough list, when there are plenty of excellent physical therapists and gynecologists who specialize in pelvic pain who are not included. The book does ask the reader to not take shortcuts and the advice is sound and up to date.

There are other consumer-based books on pelvic pain that you might find to be helpful. Here are some to consider:

Amy Stein's *Heal Pelvic Pain: The Proven Stretching, Strengthening, and Nutrition Program for Relieving Pain, Incontinence,& I.B.S, and Other Symptoms Without Surgery*. This book gets good reviews, but hasn't had a refresh in a number of years. As for "proven," maybe if you are lucky enough to be a patient of Ms. Stein's, where you and she can tap into her years of experience in evaluating your specific problem. But this doesn't mean other readers will find a cure by reading this book or any other.

Harold Glazer's book *The Vulvodynia Survival Guide: How to Overcome Painful Vaginal Symptoms and Enjoy an Active Lifestyle* is also competent, but hasn't had a refresh in thirteen years. However, Dr. Glazer is on the medical advisory board of the National Vulvodynia Association, and it's likely he would have updated the book if he felt it was out of date.

Claudia Amherd's *7 Steps to Pain-Free Sex: A Complete Self-Help Guide to Overcome Vaginismus, Dyspareunia, Vulvodynia & other Penetrations Disorders* is another consumer based book on sexual pain.

ORGANIZATIONS

For organizations, the National Vulvodynia Association is excellent. Spend time going though the information on their website at www.nva.org.

For referrals in Canada, contact the Women's Health section of the Canadian Physiotherapy Assocation: www.physiotherapy.ca.

ARTICLES

For Talli Rosenbaum's article: *An integrated mindfulness-based approach to the treatment of women with sexual pain and anxiety: promoting autonomy and mind/body connection* click on the "publications" section of her website at www.tallirosenbaum.com/en.

A SPECIAL THANKS to Caroline Pukall, Ph.D., Psychology Department, Queen's University, Canada.

CHAPTER
57
Hypospadias

Hypospadias is a condition where the urethra doesn't go to the end of the penis. In mild cases, it comes out near the end of the penis, but not quite. In more severe cases, it can come out anywhere from below the head of the penis to the scrotum.

Hypospadias is one of the most common birth anomalies there is, occurring in 1 in 125 to 500 boys. The possible reasons range from genetics and environmental pollutants called endocrine disruptors to diet. (A study released in 2008 cites diet and obesity of the mother during pregnancy as risk factors, with a vegetarian diet or a diet lacking in meat and fish showing a strong positive association with hypospadias risk.)

It makes sense that cases of hypospadias occur on the bottom side of the penis where nature left a long seam. That's because when the penis is forming in the womb, nature zips it up along this seam. The urethra goes inside the chamber of the penis that's just inside the seam. With hypospadias, the urethra gets caught in the zipper.

While it is sometimes very serious, hypospadias is usually a minor birth defect that looms far more massively in the mind of the guy who's got it than in the mind of a potential partner. There is nothing about hypospadias that makes a man any less of a aman or any less of a lover, although sometimes it results in a condition where the penis curves more than normal.

The real damage from hypospadias is usually the shame and aloneness that a man feels when he's growing up. One of the reasons for feeling so different is because he's often got to sit down to pee, given how the pee shoots out the side of his penis instead of the end. The guy knows he's different from other males, and often lives in terror that others will find out and make fun of him.

Aside from feeling like he's got this horrible secret in his pants, most men with hypospadias have a medical history where they had to have their penis repeatedly inspected and examined by this doctor and that. And not being able to leave well enough alone, surgeons are frequently called in to do what often turns out to be multiple surgeries. (While medical intervention is sometimes helpful in certain cases, there are plenty of guys who would have been far better off if their penis had been spared the surgeon's knife.)

As is the case where any kid grows up feeling his body is defective, the most important issues to deal with are often the psychological. Men with hypospadias usually feel great emotional relief when they can meet and talk to other men who have the same condition. Fortunately, the Internet is making this much more possible than in times past.

Men with hypospadias sometimes grow up fascinated by other guys' penises. This is perfectly logical when you consider how often their penis gets handled by parents and doctors, often without a helpful explanation. It also makes sense given how focused a guy with hypospadias can be about the way his penis is different from other penises. However, there is no evidence that hypospadias results in a different sexual orientation unless that's what was going to happen from the start, hypospadias or not.

As for sex and relationships, the main difference between a penis with hypospadias and one without is where the cum shoots out, and that's not going to make any difference to most women. As one female reader said,

> "I can name you hundreds of other things women are more concerned about in a man than if his pee or cum shoots out straight or from the side—most women wouldn't give a rat's ass. Only guys worry about things like that."

There is no reason why a man with hypospadias can't become a father, so birth control is just as necessary for a man with hypospadias as for any other guy. The urethral opening for men with hypospadias is sometimes a little bigger, and some men with hypospadias are prone to urinary tract infections. So drinking extra water and peeing after sex might be a good habit for them to get into.

Men with hypospadias recommend that you tell a partner about your hypospadias sometime after you've gotten to know each other but before you've got your hands in each other's pants. You can always pull out this book and point to this page if you need an ice breaker.

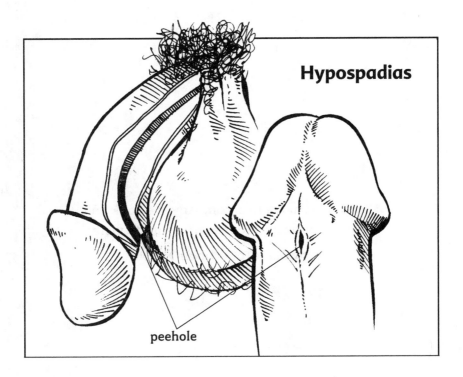

Hypospadias

peehole

Epispadias

Epispadias is when the urethral opening opens on the top of the penis. The opening can be in one spot, or it can run the entire length of the penis. While it might seem that epispadias is simply a case of hypospadias turned on its ear, it is an entirely different anomaly than hypospadias. It is also very rare. Where approximately 1 in 125 to 500 boys has hypospadias, 1 in 117,000 boys are thought to have epispadias. While they aren't sure what causes it, it is thought to result from a problem in the way the pubic bone develops.

Every once in a while, a girl will have epispadias, with it occurring in 1 in 478,000 girls. When it happens in females, the urethra will either exit higher than normal, between the clitoris and labia, or as high as the abdomen.

Resources: If you or your partner has hypospadias, an excellent resource is the Hypospadias and Epispadias Association: www.heainfo.org

For videos made to accompany the book and
frequent posts about sex, be sure to visit

www.GuideToGettingItOn.com

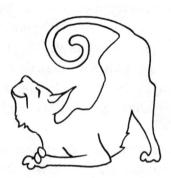

CHAPTER

58
Birth Control — Sperm v. Egg

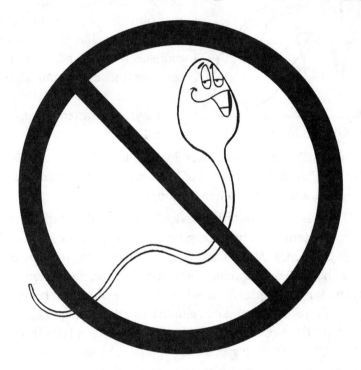

In the United States, 49% of pregnancies in women under the age of 34 are not planned or intended. The number rises to 75% for women over 40, and a whopping 80% of teen pregnancies are not wanted. Two-out-of-three unplanned teenage pregnancies happen to girls between the ages of 18 and 20.

IUDs—A Great Choice for Teens, Young Women, and Women of All Childbearing Ages

IUDs are one of the most widely used contraceptives in the world. In North America, they have the highest user satisfaction ratings among all methods of reversible birth control, including the pill, patch, ring, shot and condom. IUD's are also the most effective method of reversible birth control.

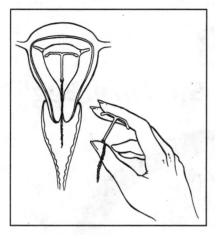

It doesn't matter if you are teenager and have never been pregnant or if you enjoy having sex with more than one guy—an IUD should work very well for you. Like most birth control methods besides condoms, an IUD won't prevent you from getting a sexually transmitted infection, but it won't make you more likely to get one, either. If you get a sexually transmitted infection, it would be your fault, not the IUD's. And most sexually transmitted infections can be treated without having to take out your IUD.

Today's IUDs are incredibly safe. More than 20% of female OB/GYNs personally use IUDs as their method of birth control. Almost 20% of women in Asia use IUDs, and 15% of women in Europe.

IUD stands for "intrauterine device." It is a small T-shaped device that is placed in the uterus to prevent pregnancy. There are three kinds of IUDs, two that have hormones (Mirena and Skyla) and one that releases copper ions instead of hormones (ParaGard). The hormone-releasing Mirena can stay in for up to 7 years. It is better for women who have crampy or heavy periods, as it helps lighten bleeding or it can eliminate periods altogether. Skyla is a bit smaller than the Mirena and releases less hormone. It lasts three years and is the first IUD that's been specifically approved by the FDA for women who have never been pregnant. It should be an excellent choice for a lot of sexually active teens and young women. The Paragard IUD is great for women who want a regular period and no hormones. It can last up to ten years.

Both the copper IUD and Mirena protect against endometrial cancer. It also appears they help prevent ectopic pregnancies, and the Mirena IUD helps shrink uterine fibroids and reduces the symptoms of endometriosis. We don't yet know about the newer Skyla.

Women who are wearing IUDs can become pregnant within a week of having the IUD taken out. IUDs only impact fertility when they are in a woman's body. Studies are showing that a woman is more likely to conceive sooner after having an IUD removed than after she stops taking the pill.

How IUDs Work: the copper in the Paragard IUD keeps the sperm from maturing once they enter the cervix. The progestin in the Mirena and Skyla

Most Effective Methods
Less than 1 pregnancy for every 100 women in 1 year.

—BEST—

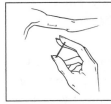 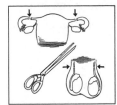 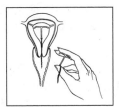 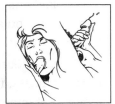

| implants | sterilization | IUDs | oral sex & hand jobs |

—VERY GOOD—

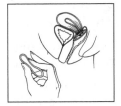 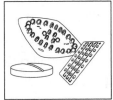 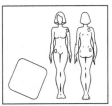

| NuvaRing | The Pill | The Patch |

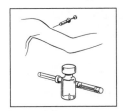 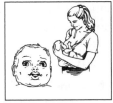

No Birth Control? 85 pregnancies per 100 women in 1 year.

| injections | LAM |

—OKAY—

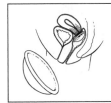 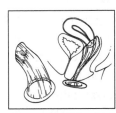 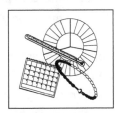 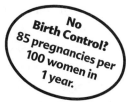

| diaphragm | male condoms | female condoms | fertility awareness |

Much Better Than Nothing ▶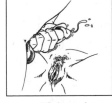

Highly Questionable ▶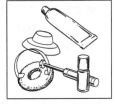

| withdrawal | spermicides |

  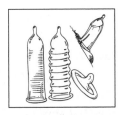 # Least Effective Methods
More than 30 pregnancies for every 100 women in 1 year.

IUDs act the same as progestin does in progestin-only birth control pills, or the implant and Depo shot. IUDs do not work by causing a low grade infection in the uterus. That is one of the unfortunate myths that some people have about IUDs.

The ParaGard (copper IUD) could be a good birth control choice for female athletes. It is highly effective, hassle free, and doesn't put out hormones that might result in water retention or soreness. (We don't yet know about the Skyla, which releases considerably less hormone than the Mirena.) The Mirena IUD might be the best control for women who have Category 5 periods with heavy flow. Some women find it eventually stops their periods.

If an IUD is going to be expelled, the time when that is most likely to occur would be during the first menstrual cycle. The chances of this happening are low, and after your first period it is very unlikely that a uterus will send an IUD packing. Once it is in place, an IUD should not cause discomfort. A woman shouldn't know it's there. The only part of an IUD that can be felt is two very thin nylon strings that hang down from the IUD. If a man is able to feel the strings during intercourse, a healthcare provider can easily snip them to be shorter.

Most women find there to be little or no pain when the IUD is inserted. Some find the pain to be moderate but manageable, and a small number of women find the pain to be terrible. If you are concerned, discuss this with your healthcare provider.

In our survey of gynecologists who insert a large number of IUDs, many felt ibuprophen an hour before insertion works well for pain management, others suggest tramadol, diazepam or misopristol as long as the woman has a ride home. All agreed that satisfaction with the IUD is high among their patients. They felt it was a great choice for younger women.

The one thing you need to be sure of is that your healthcare provider has substantial experience installing IUDs. With experience comes mastery, so ask how often the person puts in IUDs.

The initial cost of an IUD can be high, but is usually much cheaper over the lifetime of the IUD than any other form of birth control. Fortunately, an IUD is free if you fall under the umbrella of the Affordable Healthcare Act. If your insurance doesn't cover the cost of an IUD and money is a concern, be sure to shop around. Also check with your local Planned Parenthood.

An unfortunate myth about IUDs is they are not safe. This comes from what happened in the early 1970s with an IUD called the Dalkon Shield. The reason why the Dalkon Shield caused infections was because of the material used in the tailstring as opposed to the IUD itself. The material in the tail string allowed bacteria from the vagina to wick into the cervix. That kind of material is no longer used and the FDA now regulates IUDs, which it didn't in the 1970s. Even though the manufacturer knew about the problem from almost the beginning, they hushed it up and ramped up their marketing efforts to get more women to use that ill-fated IUD.

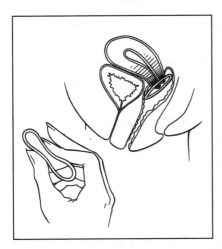

The NuvaRing

The NuvaRing is a 2" diameter plastic ring with hormones in it. A woman puts it in her vagina on day one of her menstrual cycle and takes it out on day 21. The NuvaRing eliminates the need to take a pill every day, to get an injection or to wear a patch. Aside from the Mirena and Skyla IUDs, a woman will be hard pressed to find a hormonal method of birth control that is more user-friendly than the NuvaRing.

Because the hormones absorb directly into the blood stream, the dosage of hormones a woman receives from the NuvaRing may be lower than what is in most birth-control pills. However, it still has the same side effect profile as birth control pills and other hormonal methods.

The NuvaRing is one of the few hormonal methods of birth control associated with greater vaginal lubrication rather than less, although some women finds it dries them out. Also, some women report leaving the Nuva Ring in for an entire month for period suppression, but please speak to your healthcare provider before trying this.

The NuvaRing sits in the same place as a diaphragm, only a woman doesn't need to worry if it's exactly in place because it isn't a barrier. It is fine if it moves around. One size fits all. The muscles in the vagina hold it in place, and most women can't feel it. If for some reason a woman's partner can feel the NuvaRing during intercourse, a woman can take the NuvaRing out for up to three hours at a time. If her partner can't finish doing his business in three hours, she should consider sending him to the bathroom with a jar of hand cream while she puts her NuvaRing back in.

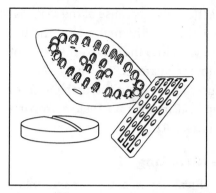

The Pill

The pill is a hormonal method of birth control that works by stopping the eggs from leaving the ovary. As a result, ovulation does not occur. They also work by causing the cervical mucus to become thicker, which inhibits the effectiveness of sperm. Women take the pills for 21 or 28 days, although a lot of pill packages come with 7 dummy or reminder pills that have no hormones in them. A woman takes the reminder pills from days 21 to 28 to allow her to have a period. This creates a 28-day cycle.

Many women find the pill to be a great birth control, while others find the side effects to be undesirable or intolerable. The side effects include a decrease in sex drive. (For a discussion of this, see Chapter 59: *The Pill and Your Sex Drive.)* There are more than fifty different kinds of birth-control pills and it can be an art to get an optimal match between patient and pill. The clinical skill of a healthcare provider and their willingness to inquire and experiment are important elements of the process. If the first brand a woman takes does not fit with her body chemistry, there are other combinations and forms of hormonal birth control. Unfortunately, not many women are aware of their choices.

As for the pill's safety, a long term study that has followed thousands of former pill-taking women for forty years. These women had taken the pill for at least four years. The women who had taken the pill are living longer than controls who didn't take the pill. This isn't to say that bad things can't happen, but they tend to be rare and the risks of taking the pill are not nearly as great as the risks of being pregnant.

If a woman is considering a hormonal method of birth control, the first thing to consider is what she wants it to do for her. Is it just for pregnancy prevention? Or is it also to help tame harsh periods or to eliminate periods altogether? A woman should talk to her healthcare provider about the advantages, disadvantages and side effects of the different hormonal methods.

A woman also needs to be honest with herself regarding her ability to remember to take a pill each day. If the mere thought of this would cause the collective jaws of her family and friends to drop, she should consider an IUD, the NuvaRing, an implant or the Depo-Provera shot instead. All it takes is one missed pill for the effectiveness of the pill to go down. Also, the effectiveness of the pill can be impacted by antibiotics and other prescriptions a woman might be using. Whenever a woman who is using hormonal methods of birth control is given a prescription for another drug, she should be sure to ask if it will impact the effectiveness of the birth control pill.

Most birth control pills contain a combination of estrogen and progestin. A woman usually takes an active pill with hormones in it each day for 21 straight days.

Progestin-Only Pills, or POPs: Progestin-only pills only contain progestins. In fact, the original birth-control pill was made of progestins only. Progestin-only pills are called POPs or mini-pills. They are used by women who cannot take estrogen, including those who smoke and are older than 35, as well as women who have heart disease, high blood pressure or are at risk for blood clotting. They can be helpful for women who have heavy bleeding or cramping during their periods. *POPs are safer than estrogen-containing methods for women who get migraines or focal neurological deficit.* They are also used by nursing mothers and women with sickle cell anemia.

There has been concern about bone density loss associated with progestin-only birth control, so women should make sure they are getting sufficient calcium and vitamin D. Female athletes at risk for Female Athlete Triad should talk about the advisability of using Progestin-only methods with their healthcare provider.

Progestin-only pills need to be taken at the same time every day. If you are more than three hours late in taking one, bleeding can start and the effectiveness can decrease. While progestin-only pills require extreme compliance, the Minera IUD, Implanon implant, and Depo shot are progestin-only methods that can be hassle free for years at a time.

If You Forget to Take a Pill: Many women forget to take 2 or 3 pills a month. Not that any guy could remember to take a pill every day, but this is not good. Skipping makes the pill less effective; considerably so. If you forget to take your birth-control pill, check with your healthcare provider or your pharmacist. Also, your pill pack info should tell you how to make up for a missed pill or visit the pill's website. *Enter "missed pill" in the search box at www.GuideToGettingItOn.com for more information.*

With most types of combination pill, if you missed only one pill, you will be told to take the pill you forgot right away and to take the next pill as scheduled. It would be wise to use a backup method such as a condom for at least a week. The exception is if the pill you forgot to take is during your week of placebo or sugar pills. In that case, no harm, no foul—get out of jail free.

If you missed two pills but remember it on the day (or night) of your second missed pill, you might be told to take both of the forgotten pills right away, and to take the next day's pill when you would normally take it. Use a backup method for at least a week.

If you missed two pills on but didn't remember them until the third day, your healthcare professional might tell you to double up now and double up again the following day. Use a backup method for at least a week.

If you missed three pills, call your healthcare provider right away! Emergency contraception might be in order, in addition to prayer.

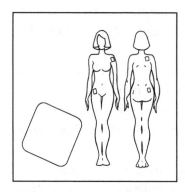

Birth Control Patch or OrthoEvra

The patch is a hormone-based contraceptive that eliminates having to take birth-control pills. It is a small 2" square that is applied to the skin. It can be placed on the hips, butt, abdomen, upper arm, or shoulder blade, but not on the breasts or extremities. Users need to replace it once a week. After three consecutive weeks with a new patch, women go patch-free for a week to have a period. The patch contains a dose of hormones similar to birth control pills. However, instead of having to swallow them in pill form, the hormones are absorbed through the skin. While the patch is not as effective for women who weigh over 198 pounds, it is still more effective than condoms. There is no research on whether the patch remains effective while swimming.

There have been safety concerns about increased numbers of blood clots being caused by the Patch. The FDA recently reviewed the data and by a vote of 19 to 5 decided to keep it on the market. They believe the benefits outweigh the dangers.

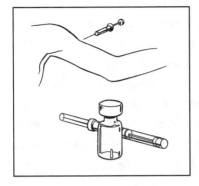

Depo-Provera
Three Months at a Shot

Depo-Provera is a progestin-only pill-in-a-shot that lasts for 12 weeks. Women seem to either love it or hate it. If you hate it, you are stuck with it in your body for 3 months. One of the main side effects of Depo is irregular bleeding. Some women bleed a lot and some don't bleed at all. Some women find that Depo stops their periods altogether for three months.

Birth Control Implant
Effective for Three Years

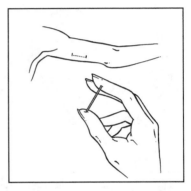

The birth control implant is a matchstick-sized rod that is inserted in the arm under the skin. It provides highly effective birth control for three years. User error is impossible. The implant is a progestin-only method that decreases or stops period bleeding in 80% of the women who use it. Yet a side effect for some women is irregular bleeding, especially during the first three months. Brand names for the implant are Implanon and Nexplanon. Since it needs to be removed at the end of three years, make sure your healthcare provider is experienced at placing it near the surface of the skin.

The Diaphragm

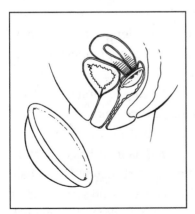

The diaphragm is a shallow latex or silicone cup that a woman puts spermicide into and then places over her cervix before she has intercourse. Diaphragms used to be as common as sex itself, but not many women use them now. They require a goop-and-insert routine each time a woman has sex. However, the diaphragm has no hormonal side effects.

The diaphragm may be a good choice for a woman who doesn't need to use birth control often, including someone who has a long-distance partner where most of the sex is on the phone or Skype. For women with latex allergies, they are finally making non-latex diaphragms out of silicone.

Fitting a diaphragm can be as much art as science. Diaphragms can also cause a feeling of pressure on the bladder. They must be left in for eight hours after the last intercourse. If a woman's lover is the kind who does a rapid reload and fire, she'll need to squirt in extra spermicide but she doesn't need to take the diaphragm out. She will need to get a new diaphragm every year or two, which should be accompanied by a refitting.

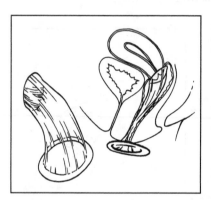

FC Female Condom
The Vagina Liner

The FC Condom is a pouch that's inserted into the vagina. It forms a thin protective barrier between the penis and the walls of the vagina. Because it sits in the vagina, the man doesn't have to pull out as soon as he comes. It is especially valued by couples where a penis is extra wide or has a foreskin that doesn't do well with male condoms. The female condom used to be known as "Reality" and was made of polyurethane. It is now called the FC Condom in North America and is now made of nitrile. Nitrile is cheaper to manufacture and it doesn't make the squeaking noises when the penis thrusts that the older model was known for. Also, the warmth from the woman's vagina passes easily through the nitrile material.

The female condom can be installed in the vagina long before lovemaking begins, so putting it in needn't interrupt the flow or spontaneity of lovemaking. It gives women more control in protecting themselves and it can even be used in water. Some women report that the ring around the outside of the condom helps stimulate their clitoris during intercourse.

A male condom should never be used at the same time as a female condom. The friction between a bagged penis and a vagina liner has the potential to cause material failures if not combustion. Unfortunately, the female condom hasn't caught on in North America. It isn't cheap and some couples find it to be strange. Like the male condom, it doesn't provide the best of birth control effectiveness. It is being used by some straight and gay couples for anal intercourse, although it's doubtful that the instructions include this small detail. Couples who use it for anal sex often remove the inner ring before inserting it into the anus. The female condom of the future will possibly be made of a gel that forms a thin mesh barrier when it mixes with vaginal lubrication.

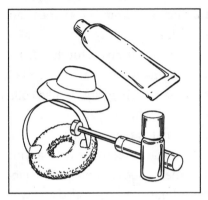

Spermicides: Sponges, Films, Foams, Gels, Suppositories & Jellies

Spermicides are chemicals that are used to kill sperm and perhaps reduce the risk of pregnancy. They are placed in the vagina before intercourse. The forms they come in include films, foams, sponges, suppositories, and jellies. Most are made with the chemical nonoxynol-9 (N-9). When used by themselves, spermicides can be much less effective than other birth control methods, including condoms. **CAUTION:** *As of press time, there was growing concern that spermicies are even less effective for birth control than was previously thought.*

Spermicides can be bought over-the-counter and they can be an alternative for women who aren't able to use hormonal methods. They can be messy and taste really nasty. The chemicals in spermicides can cause irritation in either partner, which increases the chance of getting STIs. Spermicidally-lubricated condoms can cause irritation as well.

Tubal Ligation or Essure for Women, Vasectomy for Men

Tubal ligation and vasectomy are permanent forms of birth control. They are highly popular and have a failure rate of 1% or less. Both are done on an outpatient basis. Neither procedure will cause a change in a person's sex drive, and many people report they enjoy sex

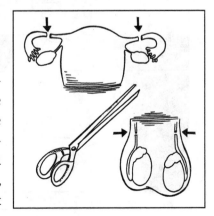

more once they don't have to worry about pregnancy. They are the best form of birth control if you are not interested in having children or more children.

In tubal ligation, a thin tube-like instrument is passed through a small incision that is slightly below a woman's belly button. The surgeon seals the fallopian tubes with clips, rings, or with electrical current. In order to see the fallopian tubes, a harmless gas is put into the abdomen. The gas is let out once the tubes have been sealed. Afterward, the eggs from the ovaries can no longer reach the womb. The total procedure takes about 15 to 20 minutes. Tubal ligation does not stop a woman's periods, but it does stop her fears about becoming pregnant. A newer method of female sterilization is called Essure. This is a non-surgical method of sterilization where spring-like coils are inserted to block the fallopian tubes.

A vasectomy begins with a small incision that is made in the scrotum. The physician reaches the vas deferens or sperm-carrying tubes with a thin instrument. The tubes are then sealed so that sperm does not mix with ejaculate. The procedure should take less than 20 minutes. There is also a newer method called the No-Scalpel vasectomy where the scrotal skin is not cut

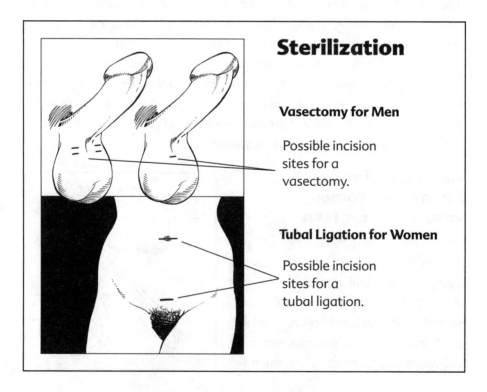

Sterilization

Vasectomy for Men

Possible incision sites for a vasectomy.

Tubal Ligation for Women

Possible incision sites for a tubal ligation.

with a scalpel. Instead, an opening in the scrotum is made with a special instrument to help decrease bleeding and pain. The rest of the procedure is like a conventional vasectomy. Since sperm makes up less than 5% of each ejaculation, the volume of semen that a man ejaculates will appear to be the same. The only thing that will be missing are concerns about pregnancy.

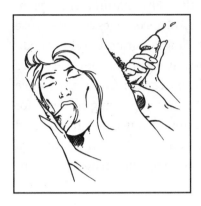

Oral Sex and Hand Jobs

If a woman uses oral sex or a handjob to satisfy her partner instead of vaginal intercourse, her chances of becoming pregnant are zero and her chances of getting a horrible disease like HIV are next to zero. She doesn't need a prescription to give oral sex and hand jobs, nor must she have the money to purchase them.

Natural Family Planning
May the Cervix Be with You

Natural Family Planning is an attempt to define which parts of the month a couple can enjoy intercourse with a low probability of conception, and which times are best to avoid. Natural family planning requires far more knowledge, planning and discipline than other methods of birth control. The

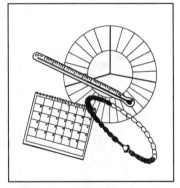

effectiveness is not usually very high and can vary greatly. There are several variations of natural family planning, including the cervical mucus method, the two-day method, the calendar method, the standard days method, the symptothermal method and the temperature method.

One of the indicators of fertility is when the mucus that comes from the cervix starts to look clear like raw egg white and is slippery and stretchy. This is the cervix's siren call for sperm. This is one of the signs that natural family practitioners look for as an indicator of fertility. When the mucus looks like this, the couple either abstains from intercourse or needs to use an alternative method of birth control such as a condom.

Natural family planning should not be considered unless the partners are monogamous and committed, and have a total understanding of what's involved. Even then, it is anything but infallible. It would also be less than optimal to practice NFP when you are younger and your ovulation is not as consistent as it might eventually be.

There are two styles of natural methods, the NFP or natural family planning and FAM or fertility awareness methods. FAM encourages couples to use a backup method such as condoms or a diaphragm during unsafe periods, where NFP is more religion based and anti-contraception. Toni Weschler's *Taking Charge of Your Fertility, 20th Anniversary Edition (2015)* is the bible of natural birth control. Also be sure to get the accompanying software for the book to help you do the best planning possible. If you are trying NFP and find yourselves having intercourse during a less-than-optimal time, the man should pull out and ejaculate on the side. However, some religious groups might not approve.

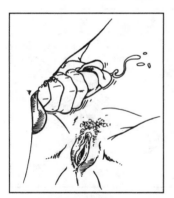

Coitus Interruptus
Withdrawal or Pulling Out

One of the problems with birth control is that people don't think they need a backup method. But what happens when you've forgotten to take your pill for the second day in a row or the condom didn't get put on in the heat of passion? Why not consider pulling the penis out before the man ejaculates, with him ejaculating to the side instead of inside? This is known as withdrawal or coitus interruptus, which is Latin for "pull it out before it spits."

Withdrawal is when the man pulls his penis from the woman's vagina before he is about to ejaculate and shoots his semen off to the side. One of the biggest problems in recommending withdrawal is that there have been absolutely no empirical studies to determine whether it works. We also know that up to 40% of men do have sperm in their precum which is mobile and capable of impregnating a partner. This could make withdrawal ineffective for these men even if they correctly pull out before they ejaculate.

Withdrawal was the only method of birth control used during the fertility decline in Europe, and was probably the only effective method of birth control used in the 1800s when the average size of the American family decreased from 7 children to 3.5. So it does work for some couples. The question is whether you want to risk having 3.5 children.

One of the world's most quoted experts on birth control recently informed us that if he were concerned about pregnancy, he would use a far more effective method of birth control than withdrawal. If he were concerned about sexually transmitted infections, he would use condoms as well.

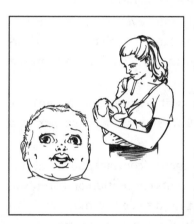

Breastfeeding or LAM (Lactational Amenorrhea Method)

Ovulation stops for six months after childbirth in women who are exclusively and consistently breastfeeding their baby. The mom must breastfeed at least every four hours and she must not substitute any other food. This assumes she has not had a period since giving birth.

Emergency Contraception And Morning-After Pills

Emergency contraception is something that is done after having had intercourse in the hope of preventing conception. There are currently three forms of emergency contraception: pills called Plan B and Ella, and the copper IUD.

Both Plan B and Ella work by preventing the egg from leaving the ovary. To be effective, they need to be taken before the egg has entered the Fallopian tubes, so it is imperative they are taken as soon as possible after intercourse. Do not wait until the next day!

Plan B works by interrupting the release of the egg from the ovary if and only if it is taken before the LH surge. If it is taken after the LH surge begins, it is not effective. Ella, the newest form of emergency contraception, contains a second-generation antiprogestin called ulipristal acetate. Ella stops the release of an egg even if it is taken after the LH surge, which is why it is more effective than Plan B.

Contrary to what some abstinence-only groups have claimed, neither Plan B nor Ella cause an abortion. This is why you need to take them as soon after unprotected intercourse as possible, because once you ovulate, they don't work. Plan B is taken as one pill, while the generic version of Plan B is two pills. You can take both of the generic pills at once. Plan B is available over-the-counter and does not require a prescription. Men can buy it as well as women. Unfortunately, you currently need a prescription for Ella.

Plan B has been shown to be extremely safe, even if taken multiple times. People often confuse Plan B with Mifepristone which causes an abortion. (Mifepristone was known as RU-486 during clinical trials, and in the US it is called Mifeprex.)

If you can't find Plan B over-the-counter, visit www.PlanBOneStep.com. *Warning: Research is now showing that Plan B does not work for women who weigh more than 176 pounds.*

The copper IUD is another form of emergency contraception that has been approved by the FDA. The IUD either prevents conception or disrupts it, depending on when it is inserted. It does not need to be taken out, and can provide several years of continuous and highly effective birth control.

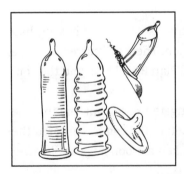

Male Condoms

For an extensive discussion about male condoms, please see Chapter 22: *Condoms— For the Ride of Your Life.*

A Very Special Thanks to Angela Hoffman, birth control and sex education expert, for help above and beyond the call of duty with this chapter. Collossal amounts of gratitude & thanks to Cynthia Graham and one of her partners in condom research crime, Bill Yarber. A big nod of appreciation to James Trussell.

59
The Pill and Your Sex Drive

"I have noticed a big decrease in my sex drive since I started taking the pill. I used to have the biggest libido and wanted to have sex at least once a day but now it just takes a lot more for me to be in the mood. I am not just randomly horny anymore and I used to be all the time. I have less sex on the pill." *female age 20*

"After a not-so-great experience with the first brand I tried, I have switched to a low-dose birth-control pill. I like it. I have no side effects at all. My sex drive is most certainly back, which is great!"
female age 19

"I used the pill and saw no effect on my sex drive whatsoever. However, my twin sister took the pill and saw a marked decrease in her sex drive. It just goes to show that everyone reacts differently— even identical twins." *female age 21*

Little research has been done on the impact that birth control pills have on a woman's sex drive and mood. The perception is that women are pretty hormonal to begin with–what's the big deal with topping off the tank?

This chapter looks at what we do and don't know about birth control pills and your sex drive. It also includes a list of questions you might ask yourself before using hormonal birth control. That way, you can have something to refer back to after you've been on the pill for a couple of months.

Fortunately, there are many different formulas of birth-control pills. So if one isn't working well for you, you can easily try others. Also, a long term study that has followed thousands of women who took the pill for at least four years has found that forty years later, the women who had taken the pill are actually living longer than women who didn't take the pill.

NOTE: It used to be that the only hormonal method of birth control was the pill. But different delivery systems have emerged, including the Nuva-Ring, the Minera IUD, the patch, the Implanon implant, and the Depo shot. For simplicity's sake, this chapter will refer to all of these as "the pill," unless otherwise specified.

Less Than 5% or More Than 25%?

"We used to use condoms until six months ago when I started taking the pill. I love the pill! I have noticed no change in my desire for sex since starting it. I was incredibly horny before the pill, and am still incredibly horny now!" *female age 19*

"I took the pill for five months but stopped because it gave me horrible side effects (no sex drive although I was a newlywed, depression, paranoia, panic attacks, weight gain, and heart burn). Now that I'm off hormones my sex drive is a whole lot better." *female 21*

A recent study suggests that sexual side effects occur in approximately 25% of the women who try the pill. Still, healthcare providers are often quoted as saying that less than 5% of women stop taking the pill due to sexual side effects. Why the fivefold disparity?

Until recently, the few studies that did inquire about sexual side effects tended to be studies of women who had been taking the pill for five years or more. But we now know that women who experience a drop in sexual desire often stop taking the pill within the first year. So most women who did experience sexual side effects would not be represented in a study of women who had been taking it for five years.

Other problems in getting consistent results have to do with the kind of questionnaires that are used (do they actually measure what the study says it is measuring?), the quality of the study design, the length of the study, and how the woman's testosterone level and other androgens are measured.

It's easy to manipulate just a few of these variables to get the results you are looking. Unfortunately, most of the studies have been funded by the drug companies who make the pills and who stand to benefit from the results.

Are Women Too Suggestible to Deserve Adequate Warnings?

"This is the third brand I have been on. The first was a three-month kind, which left me spotting for weeks, made me frustrated and took away my sex drive. The second made me very depressed with a sex drive that rose and fell like crazy. This third one has leveled out my emotions and might be making my sex drive a little stronger than before." *female age 20*

"My doctor never told me that I could have any of those side effects. Sure, I was expecting weight gain and such, but not depression and NO sex drive." *female age 21*

As long as healthcare providers are convinced that less than 5% of women who take the pill have undesired sexual side effects, they don't necessarily give warnings about possible sexual side effects. And some healthcare providers feel that to give a warning would plant the idea in a woman's mind. The trouble is, any warning can become a self-fulfilling prophecy. So why warn any patient about anything?

If women know from the start that there can be problems, but that there are as many types of pills as there are lipstick and nail-polish colors, they might be more willing to make adjustments. With the help of an astute healthcare provider, a woman might find another pill or a different delivery system such as the NuvaRing or IUD that could work really well for her.

So What's Going On?

"No change whatsoever... Still horny as a dog." *female age 21*

"The pill has totally suppressed my sex drive. I have hardly any desire." *female age 22*

"I definitely enjoy sex way more knowing that I won't get pregnant if the condom breaks or slips off." *female age 24*

One of the big crazes in drug research has been to find a pill for women who have low sexual desire, as if low sexual desire is usually a medical problem. Researchers had hoped that the answer would be Viagra, but it didn't work. It seems that women's sexual interest isn't suddenly switched on by a pill that creates the girl-version of a boner.

Since Viagra was a bust, researchers started focusing on testosterone. While testosterone tends to be associated with male arousal, having a small amount of it pulsing in a woman's veins is often necessary before she will look at a guy and think sexy things.

The reason for discussing this is because birth-control pills lower the amount of testosterone in most women. In other words, if there were a direct connection between lowered testosterone and sex drive, the pill might be a train wreck for a lot of women.

To confuse matters totally, the sexual desire of some women has either gone up or remained constant even though the pill caused their testosterone level to go down substantially. Other women's sexual desire has hit the skids with only a small drop in testosterone. So at this time, it's simply not possible to look at the testosterone level of a woman and predict whether she's having sexual problems or not.

In trying to make sense of all of this, a theory has emerged that each woman has a threshold of testosterone that is necessary for her to experience her normal sex drive. This threshold can be different for different women, and it could be that a woman won't start to experience sexual problems until her testosterone falls below her threshold.

This might explain why one woman can handle a big drop in testosterone with no adverse effects, while another woman might want to curl up with a book instead of her lover after only a small drop in testosterone.

There is also an idea that some women's sexuality is more testosterone dependent—like the male sex drive might be—while other women's sexuality depends more on relationships. So the pill-related drop in testosterone might be more of a turn-off for women whose sexuality is testosterone-driven.

Another interesting finding about testosterone is that even when women report a drop in desire, they usually don't experience a decrease in sexual satisfaction when they do have sex. That's because testosterone only impacts the desire to have sex, but not the ability to enjoy sex once the physical part of it begins. They just don't want to have sex very often.

Expectations & Our Own Sex Survey

Another factor that might influence a woman's sexual desire while taking the pill might have to do with her expectations about sex. Researchers found that women reported fewer concerns about the pill in a country where they didn't expect to enjoy sex as much as women in other countries. However, in our online sex survey, the percent of women reporting sexual side effects from taking hormonal methods of birth control has been more than 35%. While there is nothing scientific about Internet surveys, we were surprised by the high number of sex-related complaints. (On the other hand, this leaves 65% who had no complaints about the pill, with some saying they believe their sex drive is even higher now that they are taking it.)

The women who take our sex survey tend to be in the 18- to 28-year age range, with most reporting that they enjoy sex and are sexually active. Perhaps the women who go to www.GoofyFootPress.com expect more from sex than other women. Maybe they find the pill's sexual side effects to be less tolerable than women who aren't quite as amped about sex to begin with.

The Importance of Smell

If you are a woman, does the way your partner smells register in a sexual way? Do you cherish wearing a lover's shirt that has his scent all over it?

Research is showing that a woman's ability to smell a guy's pheromones, can be inversely impacted by the pill. If smell is an important turn-on for a woman and the pill is impacting her ability to sense her partner's smell, then this might contribute to her negative feelings about the pill. On the other hand, if there were something about a man's pheromones that's a turn-off, it could be that a pill-related decrease in her sniffer's pheromone detector might make sex with him feel better.

Pill Related Benefits

So far, this discussion has explained why taking the pill might lower your sex drive, but it doesn't explain why it might help increase it.

For starters, what about not having to worry about an unwanted pregnancy? It could also be that certain pills help even out premenstrual mood issues for some women, and help decrease bleeding and cramping. This might explain why some women prefer pills that pack a higher dose of estrogen: because they might result in a greater decrease in bleeding, cramping, and premenstrual mood fluctuation.

Some pills help decrease zits. This might be enough to help some women feel more sexually attractive. It could also be that certain types of progesterone in some pills can actually create an increase in sexual desire.

A Pre-Pill Inventory

You might ask yourself some of these questions before taking the pill. This kind of record can be especially helpful in six months or so, in case you're thinking something has changed but can't quite put a finger on what.

 About how many times a month are you masturbating? Masturbation reflects sexual interest that is generated from within your body and mind, so it might be helpful to see if the pill has an impact on that.

 Life events can have a big impact on how you feel about sex. So jot down a few things about how your life is going besides love and sex. How are things at school, at work, with your friends and roommates? How do you feel about yourself? Do you like yourself?

 Do a screen capture of your Facebook, blog, or Tumblr pages. This might help you recall your mood before you started taking the pill.

For a lot of women, the state of your relationship could be the biggest single factor in determining how much you want to jump a guy's bone. So if you are hitched, take a pre-pill inventory of your relationship, including what's going right, and what's not.

 If you have a partner, are you aware of his scent? Is it a turn-on, neutral, or a turn-off?

 If you've been having sex, write down how many times a month and how satisfying it is or isn't.

Are there times of the month when you feel especially horny? See if it changes after you start taking the pill.

It's perfectly normal for couples to feel less horny over time, which has nothing to do with the pill.

Different Formulas for Different Feelings?

There are many different pill formulations. There are triphasic pills, diphasic, and monophasic pills. This refers to whether they have progresterone and estrogen, or just progesterone. There are also different kinds of estrogen and different kinds of progesterone, Some researchers feel that certain kinds of progesterone might make some women more horny rather than less.

Just because the first formulation might not be the answer to your birth-control prayers, there are plenty of others to try.

More Reader Comments

"I was on the shot, the ring and the pill. The shot made me bleed for 6 months straight, the ring gave me headaches so bad that I threw up, and the pill made me cry all the time. I noticed a decrease in sexual desire. My next adventure in birth control will be the diaphragm." *female age 26*

"I use the NuvaRing, and I love it. I haven't noticed a change in sex drive, but I have noticed that I seem to be constantly wet. I suspect that it's a side effect of the Ring, but I'm not completely sure."
female age 19

"On the pill, it's harder to maintain your weight and tone even when you are eating right and exercising regularly. It fluctuates your hormones which fluctuates your water weight and feeling of attractiveness which can affect your desire for sex." *female age 22*

"I'm on the combined pill. My sex drive has dipped a bit, but that may be because we have been together for six months and the initial lust-driven 'we must have sex every night' has died down a little. Of course, staying at his parents house for two months didn't help." *female age 21*

"I think my sex drive is lower. But it is something that happens gradually, so it is hard to be sure. It definitely makes my discharge thicker, which sometimes makes it a little harder to have sex. I am not as wet and we have to use lube sometimes. I used to be on Ortho Tri-Cyclin Lo, and that had a huge effect on my sex drive. I was extremely depressed and did not want sex at all." *female age 26*

"I was on Mirena for 3 years, and I sunk into a period of low sexual drive. Also, in my 3rd year, it made me have my period every week for 3 weeks at a time. Now that I am on Ortho Tri-Cyclin Lo, I have increased sexual energy, and less problems." *female age 28*

"These days I am so horny, that I don't think it's affected me!"
female age 33

"I used to be on the pill. I feel like I have tried them all and I hate the pill. Makes me a total bitch." *female age 25*

"I used the pill in college—went through three different brands and had so many side effects. I had very little desire for sex for the most part when I was on the pill. Now I just use condoms and feel like my horny self again. *female age 25*

"When I was on the pill, both combined and pop, I found that my desire definitely waned." *female age 40*

"The pill has totally suppressed my sex drive. I have hardly any desire." *female age 22*

"I use the NuvaRing. I absolutely love it! I no longer forget to take pills, it is more reliable, and my partner doesn't feel it." *female age 21*

Thanks: Little research has been done on this important subject. We owe Cynthia Graham and John Bancroft a measure of gratitude for being among the few who are trying to do this kind of research in spite of a pharmaceutical industry that seems adamant that these questions not be asked.

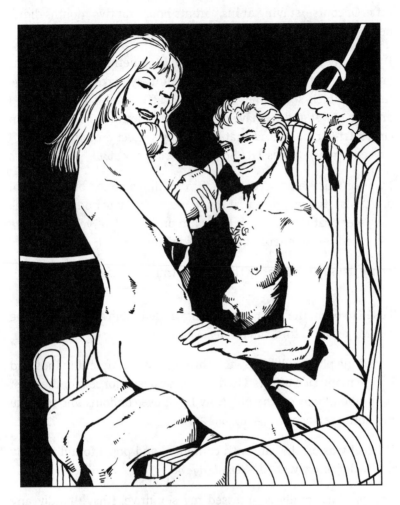

For the interesting history of this illustration, see
"About the Illustrations" on page 1084.

60
Trying to Get Pregnant

Dear Paul,
My wife and I have been trying to get pregnant, with no luck. They want me to get a sperm count. Do you know anything about this? Hank from Thunder Bay

Dear Hank,

If personal experience is of any use, here's the skinny on getting a sperm count. First, a sperm sample needs to be less than an hour old in order for an accurate test to be done. In fact, the fresher, the better. That's why they may want you to produce the sample on location—where you go for blood tests.

Unfortunately, your sperms don't suddenly appear for roll call and that's that. There's a whole procedure that needs to be followed. Like handing the proper authorization form to a total stranger in a white coat who will automatically yell in a loud voice, "Whadda ya here for?"

That's when you will become acutely aware of just how many people are sitting in the crowded waiting room less than five feet behind you. There will be a mom with a couple of kids, two teenagers, an older gentleman, and maybe even a nun—all waiting to hear your answer just like the people before them waited to hear theirs. You will clear your throat and say as quietly as possible, "I'm here for a sperm count," after which the person in the white coat will immediately say in the loudest voice possible, "SPERM COUNT?" as if for some reason you were really there for a barium enema, but said sperm count just for the heck of it.

The person in the white coat will then yell to another person at the other end of the lab, "Louise, where are the specimen cups for doing a sperm count?" at which point Louise will yell back "WHAT?" to which the person in the white coat will respond even louder, "I NEED A SPECIMEN CUP FOR THIS GUY TO GIVE A SPERM SAMPLE."

Now maybe Louise will yell back, "Top shelf in the cupboard on the right." Or maybe she'll yell "WHAT?" once again, and the person in the white coat will look up at you shaking her head, expecting you to offer a sympathetic nod.

Eventually, they will find the correct cups and hand you one. If you are lucky, they will open the door and direct you to a bathroom down the hall.

Otherwise, they will tell you to have a seat in the waiting room, where twelve sets of eyes will be staring at your face and then at the plastic cup that's in your sweating hand. And then the little five-year-old, who is sitting with his mother, will ask, "Mommy, what's a spurn count?" and the woman will glare at the child with her most intense "Don't-ask-me-that-now—OR EVER!" stare, and the little boy will protest, "But that man has to have a spurn count. Is something wrong with him?"

I am still not sure what the correct response should be when the person in the white coat finally summons you to the bathroom down the hall. Do you smile, make eye contact and say, "Thank God!"? I marvel at the man with gumption enough to look at the specimen cup and ask, "What do I do with this?" or better yet, "It won't be big enough."

Of course, if you are anywhere near to being a normal guy, harvesting your own sperm in a locked bathroom is nothing you need instructions for. On the other hand, when you are producing sperm for an official sample, thoughts may enter your mind that never have before. For instance, "How long should I take?" You don't want to return in two minutes, deed done. On the other hand, you don't want to take half an hour, because you know that Louise and the person in the white coat will be giving knowing glances to each other, as if they aren't already.

To top that, no one has ever given you a grade on what actually came out. This time, not only are they scoring you on the number of sperm you're about to produce, but your wad will be graded on how well your sperm swim and on how full you fill the cup. So suddenly you'll be asking yourself, "Is there some way I should be doing this for optimal results? Should I be squeezing my testicles at the moment of truth? How do I get the most out?" I don't know what to suggest, except if you want to save yourself the embarrassment of scoring in the lower percentile of men who have ejaculated in plastic specimen cups, save up for a couple of days. You'll never believe how large a specimen cup looks when you are trying to fill it with sperm.

Finally, when you are done, you might smile inwardly and walk down the hallway looking for the person in the white coat. That's when you discover she is drawing blood and you'll need to hand the cup to Louise. Oh God. During your entire lifetime there may have been dozens of different ways that you've delivered sperm to a woman, but never in a plastic cup and never has she held it up to the light and swirled it to inspect its contents, and never has she stared so blankly and never have you felt quite so strange.

Anyway, Hank, that's what I know about spurn–uh, sperm counts. Good luck to you and your wife.

P.S. If a couple is trying to get pregnant, it takes an average of eight months before hitting conceptual gold. If a couple is not trying to get pregnant, it only takes one night.

Dear Paul,

I've heard that couples who are trying to get pregnant are not supposed to use synthetic lubricant, and I've heard that saliva can kill those little guys who are trying to get the job done. I don't lubricate very much naturally. Are there any options that you know of besides using egg whites (eewww) as a lubricant, which I've been told might help?

Getting pregnant has not been as easy as I thought. Funny how many years you can spend trying to avoid it, then how many months you can spend taking your temperature, watching your body, etc., with no results! Sex has become a drag. I don't want to add "dry" sex on top of that. Do you have any tips to keep sex fun, after months of carefully monitored frolicking?

Mary in Virginia

Dear Mary,

It's amazing how sex can become such an unpleasant chore when you and your partner start having a menage a trois with a basal thermometer. My wife and I went there for a couple of months and decided to give it up. We became foster parents and eventually adopted.

In researching your question, I am once again reminded of how often the "science" of fertility can also be the voodoo of fertility. For instance, there are all kinds of fertility specialists pontificating about the lube question, often with different answers. One specialist who has written four books on fertility avoids the question altogether by blaming the lubrication problem on the male, saying that any woman can lubricate perfectly well if she has a partner who gives her enough foreplay. I don't think so!

Sperm, like the men who make them, can be finicky. Sperm start to croak if the pH is less than 7.0 or more than 8.5. They also start to pop if the fluid around them doesn't have enough ions in it, and they shrink like prunes if the surrounding fluid has too many ions. This should make sense if you took biology and remember what osmosis is.

Given that the pH of some store bought sex lubes is so low and others is so high, a lot of sperm might die if you use them. Egg whites and mineral oil are too alkaline. This brings me a certain amount of relief, because I feared if you used egg whites your child might come out of the womb clucking instead of crying.

As for osmosis, sperm thrive in an environment of 360 mOsm/kg. Most sex lubes have an osmolality of 1000 mOsm/kg or more, which makes for dehydrated sperm. And while saliva has an optimal pH, its osmolality tubes out at 151 mOsm/kg, which might cause sperm to explode. (Saliva can be an okay sex lube, except if you are trying to get pregnant.)

You might try a sex lube called Pre-Seed that was formulated by an andrologist (sperm doctor). It has a pH of 7.3, and an osmolality of 314 mOsm/kg. As for it being a miracle for fertility, keep in mind it's just sex lube that isn't as bad for sperm as other lubes. It's not a fix for sperm that will require Divine Intervention to impregnate an egg.

Next, you ask how to make conception-driven sex more fun. This is more important than you might think, for a couple of reasons.

It seems that stress makes the quality of a guy's ejaculation go down. They've even found that men launch a bigger and better load during intercourse than when masturbating in a cup in the bathroom of a doctor's office. If a guy is having a sperm analysis, the quality of his wad will be 2 to 3 times better if his sperm is collected from a condom (non-latex) following intercourse than from him masturbating. And here's something even more important from Dr. Joanna Ellington, who is an excellent andrologist:

"Some studies have actually shown better conception rates for couples having untimed regular intercourse as compared to couples using detailed methods to time things." She suggests intercourse 2 to 3 times a week, but with you doing it when you feel loving and horny as opposed to having a calendar and stop watch in hand. Another study has shown that women who have a regular amount of intercourse every week of the month ovulate more reliably than those who don't. Having fun in bed during your non-fertile weeks could be just as important to the bigger picture as doing it during your most fertile nanosecond.

So why not leave Mr. Basal in the medicine cabinet and get back to enjoying your lovemaking? Forget trying to engineer a Moonie-like march of sperm toward Fallopia. Your love for each other needs to be respected and enjoyed as much as the love you might have for a child that you may or may not be creating. Couples who are desperate to get pregnant sometimes forget the importance of this.

61
Sex during Pregnancy

If you hadn't noticed by now, each woman has her own unique way of looking at the world and you can't really predict how she will react to the man who knocked her up. Some pregnant women will want more intimacy than ever before, while others will want space—sometimes huge amounts of space. This can be confusing for a dad-to-be, as he is never quite sure if the love of his life wants to snuggle or pluck his eyes out. Also, don't think that the dad-to-be isn't experiencing his own set of pregnancy-related emotions. These may cause him to hesitate sexually while his child-to-be is turning somersaults half a penis-length away. The mom-to-be might be wanting to rip his clothes off, and he's suddenly prim and proper.

This chapter is about sex during pregnancy, from orgasm-related uterine contractions to swelling vulvas and fetal brain development. For most couples, anything that felt good before conception is perfectly okay after, including oral sex, anal sex, vibrator play and good old fashioned vanilla lovemaking. But no matter what you read in this chapter or anywhere else, please discuss sex during your pregnancy with your healthcare provider. There might be situations where it is prudent to alter some of the more outrageous ways that you and your partner enjoy sex.

Talking to Your Healthcare Professional about Sex

Think about this for a moment: you go to a physician, get totally naked, spread your legs apart and let your doctor put her fingers in places where even the IRS doesn't. Yet many of us are nearly paralyzed by asking the simple question "Is it okay for me to have sex while I'm pregnant?"

Plenty of physicians encourage couples to have sex during pregnancy. Obstetricians rely on people having healthy sex lives in order to keep from going broke. So do pediatricians, gynecologists, Lamaze instructors and everyone else in the healthcare industry. There is no way your physician wants you getting out of practice with intercourse as long as the possibility exists that you might have more kids. So don't be afraid to ask.

If your healthcare provider says it's okay to have sex, go to it. If the answer is "No, it's not okay to be having sex," then it is important to ask more questions. The first is "Pork hay?" which is Spanish for "Why not?"

If your healthcare provider is one of the few remaining dinosaurs who doesn't believe that pregnant women should be having sex, get a second opinion. Most physicians feel that having sex during pregnancy is completely normal, unless there are specific reasons such as a prior history of miscarriages or premature labors, the placenta is attached near the cervix (placenta previa), your water has broken or there is bleeding of unknown origin.

If your physician gives a specific reason for why you shouldn't have sex, ask two more questions:

1. "How long should we not have sex—for the next few weeks, months, or for the entire pregnancy?" All too often, when a physician says, "No sex," the couple assumes this means for the entire pregnancy, when the intent was "No sex for the next couple of weeks." If you were to ask the same question in a month, the physician might say, "It was just a precaution. Based on how well you are doing now, I see no reason why you shouldn't have sex."

2. "Does 'no sex' just mean intercourse, or does it include all sexual contact?" For instance, intercourse might pose a concern, but it's fine to have orgasms orally or by masturbating. If all orgasms are a potential problem, ask if you can still have intercourse as long as you don't have an orgasm. For some women, this would be a cruel compromise, while others might welcome the extra intimacy that intercourse allows, orgasm or not.

Urge Surge—The Mood Swing

Some women stay pretty even throughout their pregnancies, while others push the mental envelope. A feature of pregnancy-related moodiness can be the intensity of the mood and the amplitude of its swing. Some pregnant women who are horny feel so intensely horny that they find it hard to think about much but sex. They pounce on the dad-to-be the second he walks through the door. The intensity can be so great that some men feel a bit overwhelmed, while others seize the moment. Other pregnant women don't feel like having sex at all, and some might feel horny one moment and weepy the next. Also, a pregnant woman has the potential to feel hurt by comments that few women in their nonpregnant right minds would find offensive.

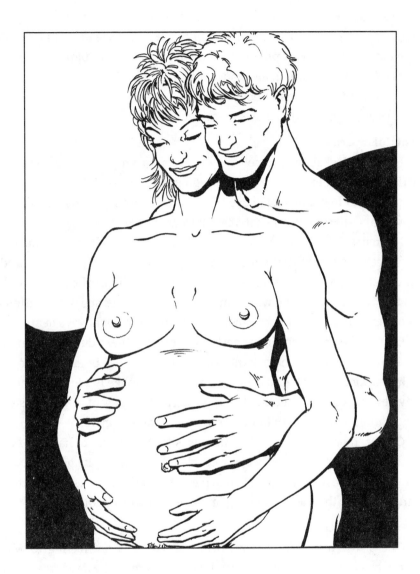

For the woman whose moods fluctuate, there might be moments when she blames the dad for her condition and other times when she feels elated about being pregnant and is ecstatic to know and love the guy who got her that way. Also, it is normal for a pregnant woman to feel moments of depression alternating with feelings of elation, and to have dreams of her child being a perfect baby as well as fears of it being handicapped.

Much has been said about the disruptive effects of hormonal changes on a pregnant woman's mood, and this might be true. On the other hand, oxytocin levels rise throughout pregnancy, and oxytocin is said to make for better moods in some situations. It also causes contractions of the uterus which may help to prepare the woman's body for labor. It is thought to be involved in a woman's orgasms whether she is pregnant or not.

Beautiful or Gross?

How you feel about yourself can be an important factor in determining whether you want to have sex. Some pregnant women look in the mirror and feel fat. Others feel they have never been more beautiful. Most women who are pregnant fall somewhere between these two extremes.

No matter how a woman feels about her pregnant self, it never hurts for her to receive loving reassurance from her partner. While a hard penis and a willing heart might be physical evidence that a man finds the mother of his child to be desirable, loving words and romantic gestures speak to a different part of her soul. Do your best to always be available if not always near.

One of the common disconnects between partners during pregnancy occurs when the dad won't ask the woman for sex—not because he doesn't find her attractive, but because he doesn't want to make her feel like she has to say yes. She, on the other hand, might interpret his lack of asking for sex as an indication that he doesn't find her to be sexy or attractive.

One of the better ways to handle this is for the couple to have an agreement that she will be perfectly comfortable telling him no if she doesn't feel like it. That will give him permission to plead and beg for sex as usual without having to worry that he is imposing on her—no harm, no foul.

The Fearless Factor

One of the nice things about being pregnant is not having to worry about getting pregnant. You can put the diaphragm in the deep freeze, keep the condoms in the bottom drawer or forget about taking pills each morning. This can make sex during pregnancy more relaxed and easy to enjoy. If pregnancy is what you wanted, there's no more "We have to do it now because my most fertile three-and-a-half minutes during the next quarter of a century is about to pass." Even if you didn't plan on getting pregnant, the fact that you can't get pregnant again for nine more months allows some couples to relax and enjoy sex in ways that they might not when consequences are a concern.

Sexually Transmitted Infection Alert! Women can get sexually transmitted infections while they are pregnant. So if you are with a new partner or are in a situation where it is possible that you might get a sexually transmitted infections, be sure to use condoms during intercourse.

Genital Swelling—Slip & Slide

Around the fourth month of pregnancy, most women's genitals begin to swell. And swell. And swell. This swelling can lead to full-time lubrication and can make some pregnant women feel very horny. The increased swelling is due to the growing vascular capacity in the pregnant woman's pelvis. As a result, her vulva often becomes a deeper color and her labia thicken.

Couples find that the added swelling may lead to a delightfully snug feeling during intercourse. Genital swelling during pregnancy can also up the intensity of the woman's orgasm. More on this in the pages that follow.

Orgasms during Pregnancy

Some women have no interest in sex or orgasms when they are pregnant. Others not only want orgasms, but report coming in awe-inspiring bursts that are more intense than their most memorable pre-pregnant efforts. Sex during pregnancy can also present a slight contradiction: even if she is more easily aroused and her orgasms are more intense, she might take longer to reach orgasm. The payoff is usually worth the extra effort.

One reason for having whopper orgasms during pregnancy might be the increased level of engorgement in the abdomen. With all the extra blood, her uterus stays hard for a few minutes after orgasm. As a result, a woman who had single orgasms before pregnancy may experience two or more at a time while pregnant. But by the end of the pregnancy, some women find that the swelling in their genitals causes a congested feeling that makes orgams feel more frustrating than relieving. Uterine contractions might also be contributing to the discomfort.

Male ejaculate contains prostaglandins, and some types of prostaglandins cause uterine contractions. However, studies show that neither intercourse nor male ejaculate induce labor. There is nothing about intercourse, oral sex or male ejaculate that will move your date up or cause you to go into labor. If you have concerns, be sure to consult your healthcare provider.

It is normal for a pregnant woman to have cramps or Braxton-Hicks contractions either before or after orgasm. These cramps can last for a half-hour or more. Some healthcare professionals believe that these cramps help improve the muscle tone in a pregnant woman's uterus. If the cramping becomes too uncomfortable, you can eliminate one possible cause by using a condom during intercourse or by having the man pull out before he is about to come. See if this makes any difference over a couple of weeks. Another approach that may help relieve cramping is for the woman's partner to give her a loving foot massage or back rub.

Another unexpected source of orgasms during pregnancy may be the prolific array of sex dreams that some women report having: "Never had one before, never had one after, but had a large number of sexual dreams during."

Breasts: Tenderness, Expansion & Leakage

Breast tenderness can happen in any phase of the pregnancy, especially during the first trimester. Breasts which used to cherish firm handling might suddenly prefer a light kiss, caress, or no stimulation at all. Some breasts that are painfully tender during the first trimester morph into pleasure zones during the second trimester. Changes like these make it important for pregnant couples to have frequent discussions about "what feels good this week."

It is normal for the breasts of a nonpregnant woman to swell when she is sexually aroused. However, when a woman becomes pregnant, her breasts may remain swollen all the time. As a result, she may get swelling on top of swelling when she is sexually excited. This might feel painful, or it may feel wonderful, depending on the woman and the stage of her pregnancy. Also, dietary salt might contribute to the swelling.

For some couples, breast tenderness will make the missionary position a thing of the past long before expansion of the abdomen does. Another problem or delight, depending on your point of view, might occur if the woman's breasts start to leak during the latter part of pregnancy. This is perfectly natural and is simply a preview of what's to come. Also, some pregnant women become highly territorial about their breasts in the name of the baby, while others are fine to share the wealth with their adult partner.

Bladder Matters

One of the biggest concerns that women have about sex during pregnancy and for up to six months after is about bladder leakage. It's one of the reasons why they don't have sex—because they are afraid of leaking while sexually excited. If this is a concern for you, then it might help to have a conversation with your partner about it, and with your healthcare provider.

Most men won't give a rip if their pregnant partner pees during sex. Most know that they'd be leaking if they had a baby using their bladder for a trampoline. So the solution for most couples is to put extra towels down and to get a pee-proof mattress-pad cover. Unlike the loud crinkly covers of old, you can't even tell the new ones are there.

What's unexpected for many women is when their bladders continue to leak after delivery. This is not unusual, and it's important to talk to your healthcare provider about it. That's because things can usually be done to help. (Kegel exercises can be helpful for a lot of women with this problem, however getting women to do them regularly can be a challenge, according to our obstetrical consultant.) Most guys are smart enough to understand that growing a baby inside of your body can require substantial recovery time. They're not going to begrudge you some pee when they are relieved it was your abdomen and not theirs that was the baby's rumpus room for nearly ten months.

Intercourse Concerns Part 1 — Fetal Concussions

It is not uncommon for couples to worry that the head of dad's thrusting penis is going to bop junior on the fetal brain and knock him senseless. Fortunately, the fetus sits in a sac filled with a fluid that absorbs shocks and provides superb protection. To make it even that far, dad's penis would have to get through mom's cervix and uterine walls. So regular sex should be fine, but hold off on rough sex until after the pregnancy and all is healed.

An important consideration during intercourse is to find positions and thrusting styles that feel good for mom and her swollen reproductive organs. If it feels good for mom, chances are the baby will be fine. As for questions about squirting the baby in the eye with dad's ejaculate, the uterus is sealed off by a mucus plug that is like the cork in a bottle of wine. The amniotic sac provides a secondary barrier that helps keep the ejaculate at bay.

Intercourse Concerns Part 2 — The Baby Will See Us

The human fetus is not taking notes and won't be emotionally scarred by the things you feel or do during pregnancy, even if you listen to rock'n'roll instead of classical music. Exceptions are drinking, smoking, or doing drugs —any of which can compromise the infant's developing brain.

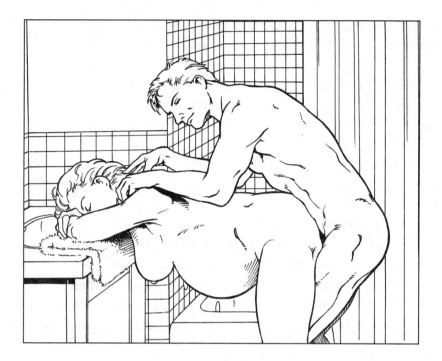

The fetal brain is not a miniature of the adult brain. Its memory units (neurons) are hardly functional at birth. There is not enough developed brain structure for the fetus to say, "Mom and Dad are having sex and isn't that disgusting" or on a more positive note, "Mom and Dad are having sex, isn't that wonderful!"

Sexy Lingerie for Pregnant Moms?

Sex doesn't stop being an expression of love and intimacy because a baby is on the way. Yet we are often given the feeling that pregnant moms are supposed to be more interested in what color to paint the baby's room than in sex or wondering what the new guy at the office looks like naked. Pregnant moms can feel sexy, and some moms and dads find pregnancy to be sexually exciting. For some pregnant women, nature turns up the horny knob instead of turning it down.

Intercourse during Pregnancy

Some pregnant women cherish the feeling of having both the baby and the baby's father inside of them at the same time. Others feel like three's a crowd. Dads, too, have their own issues about sex during pregnancy, some of which are discussed later in this chapter. If you feel like having intercourse while pregnant, important elements are a shared sense of humor and a willingness to explore. Here are some particulars to consider:

Clothes On Some couples who are trying new positions do so first with their clothes on. This helps them focus their collective energies on the engineering feat at hand, and it allows them to appreciate the humor of the situation without having to worry about feelings of urgency or declining erections. There's always time to get naked and go for it once the target positions have been mapped out and a strategy is planned.

Penetration Some pregnant women have a desire for penetration that's deep and assertive, while others prefer an approach that is more gentle. Talk it over. Different phases of pregnancy may require different styles of penetration as the pregnant pelvis becomes more crowded. Also, the swelling of the cervix and uterus can make certain types of intercourse uncomfortable. Let the woman control the thrusting depth, and if this cramps your style, be mindful that there are plenty of dads-to-be who aren't getting any at all.

Lubrication Some women seem to lubricate all the time when they are pregnant. However, there are plenty of exceptions. If that's the case for you, try adding lube.

Dizziness Some pregnant women experience dizziness or indigestion in certain positions or during some phases of the pregnancy. This can be particularly true when a woman is on her back. Doing it on her side, on all fours, or while on top might suit her better.

Romancing the Cervix The cervix of a pregnant woman often swells due to the extra blood flow. It becomes soft, and can sometimes bleed with deep penetration. Try shallower thrusting or use positions where the head of the penis romances the cervix more gently. This may be especially wise during the later months of pregnancy, when the cervix starts to ripen. If you have questions or if there is any bleeding, consult with your physician.

Third-Trimester Stretch By the third trimester, the cartilage in the pelvic region has had months of pregnancy-related hormones thrown at it. It becomes softer as part of nature's conspiracy—uh, plan—to ready the pelvic floor for the joys of childbirth. As a result, a woman may find that pressure on her pubic bone feels weird. Couples must be creative in their search for comfortable intercourse positions.

Too Much Swelling For some women, genital swelling may increase to a point where intercourse feels uncomfortable, while for others the desire for intercourse never wanes. Experimenting with positions where the woman has her legs apart might help. Be prepared to shift positions often.

Backaches & All Fours With the muscles between her ribs being slowly pried apart and her pelvic floor feeling trampled on, the pregnant female has been known to suffer an occasional backache. Some women find the rocking motion of intercourse, while on all fours, can help soothe pregnancy-related backaches. It can also soothe the throbbing between her partner's legs.

The Penile Vice (Or Vise) Grip

Some healthcare professionals think it's good for a pregnant woman to tone and exercise the muscles in her pelvic floor by doing Kegel exercises. What better way to accomplish this than by having a man insert his penis into your vagina, keeping it stationary, while you squeeze it with your pelvic muscles? Be sure to fully release your grip and totally relax your pelvic muscles before repeating. Most guys would be more than happy to lend a helping penis. This is an exercise you might keep doing after the baby is born.

When to Stop

Most physicians say it's okay to keep having intercourse until your water breaks. Some couples have intercourse until labor itself begins. There are at least four factors which should influence you on when to stop having intercourse: 1. It doesn't feel good any longer. 2. Either partner has a genital infection. 3. The woman experiences bleeding or new discharge. 4. Your healthcare provider says to stop.

Oral Sex

There are no medical reasons to stop giving or receiving oral sex during pregnancy unless the pregnancy is at risk due to other causes. There is nothing about receiving oral sex during pregnancy that will endanger the baby. The one thing a partner should never do is to make a seal around a woman's vulva with his lips and blow into it like it's a balloon.

Nipple and Perineal Massage

One of the nice things about being pregnant is that when the dad-to-be is complaining about the things he usually complains about, you have the perfect excuse to say, "Shut up and rub my nipples!" That's because as the final months of pregnancy approach, it might be helpful for a woman to have two areas on her body massaged (her nipples and perineum), or three areas if you count each nipple as having its own private domain.

Put lotion on each nipple and massage and knead it, assuming it isn't too painful. This will help condition the nipples for nursing, and it may also help release extra oxytocin into the system, which seems to be a good thing as the due date approaches.

As for the perineum, it is the space between a woman's vagina and rectum. Massaging this area helps to make it more pliable and could possibly reduce the need for an episiotomy. Talk to your doula, midwife or obstetrician about ways of massing the perinuem and base of the vagina.

Bleeding

During the first couple of months of pregnancy, bleeding may occur during the time when you would normally have your period. This is usually less reason for concern than bleeding that is random. Check with your physician when there is any bleeding, just to be on the safe side.

Touch and Masturbation vs. Partner Sex

Some women may experience a decreased desire for sex with a partner during pregnancy, but an increased need to masturbate or to receive more touch and cuddling. This can be difficult for the dad-to-be, because the cuddling and touching might make him feel extremely horny. To help him make it through these lean times sexually, his pregnant partner can cuddle beside him and caress his thighs, chest or testicles while he does himself by hand. Or he can do what guys do—masturbate in the shower.

Besides being an important time for holding and touching, pregnancy is a time for partners to reassure one another about their feelings of love and attraction, hopefully for each other.

Fears That Bubble Up from The Deep Dark Recesses of the Psyche

Contrary to how you think you should be feeling, it is not uncommon for perfectly good parents-to-be to have mixed feelings about the baby-to-be.

For instance, you may have planned for years to have this baby and wanted it with the deepest of convictions, but then suddenly start feeling, "Oh my God, what have we done?" Feelings like these can be fleeting or last for weeks. One reader says that both he and his wife were shocked to discover such feelings, given their pregnancy was better planned than the average shuttle launch. Fortunately, they did not experience their bummer moods at the same time. The one who was feeling good about the pregnancy was able to comfort the one who was feeling tragic.

Feelings can be especially intense during pregnancy and just after, when so many new demands are placed on you. These are not the sort of feelings that make us want to have sex. It can be very helpful to talk over these conflicts with a friend, partner or even a counselor if you are feeling particularly jammed by them. One reader adds: "Worries about child care, job security, and having to go back to work after only six weeks can be overwhelming."

Once the baby is born, it's not unusual for parents to feel intensely protective in ways that might leave less time or energy for sex. (The author of *The Guide* nearly met an early end when he had to take a dehydrated two-day old calf from its mom. Anyone who thinks maternal feelings don't cut across species should have seen the look of murder in that mother-cow's eyes.)

Recognizing Dad's Role

During pregnancy, attention usually focuses on the mom-to-be, which is as it should be. But this is also an important time for the pregnant woman to acknowledge the dad-to-be's role. Potential problems can occur when the woman feels that the baby is her creation alone. This can lead to problems in the relationship between father and child, as well as between the parents.

Dad's Emotional & Sexual Issues during Pregnancy

There are plenty of books devoted to the feelings that pregnant moms experience. Yet dads-to-be experience their own pregnancy-related emotions. According to researcher James Herzog, dads-to-be often fall into two groups: *more attuned* and *less attuned*. The pregnancy spurs the first group of dads onto a path of personal growth, while the latter group feels threatened by it and is not particularly fortified by it.

A factor that impacts how a man responds to his wife's pregnancy is the influence of his own father or father substitutes. Herzog noticed that during the second and third trimesters of pregnancy, a number of pregnant dads turned toward their own fathers in an attempt to reconnect with them. They felt that reconnecting with the "good dad" from their early childhood would help them be better dads to their own children. Men in the less-attuned group tended to experience a high degree of "father hunger." This resulted from having grown up without an involved and caring father figure. These men tended to act in unsupportive ways, such as becoming competitive with their wives or being sexually promiscuous; some had sexual relations with other men.

If you find yourself feeling unsupportive or disconnected from your pregnant wife, it might be a good idea to spend extra time with a friend or acquaintance whose fathering skills you admire. Tell him you are feeling on shaky ground; ask him how he manages as a dad when he's feeling uncertain or overwhelmed.

Other things that Herzog found about pregnant dads:

The Right Stuff Upon learning of the pregnancy, a number of dads-to-be feel good about themselves in a masculine and sexual way. The fact of the pregnancy may help allay fears that they didn't have the right stuff to make a pregnancy happen. With the excitement of being pregnant, a number of couples enjoy sex that is particularly intense and intimate, as though sex now has a different meaning.

Nourishment As the pregnancy progresses, some men feel as if they are nourishing or symbolically feeding their wives during intercourse, especially when they come inside of them. On some level, the dad-to-be might view his semen as a kind of milk that will help nurture both mother and infant.

Coming Harder Some men report feeling more depth to their orgasms when their partners are pregnant, with more physical and emotional awareness both before and after ejaculation. At the same time, the dad-to-be might be rethinking who he is; he is a man whose personal identity is expanding. At times, this can be exhilarating, at other times, frightening.

Dreams etc. There are plenty of ways that dads unconsciously identify with a pregnant spouse or wonder about what's going on inside of her. By mid-pregnancy, some fathers experience dreams or fantasies about being penetrated as well as being the one who penetrates. Some start to wonder more about their own inner body parts. Some put on extra weight or feel a kind of gastric fullness or upset. Some men have toothaches during this time that land them in the dentist's office. When a man has a toothache of an undetermined origin, wise dentists know to inquire if the man's wife is pregnant.

Character Evolution Being a dad-to-be can help a man shed unwanted or outdated parts of his character. The pregnancy becomes an excuse and a stimulus to mature and become more responsible. Unfortunately, not all men use pregnancy in such a constructive way, nor do all women.

Sex after Giving Birth

Some parents experience the first three to six months after the child's birth as being the most demanding and difficult time of their lives. They might not feel like having sex, or if they do, they might be too exhausted to actually do it. Other couples enjoy sneaking in quickies while the baby sleeps.

There are important considerations that affect the frequency of sex among new parents, like whether dad does his fair share of the work around the house and whether mom welcomes his help or is nervous and critical when he gets near the baby. Also, there are plenty of ways a parent can be helpful other than with actual hands-on baby care. In a few months, the baby may have grown enough that you feel more comfortable handling it.

Even with the best intention and desire, there will be plenty of times when new moms and dads are too exhausted for sex, especially if there are other children in the family besides the baby. Keep in mind that many couples struggle when it comes to adapting to their new roles as sexual partners who are parents.

Body Image & Sexual Desire

A concern that some women report during the first six months after pregnancy is feeling bad about how their body looks. Along with bladder control issues and pain during sex, this is one of the reasons why some women don't want to have sex after the baby is born. Hopefully, both partners can talk about this, and a male partner's reassurance will be enough to make it a non-issue.

Hormones & Libido

Some women don't feel like having sex after pregnancy due to a surge in certain hormones. And women who are nursing are said to produce more anti-sex hormones than women who are bottle feeding, yet statistics show that nursing mothers want sex more often than those who don't nurse.

Talking about Sex Before the Baby Is Born

Some of the best advice this book has to offer is that you talk about sex before the baby is actually born. For instance, "I've heard some new parents don't feel like having sex for a few months after giving birth. What are some of the ways we might handle it if this happens to one or both of us?" Or "What do we do if you've got a raging hard-on and want intercourse, but I only want to be held and cuddled?" Or "What if I want sex but you start seeing me as a mother type and don't find me exciting?"

One of the worst things you can do about sex after pregnancy is to pretend it is not a problem if it actually is. Nothing is to be gained by rolling over and pretending you are asleep to avoid having sex, by getting defensive, or by feeling attacked. As with other aspects of your relationship, this is a time to redefine and put things in a new perspective. Where sex was once taken for granted, it now needs to be planned or scheduled. There will be many times when sexual desire is a casualty to exhaustion. For a while, you will end up masturbating more often to help fill the gap in partner sex.

When Can We Start Having Intercourse?

It takes time for the place where the placenta was attached to heal. Until it heals, the woman is going to be vulnerable to infections. This is why it might not be such a good idea for male ejaculate and store-bought lube to be working their way up there. Also, it might take a couple of weeks for the vagina to heal after it's been stretched from here to China. Some physicians worry that intercourse before the vagina is healed can cause scar tissue to build. This is why many physicians feel it is wise to wait at least a few weeks after birth before you start doing the nasty. This is particularly true if the woman had an episiotomy, with stitches that need to heal. Don't even think about intercourse after a C-section until the doctor waves the checkered flag.

Birth Control

Be sure to stock up on birth-control products before the baby is born. Do not leave this important detail for after the birth, as you will have your hands full dealing with other things and are likely to let it slip. It is not fair to you or the new baby to have a repeat pregnancy sooner than you want. Nursing a baby during the first six months can confer a very high level of protection against pregnancy. This is called LAM or Lactational Amenorrhea Method. The mom must breastfeed at least every four hours and she must not substitute any other food. This assumes she has not had a period since giving birth. Please learn more about this before relying upon it.

IUDs are some of the best and most hassle free methods of birth control. Talk to your gynecologist or call Planned Parenthood to see how soon after giving birth you can have an IUD installed.

Lubricated condoms and condoms with contraceptive chemicals can irritate tender vaginal tissues, but your own saliva should be fine. If dryness or irritation are problems, check with your obstetrician's office for advice.

Episiotomy Repairs and the "Husband's Stitch"

Episiotomy repairs are often turned over to the least experienced medical residents, when doing it correctly requires a high level of experience and skill. You might discuss this ahead of time with your obstetrician in case you end up having an episiotomy or tearing. The reason this is so important to the future of your sex life is that the area at the bottom of the vagina is the part that stretches during intercourse. This is also where the episiotomy is made or where tearing will occur. A mass of scar tissue or a badly done repair can keep the vagina from stretching naturally during intercourse. This can lead to unnecessary pain.

Also, some old-school physicians might do a "husband's stitch" when sewing a woman up after delivery. This is essentially a tuck that's done at the opening of the vagina. The physician assumes it will make intercourse feel better for the husband. While the sentiment might be nice, the "husband's stitch" is better used in upholstery shops than on women's genitals. Tightening the entrance to the vagina makes the opening smaller and is liable to make intercourse feel painful for the woman. If a woman is concerned about vaginal tone following pregnancy, she would do better to practice Kegel exercises, which, when done correctly, can help to tighten the entire vagina rather than making the opening more difficult to get into. Please discuss this with your midwife or healthcare provider.

Painful Intercourse after The Baby Is Born?

You may need to work your way up to intercourse. If time permits, you might try taking showers or baths together and sharing a beer or glass of wine beforehand. It never hurts to have an extra tube of lube on the night stand. Some women who have never had a problem getting wet need extra lube after giving birth. For other women, it can be the opposite.

Designated Night Out

Once the baby is three months old, you might be wise to plan at least one evening a week where you and your spouse go out together for a couple of hours. There are different ways to engineer this. Willing grandparents are often at the top on the list. For instance, every Wednesday night they get the baby and you get each other. If grandparents aren't an option and a baby-sitter is either too hard to find or too expensive, call couples from your Lamaze class or find other parents with young babies and arrange to co-op the baby-sitting; e.g. they take yours every Tuesday, and you take theirs every Thursday.

Children know when something important is missing in their parents' relationship. If there is a lack of intimacy among their parents, they can suffer almost as much as the parents. Do not make the mistake of focusing all your energy on being parents and no energy on being lovers. By the time you notice something is wrong with your relationship, it may be difficult to repair.

Readers' Comments

"I had no sexual desire at all." *female age 36*

"I wanted sex more, and felt more free." *female age 44*

"I was extremely horny during my pregnancy and I felt very sexy until the last month or two." *female age 26*

"I was constantly horny when I wasn't nauseous." *female age 35*

"I viewed her expanding body as just more to love, hold & caress."
male age 41

"Intercourse can hurt toward 39-40 weeks when the baby's head is lower. Sometimes foreplay was just as satisfying." *female age 25*

"I was more horny than anything. Because of the pregnancy, we needed to start using new positions. Some worked so well that we are still using them today." *female age 25*

"We didn't do anything different, except we didn't have to use rubbers. Yea!" *female age 38*

"Don't worry about the baby. If it is firmly implanted, no orgasm will dislodge it." *female age 35*

"If anything, I admired her more for being able to 'do' a pregnancy. It's a real turn-on to feel an essential part of one." *male age 43*

"Sex felt extremely good and multiple orgasms happened all the time. They would sneak up on me. Things would feel good and if I concentrated hard I could have another and another." *female 26*

"My wife seemed to be more lubricated, which was great. She seemed more relaxed also." *male age 38*

"Be gentle, be considerate, encourage her to lead. As for sex after the baby's born, that depends on whether she's in a private room or not." *male age 40*

Sex after the kids are born?

"Sex after the kids are born? Baby-sitters, movies for kids, grandmother's house and motel rooms...." *male age 44*

"Lock the door, turn the music up, and put on *The Lion King*." *male 39*

"When you've got kids, bedtime is the most convenient time for sex, but it's not always the most exciting time for me. If I wake up early and am horny, I wake my husband up, which is something he loves, to have sex when he's just waking up." *female age 45*

"You have to make it clear they can't interrupt. Sometimes I'm very up front with what we are doing and she knows not to come in."

female age 25

Recommended:

Love in the Time of Colic by Ian Kerner and Heidi Raykeil, Collins Living. An excellent place to begin for new parents who are having trouble getting back into the sexual swing of things.

After the Stork: The Couple's Guide to Preventing and Overcoming Postpartum Depression by Sara Rosenquist, Ph.D., New Harbinger Publications, Any mom or dad struggling with depression after the birth of a child will find helpful information in this book.

Nina Hartley's Guide to Great Sex during Pregnancy. Pregnant Porn? Trust Nina Hartley to create one of porn's more intelligent and helpful videos.

A big bundle of thanks to Rachel Pauls, MD, FACOG, Urogynecologist and Director, Center for Female Sexual Health at Good Sam in Cincinnati.

CHAPTER

62
Abortion, Adoption

Alarge percentage of women who get abortions were using contraceptives at the time of intercourse. That's because even the best contraceptives occasionally fail, or sometimes a condom breaks, or sometimes we forget to take a pill. If you are pregnant and not prepared to raise a child, there are at least two options: abortion and adoption.

What If You Just Found Out You Are Pregnant and Didn't Want to Be?

There are plenty of people who will offer advice. Some of it will be helpful. One of your challenges will be in finding someone who will listen and help you think things out instead of needing to tell you what to do. In addition to talking to your partner, you might try to find a level-headed friend, family member, doctor, nurse or teacher who you trust. And call your local Planned Parenthood. They deal with this all of the time and can be helpful.

The one thing you want to avoid are "crisis pregnancy centers." These are often run by anti-abortion groups and they have a very specific agenda.

There are many people who have opted for abortion and many who have had unplanned children. Most will tell you that they did the right thing. Whichever way you decide, keep in mind that millions of people have had to face the exact same thing that you are— even though you may feel like the loneliest person on the face of the earth.

In case you are wondering about the emotional aspects of having an abortion, studies show that most women who have abortions don't report an increase in depression (as a group) for any more than a week or two after the abortion, if that. One of these studies was funded by a very biased agency that was hoping to find the opposite result. On the other hand, your own personal beliefs might not allow for abortion, in which case your options will be whether to raise the baby yourself or give it up for adoption. There are plenty of agencies that will help with the latter, but not many that will help the parent of an unplanned child who is trying to raise it on her own.

Please be aware that some of the strongest anti-abortion proponents are highly supportive while you are still pregnant, but are quite stingy and punitive when it comes to helping the unmarried mom of a toddler or older child. To many of these groups, your value is in being the vessel that is incubating the unborn child. Once the baby is born, they won't want to have anything to do with you.

Whether you choose to have an abortion or to have the baby, it's important that you make your mind up as soon as possible. Many people who are faced with unwanted pregnancies are indecisive and don't act as soon as they might. If they opt for an abortion, it is sometimes later in the pregnancy when the procedure might be more complicated. And if they decide to have the baby, they sometimes don't go for prenatal care until later in the pregnancy. This is especially true for teenagers, and it places them at high risk. Delaying prenatal care will endanger both yourself and your baby.

If you decide to keep the baby, make sure you have a support system in place to help after the baby is born.

If you have medical questions or want to schedule an appointment with the nearest Planned Parenthood, call toll-free 1-800-230-PLAN.

A Special Note on Giving Your Baby Up for Adoption

There are thousands of loving couples who can't have a baby of their own and desperately want to adopt one. These couples tend to have been married for quite a while. Most have stable homes, good relationships and solid incomes. They will give your child a lifetime of love and care. Unfortunately, many of these couples must wait as long as seven years before they can adopt a baby, since not many single parents are giving their babies up for adoption these days. Part of the problem is that younger moms are often encouraged by their nonpregnant peers to keep the baby (easy for friends to say!). Unwed moms often have the unrealistic fantasy that keeping the baby will make their lives better, or that the baby's father will want to marry them. This seldom happens.

One of the nice things about adoption in this day and age is that the pregnant mom gets to interview the couples who want to adopt her baby. She gets to decide which couple she wants to raise the baby. That way she will know her baby is being raised and loved by people she likes and who she has chosen.

63

Explaining Sex to Kids

Let's say that little Billy has gone shopping with his dad for the afternoon and you steal half an hour to lie on your bed with stereo headphones bolted to your ears, eyes closed and fingers massaging a very important place between your legs. You are all alone and the sensations begin to feel wonderful. Next thing you know, the headphones are being yanked off your head by Billy, who is asking, "Mommy, what color napkins were we supposed to get for the birthday party?"

Or perhaps you assume Mariah is fast asleep and you begin enjoying an all-too-rare moment of sex when a small hand suddenly taps you on the shoulder and you hear the words, "Daddy, how come Mommy's sucking on your penis?"

The pages that follow don't pretend to have all the answers about children and sex; they are simply a way of getting you to think about the subject before most parents do, which is sometimes too late for an effective response. Topics range from talking about genitals and masturbation to periods, sex play and porn.

Children's Sexual Development

People often think of sex as something that happens once we become teenagers. Not true. Most of us started having sexual feelings when we were babies. Each time someone changed our diapers and powdered our private parts we had sexual feelings in the most basic sense—nice physical sensations down where the Pampers go.

As children get a few years older, they often enjoy playing sex games with friends and relatives, same sex or otherwise. Sometimes they just compare and contrast; other times they enjoy doing things that big people do, like sucking on each other's genitals. Occasionally they might explore by sticking fingers, penises and heaven knows what else up each other's front and rear ends. Eventually you might encounter a third-grade child who's sitting there

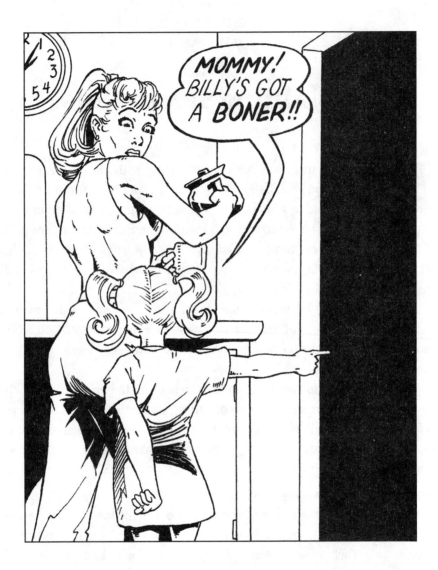

with both hands in his or her pants, happily rubbing away, while claiming how yucky it would be to ever kiss on the lips.

As children's minds grow and become more complex, so does their ability to have sexual fantasies that include others. With time, the thought of making love doesn't seem so yucky anymore. Eventually, they might even want to read books like the *Guide to Getting It On*. In the meantime, one parent might wonder if it is normal for her four-year-old boy to be playing with his penis, while another might say, "Thank heavens he's got his penis to play with. It's a never-ending source of pleasure for him!"

Telling Children about Sexual Enjoyment

Parents usually tell their children all there is to know about blowing noses and wiping rear ends, but rarely do they mention that genitals can be the source of good feelings. As a result, children learn it's okay to seek their parents' wisdom on just about everything but sexual feelings. This is unfortunate, because kids need their parents' guidance on sexual feelings as much as they do on wiping their rear ends or learning to drive a car. They will especially need it when they turn nine or ten and start watching porn.

Some parents assume that a 3-year-old who is rubbing her genitals has the same intent and fantasies as a 23-year-old. They either try to stop her or simply pretend that nothing is happening. Perhaps it would be helpful for parents to understand that their masturbating 3-year-old isn't thinking about how good her day-care bestie might be in bed! The child is simply touching her genitals because it feels good. It is perfectly normal for hands to reach between legs when a child is happy or excited, or at naptime and even when you are reading Dr. Seuss to her. All a parent needs to do is to occasionally affirm "It feels good when you touch yourself there." This gives mom and dad credibility about such matters and lets the child know it will be safe to talk to the parents about things of a sexual nature.

Boys have erections from a very early age, yet parents seldom explain to them that males get erections when they are having fun with their penis, and at other times like when they are waking up in the morning. Parents tell boys they have nice eyes, ears or even feet, but they avoid telling a boy much about his penis or saying anything nice about it. Nor do they tell a girl positive things about her genitals or let an older girl her know that her vagina will sometimes feel moist or wet. Yet girls get wet as often as boys get erections. (Parents who explain such matters to their children may need to distinguish between the sexual kind of wet and the peeing-in-your-pants kind of wet.)

Nanny Interruptus

Everyone these days is worried about nannies shaking their baby to death or kidnapping them. Few people think to ask the nanny how she will respond if she encounters your child playing with his or her genitals. What if you are trying to encourage a healthy attitude about sex, but during the nine hours a day when you are away, your nanny is slapping the kid's hand and warning of a thousand curses if your child ever touches him or herself again?

Ask about this when you are interviewing for a nanny. Discuss how you'd like these matters handled. Otherwise, much of your hard work may be for naught.

Opportunity Knocks, and Knocks, and Knocks

Four-year-old girl: Daddy, how come boys have penises?

Dad: I don't know. But I do know that boys and girls are both really lucky to have something between their legs that feels so good when they rub it!

The wonderful thing about explaining sex to kids is that you usually don't have to bring up the subject. It comes up on its own. Whether it's dogs mating in the backyard or your kid rubbing her genitals while you read her a good-night story, opportunities abound to make talking about sex a normal and natural part of growing up.

However, parents who explain sex in an open way should be prepared for nasty glares from other adults, because their children won't know it is bad to talk about sex; e.g., "Mr. Johnson, my daddy gets erections. Do you?" or "Sister Mary Elizabeth, does your vulva tingle when you feel excited?"

This kind of embarrassment is nothing compared to how it will feel if the first time you talk about sex is when your 15-year-old daughter tells you she is pregnant. (In some European countries, where children have better access to sexual information from a younger age, the rate of teenage pregnancy is way lower than in the United States. There is no downside in talking to your kids about sex from an early age.)

Playing with Themselves

Since few parents talk about masturbation, their children may regard it as a dirty secret. You can explain it to a child by saying, "Masturbation is when you touch yourself between your legs in a way that feels good." Or, if your kid loves to hump her favorite bear or some other object, you can say, "They have a special word for humping things. It's called 'masturbation.'"

If your child asks for details and you feel comfortable about it, you can make a pretend penis with a finger while saying, "This is how boys do it" or point two fingers downward and rub the knuckle part to explain how girls do it. Or you can say, "It's what you've done since you were little and you put your hand between your legs about 50 times every day." Also, it might be reassuring for an older boy to hear his father say, "I started masturbating when I was your age" or for a girl to hear her mother say, "I masturbate, too."

Keep in mind that masturbation is very common for kids between the ages of 2 and 11, and it's not unusual for a younger child to hump or rub their genitals up against anything that suits their fancy.

Public vs. Private

In doing research for this book, the author met with a class of high-school students to talk about sex. Before he had even introduced himself, one of the boys yelled, "Do you masturbate?" It's not the sort of question he is used to being asked, let alone by a punk with baggy pants and a strange haircut. Embarrassing? You bet, yet to have said anything but "Sure" would have created a serious credibility gap, and it would have been dishonest. Beyond that, it would have been inappropriate for him to have discussed details about his private sex life with the young and restless.

It's the same when you are parent. It is fine for parents to let their children know that sex is a fun and important part of their lives. But it is neither necessary nor advisable for parents to discuss the details of their private sex lives with their children.

Younger children may often need help in learning the difference between public and private. You may need to remind your 3- or 4-year-old numerous times that it's okay to play with their vulva or penis in their room, but not in the yard.

Liberal-Parent Alert For super-permissive parents who feel that putting limits on children destroys their spirits, keep in mind that children won't feel safe with their sexuality if it is allowed to explode all over the place. If a child won't stop masturbating in a public place, there is no harm in saying, "I know that feels really good, but you should consider stopping it right now if you ever want to eat ice cream again."

Also, older children who constantly rub their genitals might be dealing with emotional anxieties that have little to do with sex. You need to consider how the child is doing with the rest of his or her life. Is this one of many things that isn't going right, or is it an isolated problem that needs caring and firm guidance?

Naming Private Parts

Modern parents usually have no problem telling boys that they've got a penis and testicles between their legs, although little boys rarely refer to these items by their proper names. For that matter, neither do big boys.

Female sexual anatomy is mislabeled from day one. What you see from the outside is not a vagina, but this has become the generic term for what is nestled between a woman's legs. What you see from the outside is a vulva, which means lips. The vagina doesn't appear until after the vulva is spread open, and even then you only see the outer rim of it. It is also helpful for parents to at least mention the clitoris.

Parents should inform boys about girls' genitals. This way, girls' genitals won't seem like such a mystery. Also, it is through such talks that parents can teach boys to respect girls' genitals and to view girl's genitals as a part of an entire person as opposed to being an object for their pleasure. Otherwise, how are boys expected to learn such things? From porn?

The Difference between Cum and Pee

When you are ready to explain the concept of ejaculation to an older child, he or she might assume you are talking about pee. After all, that's what comes out of a penis, right? Kids will assume the man pees into the woman to make her pregnant. One way of avoiding this confusion is to explain there is a big difference between pee and semen. Pee is thin and mostly clear like water and there is a lot of it, while semen is white and thick, and there is less than a teaspoon of it at a time.

It won't hurt to explain that nature was very smart about all of this and made it so that a man can pee when his penis is soft and he can release semen when his penis is hard. You can say that when a man has intercourse and his penis is hard, there comes a certain point where his penis feels really good and warm and the semen squirts out. They will either think this is funny or gross.

Explain that semen is the stuff that can get a woman pregnant. Let them know that boys don't start making semen until they go through puberty, which starts to happen during middle school. Also explain that a man can't get a woman pregnant by simply hugging her or kissing her.

Child-Abuse Warnings

Now that our society is so revved up about child abuse, we've got parents and teachers telling young children, "Don't let anyone ever touch you down there!" Think about this.

In this day and age, the first time parents mention sex to children is often through warnings about sexual abuse—complete with deep, measured parental tones that barely hide mom and dad's fear and concern. Consider how dumb it would be if the first thing parents told kids about bike riding is how many scraped knees, broken bones and fractured skulls they are likely to get. At best, the child would learn to hide his excitement and questions about getting a bike from mom and dad. And if the kid did have a bad encounter on a bike, it is only natural he or she would try to hide that, too, and perhaps feel horribly guilty.

Why not establish a good rapport about sex with your child from early on? Then your child can take in your eventual warnings about child abuse with intelligence rather than guilt or trepidation.

As for an abuse prevention strategy, try giving young children a sense that their bodies belong to them and no one else. Tell them they don't need to give hugs or kisses if they don't want to. If parents respect this in their interactions with the child, then the child will learn from an early age that it's okay to say NO to unwanted physical touching. This is a better approach to preventing child abuse than the fear-based warnings that some parents give.

When your child is older and able to speak with you about sexual matters, you can say, "No one should touch you in a sexual way unless it's what you want." Inform girls that his includes boyfriends.

Let your child know that no adults should ever touch their genitals and bottoms or ask to see them undressed unless it's at a doctor's office when mom and dad are present, or it is with a helping teacher whom mom and dad say is OK. If anyone ever touches them anywhere on the body or takes pictures of them and says to keep it a secret, they should tell you anyway. Also encourage them to tell you about any kind of touching that makes them feel strange or uncomfortable. And tell them if a stranger ever asks for their help in finding a lost pet, to come straight home and get you.

Some parents tell their children there are "good kinds of touch" and "bad kinds of touch." This is too abstract and is seldom helpful, as children often confuse "good touch" and "bad touch." Any child abuser worth his or her salt will be able to turn this around to his or her advantage.

One of the greatest tools you have in combating child abuse is to spend lots of time with your child, being a real and vital part of his or her youth. Children who only get limited amounts of time from their parents (aka "quality time") are far more likely to be interested in the attention that child abusers have to offer. Child abusers are very savvy in their ability to select children who aren't getting enough attention at home or who have lots of unanswered questions about sex. They then become the involved, exciting and understanding adult figure the child longs for. They end up doing your job for you, and, unfortunately, more.

Children's Questions about Sex

Some parents overwhelm young children with biological facts about sex. A five-year-old can't understand the concept of Fallopian tubes! If a child under the age of five asks, "Where do babies come from?" it's fine to say the baby grows in mommy's uterus and point to your lower abdomen. (In your stomach? Really?) A child might want to know how the baby gets out. You can explain there's another hole between their poop hole and pee hole where the baby comes out.

When you explain sex, try to make it a "we" thing when possible. For instance, if children want to know how sperm gets from daddy's body into mommy's body, try to say, "Mommy and Daddy place Daddy's penis inside of Mommy's vagina," and not "Daddy places his penis inside of Mommy's vagina." For birds-and-bees information, you might find a book with fun illustrations and read it together with your child.

Once children ask a question about sex, they have often created a scenario or answer to the question in their mind. So you might ask your child to tell you what he or she thinks the answer is. That way, you may get more clues about what he or she needs. If there is no evidence that he or she is courting a hidden hypothesis, answer the question the best you can.

When it comes to questions about sex, or anything else for that matter, don't be afraid to tell a child that you don't know the answer. Acknowledge that it's a really good question, and say you will do your best to find the answer. Then ask a friend, find a book or do a browser search. This way your children will know you take their questions seriously and they will feel free to ask for your opinion in the future.

Keep in mind you may be asked the same question about sex ten or twenty times. It could be that young children have a profound need for repetition, or maybe they get a secret sense of joy from seeing mom and dad break down in tears after they've been asked the same question so many times. Also be aware that you will be giving a very different answer to a 5-year-old's question about intercourse than you will to the same child when he or she is 10 or 15. Just because you answered a question when your child was five doesn't mean you won't be answering the same question every couple of years, but each time in a more age appropriate way.

A Normal Five-Year-Old's Feelings about Sex

"In second grade, a little boy kept squeezing my vulva and it felt so good and tingly and warm and throbbing that I waited quite a while until I told my teacher!" *female age 23*

As part of his training as a psychoanalyst, the author of *The Guide* followed the growth of several normal children from birth on, discussing child-development quandaries with their parents as they arose.

One of those children was a 5-year-old girl whose lifelong best friend had been a boy of her own age. The girl's mother was shocked one day to find both kids buck naked with the little boy's fingers on her daughter's vulva. The mom's first thought was to break every bone in the little boy's hand, but her daughter was just as happily involved as he. So she went into the kitchen and forced herself to count to 20. She then decided the last thing she wanted to do was respond as her own mother would have. Needless to say, your author got a phone call asking for help.

The mom and he discussed how blanket prohibitions about sex often teach children to hide their sexuality from their parents. So rather than being guided by her initial response to protect her daughter, the mother asked the little girl how she felt about the way her friend had been touching her. Realizing that it was safe to answer truthfully, her daughter replied that it felt so wonderful she simply couldn't find a way to say no!

Since then, this little girl has asked her mother questions about who can touch her genitals and how to say no if she doesn't want them to. She asked these questions on her own initiative without being prompted by her parents. Few moms and dads have "perfect" answers for such questions, but just letting your child discuss it with you can be amazingly helpful. It helps the child learn how to use reason when dealing with sex.

It is likely that when this little girl becomes a young woman she will have more respect for her own sexuality than the vast majority of her peers. Her sexual decisions may even be the result of good judgment, instead of the all-too-common adolescent rush to just do it because the opportunity presented itself. Also, it seems she values herself and won't be agreeing to sleep with a boy out of fear that he will go away if she says no.

Don't for a moment think this Guide is saying to avoid setting limits on your children's sexual behavior. Parents who set no limits on their children's behavior raise obnoxious brats. Instead, why not think about strategies that might be more effective than simply yelling NO!—although there are times when a contemptuous glare and a firm "no" are fine parental responses.

When Children See (or Hear) You Having Sex

If a young child walks in when you are having sex, cover up slowly and try not to look like you were doing something bad, because you weren't. One of you should take the child back to his or her own bed and tuck the kid in. It's a good idea to ask the child in a fun voice, "What did you think Mommy and Daddy were doing?" This will help you to know what they saw and how they interpreted it; e.g., "Daddy was hurting you!" Please resist saying, "I'd be very happy if daddy hurt me like that more often!"

If the child has a negative read on what he or she saw, kindly disagree with his or her interpretation and give it a positive spin. You might also say in a reassuring voice that you and daddy were having sex which was a lot of fun and you will be happy to talk about it in the morning. Even if the child doesn't ask, try to raise the issue the next day.

Parents who make a fair amount of noise when they are making love should consider telling their young children about it, saying that mom and dad sometimes make noises at night when they are sharing sexual feelings. Explain that these are happy noises which are very different from the noises that mom and dad make when they are fighting. This is an important distinction to make.

The good thing to know about being seen by your kids is that Dr. Paul Abramson and colleagues at UCLA completed an eighteen-year longitudinal study of *Early Exposure to Parental Nudity and Scenes of Parental Sexuality.* 18-year-olds who, as kids, had walked in on mom and dad when they were having sex showed no differences from other 18-year-olds. In fact, young boys who walked in on mom and dad actually seemed to demonstrate a better long-term outcome than those who didn't.

"Why Can't I Watch You and Mommy Have Sex?"

You've worked hard to be an open, honest parent about sex and your child suddenly rewards you with the statement, "I want to watch you and Mommy have sex!" Instead of convulsing with panic, regard this as yet another opportunity to talk about privacy and sex. "One of the things that makes sex so special for Mommy and Daddy is that it's private, just between the two of us. Since sex between us is private and personal, I wouldn't feel comfortable having anyone else watching." "Well, what about that time I saw you kissing Mommy's vulva. Will you kiss mine?" "Your vulva is very sweet and nice. But I wouldn't feel comfortable kissing your vulva like I kiss Mommy's because it's a private sexual thing that I only do with her."

Nudity at Home

"Nudity was a normal part of bathing, dressing, getting up in the morning or going to bed at night. I think this is ideal. Kids get a lot of reassurance and education from the occasional observation of natural (not contrived) nudity." *female age 35*

"My daughter always felt comfortable walking around the house naked, but my teenage son is so modest that nobody can remember seeing him naked since he was five years old!" *male age 65*

Is nudity around the house good or bad? A retrospective study of college students compared how much nudity they reported when growing up with their current levels of sexual activity. There was no correlation between high levels of nudity at home and sexual promiscuity at college. Kids who reported higher levels of nudity at home seemed to report more feelings of warmth or security when away at college. Perhaps one reason for this is because it's easier for them to adjust to communal bathroom and shower situations that are common in college life. It's also possible they feel better about their bodies.

Parents' Sexual Feelings about Their Children

Our society gives parents little guidance about sexual feelings toward their children, except blanket condemnation. Children of all ages are able to evoke sexual feelings in parents, from a nursing experience that leaves a baby's mother with pleasant genital sensations, to a teenage son whose developing body gives mom an occasional sexual stirring, perhaps reminding her of the excitement she used to feel when seeing the boy's father when he was younger. The problem isn't in having occasional sexual feelings about your children; it's in what to do with the feelings.

For instance, let's say a dad is playfully wrestling with his young daughter and finds he is getting an erection. A healthy dad might think to himself, "Oops!," beg out of the roughhousing, and say to his daughter, "Why don't you grab the mitts so we can work on your pitching?" or "How about a game of Scrabble?" A less-healthy dad might keep doing the same activity over and over without adjusting to the reality of the situation.

Upon discovering their own arousal, some very good dads withdraw from all physical and sometimes even emotional contact with a child. In these cases, dad's own harsh superego can ruin a very important parent-child relationship. This can be quite sad for both parent and child, if the relationship had been a healthy one to begin with.

As for mother-son feelings, let's say that mom enjoys rubbing her teenage son's back, but finds she is starting to have a sexual response. Maybe it's time to give Junior a quick hug instead and realize it is more appropriate for him to have his back rubbed by girls his own age. Or maybe mom enjoys the way her son's teenage body looks. This is fine, but it starts to cross the line if she ends up in his bedroom when he is getting undressed. Particularly troublesome are lonely moms who encourage their sons to share the bed with them, unless such conditions are dictated by abject poverty. The same is true for lonely dads.

Problems sometimes abound in families where the parents' sexual relationship is not a particularly good one. One of the children might decide it's up to him or her to be a replacement spouse. What's amazing about this kind of mutual seduction is if a therapist suggests something might be askew, both parent and child may glare at the therapist as though he or she were seriously twisted. Especially destructive are situations where the parent alternates between being seductive and puritanical.

It's not possible to set specific rules and standards for all households. Nudity in one family might be perfectly healthy, while nudity in another family might be part of a syrupy, seductive mess. And while it might be best for parents to put boundaries on one child's sexual expression, another child might do well with the opposite kind of response. A teenager who is an exhibitionist with his or her naked body can use some limit-setting, while a highly-inhibited child who is embarrassed about his or her body might find it helpful to hear that it's okay to be naked. Another example involves a young child who enjoys masturbating before naps. This is perfectly normal. However, another child who rocks and masturbates anxiously throughout the day needs help.

It would be nice to say that common sense should prevail, but when it comes to sexual development, there isn't an abundance of collective common sense in our culture.

Explaining Puberty

"When I got my first period I was excited, but then my mother wouldn't let me climb trees or play with the guys anymore."

female age 55

"My mom had always been really open with me, so I was prepared when my body started changing. I was even glad to get my period.

female age 19

"None of my clothes fit anymore. I'd consume everything in the refrigerator and would still feel hungry. My armpits had never perspired or smelled. Suddenly, it was like someone had turned on a faucet under each one. I dreaded being called on in morning classes, because I'd often have a raging hard-on. My beard was really strange, mostly boyhood fuzz with man hairs growing through it. So I appropriated one of my dad's razors and started shaving. I didn't know why I was suddenly having wet dreams, and I used to hide my underwear and wash them myself so my mom wouldn't see the stains. I was sure I was damaging myself by masturbating, but couldn't stop to save my life. Hair started growing from my neck down. And suddenly there were zits. That's what I remember of puberty. It would have been nice if a parent or some adult had taken a moment to explain some of these things to me." *male age 44*

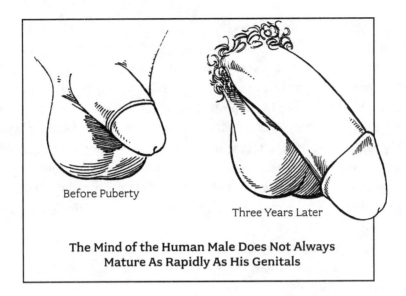

Before Puberty

Three Years Later

**The Mind of the Human Male Does Not Always
Mature As Rapidly As His Genitals**

It never hurts to let your children know their bodies will change as they get older. You will need to address the issue in different ways depending on the child's age. You can tell your 7-year-old that puberty is what happens when you stop looking like a kid and start looking like an adult—that boys get taller, their voices deepen, they start getting hair under their armpits and around their genitals. You can say that girls' hips start to get wider, they grow breasts, and their armpits and genitals get hair too.

When your child is a few years older, you can explain that puberty is a process that takes a couple of years to complete and it usually starts to happen for girls when they turn 10 or 12 and for boys when they turn 12 or 14, give or take. Mention that puberty is the time when girls start having periods and boys start to produce semen when they have orgasms, and that everyone's genitals start to look more adult-like (this is nothing they won't know from having seen porn, but it's good to hear it from you). Be sure to talk about teenage boys and unwanted erections, (see Chapter 5: *On The Penis).*

Kids can be awfully cruel toward other kids who are in the throes of puberty. Let your child know you will wring his or her neck if they make fun of another kid whose body is changing.

Period Blood

"Puberty was not a really big deal for me. I read *Are You There God, It's Me Margaret,* so I knew what my period was when I got it, although my mom never bothered to tell me." *female age 25*

"I was afraid I would just start bleeding sometime and that it might go through my clothes and I would be embarrassed."

female age 49

"My first period was a celebration. I was at my friend's house and I noticed bleeding between my legs. I rushed home to tell my mother, fully aware I was having my period. She was thrilled, and we went out to dinner to celebrate." *female age 18*

Besides warnings about sexual abuse, the only time when many parents mention sex to their daughters is while explaining menstruation. What a sad association, bleeding and sex.

As children, we learn that blood is a sign of bodily injury. We are never told that some bleeding is good for us. So when girls start having their periods, remind them that period flow is a sign of health. Periods are the body's way of giving their uterus a monthly makeover (out with the old tissue, in with the new).

Girls are now menstruating at ages 10 or 12; their grandmothers started menstruating when they were three to four years older. The bodies of girls are more developed than their grandmothers,' but their emotional development is about the same. This means they will need encouragement and support from their parents in negotiating the puberty process, especially if they started having periods earlier or later than most of their friends.

Growing Girls

Young girls tend to be self-conscious about physical changes, especially around fathers and brothers. If that's the case, don't be talking about tampons and bras when the guys are around. Hopefully your daughter won't be too sensitive, because these things are a normal part of life and it shouldn't feel strange to talk about them when dads and brothers are around. It's important for boys to learn about period gear, too.

If your daughter matures earlier than her friends, you'll need to be aware that other girls might shun her and boys might tease them. Keep reminding her that things will be fine in a year or two when everybody else has started to mature. It can help if she is involved in activities like sports or clubs, where value is placed on achievements and abilities.

Also, you can't tell your daughter often enough how the models in most magazines are *Photoshopped*. Women don't really look like that. And remind them that a lot of skinny actresses think nothing of barfing up a perfectly good meal so they won't get "fat."

Teenagers & Sex

"I used to pretend my friend Heather was another boy that I liked in school in fifth grade and we would touch each other's vulvas and breasts and have a lot of fun until my Mom found out and sent me to a psychiatrist for being a lesbian!" *female age 24*

If you ask a group of teenagers if they are emotionally ready to have sex, most will say yes. If you ask their parents whether their teenagers are emotionally ready to have sex, most will say no. Chances are your teenagers do not view sex the way you wish they would.

As a parent, you can't expect a teenager to be verbal about sex just because you have suddenly decided to offer wise counsel. Having an open dialogue about sex is an option that some parents lost when the child was 3 to 5 years old, which is why this chapter keeps harping about the importance of that. If mom and dad ignored the existence of sexual feelings back then, it might be uncomfortable for the child who is now a teenager to suddenly start talking about sex.

If there is tension between you and your teen, or if the kid is engaged in reckless acting-out behavior, you might do better to solicit the help of a favorite aunt, uncle, teacher or therapist to whom the teen is more apt to open up to. And if there are problems, you will need to become more involved in their lives than you might currently be. Also see Chapter 64: *How the Internet Killed the Plumber in Porn."*

When Teenagers Ask on Their Own

Let's say your teenager asks you a question about sex: "How do you know if you're gay?" or "What if you get so nervous before having sex that you feel like throwing up?" or "Would I have to leave home if I got pregnant?" Don't assume that she or he is thinking about being gay, is about to have sex or is pregnant. Maybe your kid heard something on the TV or radio and is putting him or herself in the other person's place. Or maybe not.

Try to respond by saying things that will help expand the question into a discussion, such as "What are your thoughts about that?" or "I'll be able to give you a better answer if you could tell me more about your question." This buys you precious time, which parents can never have enough of when being asked questions about sex, and it helps you squelch any potential screams that are about to explode from the depths of your parental craw.

You might take solace from the following words by sex educator Debra Haffner: "Like most parents, I have found myself at a loss for words when a question I never expected popped up. There have been times when I have responded in ways that I later regretted. I struggled with how to respond to my daughter when she asked about the Bobbit case, and then about Michael Jackson, and Monica Lewinsky." (Debra's kids are now grown, but there will never be a shortage of *interesting* sex stories in the news.)

Just because another actor dies from erotic asphyxiation or sex tapes start to surface of your child's favorite Disney princess, don't think you need to come up with perfect answers when your kid looks at you with his or her WTF? face. The most important thing is to provide an atmosphere where a child can ask difficult questions and know it's OK to think out loud about sex.

Wouldn't It Be Nice If...

Parents seldom talk to their children about the qualities that are desirable in a lover, or provide them with questions to ask themselves about sex with a partner. Perhaps these questions can act as guides in helping your child think about what they might want in a sexual partner.

🔦 Why do I want to have sex with this person?

🔦 Why does this person want to have sex with me? Is it for fun, romance, a personal quest? Is he or she truly interested in me?

🔦 Am I physically excited about having sex with this person?

🔦 Does having sex mean something different to him or her than it does to me?

🔦 Do I know what it feels like in my body to be sexually excited?

🔦 Do I want to have an exclusive relationship? If so, at what point should we have the exclusivity talk?

🔦 Do women and men become sexually aroused in the same way, and at the same time?

🔆Do we discuss what we do and don't want to do ahead of time?

🔆Are there ways we could please each other sexually without having intercourse?

🔆How do I say no to someone who is pressuring me to have sex?

🔆What are the most effective methods of birth control, and how do we make sure we are using one of them?

🔆What kind of stimulation does a woman need before intercourse so it feels good?

🔆Who sticks what into where when we have intercourse, and how can we do it in ways that will make it feel better?

🔆Will I feel good about myself the next day?

🔆How do I get feedback from my partner about what felt good and what didn't? How do I tell him or her what felt good and what didn't for me?

🔆What would we do if we had intercourse and became pregnant? Who do we turn to? How would we tell our parents? Would we face it together? Am I ready to be a parent? (No kid should begin dating without discussing pregnancy with his or her parents.)

The Qualities of a Sex Partner

The mere thought of asking an 11-year-old what qualities she would want in a sexual partner would send most American parents racing to the bathroom for Tagamet or Imodium. But let's think about it. If you as a parent don't introduce the notions of consent and respect in sex, where else are your children going to learn? From porn? From the other kids at school?

With kids stroking it to porn since the time they turn ten, parents have no idea how much pressure boys are placing on girls to have sex. Parents need to be talking to their children about the differences between sex in porn and sex in real life from the time their kids reach middle school.

There is nothing wrong with talking to your child about the difference between a partner who's just trying to get laid and one who is going to be a caring and loving sexual companion. Ask your kids about someone who says "I won't go out with you anymore if we can't have sex."

What are your children's expectations for someone they are dating. Here are some questions you might right by them: Are his or her friends good people? Do they drink or get loaded a lot? Is he or she responsible and caring toward family and friends? And what about introducing the expectation that a good partner is one who is trustworthy and dependable and says things such as, "How can I help?" or "I'd really like to please you. What can I do?"

None of this is going to stop your kid from shacking up with someone who is truly despicable, but it does kick into motion the idea that it's important to choose your sexual partners wisely. With enough intelligent concern and involvement on your part, your kid may even search out a sexual partner who has some of the characteristics and values that you do. Hopefully that's a good thing.

Talking about Sex in Real Life vs. Sex in Porn

Porn has become the sex educator of our young. It is having a massive influence on how young boys think sex should be in real life. Please, have talks with your pre-teen and teenage sons and daughters about the differences between sex in porn and sex in real life. If you need ideas, there are plenty in Chapter 64: *How the Internet Killed the Plumber in Porn* as well as Chapter 29: *The Fairy Pornmother* and Chapter 30: *Porndoggie's Dirty Dozen*.

Condom Advice — For Teenage Boys

Give your teenage boy a bunch of condoms and a tube of lube. Tell him these are for him to put on when he's alone to see what it feels like. If you have a straightforward relationship with him, tell him it's a good idea to try masturbating with a condom on, which is the condom equivalent of taking a test drive. Tell him to pay attention to how long it takes after he ejaculates before his penis starts to shrink and the condom might come off. That's how much time he has to pull out; otherwise the condom might stay in his partner's vagina. Tell him the shrinking-penis factor is why he needs to clasp the condom around the base of his penis as he is pulling out. Let him know that the lube is to put on the outside of the condom to help it slip and slide better when he is having intercourse. There's more about condoms in Chapter 22: *Condoms—For the Ride of Your Life.*

Condom Advice — For Teenage Girls

Give your daughter a bunch of condoms, a tube of lube and a penis-sized banana. Try putting the condom on the banana together. This should result in a number of giggles and laughs. If it doesn't, you're being way too serious. For even more fun, blow some of the condoms up as far as you can.

Explain that the condom material comes out of the center of the ring as she rolls it onto a guy's penis. Also explain that as soon as a guy ejaculates, his penis starts to shrink. This means she should clasp the condom with her fingers and push it against the base of his penis as he withdraws so he won't leave it inside her. Let her know it never hurts to put a little lube on the out-side of the condom before having intercourse. This will help it slip and slide better. Maybe you can try reading the condom instructions together.

Be sure your daughter or son have morning-after birth control pills. Dis-cuss how important it is to take them right away if something strange hap-pened with the condom, or if they are worried the condom didn't work well enough.

More Effective Birth Control Than Condoms

Condoms are way better than nothing, and they are the only form of birth control that helps prevent the spread of sexually transmitted infections. But they aren't the most effective form of birth control, and kids don't always remember to use them.

The most effective, hassle free methods of birth control that are a great choice for most teenage girls are IUDs. Many gynecologists use them for their own birth control. Please speak to your local Planned Parenthood about IUDs.

Birth control pills are more effective than condoms, but how many teen-agers can remember to take them every day? (How many adults can remem-ber to take them every day?) The effectiveness of birth control pills goes way down with every skipped pill. If your daughter forgets a pill, see our advice about this in Chapter 58: *Birth Control—Sperm v. Egg*.

Teenage girls who know what kind of birth control their mother uses are more likely to use birth control themselves.

Odds'N'Ends

If you have a son, make sure he's got a box of Kleenex next to his bed. When it's all used up in three days, don't make smart remarks like "I didn't know you had such a bad cold." Better you have to stock up on Kleenex than he be out knocking up some young thing.

Teenage girls can get major wet spots in their underwear when they become sexually excited. It's also normal for them to get wet when they aren't sexually excited. Moms need to assure their daughters this is perfectly normal and it's what vaginas do.

If your child has never helped with the laundry before and begins to hide or wash his or her own underwear or pajamas, be sure they have proper information about periods, masturbation and wet dreams.

Abstinence-based sex ed does not significantly delay the onset of intercourse. Purity rings and misinformation about sex do not work.

Let your kids know it's fine to wait until they are older before having sex with a partner and that masturbation is what you do in the meantime, which is why nature made our arms as long as they are.

Inform your kids that what they see on TV and in movies about sex is usually pretty twisted, exaggerated and outright incorrect.

A Final Word about Boundaries

Understand that good kids do not always make good decisions. If you give them enough rope to hang themselves, most will. On the other hand, no kid ever lost a friend because their parents insisted on knowing where they were and with whom. No teenager ever died because his or her parents set a curfew on weekends. No kid ever shriveled up and blew away because one parent called another parent to make sure an adult would be home when their kid was sleeping over.

Your kids will have plenty of time to do what they want once they are adults. Until then, it is your job as parents to get them there safe and sound.

HIGHLY RECOMMENDED: *The Secret Lives of Teen Girls: What Your Mother Wouldn't Talk About But Your Daughter Needs to Know* by Evelyn Resh, Hay House. As parents, we often deny our daughters' emerging sexuality or make it clear that we expect them to deny it. Evelyn Resh's book for parents of teenage girls addresses this disconnect. It offers us more effective ways to deal with our daughters' sexuality, including the use of humor to diffuse situations rather than threats or pretending it's not an issue. Ms. Resh has spent years working with teenage girls, helping to guide their growth when their parents were not able to acknowledge the sexual milestones they had reached. Whether you agree with Ms. Resh's perspective or not, this book is helpful because it frames the sexuality of teenage girls in ways that actually make sense.

Special thanks to Bill Taverner, editor of the *American Journal of Sex Education.* And to Debra Hafner's *From Diapers to Dating: A Parent's Guide To Raising Sexually Healthy Children,* Newmarket Press, for a reminder about nannies and some of the other things mentioned in this chapter.

64

How the Internet Killed the Plumber in Porn

T here's a popular saying about porn and plumbers: "Porn paints an unrealistic picture of how quickly you can get a plumber to your house." Many of us who are over the age of thirty get the joke. Yet few teenagers understand what's funny about this, and it's not because they don't watch porn.

In today's porn, a woman would never call a plumber. On the most popular sites, you don't see a zipper being unzipped or a bra being unhooked, let alone a plumber who arrives to fix a clogged drain or leaky faucet. There's no room for fantasy in mainstream porn. Instead, there's a nearly infinite supply of free videos that begin and end with highly explicit sex. Just like "Video Killed the Radio Star"—the Internet killed the plumber in porn.

Advances in technology have always had a huge impact on sex and relationships, from the invention of the telephone that changed the way teenagers engage with each other, to the creation of movie theaters that provided safe places where teens could meet and make out. But none of these technologies brought highly explicit sex to the eyes of preteens, and none of it bombarded their senses with images that would cause the jaws of a gynecologist to drop.

Parents need to understand this because it's what their eight- to ten-year-olds are watching. It's how their children are learning about sex. Many of today's male college students tell us they saw their first porn between the ages of eight and ten. For almost every child in middle school and high school today, porn is his or her primary source of sex education. For parents who think they can prevent their preteens from watching it, that train left the station years ago. So how do you talk to your kids about porn, when many parents avoid the basic birds and bees?

When children are playing video games, they can usually understand it's entertainment rather than actual fact. When children are watching the "Fast and Furious" movies, they can tell there's a difference between the way the actors drive and how their parents drive. When kids are first watching shows where people are killed, they usually have parents or siblings to tell them "They're just actors, and that's not real blood." This is not the case with porn. There's no parent standing over the shoulder of an eight-year-old who is watching porn saying "It doesn't really happen that way" or "That woman isn't screaming in pain, although I would be if someone did that to me!"

To children, porn seems like a documentary of how sex is supposed to be. So one of the first things parents need to tell their children from the time they enter middle school is "Porn is not real. Sex in porn is edited to make it look real, but sex happens differently in real life." If your kid wants to continue the conversation, great. If not, leave it until next time when you tell them the same thing again. And if your child stares at you blankly or nervously dismisses you by saying "I know that!", nod in quiet agreement, but don't let that dissuade you from saying more.

Parents should explain that sex in real life is usually part of a relationship or a friendship. Sex doesn't just happen because some guy pulls his pants down. Explain that sex is just as much about hugging, kissing, back rubs and giggling as it is about anything that's going on between your legs. And you cannot remind children enough about the importance of conversation, kindness, romance and respect when it comes to sex. These are qualities they seldom see in porn. *See Chapter 29: The Fairy Pornmother & Chapter 30: Porndoggie's Dirty Dozen.*

Never ask your children if they watch porn; this cause unnecessary embarrassment and denials. Just say "A lot of people watch porn, and they don't realize that sex in porn is way different than sex in real life." By not shaming your kids or lecturing them, you are letting them know it's okay to talk to you about sex.

Discuss how women are portrayed in porn. Porn actresses often make being degraded look sexy. Porn has a way of making it appear that women want the same thing that men want, no matter how bizarre. Porn actresses have a voracious appetite for sex the moment a man wants it, without conversation, consent or condoms.

Too often, there is pressure on middle-school and high-school girls to act like porn stars. It's not unusual for girls to send boys naked pics. Talk to your teens about how the quest for popularity and the desire to be wanted is fraught with as many perils as rewards. Help them to form a strategy for reaching their social goals without crossing lines they and you might regret.

Parents should also be aware that much of today's boy banter is inspired by porn. One of our daughters recently came home from 7th grade and told us the boys were boasting about double penetration—which is common in porn, but rarely occurs in real life. She pretended to know what the boys were asking the girls to do, but she needed her parents to explain it to her.

This type of talk at school is not uncommon today. Plenty of boys watch porn on their phones during class or at lunch, and too many of their conversations with girls are straight from the pages of porn. Most teachers and administrators turn a blind eye or offer hollow reprimands. It has become too prevalent for the schools to police. If your daughter feels uncomfortable about the conversations at school, don't assume she's being overly sensitive or that it's the usual boy boasting that's gone on since time began. It's different now. And tell your sons not to do it.

Parents should also be aware of how often Viagra is used in porn. This allows males in today's porn to achieve hydraulic perfection. There isn't any failure, hesitation, or "Oops..." Parents need to let their children know that sex in real life is full of awkward and imperfect moments, that a sense of humor is what makes sex and relationships work, and that people with average-sized body parts don't get cast in porn. In our sex survey of more than 10,000 men and women, few have complained about the size, appearance or function of their partner's genitals. Yet from watching porn, you would think that's the only thing that matters.

Remind your children that it's perfectly normal to have sexual feelings, but that there's no rush to have sex or to even think about it if they don't want to. And most important, try to be a nonjudgmental voice of moderation in a world that is far more sexualized for children than most parents know.

Hysteria about Sexual Predators Online

Much of what parents hear regarding their kids and the Internet focuses on sexual predators. The chances are good that your teenage daughter is at much greater risk of getting into serious trouble from the influence of the 21-year-old fry cook who she works with at Burger King than she is online. And if your child is going to be molested, in 9-out-of-10 cases, it will be done by someone you personally know. You have more to fear from your relatives, baby sitter, neighbors, or the people you might be dating. Far less than 1-in-100 cases of child abuse happen through a predator on the Internet.

As for risk reduction, the author's wife worked in the juvenile-justice system with teenagers. She'll tell you about a problem that is a million times more immediate for most kids than weirdness on the Internet. It's when teenage girls go to the beach, river, park, or to some unknown house with boys and get high on alcohol and prescription drugs. She's seen case after case of this, and she says the number of young girls who are in trouble with alcohol has skyrocketed. These are girls with good grades from good homes who get into cars with guys who they've never met. So if you are trying to get your harm-reduction priorities straight, drinking and drugs should be at the top of your list.

This doesn't mean you shouldn't be hyper-vigilant about what your kids do on the Internet. It just means that if you are concerned about harm reduction, there are bigger fish to fry in most kid's lives than what they face online.

Sexting, "Send Me a Hot Pic," and Dic Pics

Consider the following words from the mom of a teenage boy. She has full access to his texts and emails. She says all he has to do is text "send me a pic" and "he gets a picture of a girl topless or holding a teddy bear over her breasts, and he'll be like, 'Mom, can you believe this? I just asked her for a pic, and look what she sent.'"

So please talk to your daughters about this. As for your teenage sons, let them know that some district attorneys are not what we would call enlightened, especially if the dad of the daughter who ends up with your son's penis on her phone contacts the police, or someone finds the naked pic of an underage girl on your son's phone. If someone sends one, tell them to delete it immediately and to never, ever resend it.

Gay and Transgendered Teens Online

The Internet can be a lifesaver for the isolated gay or transgendered teen. At least on the Internet they can see that their feelings and questions aren't strange. There are a lot of wonderful resources for LGBT youth online.

We wish there were similar resources for straight males, but our society seems to have decided they should get their sex education from porn.

65

Sweet Dreams and Wet Dreams

Some people have dreams of misty-eyed romance, the kind of dreams that leave you floating in the clouds. Some people have dreams that include sex. These are the dreams that this chapter is about. And some people have dreams that combine sex and romance. These are the dreams that we dream about dreaming — the rocket-fuel variety of dream that fills the soul and tugs at the edges of who we are.

Sex-Dream Statistics

Less than 10% of American parents inform their children about sex dreams, yet the majority of young adults at one time or another have them. More than 50% of women have sex dreams, yet many women don't start having their sex dreams until they are in their twenties. With the male of the species it is different. Males often experience sex dreams as teenagers, with the frequency tending to decrease as they get older.

Sex-Dream History

In the mid-1800s, it was believed that sex dreams were caused by immoral thoughts. Some of the more fanatical experts of the day proposed bizarre operations for the penises of men who had wet dreams. Devices were patented for a man to wear on his penis at night to prevent him from having erections and the dreaded sex dreams that were thought to follow. One device was designed to wake him up by pulling on his pubic hair when he got an erection. Another machine poured cold water on him whenever he became erect during his sleep.

Dreamtime Sex Cinema—Pass the Kleenex, or Not?

During an average night of sleep, human genitals get hard or wet several times. This usually happens whenever you are dreaming, regardless of the dream's content, even if the dream is about your grandmother or someplace you once visited. A "wet dream" happens when you are actually dreaming about sex and have an orgasm.

A lot of "wet dream" orgasms are actually dry and don't include ejaculation, which makes the term "wet dream" a bit of a misnomer when it is used to describe men's sex dreams. While having an orgasm in your sleep isn't much of a problem for a woman, it sometimes leaves a guy with a sticky mess. In a more understanding world, a male wouldn't have to feel embarrassed about wet-dream stains. But wet dreams often leave a splotch on the sheets or in your underwear, and what's a boy to say? Since there is no way of predicting when you will have a sex dream, packing your shorts with Kleenex at bedtime isn't going to help.

Sex Dreams vs. Masturbation

Talk about difficult bedtime decisions. Some people assume they will be more likely to have a wet dream if they don't masturbate. They might hold out, trying not to masturbate for as many days as possible in order to force a wet dream. This usually doesn't work. Sometimes a person can have a wet dream the same night that he or she masturbates or has sex, but not masturbating doesn't seem to increase your chances by one little drip.

There is simply no way to will yourself a wet dream, unless you are good at lucid-dream enhancement, or whatever the people at Stanford are calling it these days. A seminal book on the subject of lucid dreaming is *Lucid Dreaming* by Stephen LeBerge, Ballantine. Another helpful book (except for its dumb title) is *Lucid Dreams in 30 Days* by Keith Harary and Pamela Weintraub.

Sex-Dream Complications

Not only are sex dreams a sign that you are growing up, but they are a great way of having sex when it is not readily available. Some people even have their first orgasms while asleep and dreaming. Still, other people feel upset by their sex dreams. For instance, you might have a sex dream that includes someone you know, maybe a friend, boss or teacher. This might make you feel a bit sheepish when you see that person in real life. This book's suggestion is to scope out the person from head to toe. Check everything from subtle mannerisms to what kind of clothes he or she is wearing. Then ask yourself: "Is he or she as good (or bad) in real life as he or she was in my dream?"

There can also be wet-dream downers. Wet dreams can leave you feeling frustrated when the love of your dreams doesn't want anything to do with you in waking life. This can be particularly bittersweet when the person is a former lover and is now with someone else or is no longer living. Also, it is not unusual for heterosexuals to dream about having sex with members of the same sex, or for gay people to dream about having straight sex. Gay men call these nightmares.

The Family That Dreams Together...

People sometimes have sex dreams that include members of the family. This doesn't necessarily indicate a problem. Actions that transpire in dreams are often symbols for something very different than what meets the eye, so you can't assume that the sexual partners or the sexual activity in a dream reflects what the dream is really about. Psychologists might refer to this as the manifest content versus the latent content of the dream. However, if disturbing dreams happen on a regular basis and you are bothered by them, consider seeking the help of a trained mental- health professional.

Another reason to get outside help is if you usually end up frustrated, hurt, frightened or angry in your dreams. You don't have to be Sigmund Freud to realize that repeated dreams of a disturbing nature reflect an inner struggle of major proportion. The exception is with children, since bad dreams are quite common during the younger years. It is not unusual for children who are happy and whose emotional development is normal to have bad dreams two to four times a week. If, on the other hand, the child is also struggling during the waking hours, it might be prudent to seek a professional assist.

There are no dirty words at
www.GuideToGettingItOn.com
Well, maybe just a few.

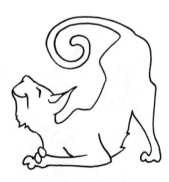

66

Dirty Word Chapter

You might be wondering why a chapter on dirty words would be in such a fine and upstanding book. Perhaps there is more to dirty words than meets the ear.

Frackin' Unbelievable

We at Goofy Foot Press probably use the word "fuck" more times each day than the Pope says Amen. The sad thing is, we mainly use our fucks to express anger or frustration. Seldom do we use them in the fun way. This is often the case with sexual slang, where swear words and sex words are often the same.

"Fuck" as an expression of anger or despair is such an integral part of our language that we have created more acceptable ways of saying it, such as "friggin'"— as if friggin' doesn't really have fuck at its core — or "frackin'" as was used on *Battlestar Gallactica*.

While people who use fuck-slang aren't always aware of the sexual connection, there's no way that texting "WTF" or saying "It's the Cylons, we're totally fracked!" have any power without a connection to sex.

Calling People by the Female Genitals

When the author was a kid, the worst thing he knew to call another person was a "cunt." He never could bring himself to use the word, but then again, he had yet to work with anyone in the entertainment industry.

Another slang word that kids often use is "pussy." While pussy is a term that refers to the female genitals, it is also an expression that boys use to taunt other boys who are being wimps, cowards, or who are using good sense and not acting on impulse alone.

Why does our culture associate cowardice with being a woman or having a woman's genitals? And why would we want to discredit the very female genitals that so many of us crave to touch and know more about?

A Fascinating Comment from Sweden

We assume that using sexual slang to swear with and insult others is the hallmark of a sexually-repressive society. This makes the following reader comment all the more interesting — when you consider that few people think of Sweden as being sexually-repressive:

> "As someone living in Sweden (and fluent in Swedish) but American, I have to say that there are plenty of sexual swear words in Swedish. One of the worst things to say is the word "fitta," which can be translated as "cunt." Many are trying to (slowly) reclaim this word. Most girls in high school will also say that "hora" or "whore" is one of the worst insults for them. "Slampa" (slut) is also another derogatory word used the same way as in English. In many cases "kuk" (cock) can be used to express frustration although it is not intended to insult a specific person."

Mother-Fucking, Titty-Sucking, Blue-Balled What?

Warren Johnson, a researcher, studied how normal eight-year-old boys and girls use slang. According to Johnson, the children's favorite expression when out of parental earshot was "mother-fucking, titty-sucking, blue-balled bitch." Johnson hadn't expected to find America's eight-year-old children capable of outswearing his former Marine troop.

Of particular interest is Johnson's observation of an eight-year-old girl yelling "Suck my dick!" to another child who was annoying her. As long as she was going to use sexual slang for swearing, why didn't the little girl yell the more anatomically correct "Eat my pussy!"? Perhaps even an eight-year-old child knows that the way to insult someone in our society is to tell them to take the woman's place in sex, with terms such as "You cocksucker!" and "Screw you!" being crude ways of demeaning a person by saying, "You're the woman in sex!"

It is difficult to understand how something as delicious as sex could be linked to anger or frustration, unless you haven't been getting any in a long time. It is equally difficult to understand why being perceived as a woman or as a woman who is having sex is a put-down. Yet these are the premises about sex that we grow up with.

When Eight Turns Eighteen

What's going to happen when the little girl who yelled "suck my dick" gets older and wants to share sex with a boy? We expect her to enjoy performing the very insults that our society has taught her to hurl at others.

Equally disconcerting is what this attitude does to boys. The message is that you either screw or get screwed, the former being associated with winning, the latter with losing.

Sluts, Whores, Virginity & Sewers

Few religions have done well with the notion of women and sexuality. According to early Christians, a virgin daughter occupied a higher place in heaven than her mother, since the mother had sex for the daughter to have been born. Around 400 A.D., Christianity's St. Jerome wrote, "Though God can do all things, He cannot raise a virgin after she has fallen" (Epistles 22). Not even God can help you when you lose your virginity, if you are a woman. It's never been a problem for men, but then again, men are the ones who wrote the scriptures.

Rigid as St. Jerome may have been about women's virginity, he was quite the feminist compared to some of his Christian and Jewish predecessors. One early church father described woman as "a temple built over a sewer," with sewer referring to her genitals. Men who made statements like these were later declared saints.

Perhaps it's no coincidence that many women who are unable to have orgasms were raised in households where the temple/sewer notion still holds sway.

To this day people still equate a woman's personal reputation with her appetite for sex: if her sex drive is too low, she is cold; too high and she is easy, a slut, whore or ho. While young men are free to strut their sexuality, young women learn to carefully regulate theirs.

Note Contrary to what makes sense, women are often the first to accuse other women of being sluts or whores. Men may have been the bozos who wrote the anti-woman theology, but women can be its cruelest enforcers. Also, if the human body was made in the image and likeness of God, as scripture says, why were church leaders so rejecting of women's genitals and sexuality? Had God been drinking the day He crafted the clitoris and vagina?

Dicks, Pricks & Morons

Why do we refer to a person who is being a total jerk as a "dick" or "prick"? A dick should be someone who brings pleasure, but that is not what our culture teaches us.

Adults will praise a young boy for his latest drawing or for making it to the toilet on time, but if he proudly displays his pint-sized boner, throats get cleared. Boys in our society are encouraged to spend eons learning how to make a baseline jump shot or to hit an A-minor flat nine on a guitar, yet they are taught to ignore their own sexuality in hopes that it will simply go away until they get older. Maybe that's why many of us grow up having more sensitivity for what happens in music, art, sports or video gaming than for what happens in bed.

Booting & Name-Calling

While our culture encourages its straight men to strut their sexuality, this doesn't mean we always do. For instance, the following story tells of how the term "faggot" is used by straight guys to deride other straight guys for preferring women to beer. It is from Regina Barreca's *They Used to Call Me Snow White But Then I Drifted*, Viking/Penguin:

"When I started my first year as a student at Dartmouth College, there were four men for every woman. I thought I had it made. Dartmouth had only recently admitted women, and the administration thought it best to get the alumni accustomed to the idea by sneaking us in a few at a time. With such terrific odds in my favor socially, how could I lose? I'd dated in high school and although I wasn't exactly Miss Budweiser, I figured I'd have no problem getting a date every Saturday night. But I noticed an unnerving pattern. I'd meet a cute guy at a party and talk for a while. We would then be interrupted by some buddy of his who would drag him off to another room to watch a friend of theirs 'power-boot' (the local vernacular for 'projectile vomiting'), and I realized that the social situation was not what I had expected.

Then somebody explained to me that on the Dartmouth campus they think you're a faggot if you like women more than beer. This statement indicated by its very vocabulary the advanced nature of the sentiment behind it. If a guy said he wanted to spend the weekend with his girl-friend, for example, he'd be taunted by his pals, who would yell in beery bass voices 'Whatsa matter with you, Skip? We're gonna get plowed, absolutely blind this weekend, then we're all gonna power-boot. And you wanna see that broad again? Whaddayou, a faggot or something?'"

Bitch vs. Faggot

The dirty words aimed at women often speak to how they regulate the space between their legs — too many penises, not good. Insults at men are aimed at a different level.

Guys are forever needing to demonstrate manliness. If we slip up, we're called a fag or queer, even if the only dick we've ever held is our own. This is particularly true among teenagers. A knee-jerk response that teenage boys have when another boy steps outside of the fragile notion of what's considered masculine is to call him a "fag."

The insults for men and women have the same premise: each likes dick too much. But a woman who is being insulted is usually allowed to remain heterosexual, albeit a slutty one. The guy, however, has his sexual identity called into question. A man's heterosexual status knows no rest. It has to be earned and re-earned or he risks falling off the stilts that define him as straight.

Origin of the Bimbo & the Stud

"Bimbo" and "stud" aren't exactly dirty words, but they achieve dirty-word status when you consider the following observation made by a female friend of the author who was sitting on the beach:

A father was standing a few feet into the surf with a young boy on his right side and a young girl on his left. The children were the same size. Whenever a wave came in the father would keep his right arm rigid. This helped the boy brave the oncoming wave. At the same time, the father would lift his left arm, pulling the girl into the air so she could avoid the splash. The boy was being taught how to face the wave; the girl was being taught to expect a man to rescue her.

Bimbo training starts early in our country. All too often, the first step is getting girls to believe that they are more fragile than boys. Then, ads in women's magazines spawn the belief that there is something unsexy about the female body unless it's plugged with a scented tampon and accessorized with perfume, high heels, and is Photoshopped.

Blowjobs & Bounced Checks

Consider the following words of an American wife:

"My husband's going to be furious when he finds out the check I wrote bounced, so I better give him a really good blowjob tonight."

This book has no problem with really good blowjobs. But when blowjobs are motivated by fear, lack of power, or manipulation, it adds to the use of expressions like "blow me" as a putdown.

Then again, after this chapter was first published, protests from female readers flooded in, e.g. trading blowjobs for money is one of the few ways women have had throughout the ages to even the score economically; trading sex for money brings far more joy into the world and is less destructive than the ways some men earn their paychecks; and what about the possibility that the wife finds the situation to be a turn on and might totally enjoy giving the payback blowjob? Husbands weighed in as well: "My bank charges $35 for each bounced check. If that gets me oral sex, let her bounce all the checks she wants!"

Rap Lyric Ho'down — Dirty Words and Then Some

No chapter on dirty words would be complete without mention of rap song lyrics. It is not unusual for rap songs to have a liberal peppering of words like "bitch" and "ho," as well as sexual references that don't always express loving intent toward women. Here are two examples of rap-song lyrics that contain the words bitch and ho:

The first is from Soulja Boy's "Crank That (Soulja Boy)." Here's one of the lines with just three words:

Superman dat ho.

Superman dat ho means to ejaculate on a woman's back when she is sleeping so she wakes up in the morning with the sheet stuck to her back like Superman's cape after the cum dries. It could be payback for when a woman won't give him sex. Soulja Boy swears this isn't what he meant, so let's look at another line in this same song:

I'm cocking on your bitch ass.

"I'm cocking on your ass" is rap for when one man says to another: "I have a gun and will shoot you with it." So why make it "on your *bitch* ass?" Soulja Boy ramps up the insult by throwing in the gender card and making it a female reference. Ramping-up insults like this happens so often in rap that we don't even notice it.

The second song to consider is Dr. Dre's "Bitches Ain't Shit." Here are three of the lines:

> Bitches ain't shit but hoes and tricks
> Lick on these nuts and suck the dick.
> Get the fuck out after you're done.

Most people would assume this is a derogatory song about women. However, the song is apparently about a fight Dr. Dre had with his fellow N.W.A. band member and former friend Eazy-E. Dr. Dre also references N.W.A.'s manager as a "white bitch."

If this is a song about men who were suing each other in a court of law, there are thousands of terms Dr. Dre could have used to express anger. So it's telling that he and other rap artists use terms that are sexually degrading to women. No wonder why some of the people who work for companies that distribute songs like these won't let their own children listen to them. They are some of the few parents who actually listen to the lyrics.

Intellectuals rationalize the negativity toward women in rap by claiming it's a cultural matter, and is not meant to degrade women. Is this what black women think? How many men would dismiss it with a smile if another man said these things about their wives or girlfriends? But give misogyny rhythm and base, and all bets are off.

Apple Computer recently paid Dr. Dre and his co-founder $3 billion to purchase their company. Do you think Apple would have bought the company if Dr. Dre had written vile lyrics about gay men instead of women?

The Sociology of Bitch vs. Ho

We usually think of "bitch" and "ho" as meaning the same thing. But that's not always the case in rap lyrics. According to sociologists Adams and Fuller, the term "bitch" in rap lyrics could be referring to a powerful woman who dominates her household and her man. They suggest that "the bitch" in rap music is a woman who has a sharp tongue and is somewhat castrating.

The "ho" in rap lyrics is a different woman entirely. She is a woman who let's herself be used, often to manipulate men into getting what she wants. She will give a man any kind of sex he might desire to achieve her ultimate goal. She is a woman whose moral compass could use a bit of adjustment. She is not well thought of in the world of rap.

A male singer can establish his street credentials by referring to the hoes he's had sex with and which of their body openings he has penetrated.

Ultimately, there is no easy answer to why rap singers use words about women and their sexuality that sound hateful. Nor is there a straightforward answer for why so many women download these songs and enjoy singing and dancing to them. But this doesn't mean we shouldn't call them on it.

End Of Chapter Notes: The Soulja Boy lyrics are from Soulja Boy's "Crank That (Soulja Boy)" from ColliPark Music/Interscope Records. It received a Grammy nomination. "Bitches Ain't Shit" is from Dr. Dre's album "The Chronic." This song is still covered today by a number of artists, including a Columbia University a cappella group composed of twelve very white young women that has gathered more than 1.5 million YouTube views. The analysis of the meaning of "bitches" vs "hos" is from an article titled *The Words Have Changed But the Ideology Remains the Same: Misogynistic Lyrics in Rap Music* by Terri Adams and Douglas Fuller, Journal of Black Studies.

There are certainly times when fuck-slang is used in a positive sense, as in "fuckin' wonderful" or "fuckin' amazing." But when the word is used this way it tends to be role-neutral and refers to the act of intercourse rather than the woman's role in it. When it takes its more usual form of "We're totally fucked now!" it's got "girl" all over it. As for the idea that the insult gets its grit from the homosexual implication, we have plenty of insults for that and few people hesitate to use them when that's what they mean to say.

Special Thanks to the writings of Ira Reiss, Paul Evdokimov, David Schnarch, Regina Barreca, Carol Tavris, the late Bob Stoller, and many others for inspiring concepts used in this chapter, and to the famous sex researchers who originally suggested that people should think of foreplay as everything that happened since the last time you had sex.

67
Barbie the Icon

This chapter is about Barbie. You might be wondering what a cultural icon like Barbie is doing in a book on sex. Perhaps the following statements by our female readers will help explain:

When you were a little girl, did your Barbie doll ever have sex?

"I had lots of Barbies. She and my giant panda bear got naked and 'did it,' and my sister and I dressed her up in Ken's clothes. Unfortunately, you can't dress up Ken in Barbie's clothes. We tried." *female age 18*

"My basement was a temple to Barbie and all her relatives. Barbie lived in a soap opera complete with abortions, sex changes, and adultery. She and Ken frequently got naked in their Laura Ashley canopy bed." *female age 24*

"Barbie and Ken had a very active relationship and 'sex' life. It's hard to say it was a sex life without any genitalia. I guess I used them to emulate the adults around me. Barbie and Ken often went skinny dipping at the ocean, and slept nude most times." *female age 35*

"My Barbie had Ken on her ALL the time. If I knew then what I know now, Barbie would have been on top more often." *female age 44*

"My friend had a Ken and we used to make them have sex by making their little plastic bodies rub against each other when they were lying in Barbie's little nylon bed. We were about ten and were disappointed that Ken's underwear was glued on." *female age 22*

"You know those parts in movies that parents were always trying to hide from younger children? I got a slight peek one day, but all I saw were sheets moving. After I saw that, Barbie and Ken made those sounds and simulated those actions. But I wasn't sure what they were really doing." *female age 22*

"She had kinky fantasies and a lot of BDSM. Barbie was a fun girl."
female age 18

"Not Barbies but definitely with my Lego men. Don't ask me why, but those spacemen certainly had interesting encounters when I sent them on missions. I was pretty inventive for a 7-year-old."

female age 19

While these women's experiences by no means represent that of most girls, it is likely they represent a significant number. (See more reader comments on their Barbie's sex life at the end of the chapter.)

Eleven Inches of Attitude

The year was 1959. The place was the Toy Fair in New York that's held every February. Mattel's new toy named Barbie was falling flat on her face, or would have if such a thing had been anatomically possible.

Since the beginning of time, toy buyers in America have placed orders for their Christmas inventory at the annual Toy Fair. It is the moment that determines which toys make it to toy-store shelves the following Christmas, and Barbie was getting the cold shoulder.

This was nearly sixty years ago, and the radical new doll named Barbie was shattering everyone's idea of what a child's toy should be. The price she paid for her uniqueness was to be ignored by toy buyers. Buyers for toy stores in 1959 were placing orders for dolls that were soft and huggable, dolls whose souls were made from rags.

Believe it or not, Barbie was cloned from a mother doll named Lilli who was made in Germany. In the late 1950s, Lilli caught the eye of Ruth Handler, co-founder of the Mattel toy company. Lilli was a sexpot of a doll who was marketed to horny German males. She looked like a German streetwalker. Lilli had been adapted from an adult comic strip where she had been a comical gold-digger and barfly.

Both Barbie and Lilli were 11 inches tall. The apples did not fall far from the tree when it came to looks, but Ms. Handler made sure that Barbie was born into an entirely different social class. Lilli was more like Anna Nicole Smith, while Barbie was Jackie Kennedy. Interestingly, Barbie's place of birth (at least the address of Mattel) was Hawthorne, California, the same city where America's other sex idol, Marilyn Monroe, was born.

Large Breasts and No Panties

In 1959, toy-store buyers wanted what they knew—dolls that reflected our society's idea of what a good girl should be and what she would hopefully become: a selfless mother, teacher, housewife, or nurse. They didn't get it when they saw Barbie, a doll who has been described by author Christopher Varaste as:

> "An 11½ inch glamour queen with exotic features in a striking black and white swimsuit. She was everyone and defiantly no one. She seemed ageless, though she was supposed to be a teenager. She was beguiling, mysterious, and yet innocent. She was a symbol of a culture struggling to find a suitable identity. As a toy for young girls, her rather severe look took some getting used to. Her Asian eyes, curly bangs, and big red lips could have belonged to a wide range of ethnic backgrounds. She was, in a word, peculiar." (From Christopher Varaste's incredible book of Barbie photographs *Face of the American Dream–Barbie Doll, 1959 - 1971*)

If it hadn't been for a stroke of marketing genius, Barbie would have gone down in flames. But Mattel's strategy for selling Barbie to the American public was as unique as their product. They were one of the first companies in history to make TV commercials that were aimed at children viewers.

From the very first commercial, Barbie was portrayed as a human with a glamorous and adventurous life. She was never described as a doll and she was never burdened with trivial limitations such as parents or a husband.

Mattel aired their first Barbie commercial during the wildly popular *Mickey Mouse Club* TV show. If parents didn't know what to make of Barbie, their American daughters certainly did. Once the summer of 1959 started, every Barbie in every toy store was bought as quickly as it arrived.

Barbie's official name was Barbie Millicent Roberts. When Ken was created a few years later, his name was Ken Carson. It is fitting and telling that Barbie and Ken's namesake was Carson/Roberts. Carson/Roberts was the advertising company that played such a dramatic role in Barbie's success.

Not Your Normal Housewife

Barbie's persona was created by two women who had both violated the housewife norm of the 1950s. One had co-founded a large corporation, the other was a tall, striking, unmarried veteran of the fashion industry. Unlike any doll before her, Barbie was created as a young woman whose life didn't revolve around a husband and a family. Her limitations were as thin as her waist and her possibilities as large as her breasts.

Early in Barbie's evolution, someone wanted to make a miniature vacuum cleaner that Barbie could use to vacuum the house. But Ruth Handler, Mattel's co-founder, refused to allow this. During the era when Barbie was born, it was automatically assumed that a woman's role was to be a housewife and raise babies. Keeping Barbie vacuum-cleaner-free was an important statement to little girls. It was a signal that they could exceed the boundaries that our culture had traditionally placed on them.

Barbie Is Nobody's Wife

Islamic leaders in Iran have described Barbie as being Satanic. They have expressed concerns that "the unwholesome flexibility of these dolls, their destructive beauty, and their semi-nudity have an effect on the minds and morality of young children." Plenty of American parents have felt the same.

However, if you read Mattel's press releases for Barbie, you'll see that when she dresses to the nines, it's not to capture the gaze of a guy or even a girl. Barbie dresses for Barbie. She has no need to please anyone but herself. This is one of the many Barbie qualities that throws feminists for a loop: they detest the emphasis on glamour, yet no one can ever accuse Barbie of coddling to the whims of a man. The Barbie that Ruth Handler created doesn't care if she goes home alone and she doesn't need the approval of a male to make her feel good about herself. That's been as much a part of her message to little girls as the big boobs and tiny waist.

Here's another part of the Barbie mystique that upsets feminists: Barbie succeeds and succeeds well in traditional male professions. Whether she's being a firefighter or a physician, an astronaut or a police detective, Barbie always pulls it off with her femininity fully intact. Some women have said this sets an impossible standard for little girls, but it also tells girls that you don't have to grow balls to have balls. Barbie has shown girls they don't have to surrender the things that they like about their femininity to compete in a man's world. Barbie has provided a way for girls to experiment with the positive messages their parents and teachers are hopefully giving them. She also provides a way for girls to be selfish and mean, as all children can be.

Mattel's Barbie has come with so few of the traditional limitations that any girl can make her do and be anything she wants.

Less Fighting, Better Play?

Researchers have studied what types of play lead to more bickering and what kinds lead to less. One thing they didn't expect to find was that girls who are playing with Barbie dolls tend to fight less and display more advanced levels of play than girls who are playing with traditional dolls. The range of activities that Barbie play provides is much greater than a doll that you simply hold, feed, and change. Barbie has friends, activities, and a whole life that's as expansive as her different outfits and hairstyles. In addition, Barbie's presence invites the involvement of mothers, aunts, gay uncles, and even grandmothers who had their own Barbies when they were growing up.

Barbie was never intended to be the *Leap Frog* or *Hooked On Phonics* of children's play. The fact that Barbie inspires a high quality of play and better language development was not Mattel's goal. Mattel's emphasis has been for people to buy more Barbies and especially more Barbie accessories, perhaps in the same way that companies who make computer printers hope to nail you for the cost of the pricey replacement ink cartridges. It is fascinating how Mattel has managed to achieve this goal without limiting the persona of Barbie.

Mattel has never married off Barbie. Yet Mattel has sold millions of Barbie wedding dresses and thousands of Dream-Bride Barbies or Wedding-Fantasy Barbies. The hitch has been that the wedding idea is all just a big Barbie dream or fantasy. Keeping Barbie from really being married allows little girls to marry and unmarry her as often as they desire. Being perpetually single keeps Barbie footloose and fancy-free.

Mattel never wanted Barbie to be pregnant, but plenty of children wanted her to have a baby. So they devised a "Barbie Baby-Sits" kit which contained an infant and other childcare objects.

As much as Barbie has been associated with fashion and glamour, she has never defined fashion nor been at the cutting edge. She has always been a year or two behind, like most women who can't afford this year's originals.

Keeping Barbie a Moving Target

Few people will dispute that Barbie has become an American icon. Given her iconic status, you would think she would appear the same today as she was in 1959. But since the very beginning, Mattel has made Barbie change and evolve. Some of these changes have been technological, like using different vinyls, skin tones, and hair. Other changes have been purely stylistic.

Barbie's face has changed as well. The first Barbie's face was a combination of her harsh-looking German mother and the Geishas of Japan, the country that first manufactured and helped to refine her. You can also see how the vinyl used in the #5 Ponytail Barbie of 1961 contained an oily compound that makes her look like she has a greasy face or is perspiring. Unfortunately, the more recent Barbies have been given a bubbly, wide-eyed generic smile rather than the more intriguing streetwalker-Geisha expression of the early years. The faces on the early Barbies were all hand-painted in Japan, while the latter ones are machine stenciled.

Barbie Torture Sessions

A study by Tara Kuther of Western Connecticut State titled "Early Adolescents' experiences with, and Views of, Barbie" clearly echoes our own readers' experiences with Barbie. When Kuther interviewed 10 to 13 year old children about Barbie, she found reports of frequent Barbie torture sessions. These included seeing if Barbie can successfully fly out of a second-story window, cutting Barbie's hair off and burning her clothes because she talked too much, making her dress up as a GI Joe, tearing off her head, drowning her at sea, melting her in a microwave, burning her at the stake upside down and attaching explosives to her.

We welcome these enterprising middle schoolers as future readers of the *Guide To Getting It On!*

A Cock-Ring Ken?

Ken was an afterthought to Barbie. He was released in answer to the demand for a Barbie boyfriend, but he was always expendable.

When Ken was being conceived, the two women who had created the persona of Barbie wanted him to have a bulge between his legs. The male executives at Mattel were horrified and embarrassed at the suggestion. They wanted Ken to have the same crotch as Barbie. The women held out and Ken got a compromise bulge, although no one would ever accuse him of holding a candle to GI Joe.

In the mid-1960s, Mattel released a "Ken a Go Go" doll, where Ken played the ukulele. Not long after that, Ken was euthanized. He reappeared in 1969 with an extreme makeover that Mattel hoped would revive his dismal sales. Then, in 1993, Mattel released the truly amazing "Earring Magic Ken." This Ken was literally swept off the shelves by a stampede of adult gay males.

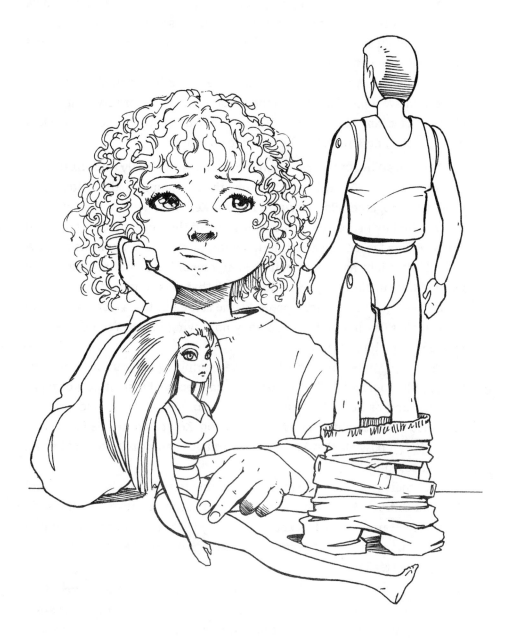

"Earring Magic Ken," also known as "Cock Ring Ken," was dressed in a lavender vest and had a necklace around his neck with a cock ring on it. The cock ring was not only the spitting image of the cock rings that men at gay male rages were wearing around their necks, but it was scaled to the exact dimensions as well. (It seems that someone in the design department at Mattel got one by the corporate brass.)

The more recent Kens have actually appeared as if they might be straight and even have a bit of a hunk factor. If Ken really is up for servicing Barbie, Mattel should consider making a Viagra Ken. That's because the average Ken has at least eight Barbies that he needs to put out for.

Ken Turned 50 in 2011—Rose from the Ashes, And Finally Had His Day

At the 2004 Toy Fair, Mattel executives announced that after forty-three years together, Barbie was dumping Ken. Poor Ken: Mattel put him into assisted living. Mattel was pushing one of their newer boytoys named Blaine. Blaine looked like a Southern California mall-rat druggie. As for how well Blaine might have been equipped, in one of his earlier packagings he was holding an electric guitar with a neck that was so long it was at least the equivalent of a nine-inch penis. Blaine came out like a lion, racking up respectable sales, but he had absolutely no staying power. You will be hard pressed to find him anymore.

By 2007, Mattel announced they were bringing Ken out of retirement. What with Viagra and all... The new Ken had received a great deal of reparative therapy, as he had a radical new hairdo, a more manly face, and he screamed "I'm straight." But as of early 2009, Ken could not be found anywhere. Was it possible that Ken had a reparative-therapy relapse, and he and Blaine hooked-up?

But then came 2010. There was the Barbie Harley-Davidson Barbie and Ken Doll Gift Set. And then came Ken's greatest moment in his almost 50 years as he starred in the blockbuster film Toy Story 3. While he didn't put to rest any rumors about his sexual orientation, Ken was the Toy Story 3 dark horse scene stealer.

Note: Just as Barbie's boys have been seriously fey, their accessories have often been quite phallic. Ken's cookout set has a long fork that is skewering a big pink weenie, his hunting outfit has a massive rifle, and his baseball outfit includes a really long bat.

Mattel Misses the Muslim Market, But Nails India

With the highly successful release of Fulla, a Middle East knockoff of Barbie, it's clear that Mattel missed what could have been a lucrative opportunity in the Muslim world. Fulla is a fine Muslim doll of Barbie proportions who comes in a bright pink box with her own prayer mat and a black abaya and headscarf. Fulla is selling like gangbusters in the Middle East.

We at Goofy Foot Press are the proud owners of a *Barbie in India* doll. The Indian Barbie comes wearing a colorful saree and ethnic jewelry. Better yet, she has a bindi, which is the traditional red spot between her eyes. We haven't undressed her to see if she might have a bindi between her gravity-defying breasts as well, but we're sure millions of Indian kids have.

Parents & Barbie

What follows is the ultimate discussion of Barbie by the parents of a young girl. It is from Margaret Atwood's piece *The Female Body:*

He said, I won't have one of those things around the house. It gives a young girl a false notion of beauty, not to mention anatomy. If a real woman was built like that, she'd fall flat on her face.

She said, If we don't let her have one like all the other girls she'll feel singled out. It'll become an issue. She'll long for one and she'll long to turn into one. Repression breeds sublimation. You know that.

He said, It's not just the pointy plastic tits, it's the wardrobes. The wardrobes and that stupid male doll, what's his name, the one with the underwear glued on.

She said, Better to get it over with when she's young.

He said, All right, but don't let me see it.

She came whizzing down the stairs, thrown like a dart. She was stark naked. Her hair had been chopped off, her head was turned back to front, she was missing some toes, and she'd been tattooed all over her body with purple ink, in a scrollwork design. She hit the potted azalea, trembled there for a moment like a botched angel, and fell.

He said, I guess we're safe.

2015 Update: Barbie Sales Go Flat!

The CEO of Mattel was recently canned following a three-year slump in Barbie sales. A Barbie doll is still sold every three seconds, so it's not like she's riding off into obscurity. But Barbie's main demographic is now 3- to 6-year old girls. It used to be 3- to 9-year olds.

Mattel is considering ways to refresh the Barbie line to make her more contemporary. A twerking Barbie? A porn-star Barbie? Hopefully these are out of the question.

Reader's Comments

"Ways Barbie impacted my femininity? She made me hate clothes."

female age 21

"Ways Barbie impacted my femininity? I dress better now."

female age 20

"My sister and I were a little obsessed with Barbie. We turned old dressers and coffee tables into Barbie mansions. I played with Barbie from the time I was 4 until I was 11 or 12. I'm not sure when Barbie and Ken started having sex (they weren't just sleeping in the same bed), maybe when I was 7, that's when I learned what intercourse involved. Mostly, I got the dolls undressed, put them in bed and twisted their bodies back and forth. They couldn't really do anything since Barbie didn't have a vagina and Ken didn't have a penis. However, once Barbie and Ken started having sex, they never stopped. Every night. That's how I thought it was done, only at night, only in bed. Several Barbies went through a sex change. I got her ready for the operation (remember Dr. Barbie?), wheeled her into the operating room, and when she came out, she'd been replaced with a Ken doll. All of Barbie's friends talked about her behind her back when she got the change–her mother (grandma Barbie) had a hard time coping. I'm being glib, but I did act all of this out. My Barbies had detailed conversations, had intimate family lives, detailed jobs, etc. There was a lot of adultery in Barbie's world which resulted in divorces, private investigators, and alcoholism. All the adultery was acted out in full detail, from Ken coming on to his secretary at work to the act itself to Barbie throwing all of Ken's clothes out the window... Barbie helped me act out my own questions about being an adult. I'm a feminist now, I have a healthy relationship, earn more than my spouse, don't wear make-up or high-heeled shoes, and my husband helps with all the housework. It's okay to let little girls play with Barbie." *female age 24*

"Ways Barbie impacted your femininity and/or sexuality: There was one summer when I was fairly obsessed with the fact that Ken had no dick. Beach Ken had a totally inaccurately placed suggestion of one, but no balls." *female age 21*

"My cousin and I were addicted to our Barbies, from as early as I can remember. I think I was 7 or 8 when our Barbies started having all sorts of high-drama romances, and there were ALL SORTS of different sexual experiences going on. My cousin and I were very creative with our Barbies' sexual escapades. I remember mine even having some homosexual experiences, which my cousin thought was weird. I actually think that my Barbies were a big outlet for my sexual curiosity growing up. When I was a teenager and no longer played with Barbies, I wondered if maybe it was odd that I made my Barbies have all sorts of sexual experiences when I was so young. But as I've gotten older, I've realized that sexually, I'm a very open and curious person, and I think it's just that I've always been that way. When I played with Barbies with my cousin though, I almost always had to play Ken. I find myself now very comfortable filling a lot of traditionally masculine roles in my relationships. The two may or may not be related." *female age 22*

"Ugh, as much as I hate to admit it, yes, my Barbies had sex. And since I also had a twelve-inch Luke Skywalker doll, they did it A LOT. I also played with a girlfriend at the time. We did sex play with our dolls." *female age 34*

Excellent Resources: This discussion of Barbie has provided only a small sketch of the truly rich and fascinating history of this cultural icon. If it has piqued your interest, you are strongly encouraged to check out at least two excellent books on the subject. One is M.G. Lord's *Forever Barbie—The Unauthorized Biography of a Real Doll,* Avon Books. One of Lord's many fine observations can be found in her discussion of Barbie's friend, Midge: "If plastic dolls could kill themselves, I'm sure Midge would have tried." Talk about having to spend your entire life playing second fiddle!

Regarding the second highly recommended book, *Face of the American Dream, Barbie Doll (1959-1971)* by Christopher Varaste, Hobby House Press, who knew that photos of the early Barbie could be so fascinating and compelling? Barbie's face and expression during this period was much more interesting than now, and Varaste does an exceptional job of capturing it.

The references for the Margaret Atwood quote: *The Female Body* by Margaret Atwood, originally printed in Vol. XXIX, No. 4, Fall 1990 issue of *Michigan Quarterly Review,* edited by Laurence Goldstein.

68
The Historical
Breast & Bra

An early reader of this chapter said, "I'd rather be flogged with my Wonderbra than do a boring chapter on bras and breasts. I'm going straight to Chapter 19 where I can learn how to give a better blowjob." Imagine that, a woman who takes her Wonderbra for granted! Before the 1920s, women were skeptical about bras. They preferred to wear corsets. As for bras being thought of as cute or sexy, that wouldn't happen until World War II.

There's hardly a woman in Western culture who doesn't have at least a couple of bras, including a favorite one or two for when she wants to feel extra sexy. She can also make a sexual statement by not wearing a bra. And what teenage boy doesn't equate success in dating with whether a girl let him put his hand under her bra?

This chapter looks at breasts and the bras that hold them up. It begins with a peek at breasts in different times and different places. It then focuses on the fascinating evolution of the bra: how it came to be in 1860, and how it eventually came to have a sexual edge.

The Ups and Downs of the French Breast

In the time of Renaissance France, it was believed that breast milk was made from blood that flowed from the vagina. This notion was handed down from the ancient Greeks, with Leonardo DiVinci eventually making a diagram of it (as shown on the following page by our own Daerick DiVinci). Since it was assumed that breast milk rose up from the vagina, intercourse was thought to curdle the breast-milk supply. Women who were nursing babies were not to have intercourse. Perhaps the French believed that a penis going in and out of a vagina was like a paddle churning buttermilk.

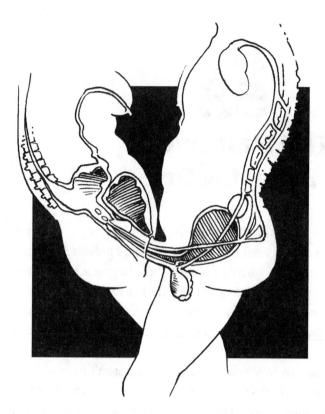

Our version of a Leonardo DiVinci drawing that was based on the belief that breast milk was made from blood that flowed from the vagina.

Given that upper-class French women would rather have sex than nurse babies, the nursing job was pawned off on the women of the lower class. This caused there to be a distinction between the breasts of the lower class and those of the upper class. Breasts of the lower class were expected to be large and lactating, while upper-class breasts were expected to be small and perky. (They must have assumed that poor women didn't like sex, so their supply of milk was safe.)

Before the revolution, women used the same kind of makeup on their breasts as they used on their faces. The goal was to make their breasts look exceptionally white. Older women would paint blue veins on their breasts to make them look like the more transparent skin of the younger girls. Unfortunately, the makeup they used on their faces and breasts was a compound that contained lead. Not only did it corrode the skin but it contributed to lead poisoning. Not to be outdone by their sisters from the past, today's runway models sometimes paint nail polish on their erect nipples as a way of keeping them erect.

In time and with the coming of the French Revolution, the heads of many upper-class French women became separated from their breasts. Eventually it became not only fashionable but a sign of patriotism for all French women to nurse their babies.

Saggy and Happy in Papua

In Papua, New Guinea, grown women parade their saggy breasts with pride. It's considered a sign of childishness or immaturity for a woman in Papua to have the kind of breasts that Americans value. In fact, when ladies in Papua are getting catty, they might accuse someone of having the taut round breasts of a younger woman.

To the traditional Papuan male, the surgically stuffed breasts of American actresses would be a big waste of time and money. And the traditional Papuan woman would think to herself, "Why would a woman want to do something crazy like that to her breasts just when they were starting to sag?"

In our culture, breasts have often been regarded as the crown jewels of feminine appeal. For whatever reason, American breasts are covered in public. But in Africa and the South Pacific, women have walked around for centuries with their breasts bare. The men in those cultures don't get much of a rise from women's breasts. Instead, it's the parts that are covered up, namely the buttocks, that the men tend to find erotic.

Imagine what a dent it would have put in the lingerie, porn and plastic-surgery businesses if women in America were always topless and breasts weren't considered sexy? The entire *Playboy* empire would have never been, and Victoria's Secret would have started with thongs instead of bras.

War Bonds and Liberty's Breasts

To see how breasts were starting to be sexualized in America, consider World War I "Liberty Bonds" posters featuring Lady Liberty.

In the first poster, Liberty is a sturdy woman with the sexual appeal of a truck driver. The only way you can tell she is a woman is by the endless yards of drapes that are covering every inch of her body except for her manly, muscled arms and her stern, angular face. After the release of this poster, bond sales continued to sag.

Months later, the next poster was released. Liberty had become less manly and she was even a bit sensual. A year later, by the time the fifth "Buy Bonds" poster was out, Liberty was quite feminine and scantily clad. She

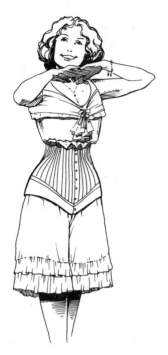

The corset has a rich and interesting history. Contrary to what you often hear, very few women who wore corsets did a practice known as "tight-lacing." Tight-lacing is a fetish where the person wearing the corset laces it up so tight that his or her waist becomes unnaturally small. Many women in the early 1900s were hesitant to give up wearing corsets. Switching to a bra or "bosom supporter" might have been like a woman today going from panties to a thong.

looked like she had been dressed by the people at Trashy Lingerie instead of being outfitted in a drapery shop. While her breasts were by no means large, they were taut and had an erotic edge. You actually had to look twice to see if any material from her nearly see-through gown was covering them. By the end of World War I, Uncle Sam was learning what it takes to sell bonds.

Twenty years later, during the second World War, American soldiers consumed six million copies of *Esquire Magazine*. Perhaps this is because it showcased Vargas girls with their massive, gravity-defying bosoms. It was during World War II that pinup girls became famous. The women who prepared the pinup models for the photography shoots would stuff the models' bras with layer after layer of felt pads. They felt this would help lift the soldiers' morale, among other things.

Birth of the Bra

For several centuries, the corset was the undergarment that supported the weight of women's breasts. The first brassiere wasn't patented until the time of the Civil War and it didn't appear in the marketplace until the late 1800s. It would be another twenty years after the end of the century before the brassiere would win widespread acceptance among American women. Several elements needed to converge for the bra to knock out the corset.

According to Jane Farrell-Beck and Colleen Gau in their excellent book *Uplift—The Bra in America,* here are some of the changes that needed to occur in women's lives for the bra to become popular:

A large increase in the number of women involved in physical activities such as bicycle riding, golf, tennis, and swimming. It is difficult to do these things while wearing a corset.

A major increase in the number of women in the workforce. For instance, there were virtually no female telephone operators in the 1880s. By the 1920s, with the explosion of telephones, there were huge numbers of female operators. These operators needed to reach across large switchboards to plug in cords to complete each call. This would have been difficult to do while wearing a corset with bones sewn into it.

The materials and design of the bra had to improve. Bras needed to fit better, have adjustable straps, be able to fasten easily, and they needed to have soft cups with underwiring to help lift and separate the breasts. The latter, when first introduced in 1910 by brassiere visionary Madeleine Gabeau, seriously clashed with the monobosom or monobreast look of the day. The monobosom look made women appear as though they had no defined breasts or cleavage. It was the bodice equivalent of wrap-around sunglasses. Needless to say, there needed to be significant changes in women's fashion for the bra to nose out the corset.

Women would need to start wearing ready-made clothing rather than having clothes custom made, and the price of the bra had to come down to fit the budget of the "new" working woman.

A further stumbling block to acceptance of the bra was the lack of a universal sizing code. It wasn't until 1933 that a bra manufacturer proposed sizing bras according to cup sizes A, B, C and D.

World War II—Bad for Adolf, a Boon for the Bra

Before World War II, many American women had never worn pants. But once women began manning America's War Machine, pants are what they wore. Most women were not prepared for this. Articles began appearing in women's magazines giving tips and suggestions for how to wear pants. With the changes brought about by World War II, American women weren't just wearing pants and bras, they were punishing them.

This is the first time in history that welders, riveters, and ship builders wore bras, or admitted to it anyway. Bra design needed to seriously evolve to accommodate the range of motion of the new female workforce. Yet the supply of bra-making materials such as rubber, cotton, metal, and rayon was now rationed and in short supply.

It required 1,000 pounds of rubber to build an airplane, 1,750 pounds of rubber to build a tank, and 150,000 pounds of rubber to build a battleship. Yet America's main supply for rubber had been through Asia—a trade route that evaporated with the beginning of hostilities. Without rubber there was little elastic with which to make bras. It was not easy for bra manufacturers to make it through the war!

Not only were bras keeping Rosie the Riveter's breasts from flopping, one bra manufacturer was given a secret contract by the government to produce special vests that carrier pigeons could wear. The vests, which employed much of Maidenform's bra technology, allowed paratroopers to parachute while holding carrier pigeons. The pigeons were used for communications when radio silence was essential, such as right before D-Day. Along with making pants a part of women's wardrobes, World War II also gave the bra, with its increasingly pointed cups, a new name: the Torpedo.

Foundations Start to Shake & Bras Become Sexy

By the end of World War II, actresses started sprouting seriously pointed breasts. It was as if the sultry Vargas Girl drawings were suddenly hopping off the pages of *Esquire* and coming to life. Books like *Peyton Place* were bringing small-town sleaze into the public eye, and the Kinsey reports on the sexuality of Americans shocked and intrigued the masses. Sex was in the air!

Shortly after World War II, the Sweater Girl started to appear. When viewed from the side, Sweater Girl actress Lana Turner's breasts came out at a 90 degree angle. This was achieved by a bra which was the latex equivalent of the Golden Gate Bridge. A similar two-cupped engineering marvel called the "Bullet Bra" sold in the millions.

1947 was the year when Frederick Mellinger opened the first Frederick's of Hollywood. Millions of Americans were seeing his sexy magazine ads and receiving his Frederick's catalogue. Frederick's teased and titillated customers with their Peek-A-Boo brassiere and half-moon stick-on brassiere.

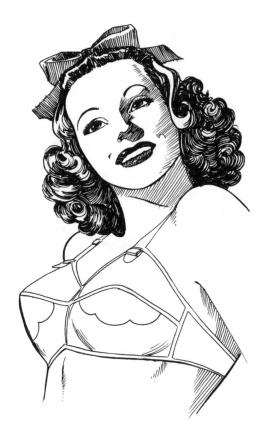

This is our illustrator's interpretation of a 1950s bra ad. The ad copy read:

"Perma•Lift, the lift that never lets you down! New, exciting, exquisite. Secretly processed Perma•Lift cushioned insets. Achieve the permanent uplift."

Sounds like an ad for car tires!

By 1949, Maidenform had begun its Dream campaign, which showed women wearing bras and flowing skirts saying things like, "I dreamed I danced all night in my Maidenform Bra" or "I dreamed I won the election in my Maidenform Bra." One of the Maidenform ads from 1962 showed a sexy young woman wearing only a bra with a bare midriff, a long tight skirt, and elbow-length gloves. She was standing next to a large bull with one hand sensuously stroking one of the bull's big horns. The caption read, "I dreamed I took the bull by the horns in my Maidenform Bra." Only a blind person would have missed the sexual innuendo of the ad. Many of today's feminists would have concerns about this notion, saying that it implied women's power was dependent on their sexuality or sexual allure. Nonetheless, like their gutsy mothers who built our planes and tanks in World War II, women in the 1960s, with their Maidenform bras were a force to be reckoned with.

The 1950s also gave birth to the inflatable bra, which gave a woman the option of pulling a tube out of each breast cup and filling it up to the desired

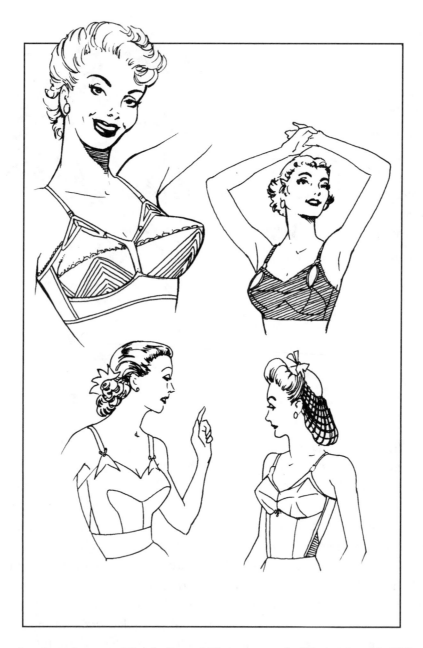

Our drawing of a 1950s WonderBra ad. The copy reads: "She's Adorable," "She's Bewitching," "She's Delightfully Deceiving," "She's Exclusively Elegant." With the way the ad is written, it is hard to tell if it is referring to the women, their breasts or their bras. Seems that if you bought the bra, you got it all!

level of allure. This was also helpful if the woman was flying in a plane and it went down over the ocean.

In 1970, Victoria's Secret emerged to grab the sexy-bra baton from Frederick's of Hollywood. Frederick's had acquired a sleazy edge, while Victoria's Secret screamed "classy and elegant." Victoria's Secret suddenly worked its way under women's blouses and into their pants. American women no longer needed to blush or make excuses to enter a Victoria's Secret as they had in the later Frederick's years. And if the thousand-or-so Victoria's Secret stores weren't enough, millions upon millions of Victoria's Secret catalogues have been read by American women and men from coast to coast. Unfortunately, there has been a price to be paid for the new elegance and sexual allure—a bra from Victoria's Secret often costs two or three times as much as a similar design from Sears or Target.

The bra is the final outpost that separates the outside world from the sensuous breast. Because of what it covers, the bra has achieved a kind of fetish quality for both men and women. That fetish quality has reached new heights in the last few decades when rock icons like Madonna started wearing designer underwear on the outside rather than on the inside. Foundations were shifting once more.

Crossing Your Heart from 1920 to Today

Bra and breast fashion has yo-yo'ed over the years, going from boy-like breasts to the Torpedo, and back again. In the 1920s, the flat-chested look was in fashion. By the 1930s, the full-busted look was back. By the 1940s, women started calling the brassiere a "bra." Bras and panties were populating underwear drawers nationwide.

During the first wave of 1960s feminism, the popular saying *Burn Your Bra* came into being, as if bras were a ball and chain placed on women's chests by male jailers. Yet women hold almost half of the bra patents that have been awarded, and women have owned a number of bra-manufacturing plants. There's never been a glass ceiling holding women back from the higher ranks of corporate bradom.

Far from holding women back, the bra was designed to hold parts of them up. It was made to help women deal with the discomforting pull of gravity. Of course, considering that breasts weigh from eight ounces to ten pounds, gravity has meant different things to different women.

Since the 1970s, some women have been trading in their natural breasts for surgically-enhanced models where the Torpedo Bra of the 1940s seems to be sewn into their chests.

The First Falsies

In case you think that insecurity about the size of body parts is a newly-acquired disease in America, some of the first falsies could be ordered through the Sears Catalogue in the late 1890s. They were called "bust pads" and were described as helping to "plump up the bosom." The same Sears, Roebuck & Co. catalogue with the bust pads also sold "The Princess Bust Developer, a New Scientific Help To Nature, If Nature Has Not Favored You." The Princess Bust Developer promised to enlarge and shape the bosom. It included a cream that was called "Bust Cream or Food, Unrivaled for Enlargement of the Bust," and a pump that looked like a toilet plunger. This sort of thing is still being advertised in magazines and on late-night TV!

For those of you who think that body-part insecurity only belonged to women, dozens of ads from the *Police Gazette* in the 1890s promised solutions for enlarging the penis.

No Room for Misfits

It is estimated that 80% of women aren't wearing the right bra. It's not like they accidently put on someone else's bra, but they might as well have. It takes a real effort to get the right bra size. Bra cup sizes can range from A to H, with stops in between at B, C, D, DD, E, F, FF, G and GG. There are also a large number of options for rib cage and back sizes.

If you compare the chests of two women who wear 36-C bras, their breasts can be shaped very differently. One woman's breasts might be shaped like eggplants, another's like cones.

Many women ignore that their breasts change size and shape over time. Just because you were a 36-B two years ago doesn't mean you are a 36-B today. Some breasts undergo significant changes in tenderness and size during the menstrual cycle. A bra that might have been just fine on day one might be uncomfortable on day 27. Also keep in mind that your breast size can increase if you go on the birth-control pill, and might decrease if you go off of it.

Bra shopping is not the sort of thing you should do by mail order, and you would be well-served to seek out a lingerie shop where the sales help has been fitting bras since the beginning of time. Avoid the sales clerk who is chewing gum and hasn't finished high school. Also avoid bras where there are bulges in the armpits or if the bra makes your breasts go out to the side. Your breasts shouldn't bulge along the top of the cups. And keep in mind that one company's 40-DD might be another company's 38-E.

Not only do you want a bra that fits and feels great through a full range of body motions, but you want one that holds up to repeated washings. It needs to support you in a way that keeps the ligaments in your breasts from stretching. Otherwise, there's not much point in wearing one.

Purchasing a bra isn't something a woman should do on the fly, and she shouldn't try to do it with two small children in tow. A caring partner will make sure that a woman has plenty of time to try on every bra in the store if she needs to.

Whether breasts are large or small, they are attached to the chest by suspensory ligaments. These ligaments are not elastic. Once they stretch they don't snap back. In her *Breast Book*, Dr. Miriam Stoppard recommends that young girls be given good supporting bras to wear, and that a woman should not go braless for long if she does not want her breasts to sag. (This would be a hard sell in places like Papua.)

NOTE: A Consumer Reports test compared a $127 LaPerla Vintage bra, a $45 Victoria's Secret Ipex demi bra, and a $11 Gilligan & O'Malley padded demi bra from Target. Of the three, the $11 bra from Target had better cup molding, more comfortable underwiring, fit well and held up better after three washings.

Highest Recommendation You will be hard-pressed to find a more interesting book on the bra than *Uplift–The Bra in America* by Jane Farrell-Beck and Colleen Gau, University of Pennsylvania Press. This book is the kind of marvel that should be—but seldom is—the staple of America's university presses. It is better researched than most of the other books on women's foundations, but it doesn't insult the reader with poor editing or incomprehensible sentences. In addition to exploring changes in fashion, *Uplift* shows the evolution of the bra within different social and economic contexts. If you want a good read about a fascinating subject, *Uplift* is a great choice.

If you are interested in more about corsets, consider the highly intelligent writings of Valerie Steele. Ms. Steele has managed to anger male corset enthusiasts because she calls their practice of wearing women's corsets a fetish. (Where would she ever get a silly idea like that?) Men who are strapping themselves into women's corsets are concerned that Ms. Steele is giving them an undeserved stigma. She's also managed to anger some academic feminists, because she has discussed how wearing corsets has had erotic associations and how the dangers have been blown out of proportion. They see her as being an apologist for the "corset torture" of women.

69

Men's Underwear
The Fruit of His Loom

What would you think if a guy phoned his partner and said, "God, honey, I start to get hard when I think about the new briefs I'm wearing." Contrast this with a woman who calls her partner and says, "God, honey, my nipples start to get hard when I think about the new bra and panties that I'm wearing."

In our culture, it's cool for a girl to get excited about her lingerie, but we would consider a man who talked this way about his own briefs to be strange. Then again, if he just spent $20 for a single pair of tightie-whities with a big name on the waistband, hopefully they would give him a rise.

Calvin Klein—The Pricey Jockey[1] in Your Underwear Drawer

In the early 1980s, manufacturers like Calvin Klein teamed up with famed homoerotic photographers like Bruce Weber to help make men look sexy in their traditional white briefs. Mind you, the men they used in their photo shoots would have looked sexy wearing a loincloth made of cornhusks. Some people might say the real emphasis of these ads boiled down to the bulge in the crotch—with all visual roads in those huge billboard ads drawing your eye to the package behind the fly. (See the illustration that follows.)

The Calvin ads had two primary targets: gay men and straight women who buy underwear for their husbands and boyfriends. Nail these two groups, and straight guys are putty in the corporate hand.

In these underwear ads, the hazy image of a penis behind the fly was sexier than if the guy had been naked or if his penis had been hanging out. With his penis behind a white cotton veil, the model was able to give attitude in a way that a man who is buck naked can't. The combination of atti-

---

[1]We think of the "jock" in *jock strap* as referring to athletes. But it comes from "bicycle jockeys" who the supporters were invented for in 1874 by the Bike Web Company. Bicycle jockeys were bike-riding messenger boys who rode over the cobblestone streets of Boston. The cobblestones made their testicles jiggle furiously.

tude and mystery about what's inside the briefs was fuel for many a fantasy. So while all roads led to the bulge in the briefs, it wouldn't have worked if the briefs had been pulled down to the hunk's knees. Women were being exposed to the same kind of "babe-in-a-lacy-bra" eye candy that's stimulated men over the ages, only with an urban contemporary edge.

Subliminal Messages?

Wouldn't it be something if a woman could buy a pair of Calvin briefs for her man and have him suddenly look like the models in the Calvin ads? And wouldn't it be amazing if a man could slip on his Calvin briefs and suddenly feel like the Calvin-Klein-version of the Marlboro Man, minus the horse and the lung cancer?

But the reality is, if one of the models in the early Calvin ads had walked into a room full of straight women, he would have had no trouble finding a place to spend the night, even if his day job had been collecting trash and he was wearing $2 briefs from Walmart.

Contemporary Girl Underwear—Finally, a Fly for Your Clitoris!

There have been a few interesting changes in the underwear scene in the past few decades. For one, manufacturers have started making men's underwear for women. This has been perceived as massively cool. The boy brief as worn by women even has a fly or the suggestion of a fly in the front.

If you are in gender studies, you might assume that girls enjoy wearing boy briefs because it's a girl's way of taking the patriarchy's penis and making it her own. Wearing boy briefs with a fly in the front makes the message even clearer. It also helps with pantylines.

But something more practical is involved. Women in our culture receive far more encouragement to explore and experiment with fashion than men do. For many women, fashion is a great adventure, and they have adopted zillions of styles throughout the ages—some were simply hideous, others were elegant. Few of these had anything to do with trying to assume dimensions of masculinity. Quite to the contrary, much of women's fashion is designed to win the awe and delight of a girl's female friends.

The road to making men's underwear cool for women to wear was much different from what it took to make women's underwear (bikinis and thongs) safe for men to wear.

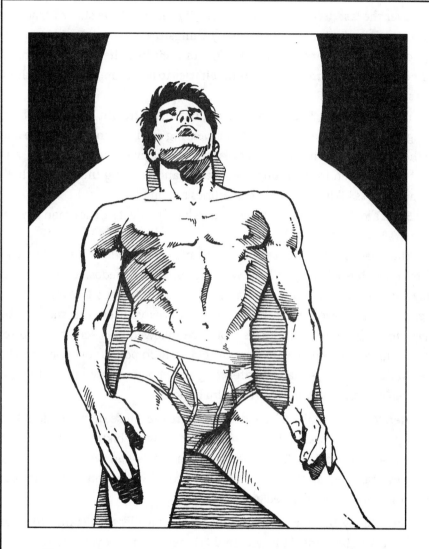

Calvin Klein Underwear

Men with Bikini Briefs, Trimmed Pubes, and Waxed Backs

Over the last decade, males in university settings have started teaching courses on men's studies. Of the many things these men worry about, trying to define masculinity is near the top of their list. They often say that a defining hallmark of masculinity is that it tries to be the opposite of anything that's feminine.

Perhaps these scholars haven't noticed that straight guys have been doing a lot of girly things lately, such as wearing earrings, and having the hair on their entire upper body waxed or lasered. Some even shave their legs, and plenty have taken to trimming their pubes and wearing underwear that's like a woman's bikini bottom or sometimes a thong.

So let's look at some of the factors that have made it safe for men to wear women's bikini bottoms.

The Speedo Coefficient Generations of incredible-looking male swimmers and water-polo players have worn nothing but Speedos, which are basically G-strings on steroids.[1] Hard as you might try to keep looking straight ahead, Speedos have a built-in device that forces your eyes to stare at the guy's crotch and butt, even if this would be followed by a scream of horror if the man in the Speedo were 60 years old and 100 pounds overweight. The Speedo Coefficient has made it safer for guys who aren't swimmers to wear what have traditionally been girls' bikini bottoms.

Men-With-Pro-Balls Effect It didn't hurt the cause of the male bikini when professional male athletes were hired to wear bikini briefs in magazine ads and on posters. These half-naked athletes had women swooning, and they reassured straight men that they could wear women's bikini bottoms and not risk being called gay.

The "Honey Do" Influence A guy would have less resistance to wearing girls' bikini bottoms if his wife said, "Honey, I do think you'll look sexy in

---

[1]**Competitive Swimming's Darkest Hour:** As a spectator sport, swimming at the Olympics took it in the shorts when the traditional men's Speedos were replaced by a cross between bicycle shorts and a wetsuit. Forget steroids, the women of Goofy Foot Press want the new suits banned. Thank heavens, the men's Speedo still rules in water polo.

these." This fact wasn't lost on the underwear manufacturers, as the ads with the male athletes in their bikini briefs were clearly aimed at women.

Penis-Over-The-Top Factor The transition to bikini underwear for men has had a good deal of practical significance. That's because when men pee, a lot of us don't pull our penis through the fly in the front of briefs or boxers. Instead, we yank the elastic waistband down and pull the penis over the top. So the fly is totally useless for a lot of men. Having the lower waistband of bikini briefs makes the process of peeing easier.

Briefs and Bras in Perspective

Publications in gender studies tend to focus on subjects like violence, rape, and the truly awful things that some people do to others. They would consider this look at men's and women's underwear superficial. However, "superficial" means "what's on the outside." In the last two chapters, we took your blouses off and pulled your pants down.

If we had a gender studies course at Goofy Foot University (a.k.a. G F-U!), students would spend the first week playing with Barbie, GI Joe, Legos, and Matchbox Cars. They would then be asked to consider the relationships between play and gender identification. The next week, they would have the option to strip down to their underwear and free-associate about what's masculine and feminine. Hopefully, one of the women would be wearing a Granny Bra and Granny Panties.

The most important lesson, however, is that a hundred years ago, no one would have been able to predict that the bra would ever be sexy. And as little as fifty years ago, no one would have been able to predict that guys would feel manly wearing women's bikini bottoms.

Think of all the effort that went into weaving these otherwise ordinary pieces of cloth into the sexual fabric of our culture. The same can be said about many of the things we consider to be sexy today.

A Note on Different Water Cultures Most male surfers wouldn't be caught dead in Speedos. The only commonality between many male swimmers and surfers seems to be water, and the water of the former smells like chlorine while the water of the latter tastes like salt.

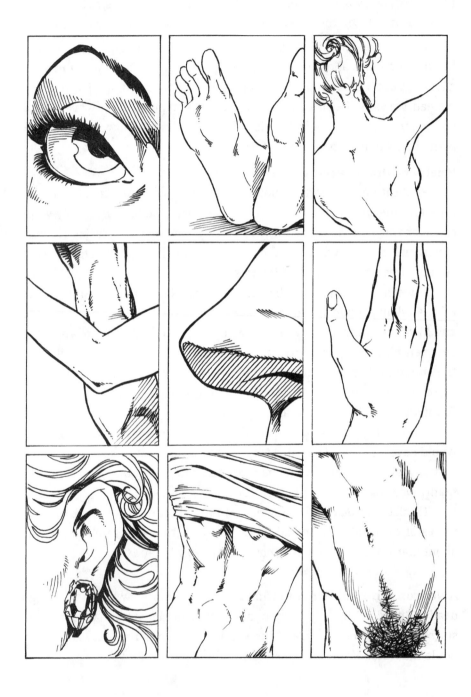

70

What's Masculine, Feminine & Erotic?

The thinking in some academic circles is that masculinity and femininity are constructed by society. Once you start chipping away at what's masculine and what's feminine in different cultures, you can't help but agree, at least a little. Men and women may arrive at sexual orientation in different ways, and our brains may process different aspects of sexuality in different ways, but culture plays a big role in determining what's masculine, feminine and erotic. This chapter takes a brief look at these matters, which can be incredibly complex.

Masculinity, Then and Now

A little more than a hundred years ago, men who didn't have much money worked in jobs that required a good deal of physical labor. Unlike today, a lean, buff man with sexy muscles did not get that way from working out at a gym. His well-defined muscles were usually the result of a low-paying job. As a result, a well-dressed man with a pot belly was a better catch for an attractive young woman in the year 1900. The big belly and nice clothes meant being able to protect your wife and children from an economy that suffered frequent and wicked downturns. They meant a woman wouldn't have to work outside the home, which was significant when the best jobs most women could get in 1900 were a domestic servant or a seamstress, working long hours at very low pay. To earn more, she might need to become a prostitute.

Have things changed just a bit? Not with the economy, but with the muscles. Nowadays, most men with buff muscles have enough leisure time to work out. A guy who has a job as computer programmer may work out at the gym in an attempt to hide the fact that his biggest physical challenge at work is opening up his laptop. And the young woman of olde who may have viewed Mr. Portly as a good catch might very well be working out at the gym today with Mr. Buff and making as much money as he is. Such an independent woman would not have been considered "feminine" just over a hundred years ago. In 1900, feigning frailty was an important element of femininity.

What Different Societies Have to Say

Each culture has its own definition of what's masculine, feminine and erotic. Here are some examples of how these definitions differ from culture to culture, year to year:

💡Women in Muslim cultures cover themselves from head to toe when appearing in public. Women in Hollywood show up wearing a few molecules of fabric, designed to tease rather than cover. The women in Hollywood claim their Muslim counterparts are sexual prisoners. The Muslim women say the real prisoners are the females in Hollywood. One female reader says that neither women are sexual prisoners, since they both use sex to control the people around them!

💡In Japan, it's a common practice for people to strip naked and bathe together. Nobody finds this kind of public nudity to be erotic or shameful, but Lord help two Japanese who kiss in public, at least until recently. In our society, it's nearly the opposite, with kissing being fine and nudity an offense.

💡Kim Edwards is a woman who taught English in a rigid Islamic country for two years and then moved to Japan. After a few years in an Islamic country, Ms. Edwards found herself at odds with her own body. When she moved to Japan, she was surprised to find herself treated as a normal person no matter what she wore. She could even bathe naked in public bathhouses, while she could have been stoned to death for doing this in an Islamic country. In Muslim countries, women are obliged to cover their bodies to live a chaste and modest life. However, within the confines of marriage, Muslim women are encouraged to enjoy their sexuality.

💡During the Summer Olympics, male gymnasts from the Russian team often celebrated good performances by kissing other male team members on the lips. Our U.S. male gymnasts wouldn't be caught dead doing that, not in public anyway.

💡In America, many straight women now wear their hair short, and many straight men wear their hair long. Sixty years ago, this meant that you were homosexual. And think of the public outcry if a 1950s professional

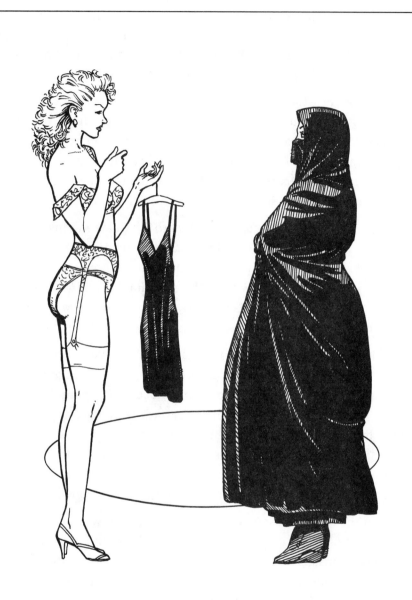

Who is the "Sexual Prisoner"?
- a. The Muslim Woman
- b. The Western Woman
- c. Neither
- d. Both

baseball player appeared in billboard ads wearing a pair of red bikini briefs; or if his 1950s beehive-coiffed girlfriend went to the grocery store wearing Doc Martens and male boxers. Or what if a straight American male wore a pierced earring before the 1980s, or trimmed or shaved his pubic hair?

💡 In America, there is nothing unusual about an unmarried 18-year-old woman having sex; but in some parts of the Middle East, India and Pakistan, such a woman risks harming the honor of her family. In rural villages, she might be murdered by her own family members in what is known as an "honor killing" to protect the family name. Fortunately, the practice is not as common as it was a few decades ago, but it still happens.

💡 Less than a decade ago, a consultant to *The Guide* was invited to India to speak on "Alternatives to Wife Burning." It seems that if a husband and his mother are unhappy with his wife, fatal "kitchen accidents" can happen with few legal consequences. What the consultant found most surprising was that it was the men at this meeting, rather than the women, who welcomed the nonviolent alternatives.

💡 In Africa, millions of women have their clitorises and inner labia crudely cut out of their bodies as children. This type of "surgery" has been considered an important passage to womanhood which many African mothers have done to their young daughters. In the West, a mother who did such a thing to her daughters would be put in prison. Of course, African women might claim that the clitoridectomy is just as cosmetic and feminine as our Western penchant for mutilating female bodies with breast implants. Who knows what an African woman might say about liposuction or labiaplasty.

💡 In the early 1800s, Americans believed that a woman's sexual pleasure was as important as men's pleasure. Then, from the late 1800s until the 1960s, it was considered unfeminine for women in our society to enjoy sex as much as men. Valuing sex became a masculine trait, and some women even believed that it was unladylike to have orgasms.

💡 In parts of the world where virginity is highly valued, family members will wait outside the newly-wed couple's door on the night of the wedding to confirm there is "blood on the sheets." The marriage can be annulled if the bride can't "prove" her virginity or if the groom fails to perform.

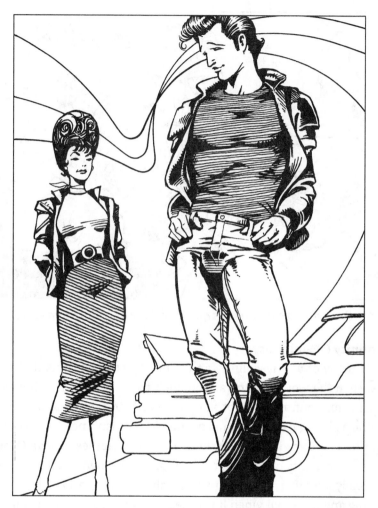

Sex roles, anyone?

💡In North America and Europe, we view a woman's sexual wetness as a good thing—the wetter, the better. Vaginal wetness is the female equivalent of an erect penis, a sign that a woman is turned on and ready to romp. But in Zimbabwe and Zaire, women traditionally worked at drying out their vaginas before a penis went in. In these countries, a wet vagina was traditionally viewed as dirty, smelly and possibly infected. It also causes embarrassing sounds during intercourse and risks being seen as a sign of infidelity. Here we use one of many brands of sex lube if a vagina isn't wet enough.

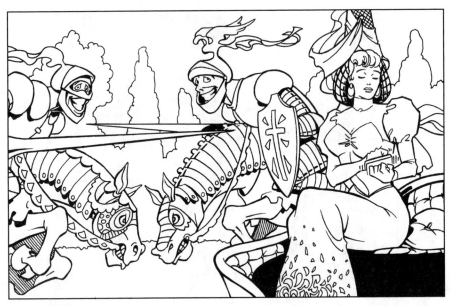

Are these sex-role differences due to biology or culture and custom?

Masculinity & Femininity

For many of us, masculinity and femininity are concepts that make all the sense in the world as long as you don't try to define them. For example, people in this country think of masculine as being rough-and-tumble and feminine as being dainty and nurturing. Yet this isn't nearly as true in pre-schools that require girls to wear the same kind of clothes as boys. Once freed from wearing dainty outfits, a lot of little girls get rough-and-tumble too.

Equally puzzling are rough-and-tumble men who become extremely nurturing and maternal when it is time to feed the baby. And if you assume that women are less aggressive or are the more nurturing sex, try talking to a random group of female lawyers, advertising execs or women in enter-tainment. While hormones may have some impact in determining male and female behaviors, what we learn from culture about our respective sex roles is clearly a large force in shaping the way we behave. That's why it is hard to talk about the definitions of masculine and feminine unless we also know the particular country, culture and year.

From this Guide's perspective, any culture's definition of masculine, feminine and erotic is arbitrary, transient and often artificial. Nonetheless, people take these definitions seriously and get really bent out of shape if you ignore their local customs.

71
God & Sex

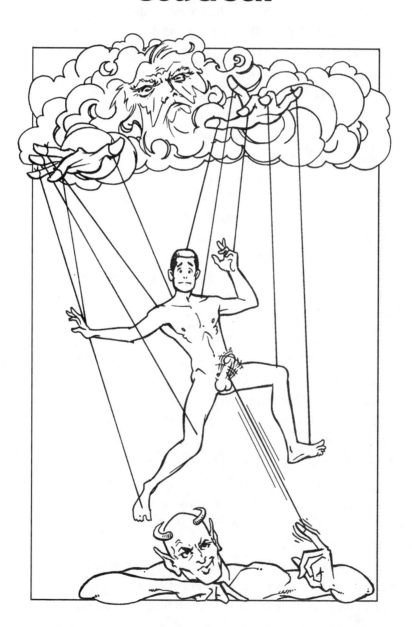

When people ask why I wrote this book on sex, I usually say it was revenge for eight years in Catholic school. But even before I went to school, I had started to appreciate the influence of religion on people's lives—both good and bad.

One of my earliest memories as a child was being at a holy-roller revival in a big tent with people waving their arms in the air and begging the Lord to save their souls. (Our family wasn't evangelical, but the baby-sitter was.) Later, as a teenager, I would revisit the revivals out of curiosity.

Revivals were like the circus. They rolled into town for a couple of days, and then rolled out in the dark of night. The county where we lived was poor, so it was interesting to see the Evangelists arrive in shiny new Cadillacs.

At what seemed like a pre-arranged moment during the revival, one of the women who had arrived in one of the new Caddys would start screaming that she'd had inoperable cancer and had been saved by Jesus. She would then crawl up the aisle to the collection basket, waving serious amounts of cash as she wept and wailed. Sometimes the preacher would lay his hands on her and she would faint, other times not. On the second night of the revival, at the very same moment, this same woman would be wearing a different colored wig and would scream that the Lord had saved her from the ravages of alcoholism and sexual excess. Again, with big bills in each hand. Many in the audience followed, admitting to their own transgressions of the flesh, and asking that Satan be cast from their souls.

The most important thing that I learned at the revivals wasn't that they were well-planned and well-orchestrated. Rather, it was their impact on the people who went to them. Even to my young self, I could see how these events put hope into the lives of people who didn't have much. It's where they went to confess and be saved, until the next time.

Maybe that's why people would show up at those revival tents and wave their arms in the air and not notice that the woman who started the parade of bill-waving sinners was a ringer from the bank of the preacher. I didn't know then—and I still don't know—if that was such a bad thing. It's hard for any of us to live our lives without hope.

As for my own personal experience with religion and hope, there was a radio evangelist by the name of Brother Popoff who I sometimes listened to on the all-night radio station that beamed up from Mexico. He was on after

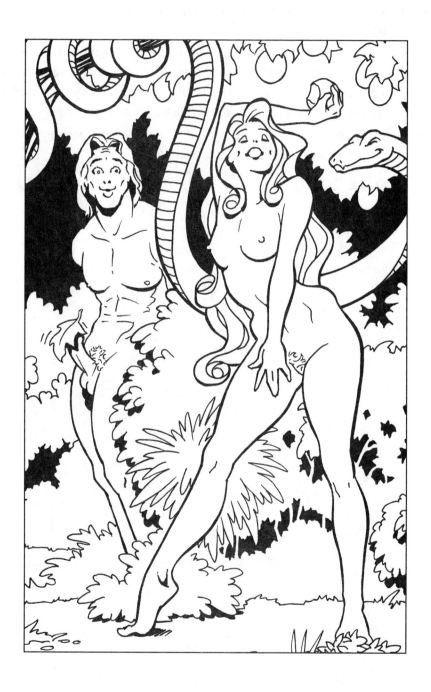

The Wolfman. If you sent him money, he promised to send you a special prayer cloth. So I taped some dimes and quarters to a card, and sent him what I had.

A few weeks later, a piece of red cloth arrived in the mail. It was about one-foot square, with no seams on the sides. The accompanying note said for me to lay it over anything that was troubling me. So I went to bed every night with that red prayer cloth tucked inside the front of my briefs.

I never did see much of a dividend, but then again, not too many people go on to write books on sex that are 1,152 pages long.

72
Sex in the 1800s

What? The longest chapter in Goofy Foot history is on sex in the 1800s? Perhaps that is because sex in the 1800s was fascinating. So fascinating that the authors of America's definitive text on sexual health included this chapter in their four-volume set.

So if you bought *The Guide* to learn how to give better oral sex, you might want to turn to the first half of this book. But if you want to see how Americans enjoyed sex during our nation's own adolescence, you've struck it rich.

In the pages that follow, you will discover how prostitution was a vital part of American culture long before men and women started dating. Time and technology would need to intervene for dating to evolve.

If you had been a young man in the 1800s, you might have had sex with prostitutes on a weekly basis. And unlike today's teenager who works at the mall or at Burger King, if you were a 16-year-old working-class girl in the 1800s, you most likely would have been a maid or seamstress who worked 60 hours a week for pennies a day, or you may have turned tricks in a brothel.

In this chapter, you will also learn about the birth of pornography as we know it today, about condoms that only covered the head of a man's penis, and about oral sex in the century of the Civil War.

Best of all, learning about sex in the 1800s will help you have a better perspective on sex today, and that is one of the things this book is about.

Many of the facts and perspectives used in the pages that follow are from the authors listed below. Without their efforts, we would know little about the incredible richness of America's sexual landscape in the 1800s:

Helen Lefkowitz Horowitz, Timothy Gilfoyle, Elizabeth Haven Hawley, Janet Farrel Brodie, Andrea Tone, Al Rose, James Morone, Sharon Ullman, Alecia Long, David Nasaw, Lewis Erenberg, George Chauncey, Alan Brandt, Anne Seagraves, Ruth Rosen, John & Robin Haller, Karen Lystra, Thomas Lowry Patricia Cohen, John Donald Gustav-Wrathall, Mark Carnes, William Cohen, Elizabeth Reis, Jan MacKell, Anne Butler, James Kincaid and Angus Maclaren.

Bicycle Seats or Live Sex Shows?

There are all kinds of ways to learn about sex, from downloading porn to taking your clothes off with someone you love. Each lights up a different part of your brain and feeds a different part of your curiosity.

Of all the ways to learn about sex, the chances are excellent you have never read about the ways our forefathers and foremothers did it in the 1800s. This chapter invites you into a lovemaking time machine. You'll get to look at how our great-great-great-grandparents got it on when they were young.

Just like today, sex in the 1800s had its contradictory ups and downs. For example, let's take a brief look at two things that you wouldn't think would be happening in the same century at the same time: live sex shows and concerns about women on bicycle seats.

Live Sex Shows: If watching live sex shows is what turns you on, it was much easier to find one in the 1800s than it is now (with "live" meaning being there in person as opposed to watching on a webcam). Consider *The Busy Fleas,* a trio of young women who made up one of New York's City's most famous live sex shows. For $5, you could stand close by and watch the three Fleas get very busy, sexually speaking. No one carded you at the door. You would watch the girls give each other oral sex, do themselves with dildos, place cigars in their vaginas and rectums, suck on each others' breasts, and lick freshly poured beer off of one anothers' vulvas while their legs were tucked behind their necks. At the show's conclusion, you might be one of the lucky audience members who would get to have sex with one of the performers while the other men in the audience watched and cheered you on. As sexually explicit as this might sound, *The Busy Fleas* sex show was tame and downright virginal when compared to the live *Sex Circus* shows at Emma Johnson's Brothel in Storyville, the legal red-light district of New Orleans.

Concerns about Women and Bicycle Seats: At the same time there were explicit live sex shows, America's professional journals were waiving flags of caution about American women who were starting to ride bicycles. A number of feminists and medical experts were concerned that the shape of the bicycle seat would leave America's women sexually aroused. They cautioned that the bicycle seat would promote "libidinousness and immorality" in the fairer sex, and that raising a leg in public to get on a bicycle might scandalize a woman of the better classes.

So how do you judge sexuality in America during the 1800s—hardcore live sex shows or concerns about bicycle seats for adult women? For that matter, how do you judge it today—abstinence-only sex education or porn-filled websites? Perhaps it's a bit of both.

"Evil Is Generally Sniffable, Don't You Think?"

Disagreements among the American people about what is and isn't sexually acceptable go back a long way. Consider the following two newspaper reviews from 1896 about a live performance that took place in one of America's popular burlesque halls. While these are reviews of the exact same performance, it would be hard to find two perspectives that differ more, down to the descriptions of the performers' legs.

"I witnessed the performance of the Barrison Sisters and never saw an exhibition in any theatre more suggestive, lewd and indecent. It was disgraceful. The whole aim of these women was to excite the base emotions of the audience. All their motions were simply vicious and libidinous. Before the curtain went up the ten legs of these Barrisons could be seen by the audience under the edge of the curtain, indecently twisting and wriggling, as they sat upon the floor. This was designed to whet the appetite of the spectators. Then they came out and turned their backs to the audience, lifting up their dresses in a vulgar and indecent manner. Their underclothes had been specially made to excite the spectators, with many parts plain to the feminine eye... A law ought to be passed putting a stop to such exhibitions, and I will make a recommendation of this kind to the Legislature this Winter." *By feminist reformer Charlotte Smith, who was no fan of the bicycle seat.*

"As Miss Lona Barrison appeared I began to sniff around for a little evil. (Evil is generally sniffable, don't you think?) Where was her beauty? That was the first question I asked myself. A complexion like boiled veal and a figure that had neither symmetry nor grace of any sort.... After she had left the stage, without any attempt on the part of the defrauded audience to cheer her by applause, she returned with the five Barrison sisters. They showed us their legs first, for they sat with them poked out under the curtain. I like a leg or two occasionally, but it must be a leg in the true sense of the word. The spindle shanks that the Barrisons betrayed were so screamingly funny and so bewilderingly emaciated that I had hard work to keep in my seat. In fact, I don't mind saying that the only things immoral about the Barrisons are their legs. They are an affront to symmetry. They should be sewn up in masses of petticoats and kept from an unfortunate public. Amputation would be justifiable.... And then the poor little Barrisons began to do what they had been taught to do for the delectation of imbeciles. They sat on the stage looking hopelessly ill at ease, and ridiculously cheap, and sang a vulgar but stupid song dealing with the physiology of generation. There was no tune to it, no metre to it, no rhythm to it, nothing latent, nothing chic, nothing clever.... The applause, like the letter, never came. Not a gleam of intelligence gleamed in their eyes. Not a wicked look was cast in any direction. Five little frumps tugging away at a cheap concert hall chason was all we saw. Such utter inanity made you feel that you might as well have left your brains at home." *By Alan Dale, a journalist and popular critic.*

While neither of these reviewers had a single kind thing to say about the performance, you would get a very different sense of sexual standards during the nineteenth century if you read only the first review and not the second.

Perhaps people in the 1800s were even more confused about sex than we are today—especially American women, given how large numbers of them were working in brothels while others were wondering what to do about bicycles. (By 1870, the second-largest industry in New York City was the selling of sex.) On the other hand, the mixed messages about sex may have seemed normal back then, just like they seem normal to us today when conservative TV networks and religious talk shows are just a click away from radio shock jocks and porn-filled websites.

Layers Upon Layers

Historians who write about sex in the 1800s sometimes present it as having different layers—with *The Busy Fleas* and concerns about girls on bikes being examples of two very different layers. Here are a few more layers that make sex in the 1800s all the more interesting:

It's difficult to know the percentage of American women who could even get on a bicycle in the 1800s when physicians were prescribing large amounts of opium and morphine for everything from headaches and depression to menstrual pain and sleepless nights. By 1872, a half million pounds of opium poppies were being legally processed in America each year, and the morphine that came from them was being used like Tylenol and Prozac are today. By 1898, a new wonder drug called heroin was being billed as a totally safe, non-addictive substitute for opium and morphine.

Narcotics were more often prescribed for women, who took them at home, while men seemed to prefer alcohol, which they consumed in more public settings like saloons and concert halls.

We know today that morphine-based drugs do a serious number on the human sex drive. We also know that between the years of 1886 and 1906 there was so much cocaine in Coca Cola that people who had a second eight-ounce glass risked a cocaine overdose. Hashish was not exactly in short supply, and amphetamines were racing their way into the drug scene. All of this while the average American man was drinking up to a half a pint of liquor daily.

So how do you discuss sex in the 1800s without taking into account how many men and women were under the influence of drugs or alcohol? We'll never have an answer, but good luck understanding sex in the 1800s without considering it. (One of the first questions a sex therapist asks a patient today is if they are taking any drugs that might be impacting their sex drive.)

And how do we handle the fact that sex-for-sale was such a central part of our culture when our country considered itself to be the home of Christian values, a fortress of fundamentalism, and site of frequent Evangelical revivals? Perhaps the drugs and alcohol helped us deal with our contradictions.

Our Sexual Desires—Shaped or Innate?

As we will see, there were many forces that shaped the sexual desires and decisions of Americans in the 1800s. Perhaps there are as many forces that are shaping our sexual desires and decisions today, but we aren't able to see them because we don't have the perspective that a hundred years can offer. We assume our sexual behaviors are determined because we are horny or in love. But what if there were other influences, such as art, religion, science, technology, fashion, television, music, birth control, the law, where you live, how much you make, what you drive, your education, your relationship with your parents, the drugs you take, whether you like your job, the cost of food, rent, and the price of gasoline?

Statistics

A writer can face no greater peril than when his readers expect sex, and he delivers statistics on population and immigration. Take comfort in knowing that sex is on the pages that follow. But first, we need to look at the population of America in the nineteenth century before we can appreciate what the population did in bed.

The Population of America's Ten Largest Cities in 1800

1. New York city, NY 60,515
2. Philadelphia city, PA 41,220
3. Baltimore city, MD 26,514
4. Boston town, MA 24,937
5. Charleston city, SC 18,824
6. Northern Liberties township, PA.. 10,718
7. Southwark district, PA 9,621
8. Salem town, MA 9,457
9. Providence town, RI 7,614
10. Norfolk borough, VA 6,926

The Population of America's Ten Largest Cities in 1900

1. New York city, NY 3,437,202
2. Chicago city, IL 1,698,575
3. Philadelphia city, PA 1,293,697
4. St. Louis city, MO 575,238
5. Boston city, MA 560,892
6. Baltimore city, MD 508,957
7. Cleveland city, OH 381,768
8. Buffalo city, NY 352,387
9. San Francisco city, CA 342,782
10. Cincinnati city, OH 325,902

It's hard to compare these two sets of figures without saying "Wow!"

In 1801, America was a small nation of 5,000,000 people. Its home was the Atlantic Seaboard. Only a few people lived west of the Alleghenies, and fewer yet had ever seen the Mississippi. Less than 10% of the population lived in cities.

By 1901, we were a nation of 77,000,000 people living in 45 states that stretched from San Francisco to New York City. Nearly 60% of us lived in cities, including millions of immigrants. Unlike our white, Protestant, old-stock settlers who arrived before 1800, English was a second language for many of our more recent immigrants.

At the start of the 1800s, America had defined herself as a small country on the edge of a boundless frontier. In 1891, the government announced that the frontier no longer existed. In less than 100 years, America had transformed from a sleepy seafaring and farming society of thirteen colonies into a major military power that produced one-third of the world's industrial output. Our rural persona was quickly becoming industrial and impersonal, especially in the North.

As we shall see, these changes resulted in a new social order that would impact our sexuality in many different ways.

Immigration & The New Sperm Glut

Today's social scientists are warning about the growing disproportion of males to females in China, where there will soon be 120 boys for every 100 girls. They worry this will cause an "inherently unstable" society with increased amounts of violence, prostitution, rape, and warlike aggression.

Imagine what these social scientists would say if they learned that between 1870 and 1910, the male-to-female ratio in some of America's largest cities may have been up to 135 males for every 100 females?

By the end of the 1800s, nearly a million immigrants were entering America every year, and most were settling in the larger cities of the North. As a result, there were almost twice as many foreign-born residents living in the big cities of the North as there were native-born citizens. The bulk of these immigrants were young, working-class males. For example, 80% of the Italians who entered the United States from 1880 to 1910 were males between the ages of 14 and 44. Our largest cities were being filled with young virile male bodies that nature programmed to ejaculate like machine guns.

Worse yet, the already high male-to-female ratio assumes that all of the potential female sperm catchers were as sexually willing as the male sperm hurlers. But think about it. Among the immigrant working class, how many Irish, Italian, German, Greek or Chinese fathers allowed their daughters to cruise big city streets that were slick with the dripping testosterone of working-class stiffs? And how many middle- and upper-class daughters of white, protestant American families during the Victorian era were willing to put out sexually for the swelling ranks of working-class males?

Good luck finding material about our cities from the 1800s that doesn't refer to them as "Satan's slums" or "infernos of vice." There are reasons for this. The demand was swelling for prostitution to flourish.

America's New Sporting Culture

Past generations of Americans who had been craftsman or farmers were suddenly living in big cities and working in large factories. Industry was becoming America's employer; cities were replacing small towns as America's bedroom. In the past, you knew who your neighbors were because you grew up with them. Now, if you were living in a large city, it was likely that your neighbor or your neighbor's parents were born in a foreign land.

A whole new "sporting culture" of young men started to emerge in America—a hard-drinking, hard-working wave of American "boyz" who craved sexual release and wild entertainment. These young men were no longer constrained by small-town mores and middle-class values. The apprenticeship system that had helped to mold young men's lives was collapsing. A factory and corporate culture had taken its place, one that provided few restraints on what a person did when not on the clock.

Men in America no longer had a desire to marry young. They were working 10 to 12 hours a day, 6 days a week. They had no traditional homes to go to. The streets, saloons and brothels became their home away from home. Whoring, gambling, fighting and public entertainment filled their free time.

The penises of millions of American men were up for grabs, and prostitution rose to meet the demand. Brothels became cheap and plentiful. They thrived in a society that believed the daughters of the better classes would face grave danger if America's men didn't have outlets to sow their seed.

Equally as important, America's economy during the 1800s was a treacherous landscape of booms and busts, pocked with financial recessions.

Brothels provided one of the few safe, high-yield investments. The rents that brothels paid were at least ten times higher than if the same building had been occupied by a home or business, and the "fees" that were collected from brothels and prostitutes kept the governments of many American towns and cities in the 1800s from going bankrupt.

A Funny Thing Happened on the Way to the 20th Century

Before 1820, when American men were often farmers, craftsmen or artisans, they worked out of their homes, and women had an important role in keeping the household together. But with the creation of factories, a number of important items like food and ready-to-wear clothes could now be bought in stores. Women were not as essential to the running of households as they had been, but it was still important for women of the working classes to contribute to the household economy.

Most of the new factory jobs needed male muscle from the working classes, and many of these jobs were dangerous. The few clerical jobs were mostly filled by males from the middle class. It wouldn't be until the early 1900s that the labor force would want large numbers of women in the form of secretaries, sales girls, clerical workers, and phone operators. As a result, the years 1840 to 1900 were often brutal for women of the working classes. The job market was so bad for these women that prostitution was often the best alternative among a small group of dismal choices.

For instance, after the Civil War, a seamstress might earn as little as 20 cents a day, with $2 to $3 a week being a good wage for a woman who was employed full time. This would hardly pay her rent. The same woman might earn more in a single night of sex work than during an entire week of domestic work. Domestic work was often unsteady, unavailable, and, according to a number of women, much harder on them than turning tricks.

Since this was the first time in our history when women needed to earn income outside of the home, there were no protections against sexual harassment. If a woman had to give in to the sexual advances of her boss to keep her domestic or seamstress job, she might as well get paid top dollar for it.

Another problem with the transition into an industrial economy was that factory jobs for men were often seasonal and lay-offs were frequent. Unemployment benefits didn't exist, and so the survival of the family would suddenly rest on a wife's ability to rustle up quick cash.

As a result, between 5% and 10% of all young women in cities like New York were probably involved in prostitution at one time or another. During harsh economic swings, the number might have been higher, and during boom times it might have been lower. (Like women today, women in the 1800s also traded sex for rent, goods and services in lieu of paying with cash. This has never been considered prostitution.)

We will talk more about prostitution later in this chapter. For now, it's important to realize there can be no discussion of sex in America during the 1800s without an awareness of how important prostitution was, both socially and economically. While prostitution is still an economic force in America today, it is not nearly as central as it was in the 1800s.

In some ways, the modern porn industry has taken prostitution's place, but it hardly holds a candle to the importance of prostitution for working class women in nineteenth-century America. Today's porn starlet has many choices for making a living besides helping men ejaculate. This is not to say the average prostitute in the 1800s would have chosen bank telling over sex work, but today's woman has a range of choices that would have made a nineteenth-century woman's jaw drop.

Honey, Who Shrunk the Family?

In 1800, a healthy, white American female had, on average, 7 children. One hundred years later, she would be having only half as many children. Among the upper and middle classes, the size of the average family would drop 50% between the years of 1800 and 1900.

There have been suggestions that the decline in family size was due to a Victorian disdain of sex. But as we look at the availability of birth control and the flow of information about sex during the 1800s, it will become obvious that this was highly unlikely.

Also, since there were no sex researchers in the 1800s to ask people what they did in bed, we can only speculate about how often couples had sex. In one of the most complete surviving diaries from the 1800s, the author put a series of Xs on the pages when she and her husband had sex. She apparently did this to help her calculate the rhythm method of birth control which was popular during the day. The frequency of her Xs throughout a marriage that lasted for several decades indicates that she had intercourse with her husband as often as married couples supposedly do today. Her writing also explained that she looked forward to having sex with her husband, and it was an important part of her married life. The love letters that were written between husbands and wives during the 1800s corroborate that physical passion was an important part of their relationships.

Abstinence Was Unnatural

There were no movies until the 1890s, and radio and TV were products of the twentieth century. Yet people in the 1800s craved information just as much as we do today. To help answer this need, public lectures became very popular, as did advice books and women's magazines.

The lectures were often about sex and birth control. This tells us that sexual enjoyment was no stranger to the masses of women and men from middle and upper classes. In the 1860s and 1870s, "Physiological Societies" sprung up where birth control and sexual knowledge were often discussed. Some of the most popular books in the 1800s were about sexual enjoyment and birth control.

One modern sociologist who has studied the availability of sex information believes that the American woman of 1860 may have known as much or more about sexuality as the American woman of 1960.

Considering all of the pamphlets, books and lectures on birth control and sexuality that were available by the middle of the 1800s, there seemed to emerge a unified voice about sexual pleasure. This voice said that sex was important to both men and women, and that abstinence and celibacy—whether you were married or not—was unnatural and bad for you.

The Cherished Victorian Sex Scandal

Even today, it is not considered proper for TV news anchors to talk about oral sex and male ejaculation. However, when an American president from the 1990s was embroiled in a sex scandal, the American people couldn't get enough of it. First-graders suddenly knew what fellatio was. A subject of frequent conversation was "that woman" and her famous blue dress.

It was no different in the 1800s, when a good scandal or trial was a cherished part of the daily headlines. America loved a sex scandal—from the 1830s murder trial of Richard Robinson, who was the moody, rich boyfriend of prostitute-victim Helen Jewett, to explicit reports from Oscar Wilde's 1895 trial in England. The more sordid the details, the better. (If comparisons to more recent American murder trials are in order, people claimed that Richard Robinson, too, had gotten away with murder.)

During the 1890s, American newspapers reported the gristly details of America's first and perhaps deadliest and most gruesome serial killer, H.H. Holmes. Medical schools had marveled at the wonderful condition of the skeletons that H.H. Holmes sold to them. These were the bones of his early victims, who he had gassed in his suburban Chicago chamber of horrors and, whose flesh he removed by hand. It was estimated that 200 men, women and children were murdered by "the archfiend" Holmes before his crimes were discovered by Frank Geyer, a Philadelphia police detective.

In addition to the reporting of the mainstream press, the 1800s had newspapers like the *Policeman's Gazette,* which was the precursor of today's popular police and crime shows. The American appetite for crime-reporting and sex scandals has always been robust. It is not a modern phenomena.

Contraception and Abortion in the 1800s

People who don't have sex don't need contraception. They don't buy contraceptives. Yet in the 1830s, America's largest newspapers had advertisements for contraceptive devices, diaphragms (womb veils), drugs to induce abortions, condoms, aphrodisiacs, and cures for sexually transmitted infections. By the 1870s, more than a third of the advertisements in America's tabloids and sporting papers were for birth control. This is not evidence of a sexually-repressive society.

But would we be able to recognize the content of these ads if we read them today? Consider the following newspaper ad from the 1800s:

Ladies. Carter's Relief for Women is safe and always reliable; better than ergot, oxide, tansy or pennyroyal pills. Insures regularity.

Today, we would assume this was to help with constipation. But after reading this ad, Americans in the 1800s weren't envisioning smoother moves in the outhouse or less time squatting over the chamber pot. They could tell the ad was for a drug that was supposed to cause an abortion, which was an acceptable form of birth control in 19th Century America. For instance, the terms "Insures regularity" and "Relief for Women" were expressions that referred to abortion. Other well-known terms for abortion included "remedy for producing the monthly flow," "ladies' relief," "cure irregularities," "ridding oneself of an obstruction," "female regulator," "female pills," "tansy regulator," "uterine regulator" or "female cure." Ads for abortion-inducing pills promised to "bring on the monthly period with regularity, no matter from what cause the obstructions may arise."

The second clue had to do with the herbs that were mentioned: "better than ergot, oxide, tansy or pennyroyal pills." These herbs were thought to induce an abortion. Abortion was legal and common in the United States until the last part of the nineteenth century. It was allowed if performed before the quickening that occurred at approximately 16 to 20 weeks after conception. Ads for abortion-inducing products sometimes contained "warnings" such as "women who are pregnant should not take them as they would surely cause a miscarriage," or "if a pregnant woman took the pills by mistake and a miscarriage resulted, it would not at all injure her health."

Women in the 1800s could also buy instruments for self-inducing an abortion. There were several different types of uterine probes (also known as "sounds") that were popular for this purpose. These instruments could easily be purchased at drug stores and through catalogues.

In addition to drugs and instruments, abortion clinics freely advertised in America's newspapers before the 1870s.

Types of Contraceptives in the 1800s

Withdrawal (Coitus Interruptus)

Withdrawal was one of the most widely practiced methods of birth control in the 1800s. There were two kinds of withdrawal: one was where the man pulled his penis out of the vagina shortly before orgasm, ejaculating outside of the woman's body. The other was partial withdrawal, where he pulled out as far as possible while still leaving the head of his penis inside the vagina when he ejaculated.

Partial withdrawal made sense in the first part of the 1800s, when two ancient theories about conception still prevailed. One was that the sperm had to be forcefully ejaculated against the cervix for conception to occur. The other was that a woman needed to have an orgasm in order to become pregnant. Partial withdrawal became less popular by the middle of the century, as the ability of sperm to swim became known.

Although withdrawal was widely practiced, some physicians and even feminists warned that it was unhealthy for males to ejaculate outside of a woman's body, as if an essential circuit was not being made, and the man's body was being unnecessarily depleted.

Douching

By the 1880s, one of the most common forms of birth control was vaginal douching. This usually happened after intercourse, but sometimes before.

Imagine what it was like for a woman in the 1800s to get out of bed on a freezing night in an unheated room to douche with cold water immediately after making love. Some of the birth control literature in the 1840s suggested that a woman could add spirits to the douche water to keep it from freezing over. Some physicians of the day—males, no doubt—recommended that douche water be as cold as possible. This echoed the Aristotelian notion that it took heat for conception to occur.

More than twenty different solutions were used as spermicides or astringents, including vinegar and bicarbonate of soda. It may have simply been coincidence, but the average pioneer family who traveled west on the Oregon Trail took eight pounds of baking soda with them.

The instructions in some of the earlier douching kits that were intended for birth control said that women should douche even if they didn't have an orgasm. This was because many people in the early part of the 1800s assumed that if a woman didn't have an orgasm, conception wouldn't occur.

Rhythm

By the mid-1800s, another "new" form of birth control became popular. It was based on the idea that there was a safe period when a woman could have intercourse without becoming pregnant. There was only one problem: modern science in the 1800s got the timing wrong. Ovulation usually occurs in the middle of a woman's cycle, and not at the start of menstruation as they thought back then.

Condoms

Condoms in the 1800s came in two styles: the full length models, like we have today, and high-water models that fit just over the head of the penis. For a long time, the caps that only covered the head were more popular than full-length condoms.

The better condoms were made from animal intestines that had been processed in lye. They were thin and strong. Large amounts of the material that they were made from, which was called Gold Beater's Skins, was imported into the United States during the 1800s. It was still being widely imported after 1873 when the Comstock laws made it illegal to import birth-control materials. Condoms made of fish skin and membranes were also available. They were considered better than those made of rubber. (The Comstock laws made it illegal to mail condoms or send information about sex or birth control anywhere in America. More on that in a bit.)

Even with vulcanization, which made rubber stretchy instead of brittle, rubber condoms were thick and inconsistent. Their only advantage was cost.

Although they were widely used, condoms were associated with prostitutes. As a result, they had a higher sleaze factor than rhythm, douching, or pills for abortion.

Diaphragms or Womb Veils

When an ad in a newspaper from the 1800s mentioned "Ladies rubber protectors" it wasn't talking about boots for rainy days. Just about any woman reading such an ad knew that it was referring to diaphragms or douching syringes that were specially made for contraception. Diaphragms were called womb veils, the French Shield for Women, and closed-ring pessaries. They became very common by the 1880s.

The diaphragm was the one contraceptive that a woman could use without her husband's knowledge. This was particularly helpful when the husband's withdrawal abilities were less than stellar, or when he didn't respect the rhythm method's black-out days. She could also use a womb veil when her husband didn't want her to use birth control.

IUDs and Nursing

During the 1800s, there were dozens of different intracervical and intrauterine devices for birth control. Many of these were popular, and women usually inserted them by themselves. It was also believed that nursing a baby kept you from getting pregnant. While nursing can be an effective form of birth control, it only works when it is done exclusively and at least every four hours. They didn't know that back then.

The Bigger Issues of Birth Control—Then vs. Now

At the beginning of the 1800s, it was beyond the consciousness of Americans to believe they could have control over any aspect of their health. Life was fragile. Even if a loved one was healthy, death could whisk him or her away at the snap of a finger. So how could you possibly control when you became pregnant? It's hard to imagine today, but accepting the idea that birth control could be a way to control pregnancy required a shift in consciousness in the early part of the 1800s.

Pregnancy had always been a concern for most women, but the option to do something about it didn't arrive in America until the 1800s. Before then, there was no difference between sex for pleasure and sex for pregnancy.

The option to use birth control was not welcomed by all. Many of the feminists during the 1800s worried that contraception would rob women of the one effective reason they had for saying no to sex—the excuse that they didn't want to become pregnant. And men in the 1800s had to digest the idea that if their wives could have sex without becoming pregnant, what would keep them faithful? What would keep their daughters chaste?

There were groups of men and women who were known as social purity crusaders. They accused women who advocated for the right to control the size of their families as being proponents of free love. Politicians accused middle- and upper-class women who used birth control of committing race suicide. Yet America's Protestant ministers—the very people who you would expect to be opposed to birth control—seldom spoke out against it.

Our concerns about birth control today are much different than they were in the 1800s. They center around cost, convenience, effectiveness and side effects as opposed to free love and suicide of the upper class.

Technology and the Presses of Satan—The Birth of Modern Pornography

The 1800s saw the birth of America's first anti-obscenity laws. Anti-obscenity laws don't just drop from the skies. There needs to be enough indecency floating around to create a fuss, and it needs to have inserted itself far enough into the mainstream to be seen by more than its intended audience. During the 1800s, these conditions were easily met and greatly exceeded.

Recently, someone tried to open a brothel in Nevada featuring male prostitutes for female customers. The other brothel owners in Nevada were upset about this, because they feared the publicity would motivate a movement to shut down all of the legal brothels in Nevada. These brothel owners were acutely aware of something that the commercial sex industry in America during the 1800s had no clue about—that vice is usually tolerated as long as the citizens are allowed to turn a blind eye to it. It seldom matters whether the sexual vice is prostitution, pornography, cross-dressing or gay sex, as long as the public isn't forced to trip over it.

Leaps in technology during the nineteenth century helped it become the temporal birthplace of pornography as we know it today.

First came the modernization of the printing press and new printing technologies. This allowed cost-effective print runs that could be tailored to fit the mass markets for mainstream porn and smaller niche markets for the kinky stuff. Then followed the technology that allowed paper to be made by machine. Before that, sheets of paper were crafted by hand. Handmade paper was often scarce and expensive.

You can't call it pornography if it isn't captured by a camera or webcam. The invention of the photograph in 1839 and the ability to mass produce it by the 1860s was what helped create the explosion of modern pornography. Next was the invention of the moving picture in 1877, and the ability to show it to large audiences in 1895.

Pornography that has survived from the 1800s is amazingly explicit and shows some of the same sexual acts that pornography does today. As for written erotica, here are just a few of hundreds of titles that were popular in the 1800s. Some of these titles were best-sellers:

Amorous Adventures of Lola Montes

Aristotle's Master-Piece (an explicit how-to)

Awful Disclosures by Maria Monk, of the Hotel Dieu Nunnery of Montreal

Confessions of a Sofa

Curiositates Eroticæ Physiologiæ; or, Tabooed Subjects Freely Treated. In Six Essays: 1. Generation. 2. Chastity and Modesty. 3. Marriage. 4. Circumcision. 5. Eunuchism. 6. Hermaphrodism, and followed by a closing Essay on Death.

Exhibition of Female Flagellants, in the Modest & Incontinent World, Proving from indubitable Facts that a number of Ladies take a secret Pleasure in whipping, and that their Passion for exercising and feeling the Pleasure of a Birch-Rod, from Objects of their Choice of both Sexes, is to the full as Predominant as that of Mankind.

Fanny Greeley: Confessions of a Free-love Sister

Marie de Clairville; or, The Confessions of a Boarding School Miss

Male Generative Organs

Physiology of the Wedding Night

Romance of Chastisement; or Revelations of the School and Bedroom. By an Expert.

Scenes in a Nunnery

Six Months in a Convent

The Amours of a Musical Student: being A Development of the Adventures and Love Intrigues of A Young Rake, with Many Beautiful Women. Also Showing The Frailties of the Fair Sex, and their Seductive Powers.

The Amours of Sainfroid and Eulalia: being the intrigues and amours of a Jesuit and a Nun; developing the Progress of Seduction of a highly educated young lady, who became, by the foulest Sophistry and Treachery, the Victim of Debauchery and Libertinism

The Bridal Chamber, and its Mysteries: or, Life at Our Fashionable Hotels.

The California Widow; or Love, Intrigue, Crimes, & Fashionable Dissipation.

The Child of Nature; or, the History of a Young Lady of Luxurious Temperament and Prurient Imagination, ...

The Intrigues and Secret Amours of Napoleon

The Lady in Flesh Coloured Tights

The Marriage Bed—Wedding Secrets Revealed by the Torch of Hymen

The Wanton Widow

The Lustful Turk

Venus' Album; or, Rosebuds of Love

Oral Sex in Another Time

In the 1800s, the medical experts of the day claimed that oral sex was an unnatural act because a woman couldn't become pregnant from it. However, oral sex was present in pornographic photos from the 1800s and it was no stranger to the erotic literature of the day, where it was sometimes referred to as "gamahuching." This rolls off the tongue as smoothly as cunnilingus and fellatio, which begs the question of how things that feel so good can sound so bad.

As for cunnilingus, references to it appear in nineteenth century erotic literature and in pornographic photos as well. Woman-to-woman oral sex was one of the favorites in the live sex-shows. If a man paid to watch one woman give another oral sex, it seems he might be inclined to try it on a woman himself, if he was allowed the opportunity.

Unlike today, a man in the 1800s who wanted to receive oral sex from a prostitute needed to find a brothel or a girl with a reputation for giving it. The buzz words to look for were "French," "French talents," "French-house," "unnatural practices" and "indecent dances and dinners." This means that when a man encountered a prostitute with the name "French Blanche LeCoq" or "French Marie," he was safe to ask for oral sex, especially if she spoke with a Midwestern accent.

In New Orleans's famous red-light district of Storyville, there was a brothel known as Diana and Norma's. This was a so-called French house, which means that fellatio was the specialty. Because blow jobs were all that Diana and Norma's offered, the rooms could be smaller (they didn't have to fit a bed) and the men didn't need to take off their shoes and pants. Due to the faster turnover and smaller space, Diana and Norma's was able to take advantage of the economies of scale and offer oral sex for the same price as intercourse. This was unusual during the 1800s, when blow jobs were considered kinky sex and usually cost more.

The best known "French House" in Storyville was that of Mme. Emma Johnson, who called herself the "Parisian Queen of America." Rather than being born in Paris or Versailles, French Emma was a native of Louisiana's Bayou country. Her oral skills were so renowned that although she was notoriously long in the tooth, she offered a "sixty-second plan" where any man who could handle more than a minute of her ministrations without ejaculating did not have to pay. Emma Johnson's brothel offered more than oral sex, including live sex circus shows where the male performer had a mane, four legs, hooves and a tail. It goes without saying he was hung like a horse.

In his 1961 interview with former Storyville prostitutes, author Al Rose recorded the following words of a black woman who had worked out of a small row house known as a crib:

> "Mos'ly for plain fuckin' on a weekday night, I use' t' get twenny-fi' cent. Ten cents in d' daytime. We chawged fifty cent, mos' alway fo' suckin' off and' seven'y-fi cent fo' lettin' d' prick come in our ass.... Good weeks I could take fo'ty dolluh, Big money dem days... Dey [black

men] come fo' fuckin'. Dat's all day hawdly done. White boys?... Shit! Dey come fo' everyt'in' else. Mos'ly dey come fo' suckin' off. Sometime' dey come fo', fi', six at one time, all jam in dat po' li'l crib an' pay me a dime to let 'em watch me suck 'em. Shit! Carrie don' caiah!"   —From *Storyville, New Orleans: an Authentic, Illustrated Account of the Nortorious Red Light District* by Al Rose, University of Alabama Press, (1978).

Another Storyville prostitute interviewed by Rose was proud to recall that the madam of the house she worked in required the girls to give oral sex only when they were menstruating. She was disgusted to say that at some of the brothels, the women didn't do much else but give oral sex all of the time!

Starting in 1933, the American Social Health Association began doing a survey of the kind of sex acts that were requested of prostitutes. Only 10% of the requests in 1933 were for sex acts other than intercourse. By the end of the 1960s, nine out of ten requests of prostitutes were for oral sex or a combination of oral sex and intercourse.

As for oral sex in New York City, during the 1880s there were a dozen brothels in close proximity to the newly-opened Metropolitan Opera House. Since a number of these brothels were "French-run," it is likely that the prostitutes performed arias the likes of which few opera goers had previously known. Anti-vice investigators reported that because the girls in the French-run houses performed oral sex, other prostitutes would not associate or eat with them. But rather than disgust at oral sex, the real reason for the rivalries was more likely inter-brothel competition, like we see in college sports today.

The Great Masturbation Panic

With many wonderful puns that were not lost on readers in the 1800s, Charles Dickens' famous novel *Oliver Twist* (1837-1839) refers often to the male body and its sexual maturation. Consider the following passage:

"I suppose you don't even know what a prig is?" said the Dodger mournfully.

"I think I know that," replied Oliver, looking up. "It's a th—you're one, are you not?" inquired Oliver, checking himself.

"I am," replied the Dodger. "I'd scorn to be anything else." Mr. Dawkins gave his hat a ferocious cock, after delivering this sentiment, and looked at Master Bates, as if to denote that he would feel obliged by his saying anything to the contrary.

The word "Prig," which was a term for thief, sounds very close to the word "frig" which was a well-known slang word for masturbation. Then we have a "ferocious cock" which is followed by "Master Bates." The puns and references to masturbation keep getting better, as Master Bates produces four handkerchiefs to clean up the mess that his name suggests will occur.

In spite of masturbation being well known and practiced in the 1800s, an anti-masturbation panic arose in the middle of the century. There are many reasons why masturbation started being described as such an evil at that time. One factor was the creation of the modern insane asylum in the early 1800s. The physicians at these harsh facilities discovered that patients often masturbated. Instead of viewing masturbation as one of the few pleasures that inmates of these dungeon-like asylums could give themselves, physicians published scientific articles claiming that masturbation had caused the insanity of the poor wretches who were under their care. In other words, the patients had masturbated themselves into the looney bins.

These reports helped fuel the fires that were being stoked by fanatics of the day like John Kellogg and Sylvester Graham, who wrote that more than 40 ounces of blood were lost during each male ejaculation. They believed that this huge depletion of blood led to horrible diseases such as cholera and the plague. In order to save a man from such a terrible fate, they declared that he was to have sex no more than once a month, and that he was to totally abstain from masturbation. This tied in nicely with religious prohibitions against any kind of sexual release that could not result in conception.

Understanding more about this panic helps us see why organizations like the Young Men's Christian Organization (YMCA) worked so hard in the 1860s and 1870s to pass anti-obscenity laws. These laws targeted any materials that might cause a young man to masturbate. There is a bit of irony in this, as it wasn't too many years later that if a young man in America wanted to find a place where he could masturbate with other young men, the YMCA was often at the top of his list.

Prohibitions against masturbation in America reached their climax in the second half of the 1800s. People today assume that these prohibitions must have scared young men and women into not masturbating. They also assume there must have been prohibitions against masturbation in America before the 1800s, and that anti-masturbation zealots like Sylvester Graham

THE NATIONAL POLICE GAZETTE: NEW YORK

1892...

...Today

and John Kellogg were giving voice to long-standing fears. None of these assumptions are true. At best, the bizarre prohibitions made people feel guilt or shame, but they didn't seem to stop many from masturbating.

Anti-masturbation fanatics like Graham and Kellogg were the first to admit that there was hardly an adolescent boy in America who didn't masturbate or know about masturbation. While the anti-masturbation fanatics weren't as concerned about masturbation among girls as among boys, this wasn't because they thought that girls didn't suffer horribly from it. It had more to do with their initial focus, which was saving the bodies and souls of white, middle-class Protestant youths who they believed were in grave danger from sexual excess of any kind, including masturbation.

The fires of masturbatory panic struck a chord in the minds of middle-class urban parents. Self-help and advice books were becoming hugely important, and the bogus medical advice of people like Sylvester Graham and John Harvey Kellogg may have found an audience among the new middle class who was consuming these books. These couples didn't take seriously the prohibitions against frequent intercourse in marriage. The only prohibitions they may have taken seriously regarded their children's masturbation. And it's unlikely that children heeded their parents' concerns about sex any more than today's children do.

Sex writers today tend to make too much of zealots like Graham and Kellogg. While these men were not without influence, especially regarding circumcision, they hardly defined the sexual climate in America during the 1800s.

Sex & The Civil War

The thirty-year span from 1846 to 1876 was one of the bloodiest in our history. It began with America's war against Mexico and ended with Sitting Bull's massacre of Custer at Little Big Horn in 1876. In between were Gettysburg, Chickamauga, Chancellorsville, Fredericksburg, Vicksberg, Shiloh and Appomattox.

Today, most Americans know about the attacks of 9/11 and the wars in Afghanistan and Iraq as images on a TV screen or computer monitor. In the 1860s, the Civil War impacted Americans in a much more personal way. Instead of fighting an enemy on foreign soil, we were fighting each other.

Among the nearly 60,000 books that have been written on the Civil War, there is only one currently available whose focus is sex.

Today, when we talk about a woman having access to the military, we mean that she is able to join and rise within the ranks. In the time of the Civil War, having access to the military meant that a woman got to sexually service men in the ranks. And there was no shortage of prostitutes who did just that. There were entire camps of prostitutes who followed the military.

For instance, much has been written about how the word "hooker" may have come from the large camp of prostitutes who General Hooker allowed to be located near his division in Washington, D.C. While General Hooker was known to have had a personal fondness for prostitutes, the slang term of "hooker" came from the 1820s, when General Hooker was five-years old.

An interesting story about prostitutes in the Civil War emerged when the Army ordered 150 prostitutes from Nashville to be placed on board a brand new passenger ship named the *Idahoe*. As was reported in the *Nashville Dispatch* on July 9, 1863: "Yesterday a large number of women of ill fame were transported northward.... Where they are consigned to, we are not advised, but suspect the authorities of the city to which they are landed will feel proud of such an acquisition to their population."

The city where the women were supposed to be let off was Louisville. The trip should have taken a few days at most. But neither Louisville nor any other ports along the Mississippi would allow the load of prostitutes to come ashore. The *Idahoe* became famous and was called "The Floating Whorehouse." Its cargo of prostitutes nearly trashed the entire boat. They were finally returned to Nashville in August of 1863.

Love letters between Civil War soldiers and their partners are often poignant reminders that sexual intimacy was seldom forgotten in the face of tragic circumstance:

From a soldier to his wife: "I anticipate unspeakable delight in your embrace and look forward to your voluptuous touch." In her reply to him, she wrote: "How I long to see you... I'll drain your coffers dry next Saturday, I assure you." From the diary of a soldier who had just returned to duty after a short leave with his wife—"We didn't sleep much last night... The reunion so buoyed up our affections that we had a great deal of loving to do." From General Weitzel to his lover—"My darling Louisa, I have pinched your picture and it does not holler. I have bitten it and it does not holler. I have kissed it and it does not return my kisses. I have hugged it and it does not return my hug. So just consider yourself pinched, bitten, hugged and kissed."

One thing we often forget about the Civil War is how the absence of men at home impacted traditional sex roles. This was studied at length during World War II, when Rosie the Riveter ran our heavy industries while men were away at war. It is likely that similar role reversals occurred during the Civil War, impacting how men and women related both at home and in the world of business. These role reversals contributed to the nineteenth century woman's growing sense of independence.

The Civil War & Proposed Constitutional Amendment

A fascinating by-product of the Civil War was a constitutional amendment that was proposed in 1863. Its wording affirmed "Almighty God as the source of all authority and power in civil government, the Lord Jesus Christ as the Ruler among the nations, and His Will, revealed in the Holy Scriptures, as of supreme authority."

You would think such an amendment would have been a backlash against so much prostitution in America. However, sexual excess was not the primary motivator. The main reason for the proposed amendment was because politicians feared that God was angry with the Union government, and that's why the North had been doing so badly in the Civil War.

A number of state governors supported the proposed amendment, and William Strong, who headed the organization that spearheaded it, was appointed to the United States Supreme Court. He would be instrumental in helping Anthony Comstock get his anti-sex legislation through Congress.

The Civil War and Rape

War is often associated with an increase in rape. While there were certainly rapes during the Civil War, the numbers were low compared to wars in Europe. Perhaps that's because the soldiers who committed rapes were often court marshaled and hanged or shot—sometimes the same day they were caught.

The rape victims of both Union and Confederate soldiers tended to be slave women. It is a sad irony that the Union soldiers who were supposed to be liberating slave women were raping some of them. But these women were the property of Southern men, and "destroying" their property may have been a way of humiliating the slave owners. Black women were also thought to have been more sexual than white women.

Slaves and Sex

For slaves, "family" had a different meaning than for most whites. The black family could be forever separated because a master wanted it that way, or because an auctioneer had placed family members in different lots. Black men were not allowed to protect their wives and children.

Sexual relations between white masters and black slave women were frequent. Some of these relationships were tender and caring, while others were rape and exploitation. The resulting mixed-race children drew particularly poor lots in life. Their presence could be a reminder to the white wife of the owner about her husband's adultery with the slave.

Before the Civil War, it was not unusual for free black women to have long-term relationships with white men. Between 1870 and 1894, it was even legal for white men and black women to marry in Louisiana. But after the Civil War, white America convinced itself that there was an epidemic of black men raping white women. Affairs between white women and black men threatened the social order and were no longer tolerated.

It is a myth to think that the North was any less racist than the South. Few people in the North were willing to tolerate the idea of blacks as neighbors or as lovers, except for visits to black prostitutes. After the Civil War, the few protections that society had afforded blacks all but disappeared.

Prostitution in the 1800s

> Here lies Charlotte
> She was a harlot
> For 15 years she preserved her virginity
> A damn good record for this vicinity.

–from the graveyard plaque of a nineteenth century prostitute in Colorado

In the bigger cities of the North, between one-in-ten and one-in-twenty women were at one time working as prostitutes. For most of these women, it was an occasional job. Some would do it exclusively for a couple of years, while others would do it only as the need arose.

Brothels were plentiful, and prostitutes could be found in almost every neighborhood of every city. Prostitutes also worked out of restaurants called Lobster Houses, concert saloons, or dance halls where they might take a trick to an upstairs room for a quick drop of the drawers. Big-city hotels were hubs of whoring, with the finer hotels having separate entrances for "respectable women" so there was no risk they would be confused with the prostitutes.

It was unusual for a man to walk down a street in a big city and not receive offers for sex. The offers came from women who appeared classy and from girls sitting half-naked in open doorways. A man could pick up a woman on the street and have sex in an alley, or he could find a prostitute working out of a small market, liquor store or cigar store.

If he were in a miner's town in the West, a man's only opportunity for sex might be to wait in a long line in front of a tent. This would get him a soggy poke with the area's only prostitute—not that his experience would be any worse than if he'd been with a prostitute in New York. Even garrisons on the frontier offered prostitutes along with food and water for your horse. There were also Native American women who danced with more than wolves.

How the Prostitutes Lined Up

Prostitution had its pecking order. At the top were the courtesans or mistresses to the wealthy. These select, educated, charm-school graduates could turn a phrase as elegantly as they could turn a trick.

Then were the Parlor Girls who worked in the upscale brothels or parlor houses. They were followed by the girls who worked in the public houses. These ladies didn't earn as much per poke, but turned more tricks per night.

Next were the cribs, which were rows of tiny shacks that were rented to prostitutes. Cribs were the horse stalls of commercial sex, often populated by former brothel girls who had grown too old or who were in poor health, or who didn't have the minimal looks or social graces to work in a brothel.

Lower yet in the ranks of whoredom were the streetwalkers. Streetwalkers were the dregs of commercial sex. They lived in sleazy hotel rooms or wretched apartments. They were not known for their cleanliness or good health. Life for streetwalkers was difficult.

At the very bottom of the barrel were the signboard girls. These girls lived on the streets and did their tricks in back alleys or behind billboards or large street signs. They didn't have a single good thing going for them.

Some of the occasional prostitutes in the cities ran in packs of teenage girls. They would hook up with men for a quick hit of cash or for a date to see the kinds of entertainment they couldn't otherwise afford. These young women became such a visible part of popular culture that they earned the name "charity girls."

Economics and Inclination

When Dr. William Sanger did his study of prostitutes that was first published in 1858, he had expected to find poverty as the main reason for why a woman would do this kind of work. What he didn't expect to find was that the second most common reason the women gave for why they were working as prostitutes was "inclination" or sexual desire. In the minds of white Christians from the better classes, this was a frightening and perplexing finding. They wanted to believe that a woman's place was in the home, with her husband supporting her. They were also trying to convince themselves that women weren't interested in sex. To realize that thousands of prostitutes were not only supporting themselves financially, but weren't exactly hating their jobs, was a curve ball that threatened their view of the world.

A Prostitute's Life

A full-time prostitute's best chance of finding friendship was from a fellow prostitute. But how many prostitutes had rewarding relationships with other prostitutes, either as friends or as sexual partners, is not known. For instance, there were plenty of brothel customers who paid to watch two prostitutes have sex with each other. Some of these situations evolved into same-sex relationships, but actual accounts are rare.

For many full-time prostitutes, the main source of companionship was their pets or their children. Long hours and boredom made for high rates of alcoholism and drug addiction. Some prostitutes did themselves in with overdoses of morphine, opium, cocaine and/or laudanum. Pregnancies were frequent, and venereal disease went with the territory as did abuse from police, pimps, customers and fellow whores. Tuberculosis, pneumonia, infected tonsils and poisoning from abortion-causing drugs were not unusual.

Prostitutes were sometimes a jealous, competitive, socially challenged lot whose only chance to feel good about themselves was at the expense of the women they were working with. Arrest records from the 1800s show that more prostitutes were arrested for public drunkenness and fighting among themselves than for pandering.

Also, before 1885, the average age of consent for American girls was ten to twelve. It was not unusual for brothels to have young girls working as full-time prostitutes. Most girls in the 1800s did not begin to menstruate until they were fifteen years of age. So a young prostitute of twelve to fifteen years of age had "the advantage" of not having to worry about pregnancy.

As for America's concern about its teenage girls, Alexis de Toqueville wrote in 1835 that there was no country in the world where he had seen girls turned out at such a young age. There was also a high demand for virgins. A virgin could get as much as $50 to $500 for her first time, which was a tremendous incentive when you consider that she might only make $1 to $2 a day for full-time employment, if she could find it.

Sex in Brothels

By the end of the 1800s, the brothel in America was a one-stop multiplex of sexual excess. To put it in perspective, there were at least as many neighborhood brothels as there are neighborhood gyms today. The main difference is in the body parts that were being exercised.

Brothels were dedicated centers of prostitution and were run by madams. They tended to be one of two kinds: private or public.

Private houses, which were also known as parlor houses, were the forerunners of today's upper-end country club. Only the wealthy could afford them. Membership was restricted to regular, well-known customers of the better classes. The furnishings were finely appointed, and everything from the food to the women were five-star. Members of private houses might be influential businessmen or lawyers, puffing on the finest cigars from Cuba and drinking the best whisky.

Public houses were the Pizza Huts of prostitution. The average stiff was welcome. There were often long, loud lines of drinking and drunken men, especially from Saturday night to Monday morning, given how this was the only time that men from the working classes had off from work.

The better of the public houses were known as dollar-houses, where men from middle class dropped their drawers. There were also fifty-cent houses that catered to the working class. These places often smelled bad and were infested with cockroaches and rats. In the working-class brothels, there might be a bench in the waiting area where men lined up next to each other. A voice from another room would yell, "Next!"

The one sex venue that a man absolutely wanted to avoid was called a panel house. A panel house was a room designed to help prostitutes rob their customers. There would be a false wall or panel that another prostitute or pimp would hide behind. Once the customer had his pants off, the accomplice would quietly relieve his wallet of all cash. Good luck finding a sympathetic policeman when you'd been robbed while paying for sex.

The Madam

The person who ran and sometimes owned the brothel was the madam. Madams were often former prostitutes who knew the business from their bottoms up.

The madam was one of the best management positions a woman could hold in the 1800s. Put in today's terms, she was a combination of hotel and restaurant manager, personnel director, head of marketing and publicity, nurse, counselor, bookkeeper and director of customer relations.

Besides being venues for sex, the better brothels were often places where business deals were made and where political wheeling and dealing occurred. When a well-known businessman or politician suffered a coronary at the brothel, the better madams would have the still-warm corpse moved to a more respectable location before the authorities were notified.

Storyville—The Sinful Sexual Sapphire of the South

"In 1897, New Orleans city officials, acknowledging their belief that sins of the flesh were inevitable, looked Satan in the eye, cut a deal, and gave him his own address."

—Alecia P. Long, author, *The Great Southern Babylon: Sex, Race, and Respectability in New Orleans, 1865-1920*, LSU Press

By the late 1800s, city governments all over the country were talking about establishing legally-controlled red-light districts. Prostitution would be allowed within these districts, but nowhere else. The most famous and longest enduring of the municipal vice districts was in New Orleans. It was called Storyville, and it was the nineteenth century's most successful attempt at harm reduction.

By 1890, the city of New Orleans was becoming a massive, municipal gumbo of sexual excess. To help save the city, a reform-minded, classical-music loving alderman named Sidney Story drafted an ordinance to create a red-light district at the edge of New Orleans' French Quarter. This was to be the only place in all of New Orleans where prostitution was allowed. The concept worked well for more than fifteen years. However, "Storyville" was the last place on earth that an upstanding man like Sidney Story would want as his namesake.

By 1900, only two years after its official creation, Storyville housed more than 2,000 prostitutes in 230 brothels and houses of assignation. It was also home to a number of dance halls, concert saloons, gambling dens and firing ranges. Particularly popular in Storyville were the brothels that promised girls who were octaroons and quadroons. These were light-skinned, mixed-race beauties. They were the product of "almagamation" or *sex between the white and negro.* An octaroon was theoretically one-eighth black, while a quadroon was one-quarter black.

Octaroons were thought to be the genetic superstars of Southern sex workers. They had just enough black in them to make them drip with a primitive, unrestrained, animal desire for sex that people believed *the negro* possessed, but with enough white to have the supposed intelligence, personality, creativity and physical features of the Aryan races. Sex with an octaroon was thought to win a man the best of both worlds, and he often paid more to fulfill his racist fantasy.

As the rest of America become aware of following hurricane Katrina, Storyville and New Orleans were built over a swamp. Indoor plumbing and sewer pipes were rare in Storyville. The streets were flats of mud mixed with excrement from freshly-emptied chamber pots and the remains of decaying rodents. The smell was putrid, but a nose for sex could ignore the wicked odors that steamed up from the streets below.

The sounds of Storyville were not tranquil. Trains ran along the main street, shooting galleries operated at all hours and music blared from the dance halls and concert saloons. A loud chorus of barkers, pimps and prostitutes wooed the wads of the passersby.

Storyville did big business during winter, when tourists from the North could warm themselves before the fires of Satan. They could gamble, bet on horses and go on sexual rampages that made the offerings of their home-town red-light districts look like church socials.

At the height of Storyville's existence, the possibilities for excess ranged from visits to expensive, elaborate brothels and bars that were the casinos of their day, to tiny, dark, foul-smelling cribs, which were little more than live-stock pens with beds. In addition to selling sex, some claim Storyville was the birth place of jazz. But jazz was born long before Storyville. What Storyville did, however, was employ as many as fifty musicians a night, including some of the early jazz greats like Clarence Williams and Jelly Roll Morton.

Jelly Roll Morton played piano at Emma Johnson's during her notorious, live sex-circus shows. In addition to tickling the ivories, Clarence Williams was a cabaret manager who invented the "Ham Kick." The Ham Kick was a contest for willing females. A ham was suspended from the ceiling, and if a woman was able to kick it, she got to take it home. But it needed to be obvious to the audience that the woman wasn't wearing any underwear.

Did the Customer Always Come First?

According to the few lasting memoirs from nineteenth-century mad-ams, the men who arrived at their brothels were often lonely. They were men who felt like aliens in a changing society that offered few comforts. Their hope was to find a moment of connectedness with a kind and caring woman. But even in the rare situations when a prostitute did pretend to be kind and caring, she was often getting ready to service her next customer before the man had finished his final thrust.

When Al Rose (author of *Storyville, New Orleans*) interviewed men who had been frequent customers of the prostitutes of Storyville, similar stories were told in different words:

"She'd take hold of your prick and milk it to see if you had the clap. I think the girls could diagnose clap better than the doctors at that time. She'd have a way of squeezing it that if there was anything in there, she'd find it.... Then she'd fill the basin with water and put in a few drops of purple stuff—permanganate of potash, it was... Then she'd wash you with it. She'd lay on her back and get you on top of her so fast, you wouldn't even know you'd come up there on your own power. She'd grind so that you almost felt like you'd had nothing to do with it. Well, after that, she had you. She could make it go off as quickly as she wanted to—and she didn't waste any time, I'll tell you. How did I feel about it?... I was never satisfied. I don't mean that I thought that the girls of the district had cheated me... They'd drain me off. I'd be depleted and enervated—but I never had the feeling of satisfaction that I was always looking for. The truth is that a man wants something more from a woman than that... No, I can't say I have happy memories of the District. I just had a weakness for those whores—and they were so easy to get."

The next Storyville veteran interviewed by Rose had frequented the more expensive brothels in Storyville and had the added perspective of comparing American prostitutes with those in other parts of the world:

"She approached me and seized my genital organ in one hand, wringing it in such a way as to determine whether or not I had the gonorrhea. She did this particular operation with more knowledge and skill than she did anything else before or after.... She washed me with some foul-smelling disinfectant and lay down on the bed, inviting me to mount her. This I proceeded to do, and the mechanical procedure that followed endured for perhaps a minute.... I've been in whorehouses all over this globe. I've been in the cheap brothels of Montmartre and in the House of Seven Stories in Tokyo. I've been fucked in Singapore, Kimberly, San Juan, Buenos Aires, and Calgary... The foreign whores, somehow, manage to feign an attitude that leads you to believe, at least for the moment of intercourse, that you have their attention and that they are interested in seeing that you have a pleasant time. While they never do it free, they always seem just a little surprised when you hand them the money—as though they'd forgotten about this crass detail... Storyville whores, no matter how well-dressed or how gaudily expensive the whorehouse, were avaricious, greedy, and uncouth.... No house in the District could, with their practices, survive for a month in Paris.... It took much time and trouble to seduce the young ladies of our social circle, though I sometimes took the time and trouble. These experiences, few and far between, were much more satisfying—but it was difficult to make the effort with the District so near."

Dating Does the Prostitute In

While talking about prostitution's decline in America is more academic than erotic, it helps us understand about the birth of dating and sex as we know it today. By the time the 1800s were over, prostitution was in decline and sex in America was starting to assume its current shape.

You would think that in the history of sexual relations in America, dating would have come before prostitution. But it happened the other way around. Prostitution was a mighty force in America from the 1830s until the end of the century, when dating started to take its place. While dating by no means boarded up the brothel door, it was one of the things that helped drive a stake through the heart of the harlot as a central figure of sex in America.

By the 1900s, the "new" American woman was becoming the standard bearer of sexual release, and she didn't work in a brothel or bear the stigma of women who did. Women now had the option of more jobs and better wages, including white collar jobs in sales and in the service sector. They were also gaining more sexual freedom.

The winds of favor that had made prostitution the centerpiece of popular culture started changing direction. Young men and women started expecting sexual enjoyment to be the reward of relationships rather than the result of pulling a dollar from a wallet. Dating and "stepping out" became the new darlings of our market economy, helping to ease prostitution into the shadows.

In the 1890s, the average age of a New York City prostitute was as young as fifteen years. By 1915, the average prostitute was twenty-five with some being as old as thirty or forty. Prostitution was no longer an entry-level position for young girls in America.

There were many reasons for prostitution's decline, few having to do with reformers, anti-vice crusaders, or sexual repression. As New Orleans Mayor Martin Behrman lamented shortly before World War I when the Secretary of War forced him to shut down Storyville, "You can make it illegal, but you can't make it unpopular."

One of the reasons for prostitution's decline was the failure of prostitutes to put the satisfaction of the customer ahead of their own greed. Prostitutes also refused to operate within socially acceptable boundaries. Prostitution in America had become like a neighbor who never turned his stereo down.

Downtowns started to grow and become centers for shopping and commerce. Good taste dictated that they needed to be protected from the antics of whores who couldn't keep from lifting their skirts in the faces of men on the street. Prostitutes in the nineteenth century knew no subtlety, not that those in the current day are models of modesty and good taste. Changes in real estate, jobs and technology were making the in-your-face type of prostitution of the 1800s a liability instead of an economic plus.

During the 1800s, brothels were the most lucrative tenants for real-estate owners. However, in the 1900s, this was starting to drastically change. Land was badly needed for skyscrapers and high-rise apartments. Factories and office buildings needed space to expand, with nowhere to go but the land occupied by brothels.

Many city governments in the 1800s would have gone bankrupt without the fees they collected from their brothels. However, with the start of the twentieth century, the revenue base of America's cities grew stronger, and politicians had their fingers in more pies than just the prostitute's. Close ties to prostitution were no longer worth the political repercussions, and politicians were finding cleaner ways to get dirty money. Due to citizen demands for reform, corruption in police forces was decreasing. Policeman could no longer collect large stashes of cash from prostitutes, and so the incentive to protect them was evaporating. All of these factors helped make the climate for prostitution less favorable.

By the 1900s, telephones were widely available. A man could phone a prostitute and arrange a meeting for sex rather than needing public spaces for the transaction to occur. The telephone also helped make gambling and numbers-running more profitable than prostitution.

There had always been a close association between alcohol and prostitution. What made the throat wet also helped to quiet the mind. It was also easier for a prostitute to relieve a drunken trick of his money than a sober one. But with the start of Prohibition, the availability of alcohol in social settings became limited to speakeasies. Prostitutes followed the shot glass, and speakeasies became America's new brothel. While speakeasy sex could be notoriously brazen, it was also hidden, allowing the rest of society to turn a blind eye.

A major source of demand for prostitution in the 1800s had been the huge waves of immigrants, led by younger males who left the old world to find their fortunes in America. However, by 1933, the number of immigrants to America had fallen to 23,000, down from nearly a million a year during parts of the 1800s. Lower male-to-female ratios no longer favored the business of prostitution.

While settling the West had often been the job of male pioneers and gold prospectors, America's railroads were making travel safer and more sensible for women. During the covered-wagon days of the 1800s, small towns often had ratios of one woman to every 10 to 100 men. These numbers started to even out by the 1900s. The long lines in front of the whore's tent were becoming a thing of the past.

With the invention of photography and leaps in printing technology, pornography was becoming a lucrative business. Resources that had gone into prostitution during the 1800s started shifting into pornography during the 1900s, to the point where adult films, magazines and X-rated websites would one day rival the market domination that prostitution had held. The porn starlet of today may have well been the parlor girl of the 1800s.

Brothels and concert saloons were the command centers of prostitution after the Civil War. But by the 1900s, movie theaters were becoming the hubs of entertainment. The new movie theaters offered social legitimacy and dark balconies—providing a new set of sexual possibilities. Rather than being haunts for beer, burlesque and whores, the movie theaters were a place to take a date, find entertainment, eat popcorn, enjoy fine confections, make out and cop a feel. They provided places where a respectable girl could go with the approval of her parents and be sexual but not scandalized.

While the whereabouts of the sporting man's penis in the 1800s was controlled by the number of bills in his wallet, after the 1900s it became fashionable for him to surrender control to his *sweetheart*. The single man's sexual expectations were changing. He and his partner were exploring sexually while keeping the head of his penis on his side of her hymen. Since intercourse was increasingly tied to serious relationships, men and women started marrying at a younger age than they had in the 1800s.

Around the time of the Civil War, sex between whites and blacks was a gray area. While people certainly noticed, their protests were often limited to searing stares and mumbled expletives. In many of the commercial sex venues throughout the country, interracial sex was not uncommon. However, by 1900, segregation was becoming the law of the land. The new segregation laws were impacting commercial sex districts, like the nation's number-one address for vice, Storyville in New Orleans. (Storyville had originally been set up as two separate, segregated vice districts, one for white prostitutes and one for black prostitutes, but this was ignored until its final years.)

A fascinating motivator for the move to close the brothels was not so much the feminist or religious outcry, but the growing sentiment that sperm was a bad thing to waste. For instance, camp whores had been seen as an important way of providing Civil War soldiers with a much-needed sexual release. But by World War I, Americans felt that prostitutes posed a great danger to our soldiers, both with venereal disease and physical depletion.

With America's approaching involvement in World War I, we believed that the best way to protect our boys was to keep their khakis on. Harsh new laws were enacted to protect our troops from the dangers they might encounter when their private parts were in a prostitute's hands—as if mustard gas and the trenches of Western Front could not compare. Cities that didn't aggressively hide their red-light districts faced losing their war-related expenditures. In the case of Storyville, the Secretary of War told the City of New Orleans that if it didn't shut down its famous vice district, they would send in soldiers to do it. Where prostitution used to be a financial lifeline, it now threatened the wartime gravy train.

Ransacked Hymens & Myths about the American Woman

During the first half of the 1800s, people believed that sexual enjoyment was just as important for women as for men. But as the latter part of the century ticked away, some very bizarre theories emerged about women's sexuality and about women in general.

In 1881, the *New York Times* claimed that the reason for the falling birth rate among the better classes was because women were addicted to the "purse-destroying vice" of shopping. According to the *Times*, promiscuous and unrestrained shopping was destroying the fabric of American life. Even the head of the Women's Christian Temperance Union cried out against "the love of finery," which she said was one of woman's greatest temptations.

A popular public-health manual warned about the physical cost to women of higher education: "Great mental exertion is injurious to the reproductive power" and "college produces women with monstrous brains and puny bodies." Not to be outdone, some of America's best-selling books in the latter part of the 1800s claimed the place of a Christian woman was in the home, where she could excel at cleaning, cooking, mending and having kids.

An editorial in America's leading medical journal in 1911 lamented the new trend of women choosing careers over marriage. America's physicians, it said, should always encourage marriage.

Medical experts began to claim that women were pure and free from sexual desire or excess. Women were starting to be described as innocent of the faintest ray of sexual pleasure, and it was said they never experienced feelings of physical pleasure or yearning.

Still, America's streets were lined with prostitutes and our newspapers were overflowing with ads for birth control, so the people who concocted the new propaganda about women's natural state of purity added the caveat that if a woman was exposed to wanton sexuality, she could easily be lost to sin and hopeless vice. Vice was apparently more robust than purity.

It is likely that these bizarre theories emerged as a backlash to the social and economic advances that women in America were beginning to make by the end of the 1800s. More teenage girls from the middle class were going to school, and they often outnumbered boys in high school. Instead of going straight home after school, the new breed of American girls socialized with each other and with boys. Instead of cooking, sewing, and caring for younger children, they were reading books and thinking thoughts that were previously restricted to men. By the end of the 1800s, a more independent, modern American woman was being born, and this was disturbing to both women and men from prior generations.

Worse yet, between 1870 and 1920, the divorce rate in America increased 1500%. The size of the middle-class American family had plummeted, and an increasing number of women were choosing careers over marriage. Women were increasingly being seen as assassins of the white, middle-class family.

As for notions of women being pure and avoiding sex, the new invention of the moving picture begged to differ. The most popular titles shortly after the turn of the century showed American women as being sassy, seductive, and very much in control.

Technology Gives America a New Nightlife

Technology can change a culture in many ways. Think of how the television changed America. And what about the car, radio, phone, record player and iPod?

The influence of technology was particularly profound after the 1870s, when Thomas Edison's invention of the light bulb may have done more to liberate American women than the day's feminists and social activists.

Before Edison brought us the light bulb in 1879, America's downtowns after dark were dangerous and scary places. They were lit by gas lights which cast dark, ominous shadows. However, the electric street light helped transform America's downtowns into places that were bright and inviting. America's women no longer needed to stay behind closed doors after dark, and our modern concept of the nightlife was being born. The scene was set for America's women and men to start going out and "steppin' out."

When we think about how the electric light helped change the way that Americans socialized, the invention of the telephone had an even greater impact. In 1848, it took upwards of a month to get a letter from coast to coast. Good luck casually checking in on a friend who lived only five miles away. Fifty years later, Americans were talking to each other on nearly a million telephones. The new telephone industry not only created thousands of jobs for women as telephone operators, but the young women who now had good jobs were able to call each other and say, "Let's go to the movie" or "Meet me at the soda shop." Modern dating began with the first generation of men who called women at the start of the 1900s to say, "Would you like to go out dancing with me?"

Technology not only changed how we spoke to each other, but how we could meet each other. For instance, in April of 1846, the Donner party began their famous journey west. If you wanted to go west, the covered wagon was the only game in town. But that drastically changed in May of 1869, when the final spike was hammered into the first of five transcontinental railroads that would connect East and West. What used to be a perilous journey in covered wagons now took less than five days by rail. By 1880, railroads crisscrossed the entire country. Not only did they provide a safe and convenient way for men, women and their families to populate new parts of the country and to visit each other, but the railroads allowed goods produced in one part of the country to be sold in another. Completing the railroads was no less of an engineering feat than putting a man on the moon—which occurred exactly 100 years after the completion of America's first intercontinental railroad.

Soon after the railroads were built, Americans turned to building public transportation in our cities. Public transit helped America's downtowns and new amusement parks become centers of social activity. Not only would young men and women have places to go for socializing after work, the new networks of public transportation would give them a way to get there.

Technology also transformed how long we lived. From 1800 to 1870, the average white American could expect to die at the ripe old age of 39. But suddenly, between 1880 and 1900, our life expectancy leapt to almost age 50. Infant mortality dropped in half. Why the sudden change? Cities began installing sewer and water systems between 1880 and 1900.

Imagine how bad our cities smelled before the installation of sewers and the diseases we suffered due to the lack of sanitation and potable water? It was the new sewers and plumbing, rather than advances in medicine that added ten more adult years to the lives of Americans. Ten more years for us to have romance and sex.

What Used to Happen in Private Becomes Public

It wasn't until the very end of the 1800s that dating and the social mixing of young men and women started becoming a normal part of popular culture. Before then, males socialized with males, and females with females. And when young men were allowed to be with young women, there was often a chaperone.

The segregation between the sexes was so great that during the last third of the 1800s, nearly one-in-every-five men in America belonged to a male-only fraternal order—from the Freemasons and Odd Fellows to the Knights of Pythias, Modern Woodmen of America and Improved Order of Red Men. These secret fraternal organizations required men to be at the lodge many nights each month for the initiation rites that were held when a member rose from one level in the fraternal order to the next. Membership in fraternal orders began to decline rapidly as technology helped transform American popular culture into a dating culture at the end of the 1800s. To survive, the fraternal organizations had to trim their elaborate initiation ceremonies.

Only a few years after the invention of the electric light bulb and the telephone, the moving picture arrived. This invention would herald in the era of the majestic movie palace, where couples could meet and date.

In 1895, there had been no amusement parks on New York's Coney Island. By 1904, three newly-built amusement parks were attracting more than 4 million visitors to Coney Island each year—many of them young couples on dates. One of the first amusement parks on Coney Island was lit up by 250,000 of Edison's miraculous light bulbs.

After the first years of the 1900s, almost every city in the country had amusement parks. Some of the new amusement parks were as amazing as Disneyland and Disney World are today. They became popular venues where millions of American couples and families would spend the day or evening.

Visitors to these story-book amusement parks could marvel at exhibits such as "Streets of Cairo and Mysterious Asia." They could see the latest in technology in the great halls, or listen to the new phonographs and view the new moving pictures. Visitors could enjoy the carnivals with their magnificent carrousels, roller coasters, skating rinks, and even "Blowhole theaters" where jets of air would blow women's dresses up into the air.

Some of the most popular attractions in America's amusement parks were their dance halls and ballrooms where single men and women could meet—men and women who didn't know each other beforehand and who were not chaperoned. Before then, unsupervised meetings of single males and females were often in sleazy surroundings, where it was assumed that the women were prostitutes and the men their customers.

Magnificent events called "world's fairs" and "expositions" began awing millions of Americans. 14 million people attended the Chicago World's Fair of 1893. By 1904, another 19 million people would attend the great expositions in Atlanta, Nashville, Omaha, Buffalo and St. Louis. These events impacted their hosting cities like the Olympics do today.

Until the end of the 1800s, much of America's nightlife had centered around the hard-drinking, prostitute-loving, sporting culture of males. The new amusements prided themselves on having no beer gardens and on quickly removing any thugs or drunken patrons. They were some of the first places in America where members of all genders and economic classes could mix and mingle, and they helped transform the way that Americans socialized. They marked the beginning of dating as we know it today.

Beyond the Boundaries of Home

During the 1800s, the American woman of the middle and upper classes had prided herself on being the anchor of the home. She provided her spouse with a refuge against a working world that was difficult and demanding. The home was where he went to escape the gambling, whoring, and bawdy street life of the lower classes.

However, as one author put it, "God Bless Our Home" never meant "God Make Our Home Happy." By the end of the 1800s, the American woman's options were evolving. It was becoming safe for women of any social class to be out in public, laughing and dancing with men they didn't know, without having to worry so much about their reputations. There were now places where young Americans could meet, and the public transportation to get them there and back.

Venereal Disease in the Time of Victoria

No discussion of sex in the 1800s would be complete without a look at venereal disease.

An interesting thing happened to venereal disease over the course of the 1800s. In the mind of physicians, syphilis and gonorrhea went from being no more serious than a headache or cold, to a social and moral plague that was worse than cancer or leprosy. The truth was somewhere in between.

It wasn't until 1837 that scientists discovered that gonorrhea and syphilis were two distinct diseases. Even then, there was little awareness that syphilis could cause blindness, heart failure, insanity and death. The more devastating forms of the disease that did not occur until years after the initial infection were not understood to be parts of syphilis until the late 1800s. Before then, physicians thought that these were separate diseases that had nothing to do with sexual infection.

As for gonorrhea, physicians believed that it was a benign infection, often resulting from too much sexual activity. Well into the 1870s, many physicians assumed it was normal for women to have gonorrhea and that there was no reason for concern. It wasn't until the latter part of the 1800s that we learned gonorrhea was a cause of sterility in women, and could cause blindness in a child who was born to a woman with an active case.

Once physicians started becoming aware of how dangerous venereal diseases could be, the pendulum swung far in the other direction. A moral panic ensued in the ranks of our medicine men. Although they had no clinical tests to confirm the presence of venereal disease, leading physicians made bold, unfounded declarations that venereal diseases caused more death and destruction than all other diseases combined. They made outrageous claims that as many as 80% of American men had a venereal disease. They declared that we could get venereal diseases from cups, kisses, pens, pencils and toilets. Cases of vaginitis among school girls were said to be gonorrhea, and people had to be especially wary of contact with America's immigrants, who, physicians warned, were naturally disposed to moral and physical degeneracy.

Once the medical community became aware of the danger of venereal disease, they did not treat it as a medical matter, but as a problem of morality. When they did provide "education" about venereal disease in the 1900s, it was fear-based and shame-based. When some states started requiring proof of no venereal disease before issuing a marriage license, it was only the man who was examined. Such examinations were thought to be disrespectful for a proper woman.

America's physicians, who were starting to view themselves as the new high priests of morality, stated that venereal disease posed an even greater threat to the American family than birth control. Perhaps, they wrote, the decreasing size of the American family wasn't the fault of selfish women who were practicing birth control, but of philandering husbands who were bringing home venereal diseases that were making their innocent wives sterile!

These ideas fit nicely with the sentiment of America's finer minds that women were constitutionally weaker than men. Not only were women's bodies being emaciated by foolish pursuits such as attending college, but America's leading physicians were now declaring that our women were being cheated from their sole purpose and destiny in life—to bear and raise children—by the venereal diseases of an immoral society.

Just how much the general population paid attention to our physicians' hysteria is not known. While popular newspapers and magazines were happy to accept paid advertisements for quack venereal-disease cures, they were terrified to actually report on the subject. In 1906, the popular *Ladies' Home Journal* became one of the first magazines in the country to publish articles on venereal disease, and it lost 75,000 subscribers as a result. As late as 1912, the U.S. Post Office seized Margaret Sanger's pamphlet *What Every Girl Should Know* because it talked about syphilis and gonorrhea. It was declared obscene under the Comstock Law.

Even if the general population did know about the physicians' fears, history shows that this might not have altered their behavior. For instance, in the 1840s, physicians started declaring that masturbation caused insanity, but there is no evidence that their dire warnings stopped a single person from masturbating. Even today, when we know that unprotected anal sex can cause AIDS, the practice of barebacking remains epidemic in large parts of the gay community. And good luck getting Americans who are having intercourse with a new partner to consistently use condoms.

It is difficult to know how extensive venereal disease was in America during the 1800s. Since the more devastating secondary and tertiary phases of syphilis were thought to be caused by other diseases, we don't know how many people died from them in the 1800s. And once the connection to syphilis was understood, physicians would often change the cause of death to protect the reputation of the family. Also, the diagnostic criteria for venereal disease was so broad that many people who did not have it were diagnosed with it.

What we can assume is that venereal disease was a significant problem and that many people died from it in the 1800s. We also know that the "cures" for syphilis were often toxic and could cause as much pain and suffering as the disease itself. However, because the initial symptoms of syphilis usually became dormant as a natural part of the disease's progression, even the strangest of the quack cures were thought to cure it.

While prostitution was often blamed as the source of venereal disease, it is unlikely that fear of catching the disease caused the decline in prostitution in the United States. The decline in prostitution started in the last decades of the 1800s, while awareness of the true dangers of venereal disease had not become part of the nation's consciousness. Even then, the newfound knowledge did not stop people from visiting prostitutes.

Anti-Obscenity Laws of the 1800s

The 1800s brought America its first anti-obscenity laws.

By the end of the 1800s, our government had given itself the authority to throw people in prison for up to ten years at hard labor for mailing information about condoms or for printing or receiving a romance novel that was declared obscene by postal inspectors—men whose sole basis for expertise was their membership in the Young Men's Christian Organization or the Society for the Suppression of Vice.

A name that has become synonymous with anti-obscenity laws in America is that of Anthony Comstock. The anti-obscenity laws of 1872 that were nicknamed after him were the most far-reaching of any in our nation's history. Yet America's first federal anti-obscenity laws were enacted in 1842, when Anthony was a mere twinkle in the eyes of his evangelical Christian parents.

These laws were part of the Tariff Act of 1842. This might seem strange, given how tariff acts are supposed to regulate foreign imports. But that was the point. Our politicians assumed that the indecent materials that were circulating in America in the 1840s were imported from abroad, particularly from Satan's country of birth, France. America's first federal anti-obscenity law attempted to stop "the importation of all indecent and obscene prints, paintings, lithographs, engravings and transparencies."

It was beyond the comprehension of American politicians that some of the erotica that was starting to flood our cities may have been homegrown. From their perspective, the new wave of printed filth must have followed the immigrant aliens from Europe who were landing on the sacred shores of our forefathers.

The second round of anti-obscenity laws were enacted in 1865. These were an expansion of the Tariff Act of 1842. Again, Anthony Comstock had nothing to do with them, as he was still a proselytizing and unpopular Civil War soldier stationed far from combat in Florida.

By 1865, the newer printing presses had the ability to mass produce photographs, particularly those of Victorians doing nasty things. As a result, dirty books were fast replacing the Good Book as the mainstay of the Civil War soldier's knapsack. Special X-rated booklets were made in smaller trim sizes that allowed them to conveniently accompany the Civil War soldier. While it was fine for a soldier from New York to kill a soldier from Virginia, our government believed it was morally unacceptable for a soldier to keep a picture of a naked woman next to his spare ammo.

The crowning jewel of American anti-obscenity legislation came in 1872. It was the brain child of the conservative power elite from the Young Men's Christian Association. This unusual legislation was passed during a last-minute, late-night session of Congress. It is unlikely that members of Congress understood its implications any more than Congressmen understand the laws they pass today. But at least with today's laws, there is usually a quorum in the House of Representatives before a vote is cast, and legislation seldom passes the Senate without the vote being recorded. Neither condition was met when the anti-obscenity legislation was passed in 1872.

Comstock's law, which was nearly identical to one written by members of the YMCA a few years prior, was quite deceptive. Its stated purpose was to close loopholes in legislation that prohibited the interstate sale of obscene literature and materials. It's title was "The Act for the Suppression of Trade in, and Circulation of Obscene Literature and Articles of Immoral Use."

But buried in the text of Comstock's law was the inclusion of "any article whatever for the prevention of conception, or for causing unlawful abortion." Not only had Comstock managed to make it a crime to send contraceptive devices in the mail, but he made it illegal to send information about birth control as well. The highly repressive laws that he and his cohorts got through Congress helped breed a number of state laws that made it a crime for a physician to even discuss birth control with his patients.

The Comstock law made it illegal to give away, exhibit in any manner, publish, write, print or have any card, circular, pamphlet, book or notice of any kind, any drug, medicine or article for the prevention of conception or for causing abortion.

Before 1872, contraception in America was neither obscene nor illegal. For the next hundred years, it would be. It was not until 1965 that the courts would declare it illegal for a state to prohibit the use of contraceptive devices, and it wasn't until 1971 that it became legal to send information about birth control in the U.S. mail.

Thanks to the Comstock legislation, the federal government now controlled the reproductive behavior of its citizens.

Anthony Comstock was rewarded for his efforts by being appointed the nation's chief postal inspector. Not only did his new law give him the power to seize material, but to arrest those sending it, as well as those who received it. That might not be such a big thing today, when many alternatives to the U.S. mail exist for sharing information. But in the 1800s, the US mail was the main artery short of telegrams for getting information from point A to B.

As America's first czar of the chaste mind, Comstock believed that the minds of the young were delicate and easily corruptible. He believed that any materials that could generate impure thoughts were obscene. This included information in leading medical journals about birth control.

Allowing Anthony Comstock to police the U.S. mails was like allowing an abortion-clinic bomber to have oversight of Planned Parenthood. Remarkably, it is difficult to find evidence that Comstock and his anti-obscenity crusade helped stem the flow of pornographic materials that might be considered obscene. He may have inconvenienced the producers of pornography, but he was unable to check them.

Comstock did his damage by stemming the flow of information about reproduction and birth control. In 1913, after searching some of the biggest libraries in America for information about contraception, birth-control crusader Margaret Sanger could find virtually no medical information about birth control anywhere in America. This had not been the case in America before the 1870s, when information about birth control had been freely available. (The stance of America's physicians against the use of contraception did little to help check Comstock's influence. Physicians, who were mostly white, male, Protestant and from the better classes, were trying to position themselves as guardians of the American family. Many of American's physicians in the late 1800s believed women should be at home, having and raising children.)

While it is easy to make blanket condemnations of people like Comstock, we need to remember that Congress and the courts could have stopped him. Instead, they usually did the opposite. It is also important to remember that the purity groups of the late 1800s occasionally had an important battle on their hands. It was not unusual for twelve-year-old girls to be turning tricks in houses of prostitution. This, and the out-of-hand nature of prostitution and pornography, was often at the center of their concern.

Fairies, Wolves, Trade and Loop-the-Loop

An important starting point for our modern categories of straight, gay, and bisexual occurred at end of the 1800s. This is when the notions of heterosexual and homosexual first got off the ground. Before then, males in America tended to socialize with males, and females with females. Men could sleep in the same bed without eyebrows being raised, and two men who had a caring relationship did not usually pay a large social price for it as long as they did not flaunt what they were doing or appear to be effeminate. And it was perfectly normal for women to live together and share the same bed for much of their adult lives. This doesn't mean that the vast majority of men and women weren't heterosexual. It just means we didn't pay as much attention to it.

Until the end of the 1800s, an American male was not usually ostracized for having sex with another man as long as it seemed like he was maintaining the normal male role in the sexual act. It was only the guy on the receiving end of male-to-male sex who was considered a "fairy," "queer," "invert" or member of the "third sex." For instance, a masculine-appearing sailor who let it be known that he enjoyed having sex with a male prostitute lost no social standing because people assumed that it was the male prostitute who was taking the "woman's role" in sex. The effeminate male was called a "cocksucker," "pogue," or "two-way artist," depending on whether he liked to give oral sex, receive anal sex, or do both.

Even when the government set up a sting operation to entrap homosexuals in the Navy in 1919, the male decoys who allowed themselves to receive oral sex and who were the inserting partners in anal sex did not consider themselves to be homosexual, nor did the Navy. Only the sailors who performed oral sex or received anal sex were charged with criminal activity.

By the end of the 1800s, same-sex activity could be found at social clubs, baths, beaches, parks, tearooms (washrooms and comfort stations where men were known to meet for same-sex activity) and rooming houses. The larger cities in America had masquerade balls where men dressed as women, dance halls where same-sex couples danced, and certain buildings and public parks that were known for their cruising and pick-up opportunities. By the time the 1900s rolled around, a young man wanting to explore sex with other men couldn't go wrong by getting a room at the local YMCA, as the Y would soon become the vortex of same-sex relations for males in America. Lesbian enclaves were forming as well by the end of the 1800s.

On the commercial side of same-sex relations, there was no shortage of "fairy prostitutes." Sailors in the 1800s had a full range of sexual possibilities, from female prostitutes who crowded naval ports, to interested males who would wine and dine sexy seamen in exchange for being able to give them oral sex or share anal maneuvers.

Only as the social order started to change in the late 1800s and early 1900s did the notions of "homosexual" and "heterosexual" come into play. Women were suddenly getting high-school and college educations, and they were beginning to compete with men for jobs in the workplace. Middle-class males found their world being invaded by women. One way these men coped with the increasing social status of women was to see themselves as having distinctly different roles from women, or to appear to be the opposite of women. This had never been necessary because men's and women's roles in society had been so different. It may have been the origin of our modern-day notion of masculinity, which rests upon the premise that a man's feminine side needs to be well-hidden. This also corresponded with a time in the late 1800s when physicians and psychiatrists were trying to invent the notion of psychopathology. Men who were attracted to men became targets for modern psychiatry, as did women who were defying the social order by choosing careers over motherhood.

Again, the percentages of men and women who were straight, mostly straight, bisexual and gay were probably no different in the early 1900s than in the 1800s or today. It's the social stigmas that were beginning to grow.

Then and Now

This is as good a place as any to end our look at sex in America during the 1800s. While it is sometimes difficult to see the forces that are guiding our sexual choices of today, that is certainly not the case as we peek under the sheets of generations past.

Whether it's 1850 or today, our sex drives have always been present. They are the engines that entice us to be naked together. But how we get there and what we do when we get there often depends on the time and culture.

Today's young couples might wonder about techniques for giving each other better oral sex. In the 1800s, there were no articles in books or magazine about oral sex.

Modern technology in the 1800s became a vehicle for delivering pornography just like modern technology has today. Consider the invention of the phonograph recording in the late 1800s. The brand-new technology of Thomas Edison and Alexander Graham Bell was soon being used to delight listeners with the sounds of vulgar conversations, dirty songs, simulated sexual encounters, and even a "secret" recording of a husband's verbal advances to the family maid.

You could fill an entire book talking about the impact of the Model T on dating and relationships in America. It was just around the corner from where this chapter stops. And what about comparing the impact of the railroads in the 1800s with the Internet today, or the obscenity laws of the 1800s with recent attempts of the FCC to levy massive fines for indecency?

As our great, great-great-grandparents were the guardians of sexuality the 1800s, we are its guardians today. While much has changed, many of the dualities remain.

Sex Slang from the 1800s

CRIB GIRLS—prostitutes who lived in tiny row houses or shacks that were known as cribs. Crib girls were often former brothel workers who had grown old or were in poor health. They often had to pay high rent to a landlord, pimp or madame.

CRUISERS—prostitutes in New York City who gathered in small groups along Broadway. If these girls had a sense of subtlety or reserve, it was hidden well.

FRENCH LOVE—when a prostitute was willing to give a man oral sex.

GAMAHUCHE—to have oral sex with, "she gamahuched me with her warm lips."

GASH—vulva

GROG SHOPS—term for bars or taverns that often had rooms in the back or upstairs that were rented to prostitutes in order to service customers (1790 to 1820), aka "slop shops" and "tippling houses"

GUIDEBOOKS—in most cities around America, small guidebooks were printed that listed the brothels and their specialties. These books were often made in a size that could easily fit into a coat pocket.

Terms for Prostitutes in the 1800s

charity girls	female Bacchanals	jezebell
cockyneys	femmes d'amour	lorettes
Corinthians	frail sisters	nymphes de paves
Cyprians or "Cyts"	gay figurantes	perter misses
daughters of vice	gay nymphs	soiled doves
dirty loafers	gay sisters	strumpet

Terms for Houses of Prostitution

brothel	female boarding house	lust palace
bawdy house	French house	palace of perdition
Corinthian haunt	house of assignation	parlour house
den of infamy	house of bad fame	public house
den of iniquity	house of infamy	

HAVE YOUR ASHES HAULED—for a man to be sexually serviced.

LEMON—stealing the money of a man when he was focused on the sexual favors of a woman.

MASQUERADE BALLS—masked balls which were often sponsored by the madams of the leading brothels. These became popular in the 1840s and remained so for the rest of the century. Dress for these often elaborate and elite affairs ranged from masks and magnificent costumes to masks and the costume you were born in. By the end of the night, the line between a masquerade ball and a drunken orgy was sometimes thin.

PANEL HOUSE—a room used by prostitutes with a false wall that an accomplice could hide behind. He or she would quietly rob the customer's wallet once his pants were off.

PUBLIC HOUSES—brothels where the average man was welcome. Often had long, loud lines of drinking and drunken men, especially from Saturday night to Monday morning.

SIGNBOARD GIRLS—prostitutes who lived on the streets and did their tricks in back alleys or behind billboards or large street signs. These were women who didn't have a single good thing going for them.

SOLDIER'S DISEASE—drug addiction to morphine by Civil War veterans. Morphine was frequently used as a pain-killer during the Civil War. A number of soldiers became addicted as a result.

SPORTING CULTURE—generations of hard-drinking, whore-loving, gambling, fighting American males who abandoned traditional mores for a social life that was lived on the streets and in the back alleys of nineteenth century America.

STORYVILLE—located in New Orleans between 1898 and 1917, the nation's most notorious and famous legally-mandated red-light district.

THIRD SEX—people who preferred to have sex with same-sex partners.

TRADE—manly or "normal" males who allowed or invited the sexual advances of "fairies" or effeminate-appearing males.

TWO-WAY ARTIST—a man who gave other men oral sex and received anal sex, e.g. "a two-way artist is a cocksucker and a pogue."

VAGINAL TENTS—diaphragms for birth control

RESOURCES

Alexander, R. M. (1995). *The Girl Problem: Female Sexual Delinquency in New York, 1900-1930. Cornell University Press.*

Becker, R., & Selden, G. (1985). *The Body Electric: Electromagnetism and the Foundation of Life. Harper Paperbacks.*

Belenko, S. R. (2000). *Drugs and Drug Policy in America: A Documentary History. Greenwood Press.*

Bleser, C. K., & Gordon, L. J. (2001). *Intimate Strategies of the Civil War: Military Commanders and Their Wives. Oxford University Press.*

Brandt, A. M. (1987). *No Magic Bullet : A Social History of Venereal Disease in the United States Since 1880 (Oxford Paperbacks). Oxford University Press, USA.*

Brodie, J. F. (1997). *Contraception and Abortion in Nineteenth-Century America (Cornell Paperbacks). Cornell University Press.*

Butler, A. M. (1987).n *Daughters of Joy, Sisters of Misery: Prostitutes in the American West, 1865-90. University of Illinois Press.*

Caren, E. C. (2000). *New York Extra: A Newspaper History of the Greatest City in the World from 1671 to the 1939 World's Fair.*

Carnes, M. C. (1991). *Secret Ritual and Manhood in Victorian America. Yale U. Press.*

Census, U. S. B. o. t. (1974). *Catalog of Publications: 1790-1972.*

Chauncey, G. (1995). *Gay New York: Gender, Urban Culture, and the Making of the Gay Male World, 1890-1940*. Basic Books.

Cohen, P. C. (1999). *The Murder of Helen Jewett (Vintage)*. Vintage.

Cohen, W. A. (1996). *Sex Scandal: The Private Parts of Victorian Fiction (Series Q)*. Duke University Press.

Hawley, E. H. (2005). *American Publishers of Indecent Books, 1840-1890*.

Erenberg, L. A. (1984). *Steppin' Out : New York Nightlife and the Transformation of American Culture*. University Of Chicago Press.

Gilfoyle, T.J. (2006). *A Pickpocket's tale: The Underworld of Nineteenth-Century New York*. W.W. Norton & Company.

Gilfoyle, T. J. (1994). *City of Eros: New York City, Prostitution, and the Commercialization of Sex, 1790-1920*. W. W. Norton & Company.

Gustav-Wrathall, J. D. (1998). *Take the Young Stranger by the Hand: Same-Sex Relations and the YMCA (The Chicago Series on Sexuality, History, and Society)*. University of Chicago Press.

Haller, J. S., Jr., & Haller, R. M. (1995). *The Physician and Sexuality in Victorian America*. Southern Illinois Univ Pr (Tx).

Hodgson, B. (2001). *In the Arms of Morpheus: The Tragic History of Laudanum, Morphine, and Patent Medicines*. Firefly Books.

Horowitz, H. L. (2003). *Rereading Sex : Battles Over Sexual Knowledge and Suppression in Nineteenth-Century America (Vintage)*. Vintage.

Long, A. P. (2005). *The Great Southern Babylon: Sex, Race, And Respectability in New Orleans, 1865-1920*. Louisiana State University Press.

Lowry, T. P. (1994). *The Story the Soldiers Wouldn't Tell: Sex in the Civil War*. Stackpole Books.

Lystra, K. (1992). *Searching the Heart : Women, Men, and Romantic Love in Nineteenth-Century America*. Oxford University Press, USA.

Marsden, G. M. (1982) *Fundamentalism and American Culture : The Shaping of Twentieth-Century Evangelicalism, 1870-1925*. Oxford University Press.

McLaren, A. (1999). *The Trials of Masculinity : Policing Sexual Boundaries, 1870-1930 (The Chicago Series on Sexuality, History, and Society)*. University Of Chicago Press.

Morgan, Lael (1998). *Good Time Girls of the Alaska-Yukon Gold Rush*. Whitecap Books.

Morone, J. A. (2004). *Hellfire Nation: The Politics of Sin in American History*. Yale U. Press.

Nasaw, D. (1999). *Going Out : The Rise and Fall of Public Amusements*. Harvard U. Press.

Reis, E. (2000). *American Sexual Histories (Blackwell Readers in American Social and Cultural History)*. Blackwell Publishers.

Rose, A. (1978). *Storyville, New Orleans : Being an Authentic, Illustrated Account of the Nortorious Red Light District*. University Alabama Press.

Rosen, R. (1983). *The Lost Sisterhood : Prostitution in America, 1900-1918*. The Johns Hopkins University Press.

Seagraves, A. (1994). *Soiled Doves: Prostitution in the Early West (Women of the West)*. Wesanne Publications.

Tone, A. (2002). *Devices and Desires: A History of Contraceptives in America*. Hill & Wang.

Ullman, S. R. (1998). *Sex Seen: The Emergence of Modern Sexuality in America*. University of California Press.

For the animal in you:

www.GuideToGettingItOn.com

73

Kink in the Animal Kingdom

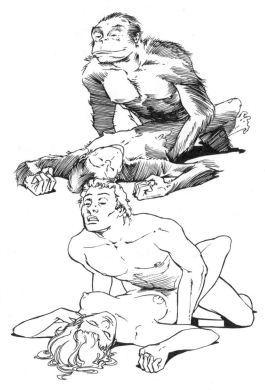

Are humans the only animals who have sex for pleasure in addition to reproduction? Are the other animals limited to having sex for reproduction and dominance only? Is there no kink in the rest of the animal kingdom? Until recently, that's what the biologists had told us. Fortunately, some biologists have been reconsidering the idea that humans are the only animals who have sex just for the heck of it. So let's pretend you are a biology professor who wants to study sex in the jungle.

Sex in the Jungle (No, Not Manhattan)

After spending years of applying for grants, you have finally gotten your project funded. Your plane is about to set down in a third world country where you hope to observe bonobos in the wild.

Discovered in 1929, the bonobo is one of the Great Apes. The bonobo's genes are closer to human genes than most other living creatures; closer than even savanna baboons and chimpanzees. It's not that bonobos are identical to humans, but they are found swinging on 98% of the same limbs of the evolutionary tree. Girl bonobos don't give birth until they are 13 or 14 years of age, reaching full maturity by age 15. When they do have babies, bonobos nurse and carry their young for up to five years. While they don't ride skateboards or have iPhones, it can safely be said that bonobos are more like humans than white mice or cows.

Your Lab in the Bush

You are finally able to set up camp in an area where you can watch bonobos do what bonobos do. You write in your notebook that you have successfully paid off the local officials, and you feel relieved that insurgent rebels haven't captured, killed or raped you.

And then it happens—your first sighting. Not only do you see bonobos having heterosexual sex, but you notice one big male has his hand on the erect penis of another male and he's giving his bonobo buddy a handjob. Eventually you see two bonobo women rubbing their genitals together. You also observe two males rubbing their penises together in a pleasurable way, and then you see a male and female having face-to-face intercourse.

After your first year of observing bonobos, you decide that while they are certainly not sex maniacs, sex appears to be an essential part of their social interactions. After spending two years in the jungle watching bonobos, you find yourself desperate for sea air, so you apply for another grant that will allow you to watch dolphins and whales have sex.

After two years at sea, you long to go back to the jungle, only this time you apply for funding to watch giraffes have sex. By now, people at the foundations are saying, "We'll be darned if we're going to give more money for that pervert professor to watch another species have sex." So instead of funding your project, they spend millions of dollars to teach sexual abstinence to students in inner-city high schools. Fortunately, your great aunt Clarice recently died and left you enough of an inheritance to return to the jungle to watch giraffes have sex.

You eventually sit down and try to make sense of all your findings. There's no way around it—your years of research tell you that the sexual encounters you have witnessed were not limited to acts of sperm competition, aggression and dominance. The same animals who one day were having a homosexual tryst might be enjoying heterosexual sex the next. And in spite of years of being told this can't possibly be, you get the sense that these animals were having sex for the mere pleasure of it, spilling sperm with a devil-may-care indifference to the theories of your fellow scientists. Good God, you say to yourself, I'll never get tenure now. So in order to make your findings more palatable to your colleagues, you report that animals have sex in order to resolve conflict, for tension regulation, and as appeasement behavior. There, you didn't use the words "fun" or "pleasure," even if that's what you've been watching for the past six years.

In spite of what's in your report, you now know that animals enjoy a full range of sexual pleasure. Males can fool around with other males without it being a newsworthy event. Females can do whatever pleases them sexually. And you never once saw animals with bibles imploring their fellow animals to take virginity pledges. That kind of behavior is only found on the highest branch of the evolutionary tree.

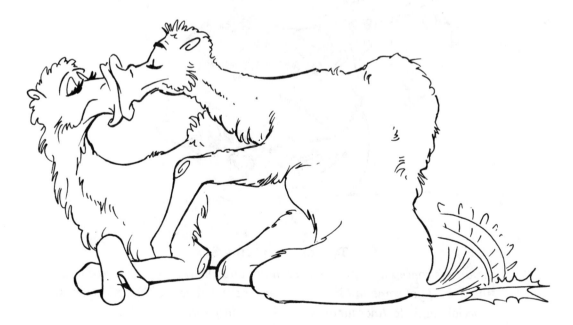

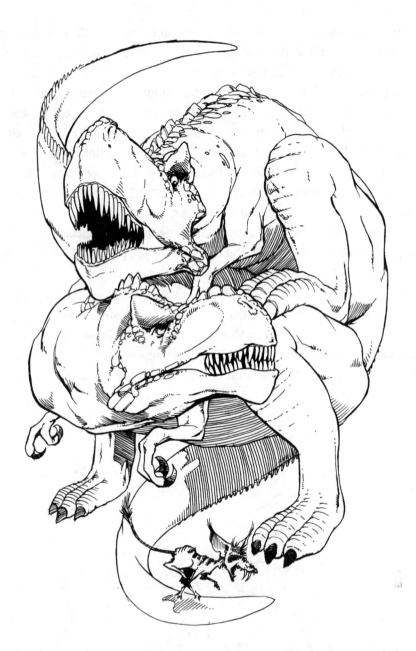

Tyrannies Having Sex

An artist's conception of how the tyrannosaurus had sex. In the Mesozoic Era, the term "I got some tail last night" was more descriptive than misogynistic. (Special thanks to dinosaur artist Luis Rey for inspiration.)

74
Orientation in Flux

Research in sexual orientation is in a state of flux. Actually, it's been topsy-turvy for the past 100 years. The latest state of flux is being fueled by new ways of looking inside the brain while people are being presented with images that turn them on. Until now, traditional research involved slapping sensors between the legs of college students when they look at dirty pictures or videos. Now we are using brain scans or neuro-imaging in addition to penile strain gauges and vaginal plesthmographs.

It used to be that people thought of "straight male" and "straight female" as being opposite sides of the same coin. Not any more. Some of the top researchers in sexual orientation were kind enough to offer readers of *The Guide* their current thinking about sexual orientation. Consider what Richard Lippa from Cal State University at Fullerton has to say:

"People come in different sexual orientations. It's part of human diversity—like variations in skin color, hair texture, mental abilities, and handedness.

Scientists are interested in figuring the causes of sexual orientation, just as they are interested in figuring out the causes of variations in handedness, personality, and intelligence. When scientists study the causes of human traits, it's not necessarily because the traits are good or bad; rather, it's because it's interesting to understand the causes of human behavior. We're still not sure of the causes of sexual orientation. However, in recent years the pendulum has swung more in favor of biological theories.

Recent research suggests that the nature of sexual orientation may be quite different for men and women. (I've conducted some of this research.) Women's sexual orientation seems to be more fluid and flexible than men's, whereas men's sexual orientation seems to be more fixed, 'black-and-white,' and perhaps biologically wired in. For example, recent studies of people's physiological arousal to sexy male and sexy female stimuli show that heterosexual men are turned on by sexy women but not by men, and gay men are turned on by sexy men but not by women (as you would probably expect). However, women—both heterosexual and lesbian—get turned on by both sexy men and women (which is perhaps not so expected).

Western society has become more open about variations in sexual orientation and more tolerant of non-heterosexual orientations and relationships. So it will be really interesting to see how the expression of various sexual orientations develops in coming years."

Here's what Michael Bailey from Northwestern has to say:

"Increasingly, people are understanding that men and women do sexual orientation differently. Men are straightforward. A man's sexual orientation results from what causes him the greatest sexual arousal, what kind of person (or animal or thing) gives him the most intense sexual excitement and the most dependable erections.

Women are different. Increasingly, it appears that women's sexual orientation is not closely linked to their sexual arousal patterns the way it is in men. I even question whether women have something called a sexual orientation, although they clearly have sexual preferences. Women's sexuality seems more fluid than men's, in that it can vacillate between different types of people, and women are known to fall in love with each other and then to revert to a heterosexual identity and life."

What Do They Mean By "Women's Orientation is More Fluid?"

When sex researchers ask women to put tampon-like probes in their vaginas that measure their blood flow, they find that just about any kind of sexual stimulus results in an increase of blood flowing around their vagina. A picture of two hippos humping would probably do the trick. But before you take a girl to the zoo hoping she'll want to have sex with you, what flows between a woman's legs and what she's experiencing in her mind can be very different. As the researchers say: *there can be a huge disconnect between vagina and cranium.*

There is also the assumption floating around that a lot of women are turned on by other women. But if you ask them what they actually feel, most women who are not lesbians will say they would rather have sex with men, unless the stars are lined up right and their chemistry with another woman is exceptionally hot. In fact, if you consider who most women have sex with, you will find that a large majority of the time it is with men.

So just because researchers are saying that female sexuality is fluid doesn't mean that waves of women are going down on each other. Perhaps a better way to put it is to say that when it comes to sex, the theater of the female mind has more potential for variety than the male mind. How much of this translates into actual behavior is another story.

Beware How the Research Is Interpreted

Just because highly sensitive probes in women's vaginas can detect an increase in blood flow doesn't mean a woman is dripping wet with sexual lubrication. In fact, we know very little about the triggers of female lubrication. This is something people don't take into account when they hear about studies that show "women are turned on by films of bonobos fucking" or "women show sexual arousal to videos of rape." There may be an increase in blood flow in the tissues around the vagina, but we still have no clue if this is related to sexual lubrication. So if you are reading studies about women's sexual arousal, pay close attention to what the women actually report in addition to what the sensors in their vaginas find.

Mostly Straight" vs "Totally Straight"

If women's orientations are more fluid than men's, it might explain the results of our own totally unscientific sex survey. Over the past years, we have received approximately 10,000 surveys from visitors to our website. One of the first questions has been, "Please state your orientation as *totally straight, mostly straight, depends on the day, mostly gay or totally gay.*" Here are the approximate results:

	"totally straight"	"mostly straight"
males	80%	15%
females	45%	45%

With great effort, we've tried to design a nonthreatening question about same-sex interest. We have tried to make the question as safe to answer as possible, since even a hint of same-sex interest can make male survey takers come unglued:

"If our society did not care or notice, and if your girlfriend and best friends thought it was perfectly normal and OK, do you think you might ever consider experimenting sexually with another guy to see what it was like?" [For the women's version of this question, change "girlfriend" to "boyfriend" and "guy" to "woman".]

The vast majority of the women replied, "Sure!" or "I've already thought about it and am wondering how to make it happen," or "It's nothing I would seek out, but if it happened, I might go with it."

It was a very different story for the male survey takers. A number of them flamed in all caps, "NO FUCKING WAY" or "I'M NOT GAY!" Around 30% did say "Maybe" or "You never know." Most said, "It's nothing that interests me." (We are pleased to report that the degree of flaming has gone down quite a bit in the last few years. Maybe society is changing, or maybe it's because there are more gay males in hit TV shows.)

As for why most males describe themselves as being either totally straight or totally gay, it could be that most males come out of the womb with an orientation that says "Seriously Straight" or "Seriously Gay" with no wiggle room. But what about males who come out of the womb sitting on the fence? Perhaps they are part of a smaller group of males whose orientation isn't set in stone, and culture and their family environment can have a significant influence on their sexual choices.

Wet Panties Have Their Advantages

If a woman becomes aroused at the sight, smell, or touch of another woman, she doesn't have to worry about being found out. If she's undressing with another woman and finds the situation to be arousing, she can smile inwardly and enjoy her feelings without having to camouflage an emerging erection. She doesn't need to think of her feelings as sexual or as homosexual.

But if a guy gets an erection in the locker room, there's going to be nastiness to deal with. If he even gets caught looking in the wrong direction, there can be repercussions. However, when he is alone, his penis will usually remind him when something is sexually arousing and will provide tactile reinforcement.

The penis is one of nature's more obvious feedback devices. Having one could possibly make sexual thinking more black and white for males than for females. However, lesbians tend to be as black and white about sexual orientation as men, and lesbians don't have a penis to guide them.

Do Social Factors Influence Women More Than Men?

Psychologist Roy Baumeister believes women are more sexually flexible than men, and not just in terms of intercourse positions. He says the reason is because women's sexuality is more influenced by social factors such as religion, education and parental pressures. Women with college educations are more likely to masturbate than women without, while a guy who is a high-school drop out is just as likely to masturbate as one with a Ph.D.

Women may be more flexible, but they often see themselves as guardians of the family and champions of the status quo. If a woman in a woman's church group is romantically kissing another woman during their annual anti-pornography potluck, she'll have hell to pay. And good luck if a lesbian takes a straight man to a lesbian-sponsored consciousness-raising seminar and looks at him longingly.

Women are also the first to call other women "sluts" or "whores." Perhaps women are more flexible about some things and more rigid about others.

Women's Crotches vs. Men's Crotches When Watching Porn

Since men watch more porn than women and women read more romance novels than men, you'd think that male genital arousal would be more visually driven and women's less so. However, women's genitals are just as responsive to porn as men's, but in a different way. Also, the blood around women's vaginas flows more to hardcore porn than to erotic stories or sex fantasies.

Straight men often get more of a penis response when porn shows female-female sex. For gay men, it's male-male sex. So if you show men either male-male or female-female sex, the chances are good you can determine whether they are straight or gay based on which kind of sex their penis reacts the most to. (All bets are off if you show them heterosexual porn. The penises of gay and straight males usually have the same response to male-female porn, but probably for different reasons.)

With women, even if they prefer having sex with men, there is an increase in the blood flow to their vaginas no matter what kind of porn they watch: male-male, female-female or male-female porn. It's difficult to tell what this means, because it is not consistent with what the women are consciously feeling.

Jerking Off Together at 12 vs. Jerking Off Together at 21

If a therapist hears about two 12-year-old boys giving each other hand jobs or oral sex, it shouldn't raise flags of concern if the kids are well-adjusted and happy. Whatever orientation they are, they are. You can't talk a child out of one orientation and into another.

If the therapist is trying to ease the minds of super-straight parents who are paying $160 an hour for the assessment, he or she might say, "Not to worry. It was *parallel sex-play;* your 12-year-old boys were really thinking about girls when they were blowing each other."

If the same boys were doing the same thing at age 21, people will automatically say, "Gay!" But if it were two girls at age 21 instead of boys, we would probably say, "Could just be a passing thing" or "Lesbians until graduation."

It is possible that young women take longer to arrive at a fixed orientation than young males. Either way, when it comes to same-sex experimentation, we tend to be more judgemental about boys than girls.

"Mostly Straight" vs "Bisexual"

Not many people would be surprised to hear that a woman who identifies as totally straight might find another woman's body to be sexually attractive. Nor would many people be surprised if a woman who identifies as being mostly straight would welcome the chance to have sex with a woman who she finds attractive.

It's different for men. Very different.

The current best estimate is that fewer than 1% or 2% of men are truly bisexual. If the number of bisexual males were higher than this, there would be dozens if not hundreds of porn sites that feature bisexual males. Yet there are only a handful of sites with bisexual males. Most porn sites go out of their way to exclude male-to-male sexual contact unless they are sites for gay males. There are many more sites that feature transgender males than bisexual males.

Men who are truly bisexual know to keep it to themselves because few people are accepting of males who have sex with both men and women.

There is another 15% or so of men who describe themselves as being "mostly straight" as opposed to bisexual or totally straight (at least on our surveys). While you might assume there is a continuum between a man who is "mostly straight" vs one who is bisexual, this doesn't appear to be the case.

Men who describe themselves as being "mostly straight" really are mostly straight. While they might find themselves being attracted to other men on occasion, they usually prefer being with women. Another man has to be seriously attractive or compelling in order for a guy who is "mostly straight" to go gay for him. Not so for men who are genuinely bisexual.

Men who are bisexual are just as attracted to other men as they are to other women. They always have been and probably always will be. It's also possible that they have a unique sexual orientation, such as being turned on by men having sex with men at the same time that a woman is involved. This is very different than most MFM threesomes in mainstream porn which is never called bisexual because the men are working hard to avoid sexual contact with each other. Even when the two men in mainstream porn are doing a double penetration on a woman, they never make sexual contact with each other.

Bisexual Men and Social Acceptance

While people are at least somewhat accepting of bisexuality in women, this is not the case for bisexuality in men. In most straight circles, it's better to say you are a serial killer than a bisexual male. In gay circles, bisexual males are accused of being afraid to come out as gay, even though males who are truly bisexual aren't gay. While an increasing number of straight people are more accepting of gay males, this would not be the case with how they feel about bisexual males. Just last year, a male student who is openly bisexual at a liberal college wrote a letter to his school's newspaper saying:

> "I am out as a bisexual male, but the degree of discrimination is worse than most know. So I don't exactly advise bi- men to be out unless they are ready and able to emotionally endure the abuse."

The abuse he is describing comes from both gay and straight students on his campus.

Your Public Sexual Orientation vs. Your Private Sexual Orientation

There are different layers to sexual orientation. There's the public layer, which is what you show to others. It's usually the orientation that your family, friends, religion and culture favor. Then there's your private sexual orientation that is innate and automatic, religion and culture be damned. It can be painful and tragic when there is a disconnect or war between one's public orientation and private orientation.

The Influence of Having a Higher Sex Drive

You would think there would be a tendency for both men and women who have the highest sex drives to also be more open to bisexual exploration. However, the research shows that this is only true for women. It doesn't matter if a male is straight or gay, he will want to have more sex but only with partners of his preferred sex.

While straight women who have a higher sex drive are more likely to want sex with both men and women, gay women who have a higher sex drive follow a pattern that is more similar to men: they only want sex with partners of their preferred sex, which is women.

Sperm-Drinking Males and The Influences of Culture

A number of years ago, an anthropologist discovered people on a remote island who believed that in order to become real men, male adolescents needed to drink the sperm of the adult males in the tribe. Given how the adult males didn't exactly have sperm spigots on their penises, the way the young boys harvested the sperm was by blowing the old boys.

Unfortunately, some of the people in the modern world who read these studies assumed that the sperm-drinking adolescents regarded their rite of manhood with homosexual glee. But the reality is, they probably did it as an anticipated experience like a teenager today looks at having to take a driving test. Passing the test means you achieve a certain level in independence, not that you want to keep taking the test again and again.

A few decades after the initial research, an anthropologist returned to the island to see what was up with the off-spring of the sperm-drinking tribe. Time had done a number on the people of the island. Many of its members had moved to a more urban part of the island, and Christian missionaries had also helped put the kibosh on any ideas that swallowing sperm confers magical properties. (Our female readers could have told them that!)

The teenage grandsons of the sperm-drinking granddads were wearing wrap-around sun glasses and listening to iPods in front of the island's equivalent of a 7-11 store. Satellite dishes meant that this was the first generation of this island's people who had grown up under the influence of prime time TV.

When the researcher inquired about rites of manhood and what the boys needed to do to be regarded as manly, they wondered if he was talking about doing extreme skateboard tricks. He eventually broached the subject of the sperm-drinking to some of the boys, who became very grossed out and said, "My granddad did what?"

Homophobia in the Homeland

Let's take a look at a study on homophobia that was done at the University of Georgia. The University of Georgia is one of the finer institutions of higher learning, and not simply because they have used the *Guide to Getting It On!* in their sex-education classes, although it does speak well of them.

Psychologists gave a questionnaire about homosexuality to a group of sixty-four men. Based upon their responses, the men were divided into two subgroups: those who were homophobic and those who were not. The testers then showed the subjects hardcore X-rated videos of men having sex with women, and men having sex with men. They did this after placing sensors on the guys' penises to see if they were having a penis response while watching the different videos.

When watching the tapes of gay guys, 80% of the homophobic men had penile arousal, while only 34% percent of the nonhomophobic men did. Yet almost all of the homophobic men denied feeling aroused while watching gay guys having sex.

Unfortunately, the penis does not always tell the truth, and studies using genital sensors can raise as many questions as they answer. It's possible that anxiety or anger caused the homophobic men's penises to briefly change size. Also, keep in mind that men who are truly homophobic don't care how they got to be that way. If they are viscerally enraged, one needs to assume they are dangerous. They might believe that their very existence is being threatened by the mere presence of a gay guy.

Happy Trails

This might be a good time to return to something that researcher Richard Lippa wanted you to know:

> There is no good or bad when it comes to sexual orientation. You are who you are. Sexual identity and sexual orientation may not be fully fixed in young people, and this may be particularly true for women. Whatever your sexual orientation is and whatever gender (or genders) you're attracted to, learn to accept yourself and enjoy your sexual feelings. Sex is always a process, but not necessarily a fixed process. So learn to go with the flow—in particular, learn to go with your flow—but do so in a safe, sane, and sensible way."

And what better way to finish this chapter than by leaving you with our two most favorite reader responses on sexual orientation:

> "I would probably be gay if I didn't find guys so damn ugly."
> *male age 23*

> "This is my first ongoing relationship with a woman. I wouldn't say it's less satisfying, but it wouldn't be able to replace sex with a man. That's because I like being dominant when I'm with a woman, and submissive when I'm with a man." *female age 29*

Note: We haven't received enough sex surveys from men who describe themselves as being "mostly gay" to say if there is a significant group of "mostly gay" men who occasionally find women to be sexually arousing. There could be, but there's no way to speculate based on our survey results.

A Special Thanks to Richard Lippa of California State University at Fullerton, to J. Michael Bailey of Northwestern University, to Ralph Bolton of Claremont College, to Ritch Savin-Williams of Cornell, to Meredith Chivers of Queen's University, and to members of SexNet for their gracious help.

75

Same-Sex
Fun & Luvin'

Most books on sex are now inclusive, which means they are written for people of all sexual orientations. But there aren't many gay men who are going to read a book on sex that has as many vaginas in it as this one, and there aren't many lesbians who are going to read a book on sex that has as many penises as this one. So what we've ended up with are a lot of books on sex that are written for everyone but speak to no one.

There's also the idea that for a book on sex to embrace sexual diversity, it needs to be inclusive of all sexual orientations and it has to use tortured pronouns that are gender and orientation neutral. Hopefully *The Guide* has proven how wrong this assumption is, because there aren't many books on sex that embrace and respect sexual diversity more than this one.

As for the following LGBT chapter, it has one goal and only one goal: to get you to think differently about one aspect of being LGBT. You pick the aspect—it doesn't matter which one.

Alice in Sexual Orientation Land

People tend to take their sexual orientations very seriously. Boundaries are staked out and rigidly enforced. So, what would happen if...

💡The head of the Lesbian Women's Caucus found herself being turned on while standing behind a cute guy at the hardware store who was on a ladder grabbing a box of screws? Is she suddenly less of a lez—as she would be the first to accuse any other lesbian who admitted to lusting over a testosterone-drenched male pelvis? And what if she had a fantasy of the hardware boy easing her down on the newly-displayed lawnchair recliners in Aisle C, as she eagerly spread her legs, clutching a Tiki Torch in each hand while he slid his bolt of a boy boner into her "women's only" area?

💡A gay male cheerleader finds himself looking up a cheerleader's skirt and suddenly wonders about something other than whether she waxed her bikini line correctly? Or he feels compelled to sneak a pair of her panties from her workout bag to see what it's like to jerk off into them? Is he in danger of having to surrender his subscription to *Out* and his 2$^{(x)}$ist coutour pouch briefs?

💡A totally straight guy gets tossed into the slammer for twenty years and has a non-exploitive, loving and tender sexual relationship with his cell-mate, Bubba? After the parole board lets him skedaddle and his choices are no longer limited by the situation, he still misses Bubba?

Would any of these people be less of who they think they are if these egregious violations of their assumed sexual identities were to occur?

Jerking Off to the Wrong Underwear Ads!

This book doesn't much care what your sexual orientation is, but in case you do and you are wondering how people with same-sex attraction learn about theirs, here's a very funny description from author Ellen Orleans:

> "At What Age Do You Know You're Homosexual? As you might imagine, this varies greatly. Guys seem to be aware of their sexuality early on. A single erection while watching Batman free Robin from the clutches of the Riddler provided many young men with their first clue. One gay friend told me that his childhood role models were Bert and Ernie. For others, it was Skipper and Gilligan.

> "Women seem to discover their sexual orientation more from personal experiences. Although I didn't realize it at the time, my first clue was when I zipped up Bobby Wolinsky's fly for him in the second grade. My teacher said this was not proper—that that was a boy's private area. At the time, I didn't see what the big deal was. Guess I still don't."—From *Who Cares If It's a Choice? Snappy Answers to 101 Nosy, Intrusive and Highly Personal Questions about Lesbians and Gay Men*, by Ellen Orleans, Laugh Lines Press

Of the various sexual orientations, which is best? We have no clue. There are times when life and relationships totally suck no matter what your orientation; being straight is no guarantee of happiness, nor is being gay. Straight is what most people think they are, and it's usually easier to be part of the majority no matter what. Easier, but not necessarily more satisfying.

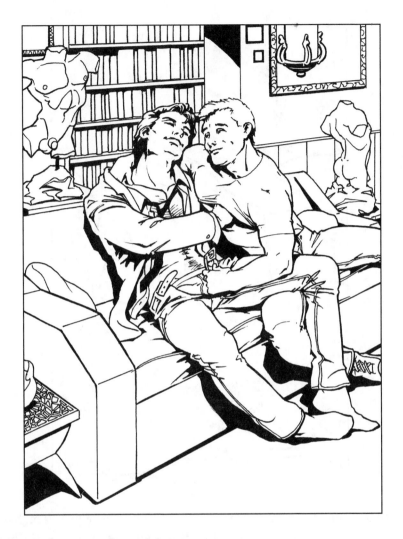

Different Takes on Male Cruising

In case you grew up under a shrub and never heard about cruising, it's where men who enjoy having sex with other men hook up on the spur of the moment to have anonymous sex. Words or names are seldom exchanged. You give or get a quick glance of approval, and one guy's dick is out and the other is on his knees or is grabbing his ankles faster than either man can say, "Thank you, Grindr!" The Internet has replaced the trailhead, with meeting locations decided online.

A lot of straight people shake their heads and say, "Gay thing." But what percent of straight males would suddenly cruise for sex if straight women

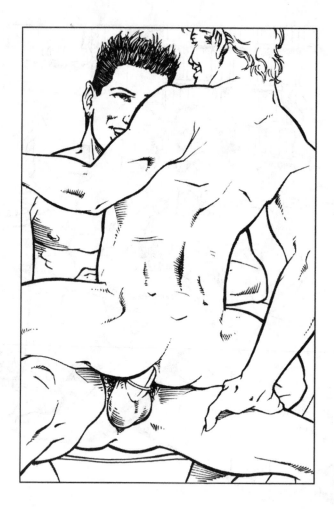

started dropping their panties for all comers? It would be just as high as the percent of gay guys who do it now. In fact, during the 1800s when the brothel was an extension of the American bedroom, the only thing that kept most single men from having sex with different women each night was how much money they could afford to spend.

"Ah," you say, "that's just proof that all males are pigs, straight or gay."

No, it isn't.

In our totally unscientific sex survey for the website of this book, we have been asking women a big "what if" question—what if they never had to worry about being pregnant, catching an STI, or being called a slut? Would they be doing sex differently than they are today?

Of the women under age 24 who are in exciting new relationships, the answer is pretty much, "No—well, maybe a little, but I'm pretty satisfied." That's to be expected at the start of anything new that is sexual. But half of the women who have taken the survey say they would be having more sex with more men if they didn't need to worry about the things that women need to worry about.

So if you take away the danger of pregnancy, STIs, needing to parent kids, and we stop calling women whores for having the same amount of sex that men have, we would not continue to see a big difference between the sexual habits of gay men who cruise and straight men and women.

With the coming of birth control for men and vaccines against STIs in the next two decades, all bets are off.

There are plenty of people who hold the heterosexual model of marriage as an ideal, and the gay model of cruising as an aberration. However, with a divorce rate approaching 50%, and with a large percentage of married couples staying together just for the kids, some people wonder whether the straight model of monogamy is all it's cracked up to be. And some experts, such as college professor Ralph Bolton, say that while plenty of gay men are monogamous, others find it rewarding and fulfilling to cruise and have multiple partners. He believes that cruising can have as much intimacy and closeness for some gay men as sex in monogamous relationships does for straights.

Straight Male Friends Can Be Important

Contrary to what some heterosexuals fear, the last thing most gay men want is to have sex with a straight guy. While there are exceptions, most gay men would be bored by the concept. And if you are a straight guy who gets hit up by other men for sex, it's quite easy to say, "Sorry, but I'm one of those boring straights." If the person is really thick and persists, you might say, "Again, no thanks, but let me describe for you how much I love licking a woman's pussy, and what it looks and feels like." If that doesn't gag the guy on the spot, be careful. He's probably an undercover cop.

Also keep in mind that there are lots of reasons why some gay men value their friendships with straight men. With straight men they are only friends and not potential sex partners, and they can have conversations about things like baseball scores and new car tires without the added postscript of who got the plague or who went home with whom after working out at the gym. Their straight male friends aren't invested in the sometimes vicious politics of the local gay scene. And the stereotype that all gay guys are fems is destructive. There are plenty of gay men who are every bit as masculine as straight men and who desire their company.

As for which sexual orientation is of concern, the vast majority of serious crimes in this country—from violent attacks, rape and child molestation to bank fraud and illegal drug importation—are committed by heterosexual males. People who are homophobic ought to think about that one.

Life As a Lesbian, As If We Had a Clue...

Gay men and women are often grouped together because they are both homosexual. This is like assuming Germans and French are alike because they share a common border. The real question that should be asked about gay men and lesbians is if there are any two groups on the planet who are more dissimilar—aside from the homophobia they receive from straights?

Even their statistics are dissimilar: while the majority of gay males in this country will have sex with dozens of different partners in a lifetime, the average gay woman has sex with a lifetime total of two to ten partners. And while less than 20% of gay males have had sex with a woman, more than 80% of gay women have slept with a man. Setting a stereotype for gay women is not possible, says sex researcher Ira Reiss. While common personality traits have been found among gay males, Reiss has found few among gay women.

Lipstick Lesbians & Dykes

People sometimes think that all lesbians ride on Harleys. This Guide is willing to bet its left foot that there were almost as many lesbians entered in beauty pageants last year as were on the women's professional-golf tour. A number of hot-looking actresses and models are lesbians.

Equally off-base is the notion that gay women make love in a delicate or particularly poetic way. Women who love women get it on with as much passion (or lack of it) as women who have sex with men.

Beyond Brown & Yale

In the past, women who preferred women still dated and married men. Women who had lousy experiences with their fathers often replaced them with equally difficult boyfriends or husbands. It was usually expected that women remain in heterosexual relationships even if they preferred being

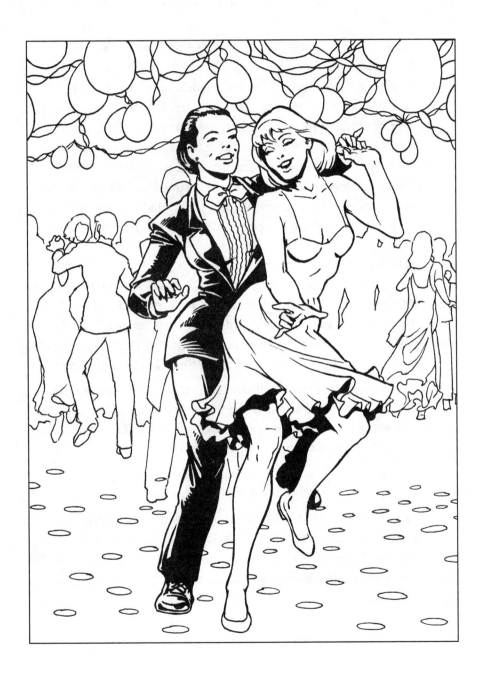

with women. There are at least five reasons why this is not necessarily the case anymore:

1. Mothers used to teach their daughters that it was hugely important to marry a man and have his children. This is not as true as it used to be. 2. Appealing lesbian role models used to be few and far between. There now exists a group of very appealing, successful, high-profile lesbian role models in sports, business, rock 'n' roll, and entertainment. 3. It is now acceptable for lesbian couples to have children by artificial insemination, spawning a whole new market for turkey basters and adoption in most states. 4. College women have sex with women at schools other than just Brown and Yale. 5. Straight women get no respect at WPGA golf tournaments.

Mistaken Identity?

Women in our society can hug, hold hands or dance together, and it is not considered a sign of same-sex attraction. As a result, they can have sexual feelings for women without acknowledging them as that. The following statements from two different women help describe how this lack of labeling can impact the ways that women think about their same-sex attraction:

"I never thought of homosexual as relating to women, only to men...." and "Our sexual relationship we kept to ourselves, and I was more excited about it than anything else. I thought it was just a delicious secret. And at the same time I had a mad crush on a guy."

—From *Women's Sexual Development,* edited by Martha Kirkpatrick, (New York: International Universities Press)

Superb Resource: No one in America who is exploring romantic attraction between women should be without Lillian Faderman's *Odd Girls and Twilight Lovers : A History of Lesbian Life in Twentieth-Century America,* Penguin. This gem provides a historical background that people today have little sense of. Anyone, gay, straight or lesbian, will learn from this book.

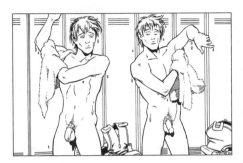

Dear Paul,

I am 17 and am on my high-school football team. I'm also gay. Nobody knows about it. It feels like I'm living a lie. I know that my dad would explode if I came out, and when someone isn't giving 100% on the football field, Coach calls him a fag. What do I do?

Mark in Atlanta

Dear Mark,

One of the books that is most often stolen from libraries is Dan Woog's *Jocks*. *Jocks* contains real stories from young athletes who struggled with exactly the same questions you are. Plenty of guys your age want to read it, but are afraid of being found out if they officially check it out.

Let's break your question down into two parts—the dad part, and the coach part. A lot of the street kids who I used to work with had been kicked out of their homes for being gay. Trust me, you don't want to ever live on the streets. So the first thing I encourage you to do is to stop worrying about "living a lie." There's plenty of time to come out later and to do so on your own terms. For now, consider where you would live if your dad kicked you out. If you don't have a safe place to go, forget any coming out for the time being.

Then there are your coach and teammates. Yes, there are stories of gay high school football players who are supported by their team. But there aren't many.

On the other hand, I recently heard from a university sex-ed teacher that one of the assignments he gave his class of mostly straight students was to write a coming-out letter to their family and friends. This was just an exercise they were supposed to hand in to him. A few months later, one of the students who was an athlete called him to tell him that his computer had a virus, and that random files had been sent to people in his address book. The "coming out" letter he had written for the class was one of the files that had been sent out.

He found out when he started receiving phone calls from his family members and friends telling him that they loved him and that they were there to support him. What surprised him the most was how supportive and loving they all were! So it could be that if you don't come out, you will be cheating your family, coaches and fellow players from the chance of rising above it all. You will also be cheating them of the opportunity to defend you if opposing players try to "spear the queer." So if you absolutely must come out while still in high school, why not wait until track season? Your chances of being accepted by your teammates would be better if you were in a sport where there are individual performances, like gymnastics, track or swimming.

I hope all of this is changing, and there are indications that it is. The NFL drafted it's first openly out player, but he never made a team.

If you do come out, you might need to deal with some of your teammates' concerns about what will happen in the showers and locker room. You can laugh and point out that nothing happened before you told them you were gay. Or you might tell them not to worry, that your standards are higher than those of their girlfriends.

Another book you might try is *Inside Out: Straight Talk from a Gay Jock* by former Olympic swimmer Mark Tewksbury, Wiley.

The Guide's Hard & Wet Steamy Fiction Reading List

Let's say you are a young adult and you would like to explore more about same-sex feelings. If you check with your local LGBT organizations, they will probably recommend one of the usual coming out books with pictures on the cover of a white kid, a black kid, a Hispanic kid, and an Asian kid, all smiling and happy. Sorry, but it didn't make our list of suggested titles.

What follows is *The Guide's Hard & Wet Steamy Fiction Reading List*. Several very smart people have helped assemble this list. The purpose is for you to have a fun time exploring same-sex feelings through the theater of your mind. One of the criteria in constructing this list was to include books that would cause a stirring in your crotch. Many of these titles manage to do just that. It was also important that the books be well-written or intelligent and fun to read.

What if you have homophobic friends and family members? How would you explain these books to them? If that's an issue, it's probably best to keep them hidden. (What else is new?) If you drive or use public transportation, maybe you can visit a library in another city. You can spend the day reading there. Perhaps a librarian will keep a book on reserve for you if you're com-

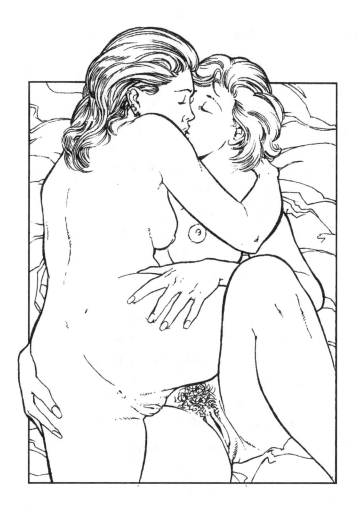

ing back in a few days. Or maybe you have an aunt or uncle you can trust, or there's a teacher or minister who will keep your secret. Perhaps they can get the book for you and you can read it at their place. Just be sure it's not some-one who is going to insist that you "come out" or that you "get help," unless you really do need help. This is about the freedom to explore without social, political or religious pressure.

There are dozens other books that deserve to be on this list. No one would be surprised if we missed some exceptional titles. Also, some of the books will be out of print. You may need to hunt them down.

Young & Wet

A list of books for girls who are exploring same-sex feelings:

Skim — Mariko Tamaki

Keeping You a Secret — Julie Anne Peters

grl2grl: Short fictions — Julie Anne Peters

Far from Xanadu — Julie Anne Peters

Annie on My Mind — Nancy Garden

Ruby Fruit Jungle — Rita Mae Brown

Fried Green Tomatoes — Fannie Flagg

Valencia — Michelle Tea

The Passion — Jeanette Winterson

Tipping The Velvet — Sarah Waters

Dive — Stacey Donovan

Strangers in Paradise — Terry Moore

Flaming Iguanas — Erika Lopez

The Wrestling Party — Bett Williams

Girl Walking Backward — Bett Williams

Dare, Truth or Promise — Paul Boock

Deliver Us from Evie — M.E. Kerr

Crush — Jane Futcher

Memory Mambo — Achy Obejas

Parrotfish — Ellen Wittlinger

As you might notice, the guy's list that follows is substantially longer than the women's list. The body of lesbian literature for young adults is a bit thin if you include the criteria of "fun and sexy." Tragic and angst-filled, no problem; boring and academic—you could fill a library. Fortunately, there's plenty of excellent panty-drenching lesbian erotica, but that could be a little intense for someone who is just starting to explore. On the other hand, the rules of "intense" have changed since the Internet became part of our lives!

If you do watch lesbian porn, be aware that there's real lesbian porn that's done by lesbians, and there's fake lesbian porn which is for straight guys and has little to do with the kind of sex that women have with women.

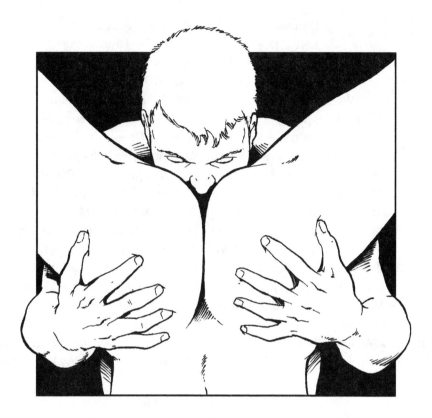

Young & Hard

A list of books for guys who are exploring same-sex feelings:

World of Normal Boys — K.M. Soehnlein

Execution Texas: 1987 — D. Travers Scott

The Milkman's on His Way — David Rees

The Front Runner — Patricia Nell Warren

The Arena of Masculinity — Brian Pronger

Sex Toy of the Gods — Christian McLaughlin

Angel, The Complete Quintet — John Patrick

Telling Tales Out of School — Kevin Jennings

Gay Olympian — Tom Waddell & Dick Schaap

Out on Fraternity Row — Windmeyer & Freeman

Entries From a Hot Pink Notebook — Todd Brown

Someday This Pain Will Be Useful to You — Peter Cameron

Dan Woog — *Jocks*	*PINS* — Jim Provenzano
Keith Hale — *Cody*	*Lawnboy* — Paul Lisicky
Perry Moore — *Hero*	*Diary of a Hustler* — Joey
Wiliam Taylor — *Jerome*	*My First Time* — Jack Hart
Will Fellows — *Farm Boys*	*Foolish Fire* — Guy Willard
Paul Russell — *Boys of Life*	*Dream Boy* — Jim Grimsley
Kief Hillsberry — *War Boys*	*Boys Like Us* — Patrick Merla
Russell — *The Coming Storm*	*Easy Money* — Bob Condron
James St. James — *Freak Show*	*Glove Puppet* — Neal Drinnan
Alex Sanchez — *Rainbow Boys*	*My Worst Date* — David Leddick
Mark A. Roeder — *A Better Place*	*The Persian Boy* — Mary Renault
William Taylor — *The Blue Lawn*	*The Boys on the Rock* — John Fox
David Levithan — *Boy Meets Boy*	*Changing Pitches* — Steve Kluger
William Corlett — *Now and Then*	*Smooth and Sassy* — John Patrick
Brent Hartinger — *Geography Club*	*Enchanted Boy* — Richie McMullen
Brian Malloy — *Twelve Long Months*	*For a Lost Soldier* — Rudi van Dantzig
James Lecesne — *Absolute Brightness*	*Harlan's Race* — Patricia Nell Warren
Richie McMullen — *Enchanted Youth*	*Blind Items* — Matthew Rettenmund
Andre Aciman — *Call Me by Your Name*	*Boy Culture* — Matthew Rettenmund

Here are some newer titles suggested
by friends of Charlie Glickman from Good Vibrations:

Choir Boy — Charlie Anders

Alanna Series — Tamora Pierce

My Fathers Scar: A Novel — Michael Cart

The Left Hand of Darkness — Ursula Le Guin

The Weetzie Bat Books — Francesca Lia Block

The Perks of Being a Wallflower — Stephen Chbosky

The Heart's Progress: A Lesbian Memoir — Claudia Bepko

Am I Blue?: Coming Out from the Silence — Marion Dane Bauer

The Man Who Fell in Love with the Moon: A Novel — Tom Spanbauer

A Big Thanks to Charlie Glickman from Good Vibrations, Matthew Torrey, Kayla Strassfeld, Dan Culliane, and Judith Rosen from PW, Eric Garrison, and to Ralph Bolton, Professor of Anthropology, Claremont College. Professor Bolton is first person in the country who the author of this Guide turns to for help with mind-boggling questions of an anthropological nature.

76

Gender Benders

We recently heard from a woman who had changed sex from male to female. She had just returned from a meeting with the managers of a company she owns. They've always known her as a man. This was their first in-person meeting since she transitioned to a female. She had been extremely anxious about the meeting.

She was overwhelmed when they told her she'd always been a kind and respectful boss, and it didn't matter to them what sex she was. Unfortunately, this is not always the reception transgendered people receive.

Transgenderism has many layers and variations. Its expression can range from when a sexy-looking girl wears her boyfriend's clothes out clubbing, to when a person endures thousands of dollars of surgery and cosmetic hell to become a member of the other sex.

Transgenderism has its own vocabulary and nuances, including words such as "packing," "tranny bois," "tranny fags," "transitioning," "drag queens," "drag kings" and "genderqueer." There can also be regional differences in how terms are used. A term that's in favor among California TGs might be considered offensive by TGs in Ohio. Even the terms transgender and transsexual are nuanced, with a transsexual being someone who wants to completely change gender by having top and bottom surgery, while transgender is more of an umbrella term that can include the girl who packs a fake set of male genitals in her jeans or a role-bending straight couple where the wife pegs her husband in the rear with a dildo.

Rather than trying to provide an overview of the transgender scene, which is still evolving and defining itself, it would be an accomplishment if you left this chapter with an appreciation of some of the different possible TG combinations and how complex it can be for those readers who live it as well as for the family and friends who love them. To that end, this chapter will focus on the transsexual part of transgenderism, which is where a person wants to change their sex.

NOTE: TG stands for transgender or a person who is transgender, while M2F and MtF are interchangeable terms that describe a bio-born male who has transitioned into a female. FtM or F2M is a term for a bio-born female who has transitioned into a male.

TG-Ball: Trading in Your Balls and Bat

Around here, when you need help explaining something fundamental about sex, you turn to baseball. What sport has donated as many sex terms such as *getting to first base, hitting a home run* or *switch hitter?* While the following quote from Yogi Berra wasn't about transgenderism, it was certainly in the ballpark: "90% of this game is mental, and the other half is physical."

So meet Clive Deacon, who spent the better part of eight seasons in the Carolina League. Given that this was the minor leagues, Clive had lots of time to think. Especially during the year when he started with the Lynchburg Hillcats and ended in Winston Salem, with stops at Durham and Myrtle Beach.

Clive Deacon was a pitcher. He was good enough to stay on a roster but didn't have the stuff to go any further. One of the things that occupied Clive's mind were his feelings in the locker room, particularly during shower time.

While the other guys would be thinking about which of the local girls were going to show up after the game, Clive's thoughts were more about being or becoming one of the local girls. You might assume that Clive is gay and wonder why he just didn't come out of the closet, but Clive knew about gay cruising and baths and gay bars. It's not like any fans would recognize him if he did any of that. He'd even had opportunities with players, but Clive wasn't homosexual. He may have done some crossdressing along the way, but Clive had no sexual interest in men. Clive was so in love with women and their bodies that he wanted to have his own vagina and female body.

As the seasons progressed, so did Clive's awareness that he felt like a woman and needed to become one. As he soaped his hairy chest and pulled his penis out to pee, it felt like he was touching the body of someone else. These were parts that belonged to a man and they symbolized being a man. Clive had less and less use for them. By the time he reached Lynchburg, it felt like aliens had stuck on the penis and had given him the hairy chest.

What's the Score?—Transgender Possibility #1.

Clive wants to be a woman. This has nothing to do with Clive being gay because Clive isn't gay. He isn't effeminate, either. Behavior wise, Clive's a guy's guy. He's always slept with women and there isn't a single straight player in the entire Carolina league who needed to worry about dropping a bar of soap when he was in the showers with Clive.

Are you starting to get the difference between gender and orientation? Being a man or a woman is about gender. Being straight or gay is about orientation. If Clive were happy being a guy and wanted to give the second baseman for the Nationals the best blow job he has ever had, it would be about Clive being gay, and that is about sexual orientation. But this is only about gender, as in being "male" or "female."

Unlike Clive, the Nationals' second baseman is 100% male in body and mind—his psychology agrees with his anatomy. He is what many of the women in town long for: a straight guy with a really good batting average. And even if he were gay, the chances are still 99.9% that he's perfectly happy being a male and that he has no desire to become a woman.

Transgender rule #1 The first question is always "What sex does the person want to be?" as opposed to "Who is the person sexually attracted to." But that will change in the next inning.

Clive's Change-up

We know Clive wants to be a woman. He feels like he's a woman. More and more, when he uses a rest room, he has to stop and consciously remind himself to go into the door with the figure of the man on it instead of the one with the girl in a dress. We won't even mention how forlorn Clive feels about his own plumbing when he passes the stand up urinals in the men's room.

This is a new inning in our game of TG-Ball and you might say, "So why not bring in a whole new pitcher?" Sorry, but the only other transgendered pitcher in the minor leagues was called up to the majors. We'll have to make do with Clive. And quite frankly, if this weren't confusing, it wouldn't be transgenderism.

In this new inning, we'll talk about how Clive is sometimes attracted to Penny, the Pelicans' scorekeeper, when he isn't thinking about changing his sex and having his own vagina. (When you are a fairly macho man who is willing to have your penis and testicles removed, the chances are good that the idea of becoming a woman overwhelms your thoughts 24-7.)

"So big whoop," you say. "Clive's a good-looking guy, nice personality, he doesn't chew—why doesn't he just ask Penny out, get her drunk like the other guys do, and have sex with her? Penny is a known resource throughout the Carolina league."

But the sex Clive wants to have with Penny doesn't include his penis. Clive doesn't even feel like his penis is his. Some mornings he doesn't know how it got there. Clive wants to make love to Penny woman-2-woman style, like two lesbians. Penny is not gay, but she might be bi. And Clive feels like he is a woman, once you get past the penis and hairy chest.

What's the Score?—Transgender Possibility #2

It's never a good idea to predict what orientation a person will be once they change their sex of origin. But the chances are good that if they were into women before, they will be into women after. In the case of Clive, who was straight to begin with, it is likely that he'll still find women sexually attractive once he no longer needs to wear a cup.

So Clive still retains his sexual orientation, which is that of a straight male who loves to have sex with women. Once he transitions into being a woman, Clive hopes to have sex with Penny girl-to-girl, rubbing his girl breasts against hers or pushing his vulva against her vulva.

Clive to the Showers, It's Barbie the Batgirl's Turn

We just traded Clive. Now our transgendered attention is on Barbie the Batgirl. Barbie is a woman of few words; maybe it's the chew, maybe it's the swagger. Some lazy evening after the Blue Rocks have been swept in three, you can buy their manager a beer and maybe he'll tell you about the night when his top reliever tried to get fresh with Barbie. They had to air lift him to a hospital in Philadelphia.

Make no mistake about it, Barbie wants to have a penis, but not in her. Barbie wants a penis hanging from her. She just can't figure why it isn't there each time she tries to whip it out to pee. And she can't figure why she doesn't have big hairy balls to scratch like the other guys. She knows they're there, she just can't find them.

Like Clive, Barbie has a thing for Penny the Pelicans' scorekeeper. But not as a woman to a woman. Barbie the Batgirl is not looking for some lesbian extravaganza. Barbie wants to make love to Penny like a man does a woman, or like they do in the minor leagues: Barbie wants to get her a little drunk and then fuck her till the Avalanche comes to town.

To the very depths of her soul, Barbie the Batgirl is a boy. She and every one else pretty much knows it. There's just that awkward problem that nature stuck the penis that Barbie wanted for herself on Clive. And Clive wishes he had been given Barbie's clit. That way, he could get off the way that feels right, by rubbing his clit instead of by stroking his penis.

Barbie wants to stroke her own penis to orgasm, while Clive wants to rub his own clitoris to orgasm. Being able to stroke instead of having to rub (or visa versa) can be a very real issue for someone who is transgendered. It's something those of us who aren't transgendered take for granted.

What's the Score—Transgender Possibility #3.

"I've got it this time!" you say. "Barbie has the gender thing going on, and gender trumps orientation. So Barbie's best bet is to load up on as much juice as Barry Bonds, get that manly muscle thing going, and become a man—a heterosexual man who wants to have sex with women." Barbie wants to make love to women as a man.

So what happens if Barbie wants to change both gender and orientation? In this case, Barbie the Batgirl becomes a man (changes gender), but becomes a gay man who wants to have sex with other gay men instead of with women. The term that is sometimes used for when an F2M woman becomes a homosexual male is *tranny-fag*.

One thing is consistent: Barbie had no desire to have sex with straight men before changing genders, and she doesn't have any desire to have sex with them after changing genders. If Barbie wants to have intercourse with a woman, she wants to have it as a straight guy who is having sex with a woman. If she wants to have sex with a guy, she wants to have it as a gay guy.

MtFs Who Aren't Players Like Clive

While each person who is TG has his or her own unique personality, situation and sexual make up, studies have shown it is possible that a number of male-to-female transsexuals might fall into one of two groups.

The first group involves the lion's share of MtFs. It's the one that best describes Clive's situation. Men in this group were seldom effeminate as children and often consider themselves to be straight. They never needed to fake being masculine, and their decision to transition into a woman often takes their former school mates by surprise.

Many of the men from this group are married and have fathered children (e.g. Caitlyn Jenner). If they decide to become women, they tend to do so later in life than males who are part of the second group. Men from this group often find themselves so entranced by a woman's *specialness* that they feel the need to become it. (It's way more complex than the old, "I feel like I'm a woman trapped inside the body of a man.")

The other group of male transsexuals were almost always effeminate as children. While they didn't start out trying to be like girls, they soon learned that they were different from the other boys and they had a lot more in common with girls. They aren't as enamoured with becoming a woman and having a vagina as are the men from the first group. If they do transition, it's often because they realize they are so feminine there's no way they would ever make it as men. They transition sooner than other M2Fs, and they worry about how well they will pass as females. Their sexual orientation is gay from the get go. They want to have sex with other males, often with men who are very masculine appearing. Unlike Clive, a number of M2Fs from this group wouldn't mind at all being sexually ravaged by one of the boys of summer.

It's unlikely that a man who is this effeminate would have been a baseball player like Clive—not even in the Carolina league. After transitioning, this group of M2Fs remain sexually attracted to men, as they were from birth. It's an attraction that feels natural for them and usually makes perfect sense.

There can also be a difference between the two groups of male M2Ts during puberty. For most straight and gay males (including Clive), puberty is when they become more masculine and start to look more masculine. However, for males in the second group, puberty does not always make them look more masculine. In fact, as teenagers, they are often confused for being girls even when dressed like guys. For these males, transitioning into a female persona is not that big of a step. They were always effeminate to begin with. However, for males like Clive, becoming female is something they might need to wing or learn along the way. They don't always transition into females with the same naturalness that men from the second group might.

Alice Novic, a cross-dressing psychiatrist and author of *Alice in Genderland* (iUniverse, 2009), offers her own perspective on these two groups:

> "In my eye, we MTFs come in two varieties: started-out-straight and started-out-gay:"
>
> "**Started-out-straight MTFs** include crossdressers and most later-transitioning transsexuals. Our hallmarks are 1) We enjoy being women (and are deeply satisfied by anything that tells us that's what we're doing). 2) We aren't spontaneously and uncontrollably effeminate. 3) We're attracted to women (whether we develop a fondness for men later on or not). 4) We gravitate toward business or technical careers."

"**Started-out-gay MTFs** include drag queens and most early-transitioning (say before 30) transsexuals. Their hallmarks are 1) They act like women and were effeminate from the start. 2) They don't automatically love being women. If they're well-received en femme, they seek it out. If not, they may be content to live more as drag queens or conventional gay men. 3) Most I've met will laugh off the idea of ever being attracted to a woman. 4) They gravitate toward people-oriented or creative careers."

For plenty of TGs, the two-camp division does not apply. Each person has their own story and each has their own journey in discovering what mix of masculine and feminine works best for them.

Orientation vs. Gender Recap

The vast majority of human males, whether they are gay or straight, are just fine with their gender. They love being guys and they love having a penis and testicles. If they wanted any changes between their legs, it would be to have more and not less. Even the queeniest of bottoms who can't be done enough each day loves being a man and has no desire to be a woman. So gender has little to do with orientation, and orientation has little to do with gender. One is meat, and one is fish.

This doesn't mean that a guy might not occasionally wonder what it's like to be a woman during sex. If some men could, they would become a woman for a few days to see what it was like to have sex. And some women would become men, e.g. a dick for a day, to see what that's like.

And what about straight couples where the woman pegs the guy in the rear with a dildo? Is this transgenderism? Not really. It's mostly a reminder that there are degrees. He doesn't want to have his penis snipped off and she doesn't want to have her vulva sewn up, and neither wants to take gender-bending hormones. Even though it's a role reversal, it's not gender bending.

Gender Benders Who Want To Remain Factory-Equipped

While sex-reassignment surgery is at the top of many transgendered persons' Christmas lists, it is very expensive and there can be nasty complications. So some TGs do everything but have bottom surgery.

There are some transgendered men who want to look like women, act like women, and be women in every way except that they enjoy their penis and testicles. Some will only take female hormones and have top surgery, opting to become a transwoman with male genitals. Some won't have bottom surgery because they can't afford it or they are concerned about how little sensation surgically-constructed genitals can have. You can look at pictures of surgically created vulvas and think, "It looks like the real thing!" but they don't necessarily feel like the real thing to the person who has had the surgery. As for a surgically-created or "after-market" penis that a FtM might have, there is plenty of room for cosmetic improvement. They sometimes lack sensation (Metoidioplasty is a type of surgery that turns the clitoris into a small penis and allows a person to pee while standing.)

One of the bigger problems with leaving your genitals intact is the law. In most cities, your gender and your crotch are one and the same, no matter how many hormones and cosmetic tortures you have endured. If you've still got a penis, you're a dude according to the law. If you still have a vulva, you are a girl. This can be a real problem when it comes to marriage, real estate, and medical and life insurance.

How Prevalent Is Transsexualism?

Somewhere between one-in-12,000 and one-in-3,600 biologically born males and one-in-27,700 biologically born females are taking hormones to alter or change their sex. So it's not like every third person in your high-school graduating class was transsexual, although you may have had your doubts.

When Transsexuals Can't Win for Losing

There are liberals who are upset by the way transgendered persons sometimes behave like caricatures of ultra-feminine and ultra-masculine stereotypes, glamorizing unfortunate gender roles. And there's nothing that will get the hackles up on a conservative fundamentalist more than a transgendered person. For them, transgenderism is an egregious assault on God's great plan that we all become breeders. Fundamentalists empathize even less with gender benders than they do with homosexuals, perhaps because there is at least hope that the demon will be exorcised from between the homosexual's legs and he or she will see the heterosexual light—not so after the surgeon has clipped off your testicles.

And then there's the world of hurt that can be stirred up when MtFs with newly created vaginas want to join groups of biologically correct lesbians. Even if a former bio-boy's penis is at the bottom of a land fill, it can be a challenge for lesbians to stop viewing an MtF as anything other than a wolf in women's underwear.

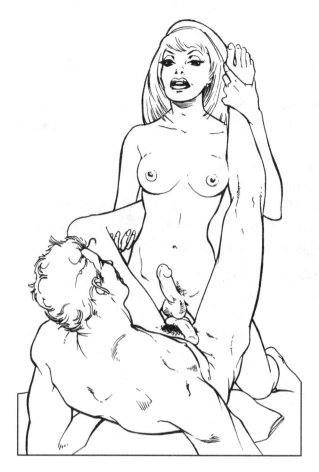

A transwoman with male genitals and her lover who identifies as being totally straight.

When a Transwoman with Male Genitals Has Sex with a Male Lover

Some transwomen are very attractive and can pass as models. They have had breast implants and take female hormones, but still have a bio-born penis and testicles. While most transwomen abhor doing sex work, some will do so in order to get bottom surgery, which is wildly expensive. According to researchers Joan and Dwight Dixon, all of the male clients of the TG sex workers they interviewed are married and identify as straight. None appeared to be homosexual.

Most men who have sex with transwomen are not interested in sex with a man. They aren't turned on by the fantasy of a homosexual experience. Nor do they show up to have sex with a woman. They are turned on by having sex with a transwoman—an attractive-appearing woman who has a working penis. The type of sex these men have ranges from wanting to suck the transwoman's penis and being fucked by her to a more traditional encounter where she gives him oral sex or he has anal intercourse with her.

Some men tell themselves that because they are having sex with a woman, they are not gay. Other tell themselves that because they are having sex with a man, they are not being unfaithful to their wives. However, most of these men are fully aware that they are having sex with a transwoman because they are highly aroused by a woman who has a penis. They know they are physically and psychologically attracted to members of what might be called a third-sex, or a woman with male genitals.

One of the challenges for an MtF who wants to keep a working penis is in getting her female hormone dose high enough to make her look and feel more like a woman, but low enough so that her penis can still become erect.

Intersex is Different from Transgendered

Our society does "male" and "female" poorly enough, but imagine if you had to negotiate it when your genitals don't look obviously male or female?

Intersex is a general term for a variety of conditions in which a person is born with a reproductive or sexual anatomy that doesn't fit the typical definitions of female or male. This differs from the transgendered who are usually born with biologically-correct genitals. A chapter on intersex is next.

Recommended books on Transgenderism:

Normal–Transsexual CEOs, Crossdressing Cops and Hermaphrodites with Attitude, by Amy Bloom, Vintage Books, New York

How Sex Changed–A History of Transsexualism in the United States, by Joanne Meyerowitz, Harvard University Press

The Man Who Would Be Queen–The Science of Gender-Bending and Transsexualism, by J. Michael Bailey, National Academies Press

Alice in Genderland: A Crossdresser Comes of Age by Richard Novic, iUniverse, Kindle edition

A Very Special Thanks to Alice Dreger, to Dr. Ray Blanchard, and to Cloudy and Kiira. (See you on the other side, Kiira. Hopefuly you are finding it to be a kinder and gentler place than this world was.) Thanks also to Joan and Dwight Dixon.

77

Intersex

When we talk about a person's sex or gender, we're usually talking about whether they are male or female. This is generally based on what's between their legs and what is in their chromosomes. We think of a person's sex or gender as an either-or thing—pull down their pants, and either a penis or a vulva will be staring back at you. While this is true for the vast majority of people, it's a distinction humans make, not nature. Nature is not constricted by pink or blue.

Nature made the sexes on a continuum, with most of our bodies falling toward one end or the other. However, there are a number of people born with an intersex condition, where their genitals don't shout "Boy!" or "Girl!"

Many people with intersex conditions look typically male or female on the outside, but inside there may be some blending of the parts we call male and female. An example is the girl who is a high-school cheerleader and who feels 100% female. Every straight guy within 100 yards gets a stirring in his pants when she walks by. But she has what's called androgen insensitivity syndrome or AIS. She has XY chromosomes like most men do but her androgen receptors did not work like those of a typical male. So she has a woman's brain and a woman's body, and her vulva looks like that of most other girls', but her vagina isn't quite as deep as that of a woman who is XX and she doesn't have ovaries. Chances are, she won't learn about her AIS until she goes to see a gynecologist to find out why her friends have started their periods but she hasn't. To say that she's in for a bit of a surprise is to put it mildly, but this doesn't change the fact that she's every bit as much a girl as any other female at her school.

Rolling Out Gender

Gender is what it means to be a man or a woman, and it usually lines up with what's in our pants.

Cultures have always assigned certain roles to one gender or another. Fortunately, some of the more confining gender roles have been falling by the wayside: we no longer assume that a doctor is going to be male or that a nurse is going to be female. We no longer assume that "the wife" does the cooking at home while a master chef in a restaurant is a man. Most people, however, continue to assume that only male soldiers should be on the front lines during combat, which is based on our gender-role idea that only men's bodies should be shot at and blown up on the battlefield.

There are other aspects of gender that are not an invention of culture.

Born With It vs. Taught

Until not long ago, psychologists assumed that we learned our gender roles as we were growing up, as opposed to biology having a strong influence. Since they believed our male and female gender roles were strictly learned, they were sure you could take a baby boy, remove his testicles, make his genitals look female, and raise him as a perfectly happy girl who would never know the difference.

And that's what they did to a lot of children who were born with ambiguous genitals. You knew a kid had ambiguous genitals when there was a painfully long silence in the delivery room while the doctor said, "It's a..... uh.... hmmm.... Can I get back to you on that?" Then it would only be a matter of time before the doctors would strongly suggest to the parents that they raise the baby to be a Katie instead of a Kyle. That's because it was easier to cut the gonads out and remove anything else that looked like a penis, and then shoot the child full of estrogen at puberty. However, there were also babies who should have been raised as girls but were declared to be boys.

While that might have worked for doctors and parents, it didn't work for the children. As it turns out, our sense of gender isn't as socially constructed as we thought.

Certain gender stereotypes are creations of culture, such as the long held assumption that girls are more helpless than boys and women want sex less than men. But whether you feel yourself to be a man or a woman— this is mostly determined in the womb before you were born. It cannot be changed by surgically altering your genitals or gonads after you are born.

So what we ended up with was a number of boys with ambiguous genitals who had been raised as girls but who never felt like girls. Once they started going through puberty, they felt even less like girls. Ditto for bio girls who were raised as boys.

Today we know to leave well enough alone. While there will be social hurdles, kids with ambiguous genitals will probably do better if their genitals are left alone. Their parents can raise them as boys or girls based on best guess, the way we were all raised. And if those kids decide to reshape their genitals later, that will be their choice. As we have discovered, only a very small percentage of intersex people who are raised this way go on to change gender or feel bi-gendered.

This is particularly important to know about, now that there are so many chemicals called estrogen disruptors in the environment. These estrogen disruptors do a number on the sexual development of the human fetus. So we should brace ourselves for more intersex babies in the future.

Teens and Young Adults with Intersex

The following thoughts for readers of *The Guide* are from William Reiner, MD, a professor of urology and psychiatry who works with children and teens who have intersex conditions:

"Often, teens with intersex conditions have been afraid of their sex organs, embarrassed by them, and they have had them examined by doctors far too many times. They tend to think that their sex organs make them freaks or weird. In fact, their sex organs are designed for pleasure just like anybody else's, even if theirs look a little different (typical penises and vaginas actually look a little bizarre anyway)."

"For teenagers in particular, how they feel about themselves and how they feel about their bodies can be very important to their happiness and sometimes even to their successes in relationships. Most typical teenagers have fears about being rejected by the person they are sexually attracted to. Teenagers with intersex conditions often have these same fears, but they may be far more than in other kids."

"Teenage boys and girls fall in love with a person (so do adults). They do not fall in love with penises or clitorises or vaginas. I try to help teenagers with intersex conditions learn how to talk about their sex organs to their lover, before they touch each other's genitals or try to have sexual intercourse. And I let them know that they must ask what makes their lover feel good. How else would you know? Sexual relations among teenagers, as among adults, is all about relating to the one you are in love with."

Intersex vs Transsexual

When your feelings of being a man or a woman don't line up with what's between your legs, you fall into the area that's called transsexual or genderqueer. The official medical term is Gender Dysphoric or GID (Gender Identity Disorder).

GID is usually very different from being intersex, given that people with gender dysphoria usually have typical genitals and the "right" chromosomes. There's nothing ambiguous about what's between their legs, and their factory equipment is just fine. It just doesn't match the gender they feel they are or should be.

Resources:

These are excellent and highly regarded:

"Intersex in the Age of Ethics" edited by Alice Dreger, University Publishing Group.

"Hermaphrodites and the Medical Invention of Sex" by Alice Dreger, Harvard University Press.

"Intersex and Identity: The Contested Self" by Sharon Preves, Rutgers University Press.

A Special Thanks to Alice Dreger, Ph.D., from Northwestern University, and to Bill Reiner M.D., Director, Psychosexual Development Clinic (Child and Adolescent), University of Oklahoma Health Sciences Center.

78

Sex & Breast, Brain & Ball Cancer

After seeing the title of this chapter, you are probably thinking, "Just the uplifting chapter I've been wanting to read!" Actually, you might be surprised.

When we have sent questions about sex to cancer experts, their responses have been along the lines of, "People with cancer are more concerned about living than orgasms!" You would think we had walked into an AA meeting with a twelve-pack of *Anchor Steam*. So if you are wondering about the subject of sex and cancer, the following account of a 37-year-old reader with breast cancer might be helpful. The readers' experiences that fill this chapter contain tips and suggestions that are far better than what's in much of the professional literature.

> I hate cancer, hate having lost a breast. I went through a horrid jealous phase, envying other women their whole breasts, their health, their fertility (treatments put me into early menopause). But that's a draining response, so I don't dwell on it. Now, I just try to appreciate beauty when I see it.
>
> Treatments for cancer can cause discomfort, fatigue and intense pain. Still, it's possible to be sexual throughout treatment, just differently than before. Self-pleasure through masturbation is easiest because you set the pace. Try masturbating even if you have a partner because then you can guide them as to what feels best. I started with self-pleasure for sleep and pain relief a few days after surgery. Later, masturbating in front of my partner also helped be a turn-on at times when I didn't feel up to active sex.
>
> Relaxing with a bath set the stage, lighting a few candles in the bathroom for mood, then a warm tub filled with epsom salts to relieve aches and detox skin. I used lots of lube for self pleasure. I started this bath ritual about a week after surgery, keeping water away from the scar area and drainage tubes until healed.

I talked with my best friend about sex and body image. She said, "You know, no man has ever pursued us for our fabulous cleavage. We both have small breasts, so we are beautiful and desirable for other reasons," and then she gave this wonderful dirty chuckle.

Imagination helps create sexuality beyond what your body is actually capable of expressing at the moment. Erotic talk and guided fantasies help me meet my partner's sexual needs. Often, I put my head on his chest and cup his balls and tell erotic tales when I don't have energy to do more. He touches himself and is happy because we are close.

Tenderness is now more important to me than carnality. My former enjoyment of raw fucking just faded away. I think my partner misses the erotic she-beast who morphed into a cuddle-kitten.

During treatment, I started using light taps and code words to signal when I needed to move, stop or pull away due to pain or discomfort. My favorite position became the couvade, or twisting my pelvis to rest on one hip for side entry, legs sandwiched around his, and supported by lots of folded towels and an extra sheet. The extra towels served another purpose. Nausea and incontinence are common responses to chemo and radiation. Having the towels there to wrap around made me feel more confident about bed play.

Lube is hugely important. Drink extra water a few hours before sex. All mucous membranes (especially the mouth) get sore with chemo and radiation, so during treatment, I added plastic condoms, even for oral sex, to help prevent any infections while my immune system was down and out. Semen made my skin burn and get rashy, so I cleaned up fast. I learned that I liked not having a bush of pubic hair so I continue to trim it even after it started growing back. Being bare makes me more responsive.

Alcohol upset my stomach, but pot soothed my nausea and made me feel relaxed enough to be sexual. I think medical marijuana should be legal for cancer patients to help sexual healing and getting a groove on as well as combatting nausea.

Lace is itchy against the scars on my chest and under my arms where lymph nodes were removed. I won't wear underwire bras anymore because they are too constricting. But I do put on cute camisoles that are soft and stretchy enough to take off without tugging.

Sexual confidence comes and goes more readily. Sometimes, I don't like being exposed, and will drape a sheet over me during sex to cover my scars. My partner has to be patient with that. If I have a hot flash during sex, I'll ask for oral sex instead, so there is a lot of back-and-forth during sex. Continuing joint pain makes me move positions a lot, so I use small pillows and bolsters for support. Yoga helps with pain management, too.

Interestingly enough, I now get aroused through massage of my inner foot arches. It's nice to have discovered a new erogenous zone to take the place of lost nipple sensation. A foot massage is a sweet way to get started relaxing and wiggling around in my partner's lap; it's fun.

My lover is an amazing partner who helped me do all the hard stuff: shaving my head when my hair began to fall out, going with me to meet the doctors when I felt afraid, or offering a helping hand to steady me as I stepped into the tub or shower. I am lucky to have such love and care.

The following is from another reader who was diagnosed with breast cancer at a very young age:

I was diagnosed with breast cancer at the age of 31. My boyfriend asked me to marry him ten days after that. Knowing that he still loved me and wanted to marry me after hearing such devastating news was so incredible to me.

I elected to have a double mastectomy which was a scary thing to do because the thing that defines you the most about being a woman is your breasts. It was strange thinking that the thing that I had criticized the most about my body was now feeling like the most precious part of it. I immediately had reconstructive surgery after my double mastectomy so I never experienced life without breasts, but the ones I woke up with were made of silicone and had no nipples. My skin was ultra sensitive, and at first I didn't want to wear a shirt let alone be touched. After a few days I had no sensation in my breast area at all.

Before my surgery I had LOVED having my nipples played with and I used nipple clamps frequently. It was so devastating to lose such an important part of my sexuality to cancer. It was hard to imagine enjoying sex as much without my nipples and the sensations they had produced in my whole body – a tingle that goes from your head all the way to your toes. I felt so ugly and disfigured. I really couldn't fathom that my fiancé would even want to have sex with me. Proving to me yet again what a wonderful man he is, we ended up having sex just a few days after I was discharged from the hospital. It was one of the most therapeutic parts of my sexual healing. Just seeing the devilish sparkle in his eyes as he looked at me with so much love and longing warmed me from the inside out!

It's been almost two years since my surgery and I feel sexy despite my cancer and reconstructed breasts. My husband has continued to be turned on by me and we've found other areas of my body that are as sensitive (if not more sensitive) than my nipples used to be. It really goes to show that being sexy is more a mental attitude than a physical trait and that facing your fears about sex after such trauma can be a very positive experience."

Dating Someone Who Has Cancer

One of the things that's different about dating someone who has had cancer is that you are with someone who has had to fight hard to be alive. Outside of combat veterans, not a lot of us know what having to fight to stay alive is like, and how it changes your perspective on a lot of things that we ordinarily take for granted.

If you are dating someone who has had cancer, they will most likely want you to know as soon as possible. This is not for some perverse kind of bragging rights, but because they don't want to have to deal with starting a relationship only to find you suddenly bailing once you find out about the cancer. This is especially important to people who can no longer have kids because of the cancer treatment or who have surgical scars or other cancer-related challenges to cope with. We live in a society where even models and athletes can be wickedly self-conscious—imagine someone who's got scars or something missing.

Outside of the effects of chemotherapy and the invasiveness of treatment, there's nothing about cancer itself that makes a person want sex any less than anyone else does. In fact, the latest study on this subject expected to find that certain cancers or certain kinds of treatments would be correlated with having less sex a few years down the line, but the biggest factor turned out to be the quality of the person's relationship. No doubt, chemo was a bitch and took a toll, and missing certain key hormones can be a challenge, but at the end of the day it was the relationship that counted most when it came to having and enjoying sex.

Advice from Anne

Sex educator and cancer expert Anne Katz recently phoned with some thoughtful reminders for readers of *The Guide:*

 Medical students get about two hours of sex education, with most of it focusing on penis problems. It's easier for many oncologists to talk about dying than sex. You, the patient, will need to be the one to ask about sex.

 Lack of desire and lack of libido can be huge in cancer patients, but it's not only from having your body nuked or poisoned. Imagine what it is like for a patient with cancer in her pelvis to lay there with her legs wide apart and a bright beam of light shining on her anus or vulva while several strangers crowd around to administer treatment? In order to cope, she learns to go somewhere far, far away in her mind. It is not always easy to come back when it's time to have sex with a partner.

 Body image issues are immense—how do you tell a perspective mate you are missing a certain body part, or you have this large scar? When do you tell a date "I can't have children"?

 With childhood cancer survivors, their whole lives have been medicalized. Some can more easily tell you their white cell count than how they feel. Many often have to face lifelong screenings for secondary cancers.

Making Adjustments

One of the things that makes sex enjoyable is that it's fun. But when you hear the word cancer, "fun" is one of the last things you think about. So the job for a cancer patient and his or her partner after the diagnosis is how to make sex fun again. This you will both need to work on!

So let's get the bad news out of the way first. A healthcare provider named Peggy McKeal, Ph.D. LMHC, who has lots of experience with sex and cancer sums it up for us. While she talks about women with cancer, what she says applies just as much to men with cancer:

"Remember, women are often the family caretakers. Nothing is supposed to happen to them. And then they need time to deal with the treatments. Imagine surgery that yanks out organs that produce the hormones that help make you want sex. And then imagine having what you are told all your life is a huge part of your sexuality disfigured. Now let's go one step farther; imagine erogenous zones that aren't erogenous anymore. Nipples that are gone and a scar left; desensitized skin, or skin that feels uncomfortably odd.

"Abdomens that have a running scar and your tummy no longer sends rushes of desire when caressed, but feels numb right down into the mons pubis. Desensitized erogenous zones all over the body due to hormone loss. (That nibble on the neck no longer makes goose bumps.) Think about body image from weight gain that will absolutely not go away due to hormone loss and cancer treatments. Think about wanting to want to have sex, be sexual, but not being interested, unable to fantasize due to hormone loss. (Yeah, that actually happens.) And then imagine trying to, but not getting turned on, and when/if you orgasm it is an incredibly quiet whisper instead of a shout. Imagine damage done to your body by radiation that makes touch or penetration painful and provokes anxiety. There are solutions that help improve things. Silicone dilators, lubricants, vibrators, time, time, time, and compassionate understanding from a partner. There are hormones that can be replaced IF your cancer is not fed by estrogen. Women who have been diagnosed with cancer and undergone treatment may be experiencing all of these things, or only some. And they feel sad, guilty and angry. They want to want. A lover who is blissfully calm, understanding, nurturing and incredibly patient is a wonderful human being."

Okay, so you see what you are up against? You'll need to both explore and find new places where touch feels good. Reread the accounts of the women at the start of this chapter. That's exactly what they did. Look at how important love and sex has been to them. The question is how the two of you approach it, your patience, and your ability to make sex fun again.

Next, if you are boyfriend or husband, get yourself a copy of *Breast Cancer Husband*. In fact, the following suggestions are from Marc Silver's rock-solid and highly-recommended book *Breast Cancer Husband, How to Help Your Wife (and Yourself) Through Diagnosis, Treatment and Beyond:*

A husband is often concerned about flirting with his wife who has cancer, for fear she will think he is pressuring her for sex. But not flirting with her can easily become a signal that she isn't sexy anymore. His hesitancy to touch and play with her remaining breast if she had a mastectomy can also become a signal to her that she is no longer attractive to him. Or he might fear hurting her if she's got drainage bulbs hanging out of an incision following surgery.

She has breast cancer, not dementia. She knows her partner's sexual desire didn't suddenly melt away with the discovery of her cancer, and the chances are, hers didn't either. At some point, hopefully sooner than later, the two of you need to talk about sex. Get your signals straight that it's okay for him to pursue sex with her, and for her to pursue sex with him, and that it's okay for either of you to say "yes" or "no" without feeling uncomfortable about it.

Adjustments will need to be made in the way you have sex, but maybe that will be one of the hidden pluses in all of this. Maybe you'll start exploring new ways to enjoy sex with each other, in addition to the old. (You'll see that in the next section, where a guy with brain cancer and his partner use sex to feel closer in times of fear and distress.)

Radiation can do a number on the skin of a woman's chest. If it feels okay, it might be a nice way for the couple to keep physically connected for her partner to rub lotion on her chest a couple of times a day. (The same can be true with radiation in her pelvis. Rubbing her vulva and vagina with lube or an oil that her healthcare provider approves of can help with tissue that's lost its elasticity.)

For some women, chemo can make intercourse extremely painful. No matter how wet she might have gotten before, have a couple of different kinds of lube handy for when you start having intercourse (each has a different feel, which is why you should try a couple of different brands). Be sure to coat both the head of the penis as well as the insides of her vagina. Otherwise, if she has painful intercourse, it might start a nasty chain reaction where her vagina automatically tenses up whenever it senses an erect penis in the neighborhood. (Semen is actually somewhat corrosive on a good day. So don't hesitate to start using a condom if that helps.)

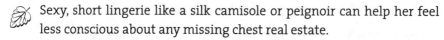 If you have access to a swimming pool, swimming-pool sex can be really nice. (As is mentioned elsewhere in *The Guide*, sex in water can actually end up being dry sex because the water can wash out a woman's natural lube. An excellent work-around is store-bought silicon-based sex lube or a vegetable oil. Coat your respective genitals with it before getting wet, so to speak.)

 Sexy, short lingerie like a silk camisole or peignoir can help her feel less conscious about any missing chest real estate.

 If she's receiving chemo and she feels like having sex (which might not be too likely) the man should probably wear a condom for the first day or two. That way, he won't risk getting a rash on his penis from any of the chemo that is in her vaginal lubrication. For the same reason, he should avoid giving her oral sex for the first couple of days after she receives chemo, unless he's got a tumor himself and you're doing couples' chemo.

Think about her physical state now compared to a few weeks before her diagnosis. If she's undergoing chemo and has had surgery, chances are she's bald and missing a big part of what Hugh Heffner tried to convince the world is the most sexy part of a woman's body. She may have scars that she didn't have and she isn't exactly feeling like she did when she was twenty and the tease of the town. While it would seem weird to her if you didn't acknowledge the new realities, this is also no time to hide your sexual desire for her. And if she's way too tired from chemo to even think about sex, ask if she'd like a foot rub or if she'd like you to massage her fingers.

 If you end up going for months when she doesn't want sex and you've been masturbating a lot, still try to keep a physical and sensual connection. This will make it easier to reconnect sexually when the effects of the chemo and/or radiation are starting to fade.

One of the biggest casualties to breast cancer can be romance. It's hard to be romantic when so many new and mostly unwelcome things are suddenly intruding on your lives. Keep in mind that if you put romance on hold during the worst of your cancer saga, you'll need to rekindle it as soon as you and she are able.

 Life can have its unfortunate contradictions. One woman who loves her pubic hair might lose it all during cancer treatments, while another who goes through the hassle of shaving herself bare every day won't lose any of it!

When there is sexual desire but little energy, think about ways to make adjustments. For instance, what if you find a comfortable position where he can have his penis inside of her vagina without thrusting while she uses a vibrator? He might then need to masturbate after she's had an orgasm, but you still get the sexual and physical intimacy without her needing to expend much energy.

If a woman is feeling bad about the way she looks and particularly unsexy, she should try not to assume that this is how her partner feels about her. And he should know that even if he still finds her to be sexually desirable, she might be so turned-off by her current condition that she assumes he is as well. This is one more example of just how important it is to talk to each other about sex.

If her vagina is too tender to handle but a minute or so of intercourse, she can get him close to coming with oral sex or by hand, or he can jerk himself off until he's just about to come, and then they start intercourse. Also, a finger on or in his anus during intercourse might help him to come sooner.

You might need to change your thrusting depth and rhythm during intercourse. Experiment and give each other a lot of feedback.

Birth control is a must for any woman who is not past menopause. Check with your physician(s), as they probably won't want you using hormonal methods.

Squeezing your breasts, sexual touching, and sexual activity will not spread cancer or impact your recovery in a negative way! Having orgasms does not alter or negatively impact your estrogen balance. Being wet sexually and having orgasms are just as good for you during and after cancer treatment as before.

From a Young Couple

We recently received an email from a young woman whose boyfriend has brain cancer. He's 20, and she's not yet. He's had multiple brain surgeries, radiation, and now chemo.

Because of his nausea and problems with stamina, she's on top during intercourse more than before. And some of the things he used to love her to do before his cancer can make him feel nauseated now. But she says as long as they give each other lots of feedback, they still enjoy sex, which shows that you can cut into a person's brain, nuke it and poison it—it won't necessarily stop them from wanting sex. In this case, his orgasms help him to feel better after chemo, assuming he's able.

She says, "Sometimes we have sex just to feel closer in a hard time like after we heard he was going to need a second surgery. It's comforting to be that close to the person you love and know that nothing is going to happen to them right then, even if outside of those moments you are living in constant fear. Sex has shifted to being almost totally focused on what feels best for him and I wouldn't have it any other way."

She didn't mention anything about her own emotional journey, but it's worth noting that modern medicine is, by necessity, so focused on the person with the cancer that we sometimes forget that his or her lover can be suffering just as much. The lover may feel way too guilty to even allow themselves to be conscious of how much emotional pain they are in. (This is a reminder to healthcare professionals, who are sometimes pretty overwhelmed themselves.) As for the details of how this couple approach sex and cancer, here it is in her own words:

"We ended up trying me on top more because he didn't have to move as much and it can be less physically trying for him. He has less stamina so it's nice for him to be able to have sex without ending up completely exhausted. I was tentatively afraid that I would cripple him if I were on top, but it turned out to be a very successful position. He actually likes it best out of all the positions we've tried.

"Communication has turned out to be key because he has sudden nausea or pain sometimes, but if sex is done correctly (with proper communication and being cautious not to over-do it) it can actually make him feel better. Sometimes we start but he needs to rest and then we keep going in a few minutes. He lets me know if something I'm doing is good or if it's making him feel worse because some of the things we did before aren't good anymore (for instance I used to kiss him on the stomach and back and he used to love it but now it can make him nauseated.) Sometimes things like that feel good and sometimes they don't.

"He has good days where he can try different positions and places and bad days where we stick to me on top and we have intercourse in kind of a soft, relaxed setting. We discuss what he would like to do that day before we even start any foreplay and then he tells me if he's changed his mind anytime after that based on how he's feeling. That way we almost always avoid nausea, and intercourse can be great even with restrictions.

"During his chemotherapy, sometimes he has close to no sex drive and then we don't do much at all sexually, but he'll still do things like finger me just pretty much to be nice, since he's not so much up to anything sexual.

"I'd say if anything has increased it would be the number of blowjobs I give him because that's another thing that gives him pleasure but lets him remain pretty much still and comfortable. We don't have as much intercourse because he's just not up to it all the time."

Cancer of the Testicles

Please see Chapter 17: *Balls, Balls, Balls* for a discussion on the nuts and bolts of cancer of the testicles.

The people who worry most about their sexual appeal after cancer of the testicles tend to be younger straight guys, as well as gay males. Hopefully, the gay males won't put up with a partner for whom only one ball would be a deal breaker. As for the straight guys, we hate to burst your bubble, but based on how women have described the scrotum when we asked them about it on our sex survey, it's hard to think that they are going to dump any man because he's one nut short of a full load. Seriously, there aren't too many women who sit around fantasizing about men's balls or scrotums. So if you are the girlfriend or wife of a guy who's just been diagnosed, please let him know that it's unlikely you'd even notice 99.9% of the time.

Unlike other male cancers, it's a rare day when a man with cancer of the testicles won't be able to get an erection after surgery. His equipment will work just fine and he'll have the same amount of semen that he had before. Believe it or not, a lot of guys who have lost a ball to cancer don't have it replaced with a fake one, and are quite happy with their decision.

As for the psychological aspects of any and all things regarding cancer of the testicles, we defer to a man who knows a bit about it from firsthand experience, Mr. Doug Bank of the amazing Testicular Cancer Resource Center: http://tcrc.acor.org:

"I would like to stress that testicular cancer is not contagious and it cannot be transmitted via sexual intercourse. There are a lot of reasons to be afraid of cancer, but this is not one of them."

"Regarding sex drive, testicular-cancer survivors we have spoken with have told me everything from having sex the day after their surgery (ouch!) all the way through having to go on hormonal therapies to re-establish their desire—which would only be the 2% to 3% of guys who lose both testicles. In those cases, supplemental testosterone takes care of everything. The desire is still there and the ejaculation is still there.

"Just as each one of us is different going in, we're going to be just as different coming out, too. If you feel different, or just out of whack, let your doctor know. They cannot read your mind, and they definitely cannot diagnose anything if you do not tell them that something is wrong!"

Highly Recommended:

Woman, Cancer, Sex by Anne Katz, Hygeia Media

Man, Cancer, Sex by Anne Katz, Hygeia Media

Prostate Cancer and the Man You Love: Supporting and Caring for Your Partner by Anne Katz, Rowman & Littlefield Publishers

Surviving After Cancer: Living the New Normal, by Anne Katz, Rowman & Littlefield Publishers

Breast Cancer Husband, How to Help Your Wife (and Yourself) Through Diagnosis, Treatment and Beyond by Marc Silver, Rodale Books. If your partner has breast cancer, get this book!

79

Bashful Bladder

Finding the right home for this unusual subject was such a struggle that we decided to provide it with its own separate chapter. It didn't fit in with the chapter on sex fluids, or with sex at all. But if you struggle with being pee shy, you will be relieved by the discussion that follows.

Being Unable to Pee in Public

You wouldn't believe the number of people who have trouble using public rest rooms, and not because they don't like the smell or have hygiene issues. Being unable to relieve yourself in a public rest room is a very real problem that can be extremely limiting. Being pee-shy can get in the way taking a urinalysis at work or for a job interview. It's a problem any time you need to pee on demand, like at the doctor's office for a physical exam. People with this problem can even find it a challenge to urinate in a private bathroom while at a friend's home or when at a party.

A college student recently wrote in who was worried because he had enlisted in the Marine Corps and was soon going to ship out for basic training. He would sometimes walk up three flights of stairs in his college dorm to find an empty bathroom where he could relieve his bladder. He had no idea how he was going to manage in basic training, where there would be next to no privacy at all.

This problem is called paruresis or bashful bladder syndrome. For readers who don't have a bashful bladder, imagine what it's like never being able to pee while you are at a concert, baseball game, or when dining at a restaurant. Imagine what it's like when you seriously need to relieve yourself and your bladder freezes up whenever someone walks into the rest room.

For millions of Americans, this happens each and every time they try to urinate when they are not in their own home. The only safe place they can go for vacation is to the beach. Or maybe someone's swimming pool.

Paruresis exists in different degrees: some people who have it can go in a public rest room as long as they are in a closed stall. Others are unable to go in a rest room if anyone else is there, and some can't urinate at all if they are anywhere but home. They won't even try to enter a crowded rest room after a movie, between classes, or during an intermission at a large event.

You might have the idea that this is a wimp's disorder, e.g. "A real man could just whip it out and pee." But plenty of guys who have this problem are tough enough to take on any and all comers. They have no shortcomings with women or sex, and are in high demand on both scores. Not only is it impossible for them to go in a public bathroom, but some need to sit when they urinate at home for fear the stream will make noise and someone will know they are peeing. This is in stark contrast to the independent and able men who they are in other parts of their lives.

The problem often starts before adolescence. Some people with shy-bladder problems can remember back to a specific event that triggered the anxiety. For instance, a kid having to use a group urinal in a baseball stadium with a bunch of grown men who are standing around him peeing six innings' worth of beer. For others, the causes can be more unconscious.

Far more men have shy-bladder syndrome than women, but few women are asked to urinate next to each other without being in an enclosed stall. Guys are expected to go where other guys can watch, casually discussing the weather with each other while whipping it out and doing their business.

The problem can be severe enough that some people need to carry a catheter in order to relieve themselves. But the best way to deal with the problem is with desensitization techniques. For most people, these exercises can provide a decrease in the severity of their bashful-bladder problem These exercises are described in an excellent book which is recommended below.

HIGHLY RECOMMENDED: *Shy Bladder Syndrome—Your Step-By-Step Guide to Overcoming Paruresis* by Soifer, Zgourides, Himle and Pickering, New Harbinger. Also try visiting their excellent website at: www.paruresis.org This website provides a great list of articles and help.

CHAPTER

80
Sex & Diabetes

You're not going to believe this, but nowhere on the website of the American Diabetic Association do they discuss whether swallowing when giving a guy oral sex impacts your blood sugar level, or if diabetic girls taste sweeter. At least they were kind enough to intimate that nobody's diabetic penis is going to get gangrene, although you might hold off on wearing a cock ring. Decreased circulation and numbness can be a problem with diabetes, and why risk making it worse?

As for aerobic activity, just about anyone who has ever done a finger stick knows about the importance of exercise. Exercise increases the number of insulin receptors in your cells. This can help your insulin work better and make your diabetes easier to manage. Fortunately, there's no rule that says exercise can't be done while you are naked at home with your sweetheart rather than at a gym. Like with any exercise, check your BG and have a snack if needed.

Unfortunately, exercise that's sexercise needs a diabetic caveat or two. For instance, one reader had a nasty experience while performing oral sex on her boyfriend. It was her first time, so she assumed the funny feeling she was having was from being nervous. She was kneeling over the boy when she fainted from low blood sugar, almost choking on his penis. At least she thinks the culprit was low blood sugar.

Checking your blood sugar before, during and after sex is the last thing anyone feels like doing. But until you understand your body's reactions while making love, especially with a new partner, taking frequent readings is the only way you will learn. Also keep in mind that the emotional part of being with a new partner can add to the blood-sugar lowering potential.

You will want to learn about your body's reactions in the minutes and hours after sex. The muscles in a horny pelvis eat up extra glucose, especially when it's been rocking back and forth. And hormones like adrenaline, noradrenaline and prolactin are released during orgasm. They can change your blood sugar, sometimes dramatically.

A healthcare provider or diabetes educator can help you with lovemaking-management strategies. Should you adjust your insulin downward? Is it a good idea to inject yourself in the abdomen instead of your thigh before a love-making marathon, or does the bunny-like thrusting of hips cancel any slow-down in the insulin-absorption rate that you might hope to gain? Should you eat something other than your partner before, during or after having sex?

Since high blood sugar and ketones are best managed by drinking lots of water and exercise, highly-aerobic sex might be just what the doctor ordered. And peak insulin times simply require a food snack before your sex snack.

It is also essential to educate your partner about diabetes, and how he or she can recognize your hypoglycemic episodes and other possible problems. They need to know how to be in charge when you aren't, and what to do. It will be much harder to explain after the fact. Since most diabetics feel good as new in a few minutes to a few hours, it won't be long after treating a low when you and your partner will be back in the saddle.

Here are a few of many other sex-matters to consider:

💡Safe sex for diabetics includes keeping a pack of Lifesavers or glucose tablets next to the condoms and lube.

💡Women should watch out for blood-sugar weirdness a few days before and after their periods. If you can find any menstrual-related patterns, make adjustments in your diet, exercise, insulin, and sexual robustness.

💡High glucose in the blood means that more glucose is available in the urine. This can trigger an infection. Plenty of women discovered they were diabetic as a result of recurrent urinary-tract infections. If you get yeast infections, avoid lubes with glycerin.

💡Sugar binges from marijuana munchies can be a problem, although some people claim that marijuana helps even out their blood sugar. There aren't any studies on this, so please discuss it with your endocrinologist. Ecstasy can make you think you have boundless energy when your body is on its way to a blood-sugar low, and people on Ecstasy tend to drink lots of water, which lowers BGL. Problems from alcohol are the most dangerous of all. Alcohol raises BGL and can also result in dehydration. Alcohol-related lows usually come from being too polluted to eat or to remember to eat. When you have been partying, others around you will assume that any unusual behavior is from being drunk or stoned. You might not get the help you need. Be sure that friends you party with know what to do, although their responses might not be 100%, either.

🔆Decreased vaginal lubrication and erection problems are common side effects of diabetes, especially in sex-crazed seniors. These problems can be due to an interruption in nervous-system feedback, problems in circulation, or a combination of both. Store-bought lube without glycerin is a great equalizer for women, and Viagra-like medications are helpful for many males. Even if they aren't, this Guide is full of suggestions for pleasing your partner without needing to have an erection. If you do take erection medicine, don't get it over the Internet. Be sure to consult with your healthcare professional, and get a prescription from him or her.

🔆Peeing before and after sex can help reduce urinary-tract infections. If you are a female diabetic who gets frequent urinary-tract infections, consider shacking up with a partner who is into golden showers. Going on your guy will be killing two birds with one stone, or stream, although women who are kinky and infection prone should only be the doers and not the receivers of the golden stream.

🔆Be sure to wear a medical ID bracelet or tag, and if you're a man who cruises the parks or trails, you might put an extra tag on the waistband in the front of your briefs where it's more likely to be seen.

🔆If you can't live without getting your love parts pierced, the chances of getting an infection are higher when your blood glucose levels (BGLs) are elevated. Infections will increase the scarring around piercing sites and they will make your BGLs shoot even higher. Get thee to a health-care provider at the slightest indication of an infection. Also, tongue piercings will make your tongue swollen and sore, which will inspire you to skip meals, which can lead to a hypoglycemic episode.

🔆We hate to mention the following little nastiness, and hope it applies to no readers of *The Guide*. But rumor has it that some girls will skip their insulin in order to keep their BGLs high. This results in decreased appetite. This kind of "weight-loss program" is dangerous and dumb.

As for inspiration, one of the founders of sex therapy had diabetes for most of his life. Management had been so difficult that he had to inject himself twice a day. His name was Albert Ellis and he recently died at the age of 93. He said that while staying on top of his diabetes had always been a pain, the bigger pain was if he didn't. Ellis had been quite the sex radical during his 93 years, and he was even a fan of *The Guide*. Out of the blue, he sent a very kind e-mail saying it was one of the best sex books he had ever read. Imagine that, still reading and writing sex books when you are in your 90s!

Diabetes doesn't mean you can't be as good or bad as anyone else in bed. As with everything else in life, it just means that you've got to plan ahead and jump through a few more hoops.

A Special Thanks to Ricky Siegel, a sex educator, therapist, and member of Planned Parenthood, and to Barry McCarthy, an author and leader in sex education who also has diabetes. Also, to Bill Taverner, for putting the word out!

81

Sex When You Are Horny & Disabled

Astory appeared on the Internet about a 22-year-old man with cerebral palsy who has virtually no control over his body's movements. He started using his wheelchair antisocially, as a ramming device. He was running over anything he could. Eventually, this young man wrote on his word-board that he was so horny he couldn't stand it anymore. Although his body has the same sexual urges and desires as an able-bodied 22-year-old, he has no ability to walk, talk or masturbate like the average 22-year-old. He can't even download porn or surf adult websites.

As quickly as they began, this young man's wheelchair tantrums stopped. The reason? A nurse's aide mercifully began giving him handjobs. But then she was caught and fired instantly. The board-and-care home threatened to file a complaint against her for sexual abuse.

Sexy & Disabled?

If you think you are fair-minded about sexual matters, consider a quadriplegic who wheels by in an electric wheelchair. The person drools a little and steers the chair with a joy stick that's strapped to his forehead. Do you think of this person as being sexual? Do you think he has the same sexual needs and desires as you? Chances are you'd wonder how good his jump shot is before you'd think of him as being just as horny as you are.

Many people not only disapprove of sex for the severely disabled, but find the concept offensive. They might even feel that we need to protect people who are disabled from sex.

Dear Paul,

I'm a paraplegic. From where I sit, I have women's rears and crotches in my face all day long. You have no idea how much restraint it takes to keep my

hands to myself. Last week I copped a feel but apologized and blamed it on my
"bad driving" and "spastic hand."

Dude from Dubuque

Dude,

There's not an able-bodied guy on the planet who could come face-to-tail with as much anatomy as you do and not want to reach out and touch some. You must consider a crowded elevator to be a gift from God, as well as one of life's great torments. **Counterpoint:** I recently received a letter regarding my response to Dude because I didn't chastise him for his inappropriate actions. "I am really disappointed that you suggest in your response that a man couldn't be expected to withhold his sexual desire and that it's fine to occasionally use a woman's body for your own purpose."

One reason why so many of us blanch at the idea of a disabled person having sex is because the advertising industry spends billions of dollars each year trying to narrow our concept of what sexual attractiveness is. Never do advertisers tell us that sexual appeal might have something to do with integrity and character, given how those can't be paid for with a credit card. Forget even existing sexually if you are missing a few fingers or an entire leg, slur your words when you talk or are paralyzed from the chest down.

A huge hurdle for many disabled people is being able to accept themselves as being sexual. If you don't accept yourself as being a sexual person, it is unlikely that others will.

Roll Models

"Prior to my becoming blind, the only person who was blind that I had seen was a beggar. I was horrified to think that this was the only option available to me as a person who was blind." From an article on women who are blind by Ellen Rubin in *Sexuality and Disability*.

One of the more discouraging aspects of having a disability is that positive role models are few and far between. If you ask people to name a famous disabled person, just as many will say the Hunchback of Notre Dame as Franklin Delano Roosevelt. Of the two, FDR was a real-life American president who provided people with a real sense of sanctuary, although he was unable to walk unaided. There were reasons why FDR tried to hide his disability. When he was a young man, disabled people were considered a success if they could get a job in the circus.

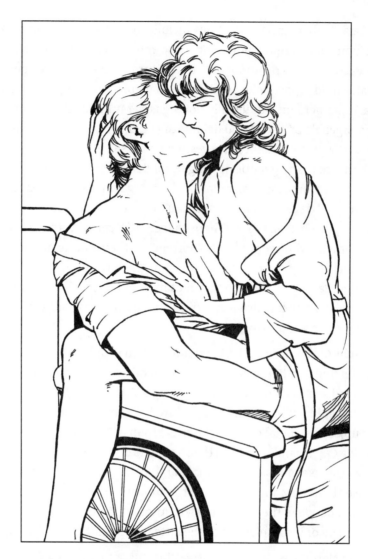

Different Ways That Disabilities Happen

When people are disabled from crashes and accidents, it is often because the spinal cord was damaged. About 85% of spinal-cord injuries happen to men, many in their teens and twenties. That's because men have a penchant for doing things that involve speed or collisions. For instance, if a boy says he needs "pads," you might assume he's talking about something to put under his football jersey. If a girl says she needs "pads," it's likely that she's referring to sanitary napkins. In addition to sports and car crashes, disabilities might come from gun wounds, stabbings, fist fights or a serious bonk on the head.

Diseases that cause disabilities include arthritis, which can make inter-course painful or cripple your fingers so much that you can't masturbate. Polio can make it nearly impossible to walk or breathe and can result in prob-lems later in life (post-polio syndrome). Diabetes can hamper an erection or vaginal engorgement, but usually not orgasm. Multiple sclerosis can be mild and manageable or severe and debilitating. Cancer and the treatments for it can impact a person's ability and desire to have sex.

There are many genetic or congenital disorders that can cause disabili-ties. Certain chromosome disorders can damage a person's physical growth and/or mental development. Congenital disorders might result in dwarfism or being top-shelf challenged. (There's a recent TV series that follows a family with dwarfism who seem just as "normal" as their tall neighbors.) Medica-tions taken during pregnancy can result in the birth of infants with severe disabilities. Parental exposure to pollutants and chemicals can cause birth defects. Disabilities can also result from strokes and heart attacks or cerebral palsy and muscular dystrophy.

Spinal-Cord Injury (SCI) Shorthand: When people with spinal-cord inju-ries are talking to other people with spinal-cord injuries, they sometimes use a shorthand such as "I'm a C-4 quad" or "I'm a T-3." This code refers to the loca-tion on the spine where the injury occurred. For instance, a C-4 injury occurs higher up on the spinal cord (in the neck) than a T-3, so it is likely that a per-son with a C-4 is paralyzed from the shoulders down (quadriplegic), whereas a T-3 has the use of his or her arms (paraplegic), and an L-4 most likely has more use than a C-4 or T-3 because the injury happened at a point on the spinal cord between the ribs and pelvis. Another factor is whether the injury was complete or incomplete, with the latter supposedly being less severe.

Quad Note: Thanks to Tom Street for this info. Tom is a C-4 quad from an auto accident in 1988. Tom manufactures a computer mouse for quadriple-gics called the QuadJoy. This special mouse, combined with extra software that Tom has written, allows the user to run the entire computer, including keyboard, by mouth. The full range of clicking and dragging happens by vir-tue of puffing and sucking on the end of the joystick. This can be particularly helpful for a quad who would like to interact with others in chat rooms or who would like to see Internet porn in PRIVATE and without the help of an attendant. Tom can be reached on the internet at www.quadjoy.com.

Chronic vs. Acute

There are disabilities that happen all at once. They don't keep getting worse. This is true of most spinal-cord injuries. There are other disabilities, usually caused by diseases, which have symptoms that worsen over time.

For some people, it is easier to have a disability that starts off worse but stays the same. For instance, once people with spinal-cord injuries are able to learn how to deal with their disability, they can be pretty sure that their condition won't worsen and they won't have to learn a whole new set of skills just to stay even. People with chronic illnesses have a more uncertain future and may have to constantly readapt as their illness progresses. The uncertainty of a chronic illness makes it more difficult to get on with your life, as you never know when your disease is going to pull the rug out from under you. Of course, you can say that none of us has any guarantees for the future, but the uncertainty of everyday life is much easier to cope with than the uncertainty of a disease that is getting worse.

Even the recovery process is different for someone with an acute injury as opposed to a chronic illness. Consider a person who had his leg amputated after being run over in the parking lot at the 7-Eleven as opposed to having a leg amputated due to complications from diabetes. Outside of not getting to finish his Slurpee, the person who lost his leg at the 7-Eleven had no pre-existing condition and must face only the problems associated with the amputation. The person with progressive diabetes has to cope with numerous problems caused by the diabetes in addition to those that are specific to the amputation. Mind you, neither situation is enviable.

Also, the treatments for disabilities or illnesses can cause sexual problems. For instance, tricyclic antidepressants are often prescribed to help with the neurogenic pain that can occur after spinal-cord injury. These drugs can decrease the desire to have sex as well as the ability to have an erection and to ejaculate. The same is true for certain cancer treatments that adversely affect the sexuality of both men and women. (See *Chapter 78: Sex and Breast, Brain & Ball Cancer*.)

Double Your Trouble

As if it weren't bad enough to have your spinal cord injured, accidents that cause the damage are often severe enough to also cause traumatic head injury. Not only does the person have to cope with possible paralysis from the spinal injury, but he or she may also experience low sexual drive, poor impulse control or unpredictable behavior from the brain injury.

Can Men in Wheelchairs Get Hard-Ons?

People sometimes wonder if guys in wheelchairs can get hard-ons, but they don't wonder if women in wheelchairs can get wet! Why's that? Contrary to what you might think, a lot of males who are in wheelchairs are able to get erections. The stimulation for the erection will often need to come from direct physical contact with the genitals rather than from feeling horny, as the link between the horny center in the brain and the genitals is often damaged. Guys with disabilities can often get good erections with the help of vacuum pumps or injections. Men with higher-level spinal-cord injuries (usually quads, not paraplegics) tend to get reflex erections. These happen when the penis is being touched and have little connection to feeling horny. They usually go down as soon as the touching stops, but some couples learn how to keep the stimulation going so they can have intercourse.

Able-bodied men often become aware of their own sexual arousal by feeling their penis grow. Men who are paralyzed have to rely on other signals to know when they are aroused, e.g. nipples getting hard, goosebumps, heavier breathing and a heart that beats faster. These aren't any different from what able-bodied men experience, but how many guys notice subtle physical clues when their penises are screaming, "Look at Me!"

Women with spinal-cord injuries may find that the sexual wetness in their vagina is decreased or absent. Using a lubricant during intercourse can be helpful. Many women with spinal-cord injuries are able to have orgasms. Bregman and Hadley interviewed a number of women with spinal-cord injuries and found that their descriptions of orgasm were similar to those of women with no spinal-cord injury. Also, some people with spinal-cord injury have orgasms that are referred to as "para-orgasms," which are different from genital orgasms but are quite compelling. Para-orgasms can be so strong that women who are injured above the T-6 level need to be aware of rapid changes in their blood pressure.

Both women and men who no longer have traditional orgasms can learn to experience a type of orgasm that is called an emotional orgasm. This kind of orgasm results in a rush of relaxation and calm in the rest of the body that's like the afterglow of an orgasm.

Whether a person can or can't have an orgasm, the good feelings that most able-bodied people get from being touched and loved are still massively satisfying for someone who is disabled. One person with a spinal-cord injury reported, "Before my accident I couldn't get enough stimulation from the waist down; now I can't get enough from the waist up!" When a person is paralyzed, areas such as the back of the neck and arms can become extremely sensitive in a sexual way. Also, plenty of disabled people report that watching a partner doing something sexual to them can be very satisfying even if they can't feel the actual sensations. The brain is able to fill in the missing pieces.

Vibrator Note: Vibrators can be a helpful sexual aid for men and women with disabilities. They can supply the necessary stimulation when a hand is unable. If you tend to be incontinent, consider getting a vibrator that's rechargeable or has batteries. Urine is a far better conductor of electricity than water, making plug-in models a wee bit risky. If your hands are too crippled to use a regular vibrator, it's possible to embed one in a Nerf ball.

"Will I Be Able to Have Children?"

This seems like a simple, straightforward question. But it is often an indirect way of asking, "Will I be able to have sex?" "Will anyone want to have sex with me?" "How in the blazes do I have sex now that I'm like this?" The answer to all of these questions is usually yes, unless the person stays in a full-time funk and never transitions out of asking "Why me?" Try as they might, nobody but God or nature has an answer to the "Why me?" question, assuming there is an answer.

Most women with disabilities are able to become pregnant. This is why most disabled women need to use birth control, even if they are paralyzed from the shoulders down. Many men who are paralyzed have problems ejaculating. Physicians are having some success helping these men to ejaculate by sticking electrodes up their rears and shocking the crap out of nerves in the prostate region. Some guys with spinal-cord injuries above T-12 are able to ejaculate with the help of a vibrator on the penis.

Born with It vs. Got It Along the Way

Unless they are in a rock'n'roll band, most people who make it to adulthood have achieved a certain level of maturity. But if a person was disabled at a young age, it's possible that this has gotten in the way of achieving the maturity to behave as a responsible and caring adult. For instance, how does a kid who is disabled at age 16 progress through the usual steps toward independence if he or she needs a parent to get them out of bed and dressed each morning? If in a rehab center, how does he or she get the privacy to explore sexually as other kids do? How do they masturbate with crippled hands?

Consider the following questions posed by a therapist who works with the disabled: "How does a young girl in a wheelchair learn how adults are sexual if her parents are afraid to be that way in front of her? How does she explore her parents' drawers when they are out and find books, movies, condoms, sponges, lingerie and so forth—as many youths do—if she cannot get into their bedroom? How can she find her brother's copies of sexually explicit publications if she cannot get under his bed where they are stashed?" [From "Performing a Sexual Evaluation on the Person With Disability or Illness" by Kenneth A. Lefebre in *Sexual Function in People with Disability and Chronic Illness*, Marca Sipski and Craig Alexander, Aspen Publishers.]

People who are disabled at a young age will become adults with the same sexual drives and desires as anyone who is not disabled. However, they may be missing a sense of appropriate ways to satisfy their sexual urges. To help fill in the missing pieces, parents and educators of disabled kids need to be more open rather than less about sexual issues.

Sex & People Who Are Developmentally Disabled

It is not likely that people who are developmentally disabled will be reading this book, although we know of one such woman by the name of Linda who loves looking at the pictures! People with developmental disabilities have the same sexual urges and desires as people without disabilities. They simply go through the stages of sexual development at a slower pace.

The developmentally disabled pose special problems when it comes to sexual training, because they may need a good deal of repetitive explanation about things that many adults feel uncomfortable saying even once. Also, in their drive toward sexual pleasure, developmentally disabled kids may be even less apt to use birth control than their nondisabled partners in crime.

If you are the parent of a disabled child, or you work with people who are disabled, you might be at a loss for finding good references to help you in dealing with your child's sexual growth. *For a helpful list of resources, put disabled into the search box at www.GuideToGettingItOn.com.*

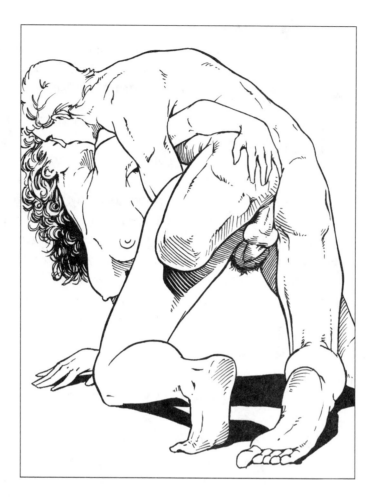

Body Image

If a person has been disabled for a long time, particularly from a young age, his body image might also include a wheelchair or braces, scars from surgeries, hands that are twisted and not particularly dexterous, a voice that slurs words, a head that doesn't sit straight on its shoulders or other features that aren't always like those of his or her peers. It may be very difficult for a person who is disabled to feel attractive and effective if they can't see themselves as separate from the devices that help them to survive. As a result, they might need plenty of feedback that you value them as a person in the same way that you do someone who doesn't have a wheelchair, braces or disfigurements.

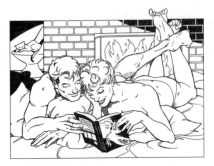

Dear Paul,

We both have spinal-cord injuries and are disabled. Yet we like watching porn that shows able-bodied people having sex. Is this weird?

Rhonda from Rolling Hills

Dear Rhonda,

None of us here have nine-inch penises, last forty-five minutes, come in buckets or have partners who like taking it ten different ways, but we like watching pornography, too. If most of it weren't so boring, we'd watch it more often! Keep in mind that pornography is a fantasy. It helps us go places in our minds where many of us wouldn't go in reality even if we could. Now here's a question for you: I'll bet you aren't worried about watching able-bodied actors in TV or movies, so why when it comes to porn do you suddenly worry about being crippledly correct?

Explaining Yourself & Educating Others

"People do have all these kinds of curiosity, and you have to find ways of making them feel more comfortable around you at first."

Steve, on the videotape *Sexuality Reborn*

Just like people who are able-bodied, people who are disabled need to learn their own sexual strengths and weaknesses and then teach a partner about themselves. For someone who has had a stroke, it might be important to lie on their affected side so they can use their active arm for caressing a partner. Likewise, they might have a "visual field cut" which causes them to ignore one side of their partner's body. The partner needs to let them know about this. (This example by way of social worker Sharon Bacharach.)

When it comes to enjoying sex, different disabilities pose different challenges. For instance, if you can't use your hands in a way that allows you to masturbate, then figuring out how to do that will be one of your first challenges. If you need help breathing but want to give a partner oral sex, you might need to alternate sucking on your partner's genitals with sucking breaths of air from your respirator hose. If you can't have intercourse, then you'll need to work out ways of pleasing both yourself and your partner without it. (This book has plenty of chapters that describe ways of doing that.) Perhaps your disability has left you with little nerve sensation in your genitals, but the opening of your anus is still sensitive; stimulating it might bring you to orgasm. Perhaps your neck, lips, cheeks or nipples are highly sensitized to touch. Maybe it helps if you take a warm bath or shower or to have a beer or glass of wine before having sex. This is just as true for able-bodied people.

Goodbye to Spontaneity

Some able-bodied couples don't like to use a condom because the thirty seconds it takes to put it on destroys the mood for them. Think of how resilient "the mood" has to be when it takes all sorts of preparations and maneuvers to be ready to have sex! Think of how resilient the mood has to be if one partner cries out in pain and adjustments need to be made in order to continue.

One of the things that people who are disabled might lose is the sexual spontaneity that able-bodied couples take for granted unless they are parents with kids who are still at home. Consider the following advice that was recently posted on the Internet:

> "Patience is truly a virtue in disability-related sex. Disability often destroys something in sex, spontaneity for one thing. Drugs, fatigue, depression, neurological impairment can also be a destructive force. Utilizing the turn-on can partially make up for what has been taken away. Sometimes erotic books, photos or videos can enhance the performance. The type and degree of disability often demands traveling that extra mile or two. "   Peter Love

Getting into Relationships

"Why would any man want this body?" "No woman's going to want this!" Some people who have disabilities feel that nobody will find them sexually attractive. As a result, they might push away people who do. Or, at the other end of the spectrum, they might offer themselves to the first person who shows interest, even if it is not someone they like or trust. A disabled person without a solid sense of self might be starved for affection or desperately need to prove that he or she is desirable. Of course, one doesn't need to be disabled to have hang-ups, but it can be extra-difficult when your physical ducks aren't in the same row as everyone else's.

Regarding the subject of dating and people with disabilities, a woman with cerebral palsy recently commented, "I think women are more accepting of differences than men. I see a lot more disabled men married or in serious relationships. I see a lot more disabled women just giving up." There are plenty of disabled men who say it's equally tough for them. Another disabled woman says one of the reasons she fell in love with her husband "was the idea that here was a person who looked and acted OK, wanting to have a relationship with me."

People with disabilities sometimes shy away from dating other people who are disabled. When you are disabled yourself, there can be a kind of hatred of other people who are disabled—an inner need to say, "I'm not like them." There can also be the added problem of social acceptance. Two people in wheelchairs humming down the sidewalk garner far more stares from able-bodied pedestrians than does one.

The Disabled Couple

Perhaps the most difficult aspect of being in a relationship where one or both members are disabled is that ultimately, the couple has to face the same kinds of fights, squabbles, disagreements and difficulties as couples who have no physical disability. As for how disability affects a couple, some able-bodied couples stay in love with each other only as long as each partner is able to mirror the other's sexual attractiveness. If one member starts to look older than the other, slows down or becomes disabled, the relationship may quickly dissolve. With other couples, there is a deep love and friendship that transcends physical change.

When there is a new disability, it is not uncommon for both partners to experience frustration, anger, fear, disappointment, and helplessness. Roles within the relationship may change. Neither the able-bodied member nor the one who is disabled should be afraid to seek help and advice from social workers and rehab staff.

When it comes to sexual intimacy, a couple with a new disability may need to learn anew. This might actually be a relief to your partner if you weren't as good in bed as you thought you were! The good news is that couples who had a rewarding sex life before the disability usually find a way to have a good sex life after.

If you are a couple whose primary expression of sexuality was through intercourse, you may have a good deal of adjusting ahead. It will be easier if you are a couple whose sexuality included a full range of sensory experiences, like enjoying the beauty of a sunset, holding hands and caressing each other.

Also, if you can afford it, it would be wise to hire an attendant to perform caretaking functions. Otherwise, a parent/child dynamic can evolve between you and your partner which can intrude on feelings of sexual passion.

With a Deaf Ear & Twinkle in His Eye

A woman who is a friend of the Goofy Foot Press works with deaf people and has also had sex with one or two deaf men. She said that she never realized how much she relies on verbal cues from a partner until she was romanced by a deaf man. Whether it's being in another room or looking down when you are having a bowl of soup, the usual conditions for connection are suddenly missing when a partner can't hear. With a deaf partner, there is no hearing without seeing. She said that the lack of verbal give-and-take is particularly noticeable during sex, whether it's oral sex or intercourse.

People who are deaf are obviously more comfortable with verbal silence during romance and lovemaking than are people who can hear. If our friend is sleeping with a man who is deaf, she lets him know that she needs more input than he might be used to giving a partner who is also deaf. She also says that it is important to have some of the lights on when you are making love to a deaf person, so they can either see you sign or read your lips. On the other hand, deaf people sometimes sign on each other's skin, or if they are in a spoons position, the person in the back can reach around a partner's body and sign in front where the partner can see.

Attacking Their Own

While many people who are disabled would welcome an increased awareness that they are just as sexual as anyone else, some clearly don't. A few years ago, when a mainstream glossy magazine for disabled people ran a story on sex and the disabled, some disabled readers were so upset that they canceled their subscriptions. You might think that the story was *Hustler*-like and included photos of the naked disabled doing things that would have pleased Caligula. In reality, the article was so tame that it could have been published in *Parade* magazine or *House & Garden*. Perhaps the subject of sex brings up huge amounts of frustration and sadness for some disabled people, to the point where they simply get angry at sex itself.

So You Won't Have to Read the "Sex during Pregnancy" Chapter Unless You Want To

Women can get pregnant in a wheelchair just as easily as they can get pregnant in any other chair. Don't think that because you are disabled or paralyzed from the shoulders or waist down you somehow can't get pregnant. Be sure to speak to each other and to your physician about birth control.

Note: Until recently, it was believed that birth-control pills, shots and implants might be unsafe for some women who are in wheelchairs. It's not the wheelchair that's the problem, but proneness to circulatory problems and blood clots that can be increased by the birth-control pill. If your gynecologist isn't used to working with women who have disabilities, check with the *National Spinal Cord Foundation* for a referral.

Attendants and Caregivers —The Good and Bad of It

Powerful feelings can develop between people who are patients and those who are hired to care for them—both loving and hateful. It is beyond the scope of this book to explore the different possibilities, except to say that it does little good to turn a blind eye to the dynamics that can arise between caretaker and caregiver.

If you are able-bodied, consider for a moment the issue of privacy. The kind of privacy that able-bodied people take for granted might not exist for someone who is disabled. This can range from bathing and completing bowel movements to preparing for masturbation and sex. It may be necessary for a disabled person to share private aspects of themselves with an attendant that some able-bodied people don't feel comfortable sharing even with a partner of many years.

Considering the level of dependency that some disabled people have, opportunities for abuse by attendants are rife. This is a huge issue, and abuse is unfortunately quite common. It is important that disabled people speak up against assistants who are abusive. If this is a concern for you, please contact your local center for independent living.

Helping the Helpers

To have fulfilling sex lives, people with disabilities need the help of several different medical subspecialities. These might include neurology, psychology, urology, oncology, endocrinology, physical and rehabilitative medicine and sex therapy. Unfortunately, getting medical specialists to work together in a collaborative effort requires that professional egos be set aside. The problem multiplies when the issue is sex, since many of the professionals who need to work together might be uncomfortable with the subject at hand.

If you are a disabled person who is struggling to get assistance with your sexual needs, maybe it will help if you give your healthcare provider a copy of this book opened to this chapter. Perhaps it will help them feel more at ease in aiding you with sexual matters. After all, it's quite likely that they, too, enjoy sex and would be more than happy to help you if they were just able to feel more comfortable.

Rehab Note: When rehab therapists get around to mentioning sex, it is usually in combination with discussions about bowel and bladder functioning. This is most unfortunate. People who are newly disabled need access to positive information about sexuality early in their rehabilitation. Even if they reject the information, it is something positive that will remain in their consciousness, to be accessed at another time.

Stroke Studies — Interesting for a Number of Reasons

Stroke survivors, as a group, experience a drop in sexual activity. Until recently, this was thought to have physical, rather than emotional, causes. However, a study of stroke survivors by Buzzellie, di Francesco, Giaquinto and Nolte concluded that "psychological issues, rather than medical ones, account for disruption of sexual functioning in stroke survivors."

It is especially significant that the researchers found no differences in the sexual functioning of people with right-brained lesions as opposed to left-brain lesions or contralateral lesions. This contradicts our modern tendency to view behaviors as coming from one side of the brain or the other. This study indicates that sexuality is neither "right-brained" nor "left-brained."

Recommended Resources

Sexuality Reborn is an excellent video in which four likeable and articulate couples tell about their personal experience with sex and disability. At least one person in each couple is wheelchair-assisted. It is very helpful for both disabled and able-bodied viewers. College instructors who use the *Guide to Getting It On!* in their classes are highly encouraged to show this to their students. A great deal of humanness is conveyed without a moment of pity or self-absorption. There is something about the honesty and genuineness of the couples who speak in this video that gives able-bodied people a more realistic and grounded perception of people who are disabled. There are parts of the video where the couples are naked and having sex, but it isn't in a way that's going to ruffle the feathers of your dean or regents. The only criticism that reviewers had was that the occasional comments by the talking-head medical specialists seemed unnecessary and detracted from, rather than added, to the video's effectiveness.

Untold Desires shows interviews about sex with people who have all kinds of disabilities. This award-winning documentary contains no nudity and makes an excellent companion tape for *Sexually Reborn*. We seriously hope that anyone going through a rehab program would get to see both videos. Included is a wonderful interview with a woman who has severe cerebral palsy. She is astute, funny, and energetic. The video provides subtitles when she speaks because her speech is so CP-involved. The interviews with other disabled people are equally valuable. As an additional bonus, there is spectacular footage of one chair-assisted man skiing down a steep mountain and a disabled dude racing down stairs and streets. Redefines the term "No Fear." Highly recommended for people with disabilities as well as those without.

Murderball is not about sex, but the next best thing: quads who play rugby. This is full-contact rugby in wheelchairs that would make Mad Max proud. They end up competing in the Paralympic Games. If people with disabilities can do this, they can make sex work.

RECOMMENDED: *The Ultimate Guide to Sex and Disability,* by Miriam Kaufman, Cory Silverberg and Fran Odette, Cleis Press. This is full of helpful suggestions and ideas, and should be on the shelf of any individual or couple who is experiencing disabilities or chronic pain.

Citations—Both quotes in the section "Getting into Relationships" are from "Dating Issues for Women with Physical Disabilities," *Sexuality and Disability,* by Rintals, Howland, Nosek, et al.

82
Snoring & Passing Gas

The best love-making techniques in the world will take you only so far if your sleeping self passes enough gas to blow the sheets off the bed, or if you snore so loudly that your partner has to check into a hotel, without you. Do both, and your relationship is in double jeopardy.

Flatulence

People with the healthiest diets tend to pass more gas rather than less, but then again, so do people who drink a lot of beer. Whether your gas is from granola or *Three Floyds Dark Lord Russian Imperial Stout,* there are things that you can do to keep your co-workers from calling you the human crop-duster.

The average bum releases from one to three pints of wind each day. But the real killer is that not all air biscuits are created equal. Some are little worse than musty turnips; others can fell men in uniform.

No matter how burly or dainty your lover is, he or she has between fourteen and twenty events a day. Pound-for-pound, girls pass as much gas as guys. It is foods full of complex carbohydrates that make the foul winds blow: everything from fresh fruit to beans and broccoli–virtually anything that's good for you. The thing that creates the ghastly odor is foods that contain sulphur.

Since the array of bacteria in our large intestines varies from person to person, a food that hardly causes a ruffle in Bob's boxers might blow Betty's dress up to the ceiling. And Brooke might be a poster child for the Milk Advisory Board with nary a bark from her bum, while anything more than a cup of milk or a single egg can cause Brianne to clear out an entire gymnasium.

If friends issue a foul-wind advisory whenever you spend the night, try to find what you might be eating that is generating so much gas. You also need to determine if your gas is a normal by product of digestion, or if it is a symptom of a medical condition that can include constipation, ulcers, gastric reflux, irritable bowel syndrome and several other things including cancer.

Only a healthcare professional can help you chase down the medical causes. There are also a number of medications that can cause an increase in gas, as well as sugar substitutes such as sorbitol and xylitol.

If you think the culprit is food, be mindful that it is often combinations of foods rather than just one food that makes a rectum rumble. Start eliminating foods on a trial-and-error basis, although we suggest you keep the chips and tequila until the very end. Also, below a certain threshold, things like onions and mushrooms might be fine, but serve yourself a second helping, and you're a poop-chute flute.

As for things like Beano, simethicone, and holistic approaches such as peppermint and ginger, don't hold your breath. What might work for one person won't stop a single toot in the next.

One of the best articles available on the subject of gas or flatulence is by Margaret C. McDonald, *The Facts About Flatulence*. It can currently be found online at www.spectrox.com/flatulence.html.

Also, there is a highly-effective carbon-embedded seat cushion that not only filters out the bad smell, but muffles the sound. It's the same material that is used in Haz-Mat operations, but packaged so well that no one at your office or sorority will know. You can fart to your heart's content while sitting on the thing, and offend no one. Their website is www.gasbgon.com, and their phone number is 877-GASBGON. Talk about a Christmas present that will blow your loved ones over! We test drove two of them here at Goofy Foot Press. We threw everything we had at 'em. Here's the official Goofy-Foot review: "Tired of your loved ones searching under your chair to make sure the cat didn't die? The GasBGon seat cushion works well enough that you don't sound like such a fool when you blame the kids or the dog. And you can take one to bed with you, much to your partner's relief."

One thing that we learned in researching this pressing problem is that there are people with serious physical problems who are unable to control when, where and how much they fart. This now explains the author's entire sixth-grade year in Sister Justina Isabel's class. Some people with serious gas problems are so mortified that they never go out in public, but that never stopped her. The GasBGone company makes carbon-embedded underwear and seat cushions that can help free people with these disorders from their gastric confinements. And if you're a guy who has trouble thrusting without kicking out some serious smells, cut a hole in front of the Haz-Mat Depends to pull your penis through. Too bad GasBGone doesn't make them with a built-in cock ring to help prevent blow-by.

By way of summary, don't let gas put a cloud of uncertainty over the future of your relationship. In the order of things in life, the fart is mightier than the desire to have sex, at least in people who you might have sex with. Fortunately, there are things most of us can do to get it under control.

Snoring

At least with gas, you get a measure of your own medicine. Not so with snoring. Snoring is on the short-list of problems that cause sexual partners to sleep in separate bedrooms. Unless the snorer has sleep apnea, he or she is unlikely to be impacted by the snoring, except for wondering why his or her partner is so cranky about it.

Snoring is an acoustical nastiness that happens when your breath collides against tissue that's inside your nose or throat. It mostly happens during sleep, because muscle tone in the throat decreases after the sandman pays a visit. The air rushing past the sagging tissue causes vibrations that can make your sleeping self sound like a drowning donkey.

Another culprit might be a blockage in your nasal pathway. This could be from a broken nose, a chronic allergy, infection, or structural defect. It can either be the sole source of your snoring (called nasal-based snoring), or it can cause you to breathe through your mouth, which gives you the snoring capacity of a level-5 hurricane.

Your tongue can also be contributing to the problem, but you don't have to be asleep for your tongue to get you in trouble.

Being overweight, drinking, smoking, and taking drugs are at the top of a long list of snoring stimulators. Hopefully, you are starting to get the idea that snoring can have an array of different causes. Until you determine the specific cause or combination of causes, you will have better luck milking a moose than finding a cure.

You might also have sleep apnea—which is at the Mayday end of the snoring continuum. This is when your breathing stops for more than ten seconds at a time. When that happens, the sensors in your brain suddenly say, "Oops, looks like we're dying!" and they generate a snort that sounds like feeding time at the pig farm. This can happen hundreds of times each night, with periods of dead silence followed by wickedly-loud snorts.

Sleep apnea is always a sign of danger and needs evaluation by a sleep specialist. It can be a forewarning of heart problems, high blood pressure, and diabetes. It can also cause extreme fatigue and depression because it interferes with REM or dream sleep. Treatment might include a special type of mouth piece or a device that blows air into the sleeping lungs, as well as dire warnings to lose weight, start exercising, and stop smoking and drinking.

There are all sorts of people who are happy to take your money for snoring cures. There are also physicians who will hack up the back of your throat in the name of curing the problem, even though there are few studies on the safety or long-term effectiveness of these procedures.

Why not get a voice-activated tape recorder and a mic to put on the headboard or wall above your head? Also, get a clock that speaks the hour. This will activate the recorder so you can learn what part of the night your snoring occurs. Conventional snorers will often start sawing logs as soon as they fall asleep, while snorers with sleep apnea tend to build steam later in the night. Sleep experts can get important clues about the cause of your snoring based upon its pitch, frequency and timing. The tape recording will help them and you to understand more about the problems.

Once a sleep specialist is able to pinpoint the cause of your snoring, research the heck out of it. UNDER NO CIRCUMSTANCES should you agree to any surgeries or throat injections without getting a second opinion by a specialist who doesn't work with the first one. Spend lots of time on snoring forums reading the posts of people who have had the various procedures.

Recommended: One snoring aid that looked promising was exercises for strengthening the muscle tone in the throat. These were designed by Alise Ojay, a singing instructor in England. They seem to be quite helpful when the problem is caused by lax throat muscles. Why not give this a try before letting a doctor cut up the back of your throat or inject funky substances into it? Read the articles on this woman's website: www.SingingForSnorers.com.

Take Heed!

If loved ones are at their wits end due to your snoring, please don't ignore them because you can't hear yourself. Hook up the tape recorder as we suggest, so you can get an idea of what has them in such a state. And then, for the sake of your relationship if not for yourself, set out to learn all you can about the problem. Put together a plan of action, and see if you can't improve the situation.

CHAPTER
83
Sex & Hysterectomy

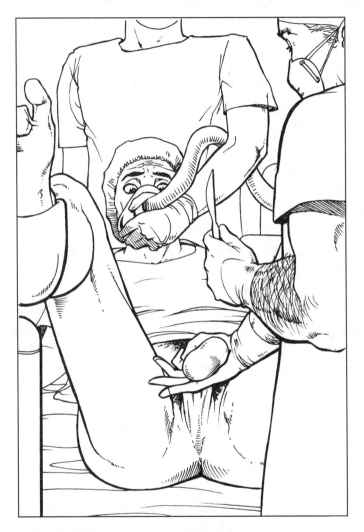

Does the Thought of This Make You Uncomfortable?

If a woman in our society has her reproductive organs removed, no one takes much notice. It's an everyday surgical event. But if a man has his testicles removed, we gasp. Are a man's organs more important?

Until the 1990s, when managed health care started taking a closer look at surgeries, approximately 665,000 hysterectomies were performed each year on women at an average age of 42.5 years. A university professor who was a second-opinion expert for Blue Cross reported, "The patients who had the recommendations for the hysterectomies either had no pathology whatsoever or had pathology that was so minimal it was inexplicable to me how anybody could have recommended surgery."

There are times when hysterectomy is necessary to save a woman's life, as in cases where cervical or ovarian cancer is found. Hopefully, if your physician recommends a hysterectomy, you will seek a second opinion. It is your body and your right.

Hysterectomy & Sex

There is nowhere near the kind of solid research on hysterectomy and sex that you would think, given the large number of hysterectomies that are done each year. To help with any decisions you might need to make, Annie Bradford, a researcher from the University of Texas at Austin, has been kind enough to offer the following perspective to readers of *The Guide:*

"If I were a woman who is preparing to have a hysterectomy, there are a few things I would want to be asked. First, I would like my physician to discuss the possibility of less aggressive/less invasive treatment alternatives—hysterectomy isn't the only option for an increasing number of diseases. I would want my MD to check in with me about my general well-being in life at that moment, because the literature shows that depression and anxiety going in tend to predict poorer outcomes. I'd also want to know that my MD cared that I had the support of friends, family, and/or significant others; this is another thing that seems to influence outcomes. If my MD suggested that I should have my ovaries removed, I would want a very good reason for it. The idea that I should remove organs that I supposedly 'won't need anymore' on that basis alone is preposterous!

"After hearing from many women about their hysterectomies, the main thing I have learned is that most of them just want information. Even if the MD can't guarantee a particular outcome, they really want to know the pros and cons of all of the treatment options. Contrary to what some paternalistic doctors might tell you, they really can handle that information! Several studies have demonstrated that patients tend to want more information, sometimes a lot more, than their doctors think they want or need. The bottom line is that women want to consent to every aspect of their treatment, and that means they understand why they're taking one approach over the other, etc. Informed consent is not just 'this is what you need, now sign the dotted line.' It's an agreement to a collaborative treatment decision (thus the word 'informed').

"The jury is still out on to what extent hysterectomy affects basic sexual physiology. I would guess that any given outcome is a combination of the surgical technique and the individual woman's composition. I've heard some women say that they have lost some sensation after hysterectomy, or their orgasms aren't as intense as they used to be, but there is no 'typical' hysterectomy experience as far as I can tell. Whether any woman would do it all over again given the chance depends on a lot of different factors. Women whose sex lives are disrupted because of huge, basically inoperable fibroids are likely to still be mostly satisfied when penetration no longer causes sharp pain, and I suspect that for many this would be true even if the cost were a slight change in sexual sensation or the intensity of orgasm. The thing is, though, we can't KNOW what that potential trade-off would mean to any individual woman unless we actually ask her! So, if I were a doctor, I would say, "Look, these are side effects that some women have reported," and summarize the latest research to give her an idea of how common the side effects actually are. It would be up to her to decide if the risk, however small, was worth the potential gains associated with hysterectomy, which themselves are not 100% guaranteed either, of course! It's a cost-benefit analysis, and even though there are a lot of women who want their physicians to make the final decision, I've never heard anyone claim that they got too much information about what might happen to them.

"I *have* heard from a few women who said that they put off their hysterectomies needlessly because of scare tactics, and this is the other side of the story. There are activist groups putting out some pretty wild claims. According to them, hysterectomy can cause asthma! They don't do women any favors with their misinformation and pseudoscience. Ultimately it's a hard decision to make, and women simply need the facts. I am fairly convinced at this point that, for an otherwise healthy, well-adjusted, well-supported woman who lives in a community or in a relationship that won't see her as losing her femininity, hysterectomy is not necessarily a bad thing for sexual function and in some cases might be exactly what she needs. If less invasive treatment options have been ruled out and the main issue is painful intercourse caused by the disease. Otherwise, the picture can be more complex. One of the most consistent findings from past research is that the worse off you are to begin with, both sexually and emotionally, the less likely it is that your outcome will be a complete success. When women ask me about their treatment decisions, I ask them right out: are you emotionally, mentally, physically, and spiritually ready for this? You'd be surprised how seldom women get asked this question.

"No matter how healthy you are to begin with, losing the ovaries IS a big deal, especially for premenopausal women, as it changes the hormonal profile and forces further decision-making about hormone-replacement therapy and so forth. The choice to remove the ovaries should be carefully justified. The medical opinion on this issue has shifted back and forth over the years, but there are many experts who would tell you that, for healthy women with no significant risk factors for ovarian cancer, the cost of losing ovaries is greater than the potential benefits. Sometimes removal of the ovaries is an easy decision because of cancer or other factors, but more often than not it should be deliberated very carefully. This is a time to get second opinions."

A Physician Gets Mad

A friend of *The Guide* from way back is one of the top sex researchers in the country. She is also a physician. Recently, she became so angry with her own private gynecologist that it appeared she was going to rip him a new— uh—vagina. She was diagnosed with cancer of the cervix, and she felt his handling of it was neither sensitive nor professional.

The reason for reporting this is not to dump on gynecologists. There are many excellent ones. It is to remind you that even an MD can become an angry and frustrated patient. So if you are feeling overwhelmed by your dealings with modern medicine, you are not alone. Don't hesitate to get a second opinion. If it appears that you will need surgery and you don't feel comfortable with your physician, find a university health center to get another opinion. That is what our physician friend recommends after her personal experience with hysterectomy.

A SPECIAL THANKS: To Annie Bradford of the University of Texas at Austin for providing some of the best advice available on hysterectomy.

CHAPTER

84

Techno Breasts & Weenie Angst

People who feel sexually inadequate sometimes focus their angst on body parts. For women, the focus is often on breast size or body shape; for men it is on the penis and sometimes height. It is silly to obsess about something that you had no say in getting, yet that is what many of us do.

When generating a physical balance sheet, it might be helpful to remember that even Man-O-War had his weaknesses. It might also help to remind yourself that sexual attractiveness is not like a steel chain, where one weak link makes the whole thing useless. All of us have weak links sexually, as part of our bodies and minds.

This offers little solace to people who are convinced their body parts are deficient. They will keep telling themselves, "Everything would be better if I just had a bigger this or a smaller that." To address such fears, this chapter offers a lengthy discourse on men's genitals, then ruminates on breast implants and ends with a few suggestions about alternative strategies.

Body Concerns: Guys & How They're Hung

While most books on sex say that penis size doesn't matter, there are two groups of people to whom it does matter. One group includes almost every male alive. The second group includes every woman who derives sexual pleasure from intercourse.

In years past, women weren't supposed to care about the size and shape of a man's penis. That is because they weren't supposed to be interested in sex. But wouldn't you notice the size and shape of something that was about to get put into your body? As for how women respond to the actual dimensions of the thing, it varies.

Some women regard the penis as a trophy—the bigger the better; others couldn't care less. Some women prefer the feeling of fullness that a beefier penis has to offer; others prefer giving blowjobs to a partner who isn't particularly well hung, and some even prefer a smaller penis for intercourse. Plenty of women get the bulk of their pleasure from what a man is able to do with his hands, heart, tongue and intellect. They view the penis as just another body part.

For some women, a lover's penis becomes her penis or a part of her body when it's inside of her. Does this mean she necessarily wants the biggest one in town? Not usually. After all, when women buy dildos, they tend to select medium or smaller units. (Sorry, but they sometimes upsize later.)

This isn't to say that women don't have their favorites. Ask a woman to tell you which lover's penis was her favorite, and she will probably be able to give a direct and clear-cut answer such as, "It was Alex's" or "There are two or three that stand out, but I'd have to say Todd's takes the prize." However, if you ask about the men behind the penises and which ones she loved the most, Alex or Todd might not be at the top of the list. Maybe the guy she was happiest with didn't have a memorable penis, but was able to put it together in other ways.

So while women might prefer one penis over the other, penis size usually isn't a deal-breaker when it comes to choosing a man. It is sometimes disappointing, but usually not the deciding factor.

Irony: While some guys grow up worrying if they are hung well enough, women sometimes grow up worrying that guys will be hung too well and might cause them pain. Maybe we humans were programmed to worry.

One More Thing Porn Has Changed...

Few women make it past age thirteen without having seen porn. So most of the erect penises that today's young women have seen are in the top 1% to 5% as far as size is concerned. The good news about this is women probably don't freak out nearly as much now as they did in the pre-porn days when a real-life lover pulls out a really big penis. The bad news is porn has upped the ante for what a lot of women assume is average. This makes sense, given that porn doesn't include warnings that say "The chances are slim that your man will be this big" or "You probably won't get to try this at home."

The Fear vs. The Reality

The Journal of Sexual Medicine recently published a review of all of the studies that have been done on penis size.

One of the most fascinating findings is that out of 414 men who complained of having small penis size, 410 or 99% had penises that were normal sized. And while only 55% of men report being satisfied with their own penis size, 84% of women were satisfied with their partner's penis size.

So, what's average? Measuring from the pubic bone to the tip of the penis head, the average limp penis is about three-and-a-half inches and the average erect penis is a little more than five inches. (This is the average of eight different studies that measured the penises of thousands of men.) The average circumference when erect is about four-and-a-half inches. When guys measure their own penises, they are up to an inch longer than when a researcher does it.

Weenie-Enhancement Techniques: Surgery That Makes Your Penis Fat

There used to be a surgical technique for penis plumping in which fat cells were harvested from the lower-stomach region and injected into the penis. The author of this book called three offices that advertised this procedure and was hit by a wave of sales pitches that he hadn't encountered since joining a health club. The heavy sales pitch, which tried to capitalize on every sexual doubt known to man, made sense given how these clinics were charging $3,000 to $7,000 for an outpatient procedure that takes half an hour.

One clinic in Beverly Hills refused to mail out information about the procedure. They claimed that a brochure had fallen into the hands of a child, resulting in great embarrassment. To prevent such a hideous event from ever occurring again, each caller had to make an office appointment where he could read the brochure and talk to a specialist. "Why an appointment?" "Because we process over forty men a day." As it turned out, the dreaded brochure contained no pictures or drawings and was embarrassing only in how it insulted the consumer's intelligence.

This fancy medical clinic insisted on getting a social-security number and health-insurance information before discussing the procedure. Each visitor was required to fill out a questionnaire about his penis. The wording was designed to make a man feel sexually insecure and blame it all on the size of his weenie. It was the forerunner for today's spam and TV commercials that promise a bigger dick with pills instead of surgery—with probably the same people being involved.

The interview was with a clean-cut salesman masquerading in a physician's coat, so he wouldn't be confused with the salesmen who populate used-car lots. None of the three offices offered any studies on the long-term safety of the procedure. They didn't agree on where the fat actually went, and none was willing to say exactly how a penis feels that is encased in a layer of fat.

The best anyone could conclude about this procedure is that a man paid $5,000 to give his penis cellulite. The biggest benefactors of the procedure have been the attorneys who specialized in lawsuits from men who had their penises surgically enhanced. Since that time, there have been ads stating that there is a "new procedure" that is vastly improved over the one used in the past. If you are considering such a surgery, remember that only a few years ago the ads for the "old" procedure used to boast about how safe and successful it was.

If you are considering such a surgery, spend some time at the library and do a search in the *Journal of Sexual Medicine* and urology journals on penis-enlarging penis enhancement surgeries. Forewarned is forearmed.

The Vacuum Pump

There is an X-rated video called *How to Enlarge Your Penis* in which porn star Scott Taylor pumped himself up with a vacuum device that is supposed to make a guy bigger. Taylor used the pump to plump his penis up fatter than a grain silo, which he then maneuvered into the apparently spacious vagina of porn starlet Erica Boyer. At no point did Scott's big salami actually get hard; he had to hold his fingers around the base to keep the pressure in. Inside-industry sources have informed Goofy Foot Press that the *How to Enlarge* infomercial took several hours to shoot. This was before Viagra, and even Scott Taylor couldn't stay hard that long.

The penis pump was first patented in 1917. Sixty years later it became popular in the gay community, both for sex play and for organ enhancement. Some pumpers started clubs where guys get together to pump. Straight men started using the pump in the mid to late 1980s. The vacuum pump is now one of the options that urologists offer male patients who are having trouble getting hard.

Pumping provides a sensation that some men find enjoyable. It also causes the penis to plump up bigger than usual. Most urologists say there is no way a guy can make himself permanently bigger with a vacuum pump and that short-term gains occur because the penis is swollen. However, the people who manufacture the pumps claim that long-term gains are possible. They say the vacuum pump expands the width of the penis by stretching the walls of the chambers that fill with blood during normal erection. The increase in penis length apparently comes from stretching the ligament that holds a third of the penis inside the body.

To achieve a "permanent" increase in size, pumpers say that a man has to pump at least a half-hour a day for almost a year. As for the safety of the vacuum pump, it has been approved by the FDA for use with erection problems, but not for use as a weenie-enhancement device, not that anyone has applied. Can you imagine the lab studies the FDA might require, with hundreds of rats having their penises pumped for hours on end?

For safety's sake, check with a physician before pumping for long periods of time. That's because there might be a difference between pumping for a few minutes to get hard and pumping for an hour to get bigger. You would think that the majority of men who pump for size would be those with smaller penises. Not so. A lot of pumpers are well-endowed to begin with.

The Bottom Line...

> "I once had a lover with an enormous penis. It was a turn-on to look at it, and an ego trip that a man that huge was my partner. But the actual feeling of it inside me didn't give me one one-hundredth of the pleasure that my more modestly-sized present partner's does. While the size of a man's penis does create different sensations, it is the relationship I have with the man who is attached to the penis that determines what those sensations mean to me." *female age 47*

Before rushing out to get either a pump or surgery, if your penis is average-sized, why do you need to be bigger? What's your problem anyway? And if your penis is closer to a finger than a phone pole, keep in mind that couples frequently have intercourse before the vagina is fully engorged with blood.

When that's the case, the penis with a bigger girth will probably fill the space better. So make sure a woman's vagina is fully-engorged before you have intercourse. It will help even the penis-size playing field.

Learn to give great back and foot rubs and become sublime at the art of loving a woman with your lips and tongue. Do this and it is likely that you will be admired by many women, assuming you are a decent human being to begin with. Also try using intercourse positions that cause the penis to be hugged more snugly. A bantam-weight penis might feel longer if the female bends her knees during intercourse. This results in deeper penetration if that's what she wants. Keeping her legs together will help it feel more snug. You might try rear-entry intercourse with both of you on your sides (aka spoons). Another position to consider is where the woman is on her back and her ankles are resting on the man's shoulders instead of around his waist.

Also try to avoid women who are confirmed size-queens. There's no sense in humiliating yourself needlessly.

As for being embarrassed in front of your locker-room buds, it's not fair to compare nonerect penises. Penises that are smaller when they are soft tend to grow more when they are getting hard than penises that are bigger when they are soft. So it's not right to compare unless all of you have hard-ons, and guys usually don't walk around locker rooms packing wood unless they are in a gay establishment.

But logic can only get you so far when it comes to feeling inferior about body parts. To put the size issue in its truest, ugliest light, if the Penis Fairy arrived one night and offered to give all men more bulge in the front of their blue jeans or an extra ten I.Q. points, a lot of us would go for the below-the-belt enhancement.

And now, for men and their partners who have the opposite problem...

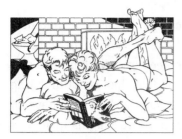

Dear Paul,

My boyfriend and I are both virgins and have been attempting to have intercourse, but we are having a few difficulties. I am quite petite, and he, on the other hand, is quite tall and "fully equipped" (8 inches, and rather large in circumference). I was just wondering if you have any suggestions as we are getting a little antsy.

Tina from Mesa Grande

Dear Tina,

Until I'd written a book about sex, I never realized that toting around a huge penis can be a liability. We're talking about guys who need to wear specially made underwear, who are forever getting stares in the locker room and at the doctor's office, and for whom hopping into bed with a woman can be a trauma. On the other hand, I interviewed a woman who was as petite as can be. Her husband's penis was in the 98th percentile for size, and she never had any problem with intercourse. So you can't predict.

Size aside, medical factors can make intercourse uncomfortable. So I am assuming you have had a recent gynecological exam and have discussed this matter with your healthcare provider. If there is a source of pain that is independent of your partner's penis, it is essential you treat it and resolve it first.

I would suggest the two of you call it quits on any intercourse attempts for the next month or two. There are lots of ways you can please each other sexually besides intercourse. As long as you are okay physically and do not have a pelvic pain disorder, you might consider working on some or all of the following:

1. Have your partner squirt a generous amount of sex lube on his fingertips (lube with silicone rather than something that will quickly dry out like KY). He can gently clasp the outer lips of your vulva between his thumb and forefinger and do a small circular massage on one area at a time. Tell him what feels good and what doesn't. He should massage as deeply as is comfortable for you, then move to an adjoining spot. His goal is not to stretch the skin, but to get the blood circulating deep inside of the folds. He should do your entire vulva, including the outer lips, inner lips and the clitoral hood.

2. Then, when you are highly aroused, he can gently insert a well-lubricated finger into your vagina and rest it there. If it feels okay, he might insert a second finger and eventually a third. Breathe deep and work on relaxing your vagina when his fingers are in. He or you should then try stimulating your clitoris while his fingers are still inside your vagina. If you can have an orgasm while his fingers are in you, it will help train your vagina to allow a penis that's bigger than it's used to.

3. If it's comfortable, you and your boyfriend can practice what the midwives and obstetricians call "perineal massage." He inserts a well-lubricated thumb into the opening of your highly aroused vagina and rests it there. His forefinger should be on the outside, resting on the skin that's between your vulva and anus. He then clasps the tissue that's between his thumb and forefinger and massages it as well as gently pushing down. This stimulates the part of your vagina that stretches wider when you have intercourse. (The ceiling of a vagina doesn't stretch very much, as the pubic bone is right above it. It's the part that's next to your bum that stretches.)

You and he should do steps 1 to 3 at least a couple of times a week until the floor of your vagina can more easily relax.

4. You might also try what's called "femoral intercourse," but it isn't intercourse at all. It is where your partner lies on his back and you lube up his penis and the lips of your vulva. You then straddle him and ride back and forth along the length of his well-lubed penis as it is lying against his belly. Think of your vulva as being like a hotdog bun, and his penis is like a Ballpark Frank. You slide up and down the length of the dog, enjoying the sensations without him trying to steal home. Be sure to use birth control. His penis is not going into your vagina, but he's going to ejaculate near the opening of your vagina and that's reason enough to call out the contraceptives. (You can also do femoral intercourse with him on top or from behind.)

It could help if you learn to give yourself orgasms this way or at least enjoy the sensations while having femoral intercourse. You are in complete control and there's no need to worry about his penis going inside your vagina as long as he agrees to not try.

5. Consider purchasing two or three penis-shaped objects or dildos that range in size from small to large. Start by lubing up your vagina and the

smallest dildo. Once you become comfortable inserting the dildo and moving it around inside your vagina, move up to the next size. But never move up to the next bigger size until you are completely comfortable with the current sized dildo. This should be done over several weeks and not all in one night. Try having an orgasm with the dildos inside your vagina.

6. Once you are comfortable with these steps, have your partner rest the head of his well-lubed penis at the opening of your vagina, but no farther. A day or two later, have him move in about a quarter-of-an-inch if it is comfortable for you. No thrusting unless you want it. Try just a little extra each time you are together, as long you feel comfortable with it. Stop if you feel pain.

If he wears a condom, it might help his penis slide more easily, as long as you coat it with lots of condom-friendly lube.

As for intercourse positions, you'll want to be really conservative. Stay with the classic missionary position where you are on your back and your legs are slightly spread. Avoid rear-entry positions and stay away from anything where your legs are flexed. Flexing your knees will compress or shorten the available thrusting space in your vagina. You almost might find that having an orgasm before intercourse helps to relax it more.

7. To help prevent pain that's associated with deep-thrusting, your BF can put a gasket around the base of his penis that can shorten his plunging depth. This is discussed on page 339 in Chapter 23: Horizontal Jogging.

If none of this helps, you might try finding a physical therapist who specializes in pelvic pain, or accept the fact that his penis isn't going to fit. Learn to have great sex by getting each other off in other ways besides intercourse. You might find you end up having a better sex life than a lot of couples who can have intercourse.

The Sound of Leaking Breasts

"I tried out for the cheerleading squad when I was a sophomore in high school. 'This isn't a beauty contest,' the advisor had told us, but we all knew better than that…. But you weren't beautiful, Julie Brown, and you knew it. Face facts. You even made a list one time, outlining your numerous faults: breasts too small, buttocks too big, teeth crooked, hair too thin, arms and legs too skinny, feet too long, four inches too tall, nose too bumpy. If you were wealthy, you could make the necessary corrections. If you had enough money, you could have the breast implants you needed, the braces, the nose job, the hairweaving, and with enough money the right cosmetics could be purchased, the ones you saw in the magazines, the ones that would render you flawless..."[1]

Men aren't the only ones who worry that body parts are too small. Women often believe the world would be a nicer place if only they had bigger breasts. Some women with petite breasts feel they would get a better job or promotion if their A-cups swelled into double Ds. Hopes like these have inspired thousands of women to have their chests packed with funky substances.

Questions have been raised about the safety of breast implants. Silicone molecules seem to leach through the plastic implant pouches. However, it is possible that this isn't any more dangerous to your health than, say, living in Detroit or Los Angeles. Saline implants appear to be safer than the silicone, but less so than the original equipment that nature saw fit to provide.

Breast Implants Are Not Permanent

Twenty to twenty-five percent of women who have breast implants will need additional surgery within only five years. Within thirteen to fifteen years, eighty-five percent of breast implants will fail.

Even the saltwater implants make it difficult to screen for cancer. On the other hand, implants are truly a godsend if you have had cancer and get them after a mastectomy.

Breast-Reduction Note Some women have breast-reduction surgery because it can be severely uncomfortable to lug huge breasts around 24/7. If this is what you are considering, be sure to consult at least two surgeons who specialize in breast-reduction surgery. This is not a simple operation and can leave permanent scaring or disfigurement.

---

[1]By Julie Brown, published in "Beauty" pages 68–70, *Michigan Quarterly Review*, edited by Laurence Goldstein, Vol. XXX, No. 1:91.

Microchip Melons — A New Generation of Breast Implant?

Unless there is a major shift in the consciousness of American men and women, it is likely that the medical world will find new ways to surgically enhance women's breasts. As long as that is the case, this Guide suggests that the next generation of breast implants contain WiFi and a couple of HDMI ports. Perhaps breast-implanted gaming displays might help the female chest become a full-fledged entertainment center, which is what some men and women expect it to be.

Labiaplasty

Labiaplasty is cosmetic surgery to help a girl's inner lips look like those of a porn star. Think of it as a nose job for your puss.

A lot of people are critical of labiaplasty, but buy teeth-whitening products, get botoxed, have their hair colored, have moles removed that they consider to be unsightly, and have their sons circumcised. Given how this book has wailed and ranted against breast implants with absolutely no impact, maybe it's best we simply give you the info you need, and leave the rest up to you.

Women should be aware that the labia minora or inner lips are made from the same tissue as the head of the penis. (That's the head of the penis, not the foreskin.) The inner lips swell during sexual arousal and their edges are packed with nerve endings. They move with each thrust of intercourse. Have them pruned at your own risk

Women who want to have labiaplasty should look at pictures of different labia and see how normal it is for labia to come in many different sizes and shapes. If the woman still wants the surgery, she needs to find a surgeon who specializes in this procedure and has performed many prior labiaplasties. It is not a simple matter of snipping a bit here and there. The woman should be sure her surgeon knows the different techniques and can describe the difference between oversewing the edges, wedge resection and 90-degree Z-plasty.

WARNING #1: *If your healthcare provider suggests you have labiaplasty, it might be more to improve his cash flow than to improve your crotch. There are now seminars for gynecologists on how much extra money they can make*

each year by trimming their patients' labia. So if your healthcare provider suggests you have labiaplasty, please get a second opinion.

WARNING #2: *Reports are beginning to surface of women who have had labiaplasties and who are experiencing pain and discomfort during intercourse as a result. Given their role in sexual arousal, it appears that labia might not be the best candidates for cosmetic surgery.*

Alternatives for Both Men & Women

American advertisers spend millions of dollars to make us think, "If only I had this or that, I'd be sexier and happier." It is easy to see why many of us fall for these traps. The thought of instantly having bigger, smaller, hairier or balder body parts can be terribly seductive.

If cosmetic surgery is what you need, please choose carefully. You might first read Virginia Blum's book on the subject: *Flesh Wounds, The Culture of Cosmetic Surgery.* Blum has had plastic surgery and has interviewed surgeons and patients. What would it hurt to read some of the information that you won't find in the glossy brochures at your plastic surgeon's office before making such a big decision?

For alternatives to cosmetic surgery, think about getting your body in good physical shape or dressing better. Breasts that sit on well-developed chest muscles sometimes look bigger, if that is what you are trying to achieve. At the very least, being in good shape makes most people feel and look sexier. A smaller penis will often look bigger if it isn't being dwarfed by a pot belly, or if the eyes are drawn to nicely developed shoulders and pecs. Also, why not find ways to expand your mind's creativity and intelligence? These are the kinds of measures that will make you a better and sexier person.

As for sexual performance, some of the best and most eager lovers are those without ideal dimensions. Since they have less natural endowment to fall back on, they sometimes learn to be extremely attentive in bed.

85

Basic Brain Weirdness

his chapter is about the mental landscape and parts of it that can get in the way of having a good sex life, or just having a good life. Some people would call these unusual glitches; others would say they are a normal part of the human condition.

Shyness

Shyness is a funny thing. Sometimes it sits like a shroud over everything you do. Other times it is highly selective, making only certain parts of your life sheer hell. Shyness can take many forms and can be a great deal more mysterious than people give it credit for. Shyness can make you babble like a fool and say really stupid things or it can make you seem cold and aloof when you're really not.

To illustrate what happens when shyness gets the better of you, consider the following true story of Andrew. Andrew is now really old, but he used to be really young.

It was a beautiful spring day about a month or two before the beginning of a somewhat magical time that later became known as the Summer of Love. Unfortunately, Andrew had never even put his hand up a woman's shirt.

None of this stopped him from having an overpowering crush on a very popular young woman who was a senior when he was only a sophomore. Among other things, this female heartthrob was the homecoming queen. She was so special that he was too embarrassed to tell even his best friend about his lick-the-mud-off-her-shoes-if-that's-what-she-wants crush. Instead, he focused his energies on trying to act cool whenever she passed by.

To make matters worse, the young goddess was constantly surrounded by senior guys who had their own cars, lettered in football and baseball, and got drunk and never threw up. He, on the other hand, saw himself as just another soph-moron with less than a snowball's chance in hell of attracting this woman's interest.

One day about an hour after school, some strange and peculiar force caused this special woman to toss her pompoms into the back of her car and aim it for the very address where this young man lived. When the doorbell rang he figured it was probably Jehovah's Witnesses with "The Watchtower." When he saw who it was his knees turned to Jell-O and it seemed like forever before he was able to take a breath. All things considered, he did well to maintain bladder control.

He just stood there staring. He felt so paralyzed that he couldn't even mobilize the words to invite her inside. After about twenty awkward minutes of trying to deal with the situation, the young goddess blew the baffled boy a puzzled kiss and drove away, never to return. Many years have passed since this fellow botched the Summer of Love. For much of his life, he continued to feel clumsy and awkward whenever he met a woman who he was attracted to. Shyness can be that way.

On Being a Sex Object

People usually associate "being a sex object" with being a woman. However, this is about a guy named Steve who women treated as a sex object. Steve was tall, blond, blue-eyed and had a perfect body. In addition to being a fine surfer, he was a male model who was actually straight.

Everyone was thrown into total shock one night at Steve's tearful lament that he wished women would stop wanting him just for sex. It was a problem none of us could relate to. Steve was in a total funk because women were constantly diving for his crotch.

It's difficult to imagine that physical attractiveness can get in the way of leading a happy life, but people who are physical 10s are sometimes lonely. Friends of the same sex are often envious and sometimes feel threatened by the attention that the 10s seem to get. Members of the other sex often stare or act bizarrely. People who are extremely attractive sometimes marry simply for protection.

What's Wrong with This Picture?

The opposite problem of being a 10 is when you are less than beautiful and have someone who is drop-dead gorgeous show a romantic interest in you. Instead of responding romantically, you might be saying to yourself, "Naw, can't be true. Big mistake here." While the physical 10 may be begging for romance, the less-than-10 is turning a great opportunity into a self-fulfilling prophecy of doom. Sometimes other people can see beautiful things in you that you have no idea even exist.

People Who Claim "The Opposite Sex Is Worthless"

Some people choose sexual partners who can't supply any of their emotional needs. It's as if they would be horribly overwhelmed to find a partner who could be both a friend and a lover, and therefore not quite so "opposite." Perpetual victims such as these claim that they are more mature and able to love more than their partners.

The fact is, people who have a healthy self-regard do not suffer the presence of fools and jerks, let alone sleep with them. The perpetual victim is just as immature and has as many problems with intimacy as does the jerk whom he or she dates or marries. Neither has much to brag about.

Giving Friendship a Chance

Platonic male-female friendships are a wonderful thing, but they sometimes become endangered if one person starts to feel sexual and the other doesn't. A lot of male-female friendships never happen because people are unable to work it out when one of them wants sex or romance and the other just wants friendship. Knowing that a friend wants romance when you don't can be uncomfortable. However, if he or she were given the time and understanding to cool his or her jets, the nonsexual friendship might flourish for years to come.

As for the person who feels smitten and then bitten, keep in mind that a platonic friendship often lasts for years, while that is not always the case with romantic affairs. You might be losing out on something special if you aren't able to accept the person as a friend instead of as a lover.

Another factor that often destroys male-female friendships is the jealousy of spouses or partners.

Initiating Sex When Holding Is What You Need

Some people find it hard to acknowledge that they need to be held. Asking might make them feel weak or vulnerable. So they sometimes initiate sex when what they really may have wanted was physical tenderness and comfort. Fortunately, the desires for sex and tenderness often overlap, which allows us to receive both at the same time. But sometimes we need more of one than the other. Hopefully you can evolve a set of signals that will help your partner know what you need, assuming you know yourself.

In Love but out of Sync

It's the saddest thing in the world when people have powerful feelings for each other but can't make their relationship work.

One of you might become more settled and grounded earlier in life than the other. You may feel like putting down roots or becoming established while the other is still an emotional tumbleweed who needs to experience the outside world and soak in whatever it has to teach. The lack of synchrony forces a breakup, or maybe there's a missing level of sensitivity or maturity that one partner won't have for several more years. While you may not have any desire to get back together, there might always remain a place in your heart for the other person.

Breaking Up

Breaking up is the sort of thing that should have its own book. Otherwise, you risk sounding trite about a phenomenon that can leave the strongest of hearts totally shattered.

Contrary to what you might think, breaking up isn't always accompanied by a big fight or a hell storm of hostility. In fact, sometimes you spend your last hours together holding each other tight, with a kind of desperate, profound sadness in your hearts. Even if you are the one who is doing the leaving, the final steps toward the door can sometimes feel horrible. Necessary, but horrible.

And in case you've been there, a lot of casual sex ends up being with an ex rather than with a random hook-up.

Stupid Mistakes — Young vs. Old

If anyone ever tells you that making stupid mistakes is from being young and will pass as you get older, don't make the really stupid mistake of believing them.

True, you usually don't make as many mistakes as you get older, but that's only because your brain doesn't work nearly as fast. As your brain slows down, you simply don't have the opportunity to make mistakes with the same lightning speed that you once did.

Forgiving Yourself

Every once in a while we say or do something so stupid that even friends talk about having us committed. This can be particularly devastating when it results in the loss of friendship or love.

The best thing you can do in these situations is to figure out how and why you messed up. Then do what you can to mourn the loss and get on with your life. While there is much to be gained from introspection, there is little to be gained from beating yourself up. On the other hand, if you suffer from a perpetual case of foot-in-mouth, it is possible that there is a chronic confusion or anger in the depths of your soul that prevent you from using good sense. In that case, the input of a respected friend, teacher, colleague, relative or therapist might be an important thing to seek.

The Fantasy of Love & Commitment

When you feel particularly empty inside, it's easy to have the illusion that things will be better if you can just find someone to love.

Love is a special way of sharing friendship that can bring tremendous joy. It allows you to think and worry about someone other than yourself, which can be a much-needed relief. It also lets you know that there is some-one who believes in you when you don't believe in yourself. But in spite of all its pluses, it's unlikely that love will take away your fears and insecuri-ties, organize your chaos, cure your bad habits, help you to lose weight, stop smoking, get in shape, or turn you into a better human being—not in the long run anyway. Our personal demons are things we usually need to con-quer on our own.

The Dark Side — Nights of Quiet Despair

Sometimes you get hit by a certain mood, one that's a quiet mix of frus-tration, hopelessness and despair. It's when something deep inside you isn't working right, something incredibly human, but you can't put a finger on it.

Sometimes it becomes a contest between you, the despair and the beer, pills, sleep, food, sex or whatever it is that helps make you feel better. Presi-dents' wives tell you to just say no, the disc jockey on the all-night radio station never plays the song you need, and a river of pain cuts your heart in two.

Nights of quiet despair sometimes go away by morning.

Dear Paul,

Ever since I graduated from college my sex life has taken a big nose dive. I have had sexual intercourse ONCE between then and today! I had a healthy sex life in high school complete with true love and several short-term physical relationships. That was when I wasn't even an adult. Now I am almost 30, and for most of my 20s my sex life has been NO life at all. I am not at all physically unattractive, although I am somewhat shy and keep very busy. I think my problem is not meeting women. I dislike bars. I do not feel my sex life is representative of a mature, healthy adult male, and the lack of physical intimacy bothers me considerably. Both of my house mates have the same problem, and I know many other guys do. Paul, what is up with this problem, and besides offering your own suggestions, can you direct me to some resources that might help me locate and meet available women?

Blue in Boulder

Dear Blue,

Regarding your question about helping you to locate and meet available women: the odds in Internet dating are stacked way towards women. But if it provides a safety net, see if you can make it work. Also, given your age, a lot of single women are going to have children. If you are good dad potential, don't forget to mention that, but in the current environment, you'll need to do it in a way that doesn't sound like you're trolling for children. Maybe saying you hope to have a family some day will put out the right signals.

As for the other matters you listed, here's my personal take.

High school and college may not fill our lives with happiness and bliss, but they do provide an important social safety net. I can remember my own horror at finally having to leave college. I hadn't gotten into medical school, I didn't feel like doing grad work, and my girlfriend had just given me the boot. I didn't know it was possible to feel so awful. I got a job waiting tables—which is the equivalent of leaving school but not really. I wrote and floundered for a couple of years until I finally went back to graduate school when I was about your age. I didn't get laid much during that time. I also made the huge mistake of doing what you are doing—trying to find ways of meeting women. There is no shortage of books on that subject. But I'm not so sure they will help, and I don't know if they are what you need. In fact, I strongly encourage you to do something else with your time besides focusing on how to meet women.

Please take a moment to imagine that you only have a couple of hours to live. I am willing to bet that even if you had been a stud lover and had created wet spots on mattresses all over Boulder, memories of your love life wouldn't bring you tremendous amounts of solace in the face of death. I don't think it's sex that would make you feel like your life had been worthwhile. What's more important are the contributions that you've hopefully made in life.

For instance, if you had volunteered in a program where you helped people learn to read, or helped make your community a better place, you would have something to look back on with pride, not that being good in bed doesn't help a community be a better place. Or what if you helped build a park or coached a soccer team—not that an affair with a bored soccer mom wouldn't do you both a world of good. (Am I saying you'll find more women by coaching their kids than by hanging around bars? Hint, hint.)

Instead of wasting your time trying to find a bed partner, why not do things that will make you a better person? Please, don't think I am suggesting that you take part in altruistic events as a thinly disguised sham for meeting women. There is nothing more obnoxious than people who volunteer for things with the ulterior motive of trying to find love or sex. But do try to improve yourself, and maybe love will come. Maybe it won't. People who are vitally involved in life tend to have an energy that attracts others.

Counterpoint I can't tell you how many dying people I've heard from who have begged to differ—not about the solace that living a meaningful life can offer, but about their thoughts as the end was approaching. For instance, I received an e-mail from a dying man who said the thing he was enjoying most in his waning moments was his memories of sex. And I received this:

> "I'm a 58-year-old widower who was married to a supernova of a wife for 25 years. I was a horrifically shy young man. She was the second woman I'd been with. As she was leaving life with stunning poise and bravery, one of the aspects of her life that she specifically named as being valuable and memorable was our love life, so don't be so sure about how inconsequential this is."

I stand corrected!

Dating a Single Parent

There is an amazing pool of women to date that some guys don't realize exist. However, these women come with strings attached besides the ones on their IUDs—kids!

While plenty of single moms are only interested in long-term relationships, others will say it's the last thing they want. Having a trustworthy guy to meet for sex and conversation could more than fill some single mom's bills.

While a man who dates a woman without children should be aware of things like restaurants, movies and condoms, a man who dates a single mom needs to know about babysitters. No babysitter, no date, unless it's a family date or the kids are at their dad's. So learn about baby sitters. The first words out of your mouth after a single mom agrees to go out with you should be, "Can I help pay for the sitter?" and "This isn't the time for me to be meeting your kids, but I can pick up a pizza for them."

The next thing you need to know when dating a single mom is how kids can suddenly spike temperatures or start throwing up, especially when they don't want their mom to go out. And you won't believe the nasty array of colds, coughs and flus that kids bring home from school. So you will need to have the patience of Job, and a strong hand that you can go home to jerk off with. No matter how important you might be in a woman's life, you are not going to come between her and her kid's viruses. And if you do, then you might wonder about her character and take heed.

Until you've been dating for a while, think twice about getting super-expensive tickets for events. It will just make her feel like crap if she has to cancel at the last minute, and it will bother you more than if the casualty were only dinner and a movie. If she suddenly has to cancel because of Junior's croop, you won't be anybody's chump if you leave a bouquet of flowers at the door with a note saying how much you look forward to seeing her soon. Yes, some women are flakes and will use their children as an excuse, but you'll be onto that soon enough. Plenty of women without kids are flakes as well.

Do not try or expect to meet her kids for a long time. It's not fair to them if they become attached to you and you suddenly end up out of the picture. But you can still help. If time and money are in short supply, ask about the things her kids like to eat. The 12-box carton of Mac'n'Cheese and frozen chicken-pot-pies from Costco might be calling. At the end of a date, ask if she needs to stop by the grocery store on the way home. If that's the last thing she wants to be reminded of when she's out with you, she'll let you know. If you do meet the kids, don't go sticking your tongue down their mom's throat when they are around. Don't try to buy them off with gifts. Your friendship and concern about them is more than enough. Do introduce yourself as one of their mom's friends, but nothing else. From their experience in school, they will understand that some friends stick around and others move away. And if the two of you start having sex, keep in mind that you'll need to become logistical wizards. It's that way when kids are around. And don't assume she remembered birth control just because she is a mom.

The Guide is also available in
a spectacular color eBook version for
your iPad, Kindle or Nook.

CHAPTER

86

Rape & Abuse
Good Sex after Bad

Some kinds of sex are wicked. Some sexual acts are uninvited and forced, leaving confusion in their wake, especially when the person involved is an otherwise kind and important figure in your life. This chapter looks at the aftermath of rape and abuse with an eye on learning to have good sex after bad. The information it provides is a small drop in a large and sometimes difficult bucket. There is no shortage of information for people who have been raped or abused and hopefully you will seek it out. Some is recommended in the pages that follow.

While sexual assault is not unique, you are. What works for someone else might not work for you. Be diligent in finding information that is helpful and be cautious when self-described experts tell you what you should do instead of giving you a wide platter to choose from.

The first part of this chapter assumes that the person who experienced the assault or abuse is female and that the perpetrator is male. That's how it usually is, but not always. The last part of the chapter is for straight guys who have been raped by other men, although gay men get raped as well. If the person who abused you was a woman or if your situation is not described here, rest assured you can find plenty of material on it with the right search terms.

Rape Versus Abuse

Rape and abuse are often lumped together, as if the experiences are the same because they are both sex crimes. Depending on who you are and what happened, this may or may not be true. Let's consider two women whose only similarity in life is that both had sex forced on them.

The first woman grew up in a safe and loving home. Her parents were there for her from day one. The men she chose for lovers were respectful and decent. The chemistry in her relationships wasn't always the best, but the problem was not because the men lacked character or concern. In times of stress and tumult, this woman's family was a resource she could fall back on. When she was raped at age 24, her family and friends circled the wagons and stood by her. When she was trying to rebuild her sex life after the assault, she had the memory of many satisfying nights with loving men to help her recall that sex could be wonderful as well as wicked.

The second woman had a very different family and childhood. The man her mom remarried had sex with her from the time she was 8. When her grades began to drop and she started to become isolated at school, her mom chalked it up to "growing pains." Signs that a less-chaotic parent would have picked up on went ignored. While the house was well-maintained and she was fed, clothed and clean, home was not a safe place. As the little girl grew into a young woman, her choice of sexual partners reflected the chaos she grew up in.

In telling about these two very different women, it might give you a sense that the challenges sexual-assault victims face are not the same. For the second woman, there is an emotional abandonment that's part of the mortar that binds her entire psyche. She has no memories to fall back on of sex being wonderful and loving. That is very different from the first woman's challenge regarding her rape, which is to deal with the kinds of issues that one might address after a terrorist attack.

There is also no way of predicting which victims of abuse or rape will have sexual and relationship issues. Some of it has to do with a person's temperament and constitution. It might also have to do with whether she had something good that she could hold onto in her mind.

Sexual Confusion in a House of Abuse

For some women who experienced childhood abuse, the times they were abused might have been the only times they were treated with tenderness. Talk about confusing! For other women who experienced childhood abuse, the family member might have otherwise been an important and loving part of her life. This can make sorting out things incredibly difficult and confusing.

Equally difficult are situations in which the girl's own mother was jealous of her, as if she were competition for the woman's husband or boyfriend. Imagine if you grew up in a household where you got treated better for being "daddy's favorite" and your mom was jealous? The idea of having sex for intimacy and enjoyment would be as foreign as wearing a burka would be for a girl who grew up in a beach town with a closet full of bikinis.

Non-abused sons who grow up in situations where a girl is being abused can find it just as difficult to process what is unfolding around them. Some are isolated and depressed. Others grow up finding it a challenge to respect the sexual rights and emotions of others.

Learning to Have Good Sex After Bad

Women who have been raped or abused sometimes report that their bodies are betraying them. Perhaps it's just that their bodies are trying to protect them, and the nerves and muscles beneath their skin have no way of knowing that the danger has passed.

Think of what happens in your body when the man of your dreams is tenderly kissing the sides of your neck. As you are becoming sexually aroused, your heart beats faster, you breathe more quickly, and your skin starts to perspire. You might not be consciously aware of it, but your hearing and vision also become more acute.

A woman with no experience of abuse might experience these body sensations as a sign of the good things to come. But for a woman who has been assaulted or abused, her body is apt to confuse these signs with danger. Far from trying to betray her, her body is most likely trying to protect her. Her nerves and muscles are still preparing for combat rather than for relaxation and pleasure. The retraining process can be slow. So one of the first things a woman might do is to become aware of sexually-charged situations that cause her body tone to go from "Oh boy!" to "Yikes!" or those that make her feel numb or disassociated.

For one woman, the trigger might be a quick, admiring glance from a man in a restaurant. Another woman's body might be totally into having sex until she feels her lover's penis on her outer labia.

As a woman begins to recognize these triggers, she can take any number of actions. One woman might find it helpful to stay with the bad feeling and observe how it unfolds within her. Another might remind herself the situation isn't the dangerous one that her body is confusing it with. If it happens during lovemaking, she and her partner might have a signal so they change positions or automatically stop. A woman might find it important if her lover says something to her, or maybe they switch on a light so she can physically see his face in addition to hearing the sound of his voice. It might also be helpful for her to have environmental cues going on from the start of their lovemaking, such as certain music or a particular light, or having a special object that she can feel or grasp—a good transitional object that helps her feel safe enough to stay in the here and now.

> "Initially, my now-husband had to learn how to stop and comfort me when I had flashbacks during sex. Thankfully those no longer occur. I really need to have music on, or something to concentrate on that adds to the sex. If it is silent, or we have relaxing sex without music or awesome satin sheets or something that provides other sensations, then I will have a lot of trouble not disassociating."
>
> *female age 27*

Masturbation to the Rescue

For some women who have been sexually abused or assaulted, masturbation can provide an important bridge to healthy sexual enjoyment. When she masturbates, she can retrain her body to associate a good sexual outcome with the increased breathing and faster heart beat. For a woman who has never had a good sexual experience, masturbation can be the first step in learning how good sex can feel. For a woman who has had good sex in the past, it can be a safe way for her to remember how good it used to feel.

If she has a trusting, loving relationship with a partner, it might be a huge step for a woman to pleasure herself while he holds her. Hopefully, he can understand how big of a step this can be for her, and not to feel like she's rejecting him because the sight of his hard penis throws her into a panic. All things in good time.

Her partner will also need to be comfortable with masturbation himself, as there might be times when she suddenly needs to put the brakes on during lovemaking. While this might be her need, it could feel like punishment for him. He needs to have the option of getting himself off by hand. Hopefully they can talk about this, and she can appreciate and respect his need to get off, and he can appreciate and respect her sudden need for space.

> "Masturbation had lost a lot of its fun. Isn't that terribly sad? I'm finding it again now, and it makes me proud of myself.
>
> *female age 27*

"I was a frequent masturbator before the rape, but for a while after I didn't really want any sexual things at all. But masturbating helped me to start enjoying my body again." *female age 19*

[After being raped at age 12] "I was 14 and my older friend was telling me about how she could have orgasms in the shower. I tried it, and the experience was so amazing and so all-my-own that I began to feel a lot better about what sex and sexuality should be."
female age 18

"Fantasy men were always nice to me—patient, kind, concerned about me, etc. Not like in real life. In a weird way, it taught me what and who to look for in real life." *female age 30*

What Some Women Have Found Helpful

There isn't a right way or a wrong way to have sex after you have been raped. There are many different options, and only you can decide what's right for you. Here are some things that other women have found to be helpful:

Setting Limits & Feeling Safe: If the places and situations where you used to date and have sex no longer feel safe, see if it helps to treat yourself like the nervous parents of an attractive and sweet 15-year-old. Set the kinds of limits you would for yourself that they would for her. Should you be home by 10 or midnight? What about only double-dating with a trusted friend? Don't go to a party without a friend. If you are in a social situation and start to feel unsafe, don't stick around. Go home. If a guy you like asks you to have a beer, there's no reason why you can't say, "No, but brunch on Sunday would be really nice. I know this fun (and really crowded...) restaurant." Decide ahead of time how much physical contact you are going to allow—a handshake, a kiss, a feel above the waist, a feel below?

Note As the women of the Seattle Institute for Sex Therapy so aptly note, if you discover that you are exclusively selecting men to date who you feel safe with, but who you don't feel sexually attracted to, or it's been a long time and you're still not able to get as sexually excited as you used to, it might be a good idea to seek some counseling.

Re-Virginization OK, it was bad enough being a virgin the first time... If you are planning on having sex with a guy and think you might need to stop groping each other midway, or will be needing special reassurance, then it's probably best to tell him that you had been sexually assaulted. Otherwise, he might rightfully think you are a bit strange. Most guys will be very understanding and try to help in any way they can, especially once you have given them permission to be something less than he-men. It's perfectly fine to say, "The old me might have been pulling your pants off by now, but with the new me, it could be a couple of months before you even get to feel under my bra. I have no idea how it's going to go, but I need to be able to totally trust that if I say stop, you'll stop at that very moment."

You should also warn him that you might have days when you can't get enough of him sexually and other days when you have the sexual sensibilities of a 90-year-old nun.

On the days when you need to send him off to the bathroom with porn, let him know that it still might be really important that the two of you do something romantic together, like taking a walk, or going to the bookstore or to a movie, or flying a kite, or doing any number of things together that couples like to do. And on those days when you need physical contact but want him to keep his penis in his pants, talk to him about cuddling together, holding hands, or exchanging back or foot rubs. If it's not too much for him or you, a warm bath together or dip in a hot tub might feel great.

No matter how passive you might have been before being sexually assaulted, you now need to call the shots. Perhaps it's something you will keep doing as one of the few helpful lessons you learned from an education that you paid way too much to get.

If You Have a Partner Your partner isn't the man who raped you, but he can be almost as affected by the rape as you are. First is the little matter that he might try to kill the rapist. That's to be expected when someone intentionally harms a loved one. Then there's the possible "guilt by association" that he might have to deal with from you, by virtue of the fact that he has something similar between his legs as the rapist. Even though you know he wasn't the one who harmed you nor would he ever want to, he is a guy, and guys might not be at the top of your most-favored-sex list right now. He will need to be aware that for some women, it might take months before sex returns to normal. For others, things will return to normal much sooner. You can't predict, and you can't tell. Hopefully, he will read all he can and educate himself about the reactions that victims of sexual assault can have, and learn how to be an ally of the healing process. Patience will have its rewards.

Flashbacks Some women who have been sexually assaulted have flashbacks; others don't. You and your partner need to be aware that flashbacks sometimes happen when you are at the peak of sexual excitement and are orgasming left and right. Your partner needs to understand that flashbacks are not because of anything he is doing that's wrong. Learn about the things that trigger flashbacks and come up with a strategy for dealing with them. Have faith that they will decrease with time.

Don't Confuse the Female Body's Protective Mechanism with Being Turned On

Researchers have discovered that there is a difference between what makes a vagina lubricate and what turns a woman on mentally. It is not unusual for a woman's vagina to lubricate in situations where she is frightened or terrified. This will protect her vagina from tearing if intercourse is forced upon her.

This primitive reflex can be very confusing for a woman who has had sex forced on her. For instance, if she had an orgasm while being raped, she might wonder if she has a secret thing for violence and somehow invited the rape. She should understand that other women who have been raped have had orgasms, and those orgasms are the product of a body in terror that's spewing out a flood of adrenalin while physical pressure is being put on her genitals. This kind of reaction is not limited to women. Erections are no stranger to the gallows. It's been known for many centuries that men who are executed by hanging often die with erections, and some even ejaculate. While this may have something to do with the body's response to asphyxiation, terror also plays a role in it. These men were no more sexually turned-on by being in the gallows than is a woman in a violent situation in which sex is being forced on her.

Ways to Help Prevent Rape

Before you read about ways to prevent rape, keep in mind that women who have been raped sometimes go overboard in trying to avoid situations that cause them anxiety. The problem with this is that avoidance merely reinforces anxiety and stress disorders. So it is important for those who have been raped to conquer the temptation to avoid too much. The key is in using your good sense.

Common-sense ways to prevent rape include not jogging or walking alone, especially at night. Never hitchhike or pick up a hitchhiker. Lock your doors and windows, even if you are going away for a brief time, and do not open your door unless you are certain you know who is knocking or ringing the doorbell. Don't lend your keys to anyone, and do not put your name or address on your keys. Avoid being alone in underground garages, apartment laundry rooms, or offices after hours. Park in areas that are well-lit, and lock your car doors even if it's a quick stop. Lock your doors when you drive, and try not to drive with less than a quarter of a tank of gas.

At parties, open drinks yourself, avoid the punch bowl, don't accept drinks from anyone else or share them, and don't leave drinks out of your eyesight. Even more importantly, never get drunk or stoned outside of the safety of your own home or that of your sexual partner's.

Strategy

According to interviews with incarcerated rapists, they do not pick a victim based on how she looks or how she is dressed. The first criteria is not getting caught. So what he is looking for is a highly vulnerable victim. Can he easily isolate her from others? Can he commit his crime without her noises drawing the attention of others?

Those who target children can be good con artists. They may have a well-honed approach that gets victims to suspend their sense of suspicion. They seem to know just what to say that makes you feel good. They can often sense loneliness and the need for attention and approval. They excel at flattery.

The sex offender's goal is to find ways to control a victim. He is good at getting women to engage in light forms of romance or sex play, not so much at their invitation, but in a way that she doesn't think to scream "STOP IT!" He manages to take her off-guard, doing things that feel good enough so she gets confused. Then, after it's too late, he's managed to physically isolate her and emotionally confuse her. She is suddenly wondering, "Did I invite this?" If she didn't put a stop to it immediately, she is pretty much a goner. He will have invaded her personal space and personal boundaries, and then there's no stopping him.

After committing his crime, his next goal is to not get caught. If you are a friend or acquaintance, he might try to catch you up in the confusion of whether you invited the assault, until you start thinking, "I shouldn't have let him start fooling around with me." Depending on the situation, he might also be able to control you with bribery or threats. And if you are child, he might act convincingly that nothing really happened. You end up distorting your own awareness of what went on.

Date or Acquaintance Rape

An agreement to kiss is not an agreement to have intercourse. It never has been. Fucking requires a separate level of consent than making-out. Likewise, feeling each other up and finding a vagina to be wet is not consent to put a penis in it.

Do not assume a woman is playing a game when she hesitates or says "No." And never, ever try to win her over with pressure or persuasiveness. The courts have made it clear that this will not be tolerated. In the absence of a woman making it completely clear that she wants sex, a man needs to assume that sex is neither desired nor is it legal.

Please see Chapter 13: *Consent* for a full discussion of mutual consent.

If You Have Been Raped—the First Hours After

The thing you don't want to do is to disturb any of the evidence, and unfortunately, the evidence is on you and in you. Much as you might want to, do not shower, douche, wash your hands, change your clothes, drink anything or even brush your teeth. Saliva can be used to identify a rapist as well as his semen. Try not to pee. If you think you might have been drugged and you have to urinate, do so in a bottle and take it with you to the hospital. Be sure to tell the doctor about any suspicions of being drugged. The way they find out if you have been drugged is through testing your urine, and some drugs pass through your system quickly. (In some states, the threshold of evidence is lower if it is discovered that the victim was drugged.)

If you are a minor, you don't need to have a parent's permission to have a "rape kit" done at the hospital. So there's no reason to fear going to the hospital if you've been doing something that would make your parents want to kill you.

You should take extra clothing that you can change into after they have collected all the evidence at the hospital. If you can, ask a friend to go with you or to meet you at the hospital. If you live in a dorm, ask a resident advisor to go with you as well. It's OK if the friend stays with you during the exam and during your entire hospital visit. Your friend can be your ears, eyes, and brain in case your own are feeling fried. If you or your friend has it together enough, call RAINN (800-656-HOPE). See if there is a victim advocate who can meet you at the hospital.

As a victim of a sexual assault, you have priority over just about everything other than life-threatening illnesses. So unless you see people being wheeled in with panicked-looking doctors hovering around them, you should get in sooner than later. If a long time has gone by, ask your friend to remind the person at the desk that you are a rape victim and haven't been seen. If you prefer a doctor of your same sex, let them know. If they can, they will get you one, but it may take more time.

Going to the hospital doesn't mean you need to speak to the police or press charges. But it's essential to go to the hospital for a couple of reasons. If at some point you do decide to press charges, they will have the necessary evidence. It will be much harder otherwise. The people in the ER can give you the morning-after pill to help prevent pregnancy, and they can tend to any physical trauma. Going to the hospital right away greatly increases your chances to receive victim's services if you should need them, and in a lot of states, the state will pay for your expenses. The people in the ER should be able to explain your options and connect you with counseling and other help. It is a very, very good idea to visit a hospital emergency room right away. There are virtually no downsides. As with a car accident, you have no idea of the kinds of emotional or physical trauma that might present itself in a couple of days or weeks. Having everything on record at the ER will make it easier for you to get free services if you should need them in the future.

How People Act after Being Raped

There is no manual for how to act after a sexual assault. Some people will be hysterical while others will be unusually calm. Some will be agitated, others will be numb. It is unwise to judge a person's emotional experience of a sexual assault based on their behavior following it.

Rape in Marriage

People have the idea that rape in a marriage isn't really rape, and it's less serious than if the sexual assault is caused by a stranger. But given all the baggage and history of a married couple, it makes sense that spousal rape might be even more devastating than stranger rape. The stranger never said,

"To have and to hold, to love and to cherish, till death do us part."

Women who are raped by their husbands are likely to be raped a number of times before finally leaving. The rape can be oral, anal and vaginal. Dealing with it can be a particular challenge when the wife lives with the rapist.

Further Humiliation

Some rapists will force their victims to pretend they are enjoying the rape. Rape experts indicate that it's is a good idea to go along with the rapist on this one if he is so inclined. It seems that if the rapist is unable to complete the act, he is more apt to seriously injure his victim. Think of how seriously imbalanced he is mentally if he wants you to pretend you are enjoying the experience.

Whether to Report—If It's Child Abuse

While it is important if a child who is being abused can find a trusting teacher, counselor, minister or parent to tell, it's an unfortunate comment on our society to say that reporting doesn't always improve the situation. For some girls, it makes it worse, as dysfunctional families will often try to make her the problem. There is also the reality that while some state protective services agencies are top-notch, others are as dysfunctional as the families they are supposed to be protecting children from. Between failures of the criminal-justice system and an overwhelmed social-services system, good outcomes are sometimes the exception rather than the rule.

If you are an adult who suspects a child is being abused, you are often legally required to report to your nearest child-protective-services agency. Unfortunately, you wouldn't believe the number of grandparents and relatives who suspect abuse is occurring, but don't report it, and not because they are concerned about how well the system will or won't work. They will be the first to tell you what a shame it is the child is being abused, but in these cases, blood is thicker than semen. They wouldn't want to upset the family.

Equally disturbing are the number of divorces where one angry parent accuses the other parent of abuse out of revenge. If they are so sure the other parent was abusing the child, why didn't they say something about it before the divorce? This shouldn't be confused with situations where the divorce came as a result of learning that a child was being abused.

Whether to Report—If You Are an Adult and It's Rape

It's no secret that few rapes are actually reported, and that the percentage of reports is even lower in rapes where the victim knew the offender prior to the sexual assault.

There are reasons why women don't report. A common one is if the rapist is an important member of your social circle or your mother's favorite cousin. Or if he's your sister's husband or a popular guy at work or school.

Aside from social realities, it's hard to talk about a sexual assault. Other reasons for not reporting include fears that you won't be believed, fears that you will be blamed, and fears that the accused will somehow retaliate. Some women believe that if they didn't put up a fight, the state won't consider it rape. This is not true. Not fighting may have been the best way to prevent further injury or death. The fact that you are still alive indicates that you did the smartest thing that you could have. While fighting may have stopped the rape, it could have just as easily ended up in you being killed or seriously injured beyond any sexual trauma.

So why should you report? There are three very good reasons:

1. Rapists tend to be bullies who may see your failure to report as an indication that you liked what they did, or that you are an easy mark for a repeat offense. Reporting a rapist tends to protect you from re-assault rather than putting you in harm's way.

2. One of the greatest regrets among women who don't report is knowing that their lack of action may have made it possible for the rapist to sexually assault other women. This fact, even more than the rape itself, is what haunts some women the most.

3. Even if the man is not convicted, your report puts him in law-enforcement radar. It makes it much less likely that he will get away with it the next time. Even if he is not convicted, your reporting is what might save his potential victims.

Reporting—If He's In Your Social Circle

Reporting is socially easier if the rapist isn't part of your social circle. If he is, be prepared for people taking sides, and not necessarily yours. On the other hand, if you don't report, he will know you are an easy target, and you will have to live with letting him get away with it and with victimizing others. Don't waste time trying to warn him or threaten him. Your actions in not reporting him are all he will hear.

If you have reported someone from your social circle, it's probably best not to discuss it. Don't try to defend yourself or to say anything negative about him. The only people you should be speaking to about it are the police, the DA and your healthcare provider or counselor if you have one. Keeping these boundaries will probably make it easier for you in the long run.

Reporting—If You Are in a Sorority

Hopefully things in the Greek system have evolved and justice is more important than keeping quiet to maintain the social order. But understand that if you were raped and report a fraternity member to the police, his house brothers will likely feel that you have reported them—all of them. And the sorority sister of yours who had a secret crush on the guy? Get ready to meet your new worst enemy.

You won't read this advice in the "Welcome To Our Wonderful College!" booklets, but if you've been raped by a fraternity bro and decide to report him, get thee to the psych library and read about what happens in dysfunctional families when a child reports that she's been abused. Knowing how strange it can get will help you maintain a sense of irony and perspective that could be necessary if a psychodrama were to unfold around you. People join fraternal organizations with the hope of being a part of something that's bigger and better than they are. In accusing a fraternity man of rape, you are not only threatening the relationship between your sorority and his fraternity, you are taking to task the very system that has been the spawning ground of presidents, senators and supreme-court justices.

Does this mean you shouldn't report? Heck no. But it does mean that you will be standing out as an individual in an organization that is not exactly the Walden Pond of free thinking. The priority of some sorority sisters is to party with boys with pedigrees. They are as likely to see you, rather than a fraternity man who takes uninvited liberties with his penis, as the problem.

If you are in a sorority and you report a fraternity man for rape, or if you are in any tightly-knit organization and report a fellow member, be prepared to move out and move on. But think about it—in a world where people are tortured and killed for speaking the truth, is having to find new friends such a huge price to pay for doing the right thing? Is it such a huge price to pay for helping to protect other women this person might victimize throughout his life, because that's who will suffer if there is no price to pay for sex that is forced. In the long run, wouldn't you rather be known as a woman not to mess with, rather than as an easy target for forced sex?

If you are raped by a fraternity member and your sorority sisters stand by you, understand that you have found something that is truly precious.

When Straight Men are Raped by other Men

Most of us believe that rape happens to only women and gay or imprisoned men. We assume that any man who doesn't want to be sexually assaulted is able to defend himself and fend off the attacker. But just because you are a guy, it doesn't mean you should be able to win a barroom fight, thrash a mugger or fend off a rapist.

Rape is first and foremost about violence, power, sadism and hatred. The rapist didn't choose you because he thought you had a cute butt. He chose you because he thought he could.

When you've got a gun to your head or a knife to your throat, you suddenly have other priorities than saying, "Excuse me, Mr. Rapist, you've got it all wrong. I like girls!" Your job is to survive, and even if that means having to go down on the guy, you should do it and not think twice. Think of how many girls given you oral sex—and hopefully lived.

In addition to being blind-sided with a lethal weapon, a man can be sexually assaulted by a group of men he doesn't stand a chance against. Sometimes the rape can be the result of blackmail or of being drunk or stoned. The last thing a guy who is drunk is going to be able to protect is his rear end.

Male rape can happen in other ways, as well. Not too long ago, a former National Hockey League Player revealed that he was sexually assaulted by one of his coaches when he was a teen.

Unfortunately, a man who has been raped has fewer options than even a woman who has been raped. Think about it: how many guys are going to find it cathartic to tell their friends they were raped? Sad but true, the chances are good his drinking buds will be doing all they can to keep from giggling.

If you are a guy who has been raped, call a rape-crisis center or, even if you are the epitome of straightness, consider calling a gay-men's health center. They tend to be understanding and helpful about sexual violence against men. The advice they give you will most likely be the best to follow.

One thing that can be really confusing is if you became hard or came when you were raped. The truth is, it is not unusual to have an erection and orgasm when the body is under extreme stress or panic. As mentioned earlier in this chapter, plenty of guys who go to the gallows meet their maker with an erection and ejaculate in their pants, and not because they thought it was sexy to have a noose around their neck.

Some rapists are aware that you might get an erection. They will intentionally stroke you to orgasm just to mess with your mind even more. So what's the big deal if you did get hard and came? The important thing is in understanding that you were violently assaulted. We should all have erections and orgasms in such situations. At least you lived to think about it, which is a very good thing.

Men who are bisexual or gay sometimes worry that being raped or abused is what gave them their same-sex orientation. Or if you are a straight guy who was sexually assaulted by another male, you might wonder if this will impact your sexual orientation. Studies have never shown that sexual abuse or rape influences a person's sexual orientation, yet this is a myth that persists.

While you might want to keep it all inside, it could be that the rape has been causing you to deal with others–especially intimate others–in strange ways. What do you have to lose by speaking to a counselor about it for a session or two? As for reporting, the big issue is how strongly you feel about the guy being able to do this to other men, because it is likely that he will if he can.

Stephen Braveman specializes in the sex abuse of men. You might spend some time reading the articles on his site: www.bravemantherapy.com

Resources:

National Center for Victims of Crime
(800) 394-2255

Rape, Abuse, and Incest National Network
(800) 656-4673   (800) 656-HOPE

National Domestic Violence Hotline
(800) 799-SAFE

Your state or county may have excellent resources as well.

Recommended Reading:

Evicting the Perpetrator by Ken Singer.

Principles of Trauma Therapy: A Guide to Symptoms, Evaluation, and Treatment by John Briere and Catherine Scott.

Child Trauma Handbook: A Guide For Helping Trauma-exposed Children And Adolescents by Ricky Greenwald.

Treating Nonoffending Parents in Child Sexual Abuse Cases: Connections for Family Safety by Jill Levenson and John Morin.

Just Before Dawn: Trauma Assessment and Treatment of Sexual Victimization by Jan Hindman.

Readers Speak

"I was seriously dating one guy for four years (I was 16 when it started). Over time he became more and more thoughtless during sex until the point where it had crossed the line into violence. If sex was painful he would not stop, and there was emotional violence. We started out using porn to enhance our sex lives, but after a while he would position us so he could ignore me during sex and just watch the screen.

"I did two years of being single without sex after that to pull myself together. When I began having sex again I had flashbacks and would panic. I used to be so sexually outgoing and playful. I would enjoy oral sex. Now I don't do any of that anymore. For a long time I could not joyfully give my partners oral sex because of the negative associations with it, and sometimes I still have trouble not choking, even when it is barely in my mouth. Things are slowly improving, but I am worried it will never have that carefree way about it. It is hard to relax and not over protect myself. I've been married for a year now to a wonderful and gentle man that I've been intimate with for five years.... That's how long it's taken." *female age 27*

"I have been raped twice in my life by two separate men. The first was during my 16th birthday. After the party I went to my friend's spare bedroom to sleep. My then-boyfriend came in and lay next to me. We started fooling around but things started going too far. I asked him to stop but he didn't. He kept pressuring me, saying he wouldn't do anything serious. It ended with him just shoving himself in me while I was sobbing. That was how I lost my virginity. The saddest part is that I stayed with him for two more months.

"The second time I was at a friend's house. Drinking and playing Dungeons and Dragons. (Yes, girls are nerds too.) I drank far too much and lay down on a mattress that was sitting in the middle of the living room. All my friends went into the den to watch TV while this guy lay next to me. I should have figured it out then, but I was really drunk. I asked him to leave me because I was too drunk to be near anyone, let alone a guy with 'intentions.' He didn't leave. He started with the foreplay. I alternated between liking it and asking him to go away. It ended with him on top of me while I told him to stop. I suppose this one was partially my fault. Needless to say, the friendship ended there.

"Sex since then? I've never orgasmed. That may be due to the fact that I can't trust men. I'm never comfortable being naked around anyone. And to be completely honest, I don't really like sex. I think I'm just expecting men to mistreat me after having it. To just use me. Recently I have been in a relationship with a man who was a virgin before we had sex. His love and trust have gone a long way toward helping me believe that a guy might like me for more than just sex. It's helping me to enjoy myself more." *female age 20*

"I was continually abused growing up (emotionally, spiritually, verbally, mentally, sexually), so much so I don't remember much of it. I continued the abuse voluntarily by getting involved with men who abused me. For instance, I have two kids as a result of 3-a.m. encounters when I was three-quarters asleep. I'm still pretty badly messed up and have a hard time seeing when someone is trying to be decent. I have never had normal sex. I discovered recently (in the past two years) that what I thought was normal was far from normal. I never knew that you were supposed to have feeling inside. I thought it was normal to be numb inside. My former partner could stick any number of fingers up inside me, and I could never tell him how many there were. He could even put a whole fist inside, and I didn't know. He could scratch and wiggle–nothing, nada, zip, zero, zilch. Still have that problem. Maybe I'll figure it out someday."

female age 31

"When I was in middle school, and my body was just starting to mature, my step-dad was going through a rough time with work. He was pretty stressed. My mom was around, but she had a job as well, so obviously I was left alone with a man who I wasn't exactly fond of. He started getting a little too close and intimate for comfort. I told him I didn't like it. When he didn't stop, I told my mom. She didn't want to believe me. One night while she was out with her friends, I woke up and he was on top of me. I tried to scream. He stifled me. "It'll feel good, I promise," he told me. It didn't feel good. I screamed and flailed my body until I could get away. I ran and tried to hide. He found me and hit me so hard that I don't remember any more of that night. I was 12.

"I was ashamed of my body for a long time after that. But at the same time, I still really wanted the fellas who were my own age to take notice of me. I think I was looking for someone who would try to protect me. Eventually, I found myself in a good relationship that was much more about the emotional connection than a physical one. When we finally did get to that point, I felt so at ease with him that it was completely natural, pure and honest [and way good!]."

female age 18

"I was 9 years old. My karate instructor gave me a lesson in oral sex and other such matters. This was 32 years ago. I was not in a huge hurry to lose my *official virginity.* But then I had a great boyfriend for my *first time,* so it worked out. Get someone to talk to—a professional—and don't stop until you find one that helps you to release the pain or anger. It's not only possible; it's probable for good sex after bad IF you take it slow and find the right person. I think about sex not as something that is being done to me, but as something that I am giving to someone else." *female age 41*

"I was molested by my dad & younger brother. It took years of therapy to overcome self-destructive behavior. The abuse took a seemingly wholesome, enjoyable act, and made it ugly. I became psychotically self-destructive with sex, alternating between frigidity and promiscuity. I was able to find good therapist and a good man who loves me. I can finally breathe and trust, relax, have fun, and enjoy sex. (We're getting married later this year.)" *female age 30*

"It was seven years ago. In my room. My cousin's husband attacked me while I was sleeping. I never had sex before then. I look at sex as something that I don't need. Sometimes it just brings back the night of the bad. My advice? Take control next time. You'd be surprised at how much better it can be the next time that way! If it's happened to you, don't hesitate to tell someone else. I didn't, and I'm still paying for it. It took me four years to come to the reality of it. Don't hide anything. If you've been raped, don't think of sex as bad. Think of it as a way to better yourself." *female age 20*

"Recognize and accept what you can morally live with. If I'd had someone to turn to/talk to when I was a kid, things may have turned out differently. Now'days there are people, places, and/ or Websites you can contact to help you adjust. It's not your fault. Masturbation has been the one saving grace which has helped me adjust to my sexuality." *male age 68*

"Report it right away. My biggest regret is that I never did. The man who raped me raped others. Maybe if I had said something, they would never had to experience that. And get counseling. Don't just sit there and blame yourself. Always remember it wasn't your fault, and it doesn't make YOU a bad person." *female age 20*

"When I was about 7 or 8 years old, I was masturbated by an uncle. He gave me a dollar to "not tell." I never did. I began having sex at age 13 and was quite promiscuous. I believe I've had about 50 sexual partners, but only 6 or 7 of those in the past 10 or 12 years. I now realize that my behavior probably has something to do with the experience. I've learned to forgive, and to realize that people are better than their worst moments." *female age 33*

"I can't imagine a single situation in which rushing out and boning the first willing, semi-attractive person with a pulse is a good idea to help you overcome an unfortunate sexual encounter."

female age 18

"Relax and take your time. My fiancee & I weren't exactly rockin' the first few times. I needed to build trust and security, and then I could relax and truly enjoy myself." *female age 30*

"When I was 6- to 8-years-old, my best friend's dad molested me. He would make me give him oral sex, and touch him, and he'd touch me.... I try not to make too big of a deal about it. I have good relationships with women and like to think I am a relatively emotionally stable person. You can't let yourself be a victim. However, I still have frequent dreams about him abusing me, and sometimes I have sex fantasies about him as well. These disturb me because he abused me. I was so young that I think I repressed most of the negative thoughts. All I can remember are the way things felt."

male age 21

A Very Special Thanks to Dr. Robin J. Wilson, David S. Prescott, and to Alessandra Rellini at the University of Vermont and Cindy Meston for making the introduction!

87
Vaya Con Dios!

Hopefully, some of the beauty and magic of sex have been captured in the preceding pages for you to enjoy and share. And hopefully, *The Guide* has conveyed a sense that there's way more to sex than huffing and puffing while the bedsprings squeak.

This book doesn't pretend to have many answers, but it is a more evolved view of sex than many of us had when we first started getting it on. Thank you for being patient with its efforts to be more than just another how-to book on sex.

Whatever role sex has in your life, try your best to approach it with the respect and awe it deserves.

Vaya Con Dios!

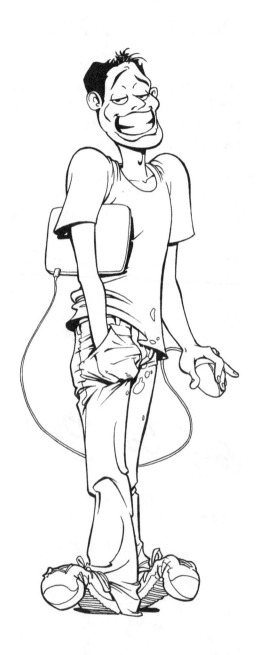

About the Illustrations

While readers usually ask for more illustrations, some have asked why the characters in the illustrations look so buff and nearly perfect. So here's some background about the illustrations.

The line-art in *The Guide* is extremely challenging to do because the illustrator has so little to work with—a simple black line on white paper. He doesn't use any of the usual tools that bring art to life: shadows, texture and colors. As a result, to give the line-art its feeling, the illustrator has to be a master of exaggeration. Without the exaggeration, line-art becomes flat and boring.

Notice how cut and buff the males in the book's drawings are, while the women are soft and smooth? These are exaggerations; without them, it's difficult to distinguish males from females in line art. Plus, there's the comic-book tradition where the males were werewolves, monsters and Supermen.

One of the challenges is balancing the exaggeration so the illustration is fun and comes to life, but doesn't put you off because it seems so outrageous. So each illustration is often worked and reworked, with a lot of give and take between Daerick, the artist, and Paul, the author. Here's an example:

> **Paul:** Her breasts are humongous and his penis looks like it's 16 inches long! And can't you put some weight on her? She looks like she hasn't eaten in two years.

> **Daerick:** OK, but you're going to hate how this one looks if I make them normal.

The Anatomy of a Drawing

While the concept sketch on the next page looks promising, it is still in sketch-form where the illustrator has used shading to deliver the concept. Getting it from there to line-art form can be fraught with peril. Fortunately, *The Guide's* illustrator is one of the finest in the world. If anyone can make it work, it's him. Sometimes just a tiny tweak at the edge of a character's mouth can be the difference between an illustration that works really well and one that doesn't.

An extra benefit in working with Daerick Gross Sr. is the humor, parody and detail that he is able to create within his line-art drawings.

1 THE CONCEPT

Paul to Daerick: I'm looking for a commentary on the couple who is certain the world will end if they aren't checking for messages. So I'd like you to try creating an illustration with a couple having intercourse doggie style–she's on her elbows and he's kneeling behind her. She has a laptop open on the ground in front of her, working the keyboard with the fingers of one hand, while perhaps texting on her phone with her other hand. Her male partner has his laptop open on her back while he's texting someone with a phone in his other hand.

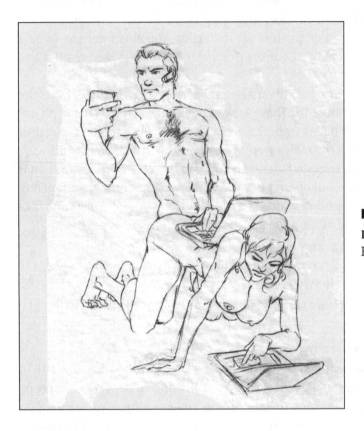

2 FIRST DRAFT

Daerick to Paul: How's this?

3 CRITIQUE OF FIRST DRAFT

Paul to Daerick: Fascinating—if they weren't using laptops and headsets, it would be obvious they were having sex. But adding the technology makes it confusing. The sex needs to be more obvious; perhaps more of a sideways POV. Also, can you reel in her breasts?

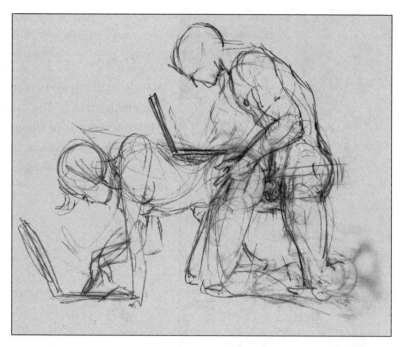

4
SECOND DRAFT
Daerick to
Paul:
Okay...

5 **CRITIQUE OF SECOND DRAFT**
Paul to Daerick:
Bingo. Ink it!

6 **VICTORY!**

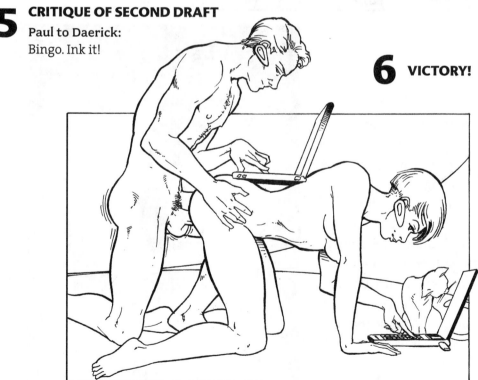

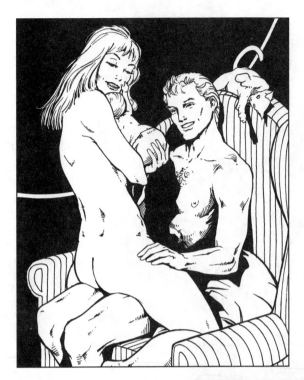

Here's an illustration from the 2nd edition of *The Guide.* The concept was to show that sex brings more than just orgasms, including hope and new life.

Naturally, someone claimed we were showing a couple having sex while holding a baby.
So for the 3rd edition, Daerick moved the mom back and crossed her leg over in front to remove any doubt. Since then, Paul said "I miss the original!" and so the original is back.

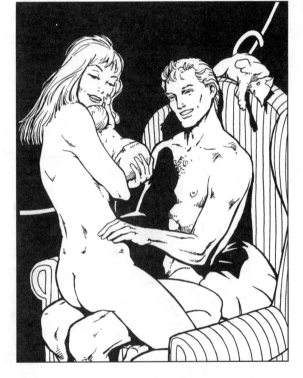

Thanks! Thanks! Thanks!

Mr. Jed Lyons, George "Chip" Franzak, Spencer Gale, Jason Brockwell, Kim Flowers, Vicki Funk, Karen Mattscheck, Michael Sullivan, and everyone at National Book Network. To the incredible staff of McNaughton & Gunn (present and past) including Renee Lane, Vickie Jedele, Jill Esch, Carleen Rogers, Tiffany Voorhees, Kerwin Leader, J.P. Stando, Dave Hite, Dave Fleming, Mike Vezo and Jeff Ochs. And to all at Publishers Group West who helped the book grow and thrive through its first five editions.

Karen Vail-Smith, Brian Cavanaugh, Janet Minehan, Marian Shapiro, Richele Frabota, Michele Sugg, Melissa Wittmayer, Dan Poynter, Jeff Harris, Tom Hunt, Neil Levin, Tracy Fortini, Kidder Kaper, Bill Hazeltine, Liz Brody, Cory Feldman, Kim Wylie, Sheri Lent, Rich Freese, John Cabral, Sarah Rosenberg, Heather Cameron, Melissa Fonseca, Kevin Votel, Elise Cannon, Cathy Vancik, Judi Baker, Mary Skiver, Kent Anderson, Sue Ostfield, Charles Gee, David Dahl, Eric Green, Keith Arsenault, David Ouimet, Kat Mulkey, Bill Richter, Michelle Fisher, Andrea Tetrick, Betty Redmond, Bill Getz, Eric Kettunen, Cindy Heidemann, John Masjak, Jon Mayes, Kristen Keith, Mike Katz, Ron Shapiro, Roy Remer, Graham Fidler, Sarah MacLachlan, Jill Kamada, Chris Schrader, Sabrina Young, Lance Tilford, Charlie Winton, Jerry Delaria, Becky Kaapuni, Cyndy Perlich, Chris McKenney, Sandra Patterson, Betty Redmond, Patricia Kelly, Harry Kirchner, Matthew Chilcott, Lina Hines, Roni Gallimore, Paul Rooney and Gary "who got the whole thing rolling!" Todoroff.

Bill Taverner, Melanie Davis, David Ley, Ken Haslam, Maureen Wehlihan, Adam Safron, Stephen Snyder, Steve Schrader, Marian Shapiro, Angela Hoffman, Kara Wuest, Bob Francoeur, Sue Palmer, Joe Marzucco, Rich Siegel, Jennifer Ashley, Theresa McCracken, Scott McCann, Regina Seitz, Leonie S.

Ralph Bolton, Bev Cutler, Cyrus Farivar, Kayla Strassfeld, Adrienne Benedicks, Inger Klekacz, Ryan Hanson, Todd Hawley, Dan Cullinane, Trena Jayne, Leslie Rossman, Michael Meller, Franka Schmidt Zastrow, Anke Vogel, Dmitri Siegel, Denise Westmoreland, Harry Gilmartin & Karen Kummerfeldt, Janet Hardy, Jay Wiseman, Matt Torrey, Dan Culliane, Kirk Groeneveld, David Hoffert, William W. Young, Claire Yang, Alessandra Rellini, Marca Sipski, Marilyn Milos, Stanley Althof, Violet Blue, Annie Bradford, Joe Pittman, Ricky and Larry Siegel, Braxton Sherouse.

Matt Comito, Rose Reed, Janice Hamilton, Larry Hedges, Barbara Keesling, Debra Hanson, Steven Wales, Avedis Panajian, Bill Young, Rob Hill, John & Miss Kelly, Nancy "Professor B" Carmel Eyes, Carol Bee, Ron, Steve, Linda & Jeanette at Old Town Printers (RIP), Martha and the staff at the Newport City Library. Ellen Barnard, Myrtle Wilhite, Monica Stone, Jamye Waxman.

Jon Westover, Morgan & Burce Yarrosh, Suzanne LaPlacette, Mike Fischler, Wanda Moore, Veronica Monet, Monte Farrin, Dixie Marquis, Mike Conway, Karen Saliba, Carol Tavris, Michael Kogutek, Katherine Almy, BJ Robbins, Ken Sherman, Bob & Kim Otto, Duncan Rouleau, Bill Applebaum, Nancy Reaven, Bruce Voeller, Andre Deuschanes, Meridith Tanzer, Roan Singh Sidhu, Evan Rapostathis, Kenny Wagner, Ross Rubin, Paula Samuels, Daphne Rose Kingma, Cathryn Michon, Diane Driscoll, Billy Rumpanos, Ben Fiorino, Ray Calabrese, Diana Heiselu, Judy Seifer, Randi Lockwood, Breta Hedges, Brent Myers, Ron Goosen, Pat Lincoln, Alison Rosenzweig, Marty Gilliland, Val Littou, Mat Honig, Sheryl Palese, Chip Rowe, Kathy Herdman, Jack McHugh, Pat Patterson, Dana Smart, Laura Corn, Elizabeth Olsen, Pam Winter, Judy Linnan, Theresa Benedick, Joe Sparling, Carol Queen, Lily & Bill & Louie at Sir Speedy, Monte at Input/Output, Joe Marsh at the Earthling (RIP), JuliannPopp, Jason Aronson, Bill & Beryl Johnson, Karen Seemueller, Christianna Billman and Lisa Blai , Glenn Knight, Emily Gudhe, Barbara Seamen.

Connie Overholser, Phil Bruno, Pam White, Jan Nathan, Terry Nathan, Peter Handel, Carol Fass, Eda Kalkay, Leslie Rossman, Patricia Holt, Adrienne Benedicks, Heidi Cotler, Babs Adamsky, Kevin Samsel, Mark Collins, Vince Darkangelo, Jon Cooper, Kris Lorret Rourke, Ben Saltzberg, Whitney Thomas, Stacie Herndon, Genanne Walsh, Rachael Cart, Joanie Blank,Constance Claire, Gretta, Christophe and Heather Shaw from Blowfish, John Davis, Leonore Tiefer, Marian Dunn, Michael Metz, Julian Slowinski, Katherine Hall, Helen Fisher, Dodie Ownes.

Andrea Best, Adam Moore, John Money, Rob Hardy, Kristen Kemp, Nooshin Thorpe, Carol Briezke, Esther Crain, Julia Gaynor, Carol Edington, Paul Harrington, Ed Alcocer, Diane Morrison, Elizabeth Lee, Verne Graham, Brett Miller, Joe Casella, Anne Katz, Donna Coomer.

The book would never have been completed without the friendship and psychological support of William Erwin. Thanks also to Donald Marcus,

Glossary of Sexual Slang
in Popular & Unpopular Culture

A2M—means ass-to-mouth. Sucking on a partner's unwashed penis after it has been up her bum. Way more popular in porn than in real life.

AC/DC—1. a bisexual; enjoys bedding members of either sex; ambisexterous, switch-hitter, or versatile. 2. heavy metal geezer band.

ADULT GRAPHICS COMMUNITY—3-D adult erotic art, comics and animation created by graphic artists in programs like Poser, Daz Studio and Photoshop. Premier website: www.renderotica.com.

AFRODESIAC—sexy-looking black man.

AFTER MARKET—a biological female whose genitals have been surgically constructed to appear male, as opposed to factory-equipped or original equipment; aka: F2M transsexual.

AFTERNOON DELIGHT—sex in the afternoon; a nooner.

AGE PLAY—sexual role-playing where one partner pretends to be older and in control while the other pretends to be much younger.

AIRHEAD—in a discussion on the effects of global warming, an airhead would want to know how it would affect his or her tan lines.

AIRPLANE BLOND (US) OR AEROPLANE BLOND (UK):—a woman who has dyed her hair but still has a black box. When the carpet doesn't match the curtains.

AMATEUR—a genre of porn that's supposed to be the real deal, allegedly created at home by horny housewives, hubbies with hard-ons, naughty neighbors, slutty sorority sisters and average guys in college dorms who just happen to have 9" penises. Prides itself in being free of the gloss, glitter and high production values of studio porn. Sure.

AMBIEN SEX—the website of the prescription sleeping pill Ambien warns that individuals who are taking Ambien have been known to engage in complex behaviors (e.g., preparing and eating food, making phone calls, or having sex) while not fully awake. You'd think this would be like having sex with a zombie, but spouses have claimed their Ambien-taking partners become very uninhibited and initiate intense and wild sex after taking a normal dose. While the person might seem totally awake, they often don't remember a thing about it the next day. Small doses of Ambien after a glass of wine have resulted in the same kind of uninhibited sex with no memory of it. So if your partner initiates sex after taking Ambien, she is not able to legally consent and you could possibly be

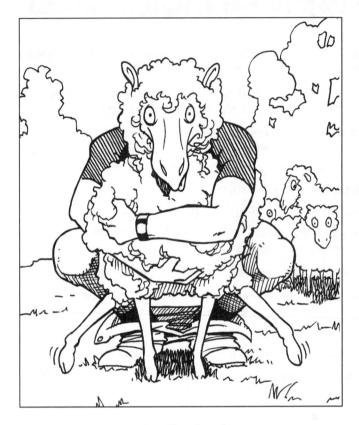

animal husbandry?

charged with sexual assault. Why not discuss it with her the next day and ask for guidance if it should happen again? Some women will say it's rape, don't you dare; others will tell you to go for it but lament they won't be able to remember the great sex they were having. Is it no wonder Ambien has become a leading date rape drug?

AMERICAN CULTURE—refers to traditional, missionary-position intercourse.

AMPALANG OR PALANG—a horizontal piercing through the head of the penis.

ANAL STRETCHING—what people do when they are into body modification and want their anus to achieve a much larger diameter than is normal. Or when a person uses a butt plug or dildo to help accommodate a penis.

ANAL—a blanket term for anal sex, anal play and rimming. May also refer to a person who struggles with orderliness and perfectionism to a point of not being able to complete things. Tends to be rigid and stubborn. People need to be somewhat anal to succeed in life, but more than that and they risk driving everyone around them crazy.

ANAL BEADS—worry beads for the rectum, to be pulled out as orgasm is beginning. Since the anus has an extreme number of nerve endings, pulling out the beads can help intensify the feelings of orgasm. Anal beads come in many sizes and configurations; pearl string.

ANAL BLEACHING—When a porn actress or actor slathers skin fade cream on their anal openings to make them look pink instead of brown. Makers of age-spot creams haven't included anuses on their list of body parts that are safe to bleach.

ANALINGUS—kissing or licking ass; rimming.

ANDRO DYKE—a lesbian who is neither butch nor fem, butch lite.

ANDROGEN INSENSITIVITY SYNDROME (AIS)—a genetic anomaly where an embryo with XY chromosomes is not sensitive to androgens. Androgens are the masculinizing hormones that push a male embryo out of its female-like state and result in male genitals and a masculinized brain. There are different kinds of AIS, including complete, partial and mild. With complete AIS, the baby is born a female, with a feminized brain and a vulva. Her vagina can be a bit short, and she doesn't have a cervix or uterus. As for appearances, she can be as plain or striking as any other woman, and she is a woman in almost every way except for a short bit of code on one of her chromosomes. A lot of women with AIS don't find out until their late teens, when they go to a gynecologist because their periods haven't started. AIS is an intersex condition.

ANDROGYNOUS—not really masculine or feminine. Boy bands often have an androgynous look.

ANIME—animated art or cartoons from Japan with a distinctly Japanese style. It is sexualized and is aimed at a more mature audience than American cartoons; characters have large eyes and wild expressions; women have multi-colored hair and breasts so big they look like they are going to pop. Often has nudity and violence, but stops short of being considered porn in Japan; Japanimation. Anime that crosses the line into porn is called hentai.

APADRAVYA—a vertical piercing through the head of the penis.

APHRODISIAC—substance that is given (or taken) to increase sexual desire. Be wary of anything called an aphrodisiac because it is usually people, and not substances, that turn other people on.

ARSE—British for ass, e.g. piece of arse, up your arse, arse wipe, Tom's an arse, arsing about, arse-over-tit (a bad fall), or tight as a duck's arse.

ASS BLOW—sticking your tongue into the anus; rimming, tossing salad.

ASS PLAY—sexual stimulation of the arse, especially focusing on the anus.

ATROPHY—1. scientific term for use it or lose it. 2. a fear that many guys have concerning their penis, especially when they haven't had sex for an epoch or two. Atrophy happens to muscles; the penis is not a muscle. The penis often gets a better workout from masturbating than from intercourse, so if you are concerned about atrophy...

AUTOFELLATIO—to suck one's own penis. Requires a long penis and a very nimble spinal column.

AUTOPEDERASTY—when a male can stick his partially-erect penis into his own anus; not the sport of short-dick men. Pederasty is when an old guy has sex with a young guy, so why this is called autopederasty makes no sense.

AVN—Adult Video News, official organ of the adult-video trade. Also refers to the annual trade show of the adult entertainment industry which is held every January in close approximation to the Consumer Electronics Show.

BABE RATIO—ratio of people you find sexually attractive to the total number of people in the room.

BAD LESBIAN—among politically stiff lesbians, a bad lesbian is a gay woman who has sex with a man or fantasizes about it. Writer Carol Queen attributes this kind of rigid thinking to the lezzie thought police.

BAGGER—male who attempts to partially asphyxiate himself while masturbating. Has resulted in deaths that are mislabeled as suicides.

BALL—noun: a testicle. verb: to have intercourse with; past tense is balled.

BALL GAG—a BDSM device which has nothing to do with the testicles. It is a strap which runs through the center of a rubber ball. The ball is placed in the mouth of the person being gagged and the strap goes around the head to hold it in place. The BDSM version of Croakies, with a rubber ball where the glasses should be.

BALLS TO THE WALL—a state of mind where one powers through a situation with tenacity and courage; origin: the Air Force.

BANGER—British for sausage or penis, with a banger hanger being a vagina.

BAREBACKING—anal intercourse without a condom.

BARE-BALLING—when a guy isn't wearing underwear. Also commando.

BARTHOLINS GLANDS—two small glands at the bottom of the vaginal opening which help secrete lubrication; explains why you should reach to the bottom of the vaginal opening to bring lubrication up to coat the clitoris.

BASHFUL BLADDER SYNDROME (PARURESIS)—when you can't urinate in a public bathroom or when someone else is present. Can be very debilitating. Shows how severely the mind can mess with the body; pee-shy.

BATTERY-OPERATED BOYFRIEND—a vibrator.

B-BOY—short for butt-boy, a man who enjoys taking it up the rear.

BBW—means Big Beautiful Women.

BDSM—umbrella term for erotic power play including bondage, discipline, spanking, and certain types of fetish play. The term BDSM started online, and encompasses the older acronyms of BD (bondage & discipline) and SM (sadism & masochism) and DS (dominance & submission). While BDSM is sexual, genital orgasm and stimulation is not its focus.

BEAR—large, mature male with masses of body hair and a fondness for other males. Used in gay porn and ads for sex or dating to describe big hairy guys.

BEARD—date or marriage arranged for a person who is gay to make them appear straight. Important for when mom and dad are in town, or when you are in the military, where a beard is known as a stunt babe.

BEARD BURN—inner-thigh hazard to women who receive oral sex from men with five o'clock shadow. Can be prevented by draping the woman's thighs with towels or plastic wrap, or by a quick shave on Thor's part.

BEER GOGGLES—alcohol-impaired vision that casts a beautiful glow on all that walks, often accompanied by feelings of dread in the morning.

BEAT OFF or BEAT YOUR MEAT—male masturbation; wank, jerk off, fap.

BEAVER—someone who attends Oregon State University. Refers to the female sex Oregons.

BEEFCAKE—idealized nude male body in photos and drawings in muscle magazines whose stated purpose was to extol the virtues of exercise and nutrition. The giants of the beefcake magazines were Bernaar MacFadden's *Physical Culture*, started in 1908, and Bob Mizer's *Physique Pictorial* which he founded in the 1950s. Its brother publication, *Athletic Model Guild* was wildly popular from the 1960s until 1993. Tom of Finland's famous drawings were highly stylized and overtly gay versions of the beefcake.

BEN WA BALLS—a pair of metallic balls that are inserted into the vagina for sexual pleasure while the woman rocks back and forth or squeezes her thighs together; more hype than reality since they don't work for most people.

BESTIALITY—when your sexual partner has four legs and a tail; farm sex, K-9 and animal training. The Spanish called it the Italian vice.

BICURIOUS—someone who is interested in exploring sex with a member of his or her own sex, but hasn't gotten around to it yet.

BIDET—oval-shaped porcelain bowl that is plumbed with a fountain of water over which a person squats to clean and sometimes stimulate the genitals; found in traditional European bathrooms; can also be used for anal hygiene.

BIKINI—a type of low-cut panties or swimwear that were originally for women. The bikini has been a fashion staple of the Western world for the past fifty years. The modern bikini was born in 1946. It was named after the island Bikini Atoll, which is part of the Marshall Islands in the Pacific Ocean where nuclear-weapon tests were done. It was so daring that the only model who would originally wear it was a nude dancer. It did not become popular in the U.S. until Brian Hyland's song *Itsy Bitsy Teenie Weenie Yellow Polka Dot Bikini* hit the charts, and women suddenly started gearing up, or down, in bikinis.

BIKINI LINE—how women in America often define their genitals.

BINT—insulting term for a woman in the UK, originally Arabic for daughter.

BIO-BOYS—transgender term for males who were born as males and who remain males.

BIOLOGICAL CLOCK—refers to a procreational urge or crisis that overwhelms some people between the ages of 35 and menopause.

BISEXUAL—person who is able to feel sexual arousal for both sexes.

BLADDER INFECTION—when bacteria with a painful kick establish residency in the human bladder; cystitis. A person so affected would be willing to pawn her grandmother's wedding ring for a hit of antibiotics. Bladder infections are more common in women because the passageway from the bladder to the outside of the body is much shorter, allowing bacteria easier access.

BLENDED ORGASM—popular-culture term for an orgasm that is thought to be from both clitoral and G-spot area stimulation.

BLIND DATE—aptly-named social event where two people who don't know each other have been set up by others.

BLOOD SPORTS—extreme BDSM play where the skin is broken and/or blood is drawn, such as piercing, whipping, cutting and vampire games.

BLOW—cocaine.

BLOWJOB—oral sex that's done on a guy; hummer, give head, go down on him, fellatio.

BLOW'N'GO—a quick blow job, can also refer to cruising.

BLUE BALLS—refers to a condition where a male has been sexually stimulated but not to orgasm. Sometimes hurts and is rumored to cause a blue tint to shroud the scrotum. Is easily cured by jerking off. At one time, blue balls was thought to cause physical damage, but evidence does not support this fear.

BMS—acronym for baby-making sex.

BODY SHOTS—when doing tequila shooters, suck the salt from whatever part of your lover's body he or she puts it on, and then suck the lime from his or her mouth. Somewhere in between, gulp down the tequila.

BODY MODIFICATION—things people do to change their bodies in primitive ways, including piercing, tattooing, branding, binding, cutting, castrating, nullification or corset training. The Rome of bod mod is www.bme.com.

BOFF or BOINK—to have intercourse.

BONDAGE—when someone gets a sexual high from that which the rest of us try to avoid.

BONE—a less than delicate reference to intercourse; e.g., to bone a babe. Also the dominant partner in a prison relationship, or a penis.

BONEYARD—area in prisons where conjugal (sex) visits occur with spouses.

BOOT BOY— a male submissive or an intern in a law firm or big corporation.

BOOTH TROLL—a male who cruises for sex with other men in the video booths at some adult sex stores. If successful, anonymous sex occurs, often while viewing straight porn flicks to give the appearance of being straight. Has the added excitement of potentially being busted by the vice squad.

BOOTY—means rear end, bum or caboose. Can refer to having sex, but not anal sex; go figure.

BOOTY CALL–late-night text message or phone call for sex, often cryptic, as in R U busy?

BOOTY CHECK—prison slang for rectal cavity search; finger wave.

BOTTOM—means sexually submissive, a BDSM term; Can also be the receiver of the penis during anal intercourse; catcher.

BOTTOM'S DISEASE—BDSM term for when a submissive takes the role too far.

BOTTOM SURGERY—when a transgendered person has their genitals surgically reassigned, as opposed to top surgery which refers to everything else.

BOXERS OR BRIEFS?—a question every guy ponders at one time or another.

BOY SHORTS—women's underwear. Low rise briefs with the start of a leg that offer full coverage but don't look like granny panties.

BRA HOOK—no single device known to humankind has caused more men (and some women) more angst than the hook of the bra. Legend has it that

Obi-Wan Kenobi originally taught Luke Skywalker about the force to help him unhook Princess Leia's bra. Given how they turned out to be brother and sister, it's fortunate that Leia's bra hook proved even tougher than the force.

BRANDING—when that which is done to a cow is done to a human. An extreme form of BDSM.

BRAZILIAN—differs from a usual bikini-area waxing because it goes all the way back to the tail bone, including deforestation of the anus. People mistakenly think a Brazilian has to do with the entire vulva being bare, but the key element in a Brazilian waxing is that the perineum and anus are plucked, as well as the sides of the labia. The mons pubis is the wild card: it can be bald or left with a landing strip, as long as whiskers don't hang out the sides or top of a thong.

BREATH PLAY or BREATH CONTROL—erotic asphyxiation. When the oxygen supply is cut off as part of a sexual turn-on. It is done during masturbation or couple's play, but is a health hazard and should never be done under any circumstances. The danger cannot be controlled or minimized, even if a cardiologist were monitoring the act.

BREEDER—a gay term for a straight person.

BREMELANOTIDE OR BREMELANOTIDE PT-141—a melanocortin agonist originally tested as a sunless tanning lotion. Imagine the surprise when men who were test subjects got erections in addition to tans and women test subjects wanted to jump the male test subjects? Development was stopped due to side effects including high blood pressure. The company then found that injecting bremelanotide subcutaneously (into the fat layer under the skin rather than into the muscle) does not appear to cause the elevated blood pressure side effects of the original nasal application. As of 2015, the company was doing phase 3 trials to test the safety and efficacy of the drug for female sexual dysfunction. According to one user, it won't make you want to have sex, but it will make things easier, and once things are going, it will keep them going. Do not use versions of this drug that are available on the Internet! On the street, PT-141 has been layered with erection drugs, which could be quite dangerous given the possible cardiac risks.

BRO JOB—oral sex between two males who consider themselves to be straight, often alcohol aided.

BROKEBACK MOUNTAIN—closeted cowboy extravaganza. As for the anal scene in the pup tent, according to www.NightCharm.com, no self-respecting gay man is going to throw spit on his penis and shove it up the bum of some cowboy who hasn't had a shower in years and has been eating nothing but beans by the campfire. Butt-fucking requires preparation and lube, or at least some bacon drippings. So the pup-tent scene in the movie was just symbolic.

BROWN SHOWERS—when being defecated upon is a sexual turn on as opposed to being a part of everyday life; scat, coprophilia, brown session.

BROWN SUGAR—refers to a sexy black woman or to having sex with her.

BUCK WILD—rap term, meaning to have wild sex or to act crazy; buckwildin. An example of proper usage is provided by *Body Count:* Get buckwild with the white freaks, show 'em how to work the white sheets.

BUDDY BOOTH—booth in an adult sex venue where there's a window to the next booth that has curtains and a button to raise it. This lets you watch the person in the next booth put on a show.

BUDDY SEX—see fuck buddy.

BUFF—having well-developed muscles, often the result of spending hours at the gym. While the buff look on men is sexy today, this might not have been the case in the early 1900s, when buff men were members of the working class and got their muscles from slaving at factory jobs. Back then, the pot belly may have been an indicator of opulence and sexual desirability.

BUGGERY—an academic tradition. Anal sex that's done to boys and young men in boarding schools as well as other places where men are warehoused.

BUKKAKE—a Japanese term that refers to showering the face of the receiver with the ejaculate of many men. Legend has it that in ancient Japan, a woman who was unfaithful was tied up in the town center where the male citizenry ejaculated on her face to show their distaste. Perhaps they were angry because the adultery happened with some other Samurai and not them. Has since become a fetish with some Japanese porn featuring it; aka facial.

BUM—British term for rear end.

BUNK-BED SEX—an agony forced on college students and some members of the military. Sex is the main reason to avoid bunking your beds. Get the bottom bunk if you have no choice. Imagine being drunk and trying to get you and a hook-up to the top bunk? And with the way a lot of bunk beds shake, it will be like trying to shag while sitting on top of an ocean buoy. If one of you falls out of bed from the lower bunk, we're only talking a broken clavicle at worst. Fall out of the top bunk, and all bets are off. A downside of being on the bottom bunk is the whole thing will shake when your roommate in the upper bunk is masturbating. And no matter if you get the top or bottom bunk, beware of overhead clearance. Will your partner need a helmet if she's doing a reverse cowgirl?

BUSH—refers to female pubic hair or to women's genitals.

BUTCH—a lesbian who has adopted the male role and runs with it. Formerly associated with short hair, Bermuda shorts and a T, and preferring to shop for clothes in the men's department. Now it refers to women more like Rachel Maddow, Ellen, Wanda Sykes, Julie Goldman or Megan Rapinoe. The term can also refer to an exaggerated form of manliness.

BUTCH-FEMME—an alluring woman who combines the no-nonsense strength of a stone butch with the steamy make your crotch drip and throb attraction of a femme fatale. This is a woman who can ride into town on a Hog wearing tattoos and leather, and ride out with men and women tripping over themselves to get her in bed. She blurs sex and gender boundaries, yet you would never use the word androgynous to describe her. The butch-femme was played well in some movies by actress Angelina Jolie. Butch-femme also refers to the community of women who describe themselves as being butches, femmes, stone butches, stone femmes, TGbutches, transmen and FtMs.

BUTT PLUG—toy for the rectum that's diamond-shaped or shaped like a Christmas tree with a stand, minus the holiday cheer. The base is specially flared so the anus can grasp and pucker around it, while the stand-part keeps the rectum from sucking it all the way inside. Gives a feeling of fullness. Can be made of silicone, rubber, metal, tempered glass or acrylic and sometimes vibrates and shoots fluid.

C2C—when used as a sexual term, it means cock-to-cock, as in two men rubbing their erect penises together. Also a British train company.

CAMEL TOES—when a woman's clothes (pants, shorts, bikini bottom) dig into her crotch and you can see her labia bulging along the sides of the crease; crotch cleavage.

CAMGIRL/CAMBOY—someone who spends from a few minutes a day to fulltime broadcasting images of themselves or their living space in front of a webcam. The vast majority of people who are doing this throw in a lot of sex and personal diary entries, enticing viewers to ante up a monthly fee for the privilege of watching. Now, it can include anything from exhibitionists to lifecasters to kids from Japan who spend a few seconds a day live but pull in hundreds of thousands of viewers; camwhore. See the discussion of Jennicam at the end of Chapter 4: *The Importance of Getting Naked*.

CAM WHORE—person who spends hours in front of his or her webcam, sometimes with clothes on, sometimes with clothes off.

CANDIDA ALBICANS—a yeast growth or yeast infection.

CAN ENTERTAIN—swinger term, signifies you are able to host the sexual activity in your home.

CASTING COUCH—entertainment-industry term referring to a process where a director or producer receives sexual favors in exchange for casting an actor/actress in a production or show.

CATHETER—in medicine, a tube that goes up the urethra to allow the draining of urine from the bladder. Used for sexual play in some parts of the fetish/kink/BDSM world; part of urethra play.

CAT 'O' NINE TAILS—the Mercedes Benz of flogging devices. Were first created by unbraiding rope used on ships in the British Navy which resulted in nine tails, which where then used on the backs of British seamen as a motivational device.

CBT—cock'n'ball torture.

CERVICAL CAP—birth-control device approximating a small rubber beanie that sits on the cervix to discourage male ejaculate from entering. Differs from a diaphragm in several ways: it is smaller, stays in longer, is usually not filled with birth control jelly, and is not as effective, especially for women who have had prior pregnancies.

CERVIX—the bottom part of the uterus found in the back of the vagina. It can be as small as a cherry in a woman who has not delivered a baby through her vagina, or it can be much bigger. Mucus passes through the cervical opening (os) and bathes the vagina. So does period flow. Sperm enters the uterus through the os of the cervix. The cervix feels softer during ovulation and its secretions change at that time. This is an important indicator for couples practicing natural birth control. The diaphragm birth control device works by making a dome over the cervix to prevent sperm from passing through it.

CFNM—means Clothed Female, Nude Male. Refers to situations where male strippers walk around naked and clothed female party goers grab their penises, give them oral sex, etc. a bachelorette party gone wild. Can include domination and submission, and can occur in a variety of sexual venues or situations. To find CFNM websites, enter the four letters in your browser.

CHAKRAS—an eastern concept (India, not New Jersey). The fuse box of the body whose seven points are said to regulate energy.

CHASTITY BELT—according to popular mythology, chastity belts with locks were popular in the 1100s. Crusaders who were leaving for war were said to have locked chastity belts on the pelvises of their female partners to assure the women would remain chaste during the years when they were off fighting the Pope's wars. Despite the myth, no such things existed in the 1100s, nor would they for another six- or seven hundred years. Chastity belts were a literary illusion dreamed up by Renaissance poets in the 16th Century as a way of saying "let us be true to each other," not that any of the poets offered up a male version of the chastity belt. The first real chastity belts weren't created until the 1800s, and they weren't for keeping women from straying sexually. The first chastity belts appear to have been crude devices designed to keep boys and girls from masturbating. There may have also been something akin to chastity belts in the 1800s at the dawn of the Industrial Revolution when women were beginning to enter the work force and sexual harassment was a serious problem. Some women may have devised their own versions of chastity belts to help keep them from being raped or molested while in the workplace. The most popular use of chastity belts throughout history is probably today in the BDSM community.

CHERRY—virginal or like new. Also refers to the hymen or maidenhead (for fans of Shakespeare).

CHEW TOY—refers to a person you are having sex with, usually on the Q.T., aka friends with benefits.

CHICKEN & CHICKEN FOX—a chicken is a boyish-looking younger man who wants to be cruised, cared for, or paid for by an older man or chicken fox.

CHICKEN OF THE SEA—a young gay sailor.

CHICKS WITH DICKS—persons who appear to be women except for the genital region. Usually a gender-bending or transsexual MtF man who would like to have bottom surgery but hasn't, or he loves his breasts, estrogen, female exterior in addition to his penis; she-he, she-male or he-she. Could possibly be a woman whose clitoris was enlarged prenatally due (an intersex condition), but that's not how the term is usually used.

CHIGGER—a small mite. You tend to get them from walking through infested areas rather than from sex. Can cause reddish welts and intense itching. Unlike scabies, they don't burrow into the skin and they don't drink blood. Their saliva causes a small wound in the skin, which becomes a welt. The chigger then drinks the body fluids which are in the welt. They usually drop off the skin in a couple of days. Under a microscope, they look like a small spider as opposed to scabies which look like small June bugs or tiny sand crabs. They are not as much of a medical problem as scabies. See scabies.

CHLAMYDIA—a sexually transmitted infection that is caused by a bacteria. You can get chlamydia in your vagina, penis, anus or mouth. It is one of the most common sexually transmitted infections, with almost 3 million new cases in the United States each year. Chlamydia is called a silent STD because most people who have it don't have any symptoms. See the chapter *Gnarly Sex Germs* for more information about Chlamydia.

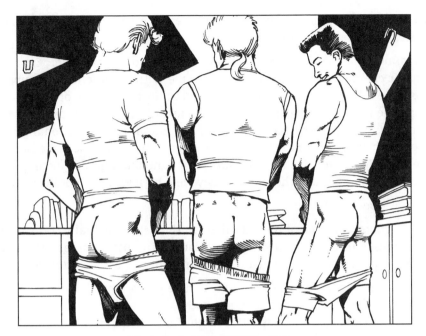

Circle Jerk. Boys Will Be Boys

CHOCOLATE—one of the few substitutes for sex. Traditionally used in the wooing process, chocolate lights up the same part of the brain as heroin. May have anti-depressant properties for women.

CHODE—slang term for a penis that is wider than it is long. In a different context, refers to the taint or perineum (area between the anus and genitals).

CHORDEE—downward curvature of the penis, congenitally caused.

CIRCLE JERK(S)—guys masturbating together. Also a semi-notorious punk band.

CIRCUIT OR THE GAY CIRCUIT—a series of same-sex dance parties. A cool concept in its early years. Some say the circuit still sizzles, others say it has become commercialism at its worst, catering to the cookie-cutter masses.

CIRCUMCISION (GOYIM)—an often unnecessary medical procedure where the foreskin of the penis is sliced or chopped off. The foreskin comprises up to a third of the skin on the entire penis. It was originally done in this country to prevent masturbation. It makes little (if any) medical sense to routinely circumcise young males. See Chapter 27: *Fun with Your Foreskin*.

CIRCUMCISION (JEWS)—the way a Jewish mother lets her son know who's in charge—jmw. What if Jewish males were required to wait until they were old enough to phone the mohel themselves so it could be a young man's conscious expression of his faith?

CISGENDER—gender-speak for someone who is not transgender. Cis is an organic chemistry term meaning a molecule with its functional groups on the same side. Trans means the functional groups are on the opposite sides. So people who are transgender have come up with the term cisgender when referring to people who have no gender dysphoria. Their functional groups (feeling they are male or female) and their genitals are on the same side. For the TRANSgendered, it's the opposite: their functional groups (feeling they are male or female) and the genitals they were born with are not the same.

CLAMPS—see nipple clips.

CLAP—gonorrhea. One of the old timers in the field of sexually transmitted infections. Can cause a burning sensation during urination as well as an unusual discharge. Is easily treated, but can do damage if not attended to.

CLITORIS—1. Latin for darned thing was here just a second ago. 2. The only organ in either the male or the female body whose sole purpose is pleasure—which from a biological perspective might indicate that female genitals are more highly evolved than males'. 3. Sometimes regarded as the Emerald City of women's orgasmic response. 4. Not to be approached in haste. 5. Sometimes wants to be caressed with vigor, other times can hardly tolerate being breathed upon. 6. While the clitoris is a fine organ to lavish huge amounts of attention upon, qualities such as tenderness, playfulness and respect also contribute largely to orgasmic response. 7. In Ebonics, it is called a click. 8. UK slang for an aroused clitoris includes the term budgie's tongue.

CLITORAL PUMP—a suction device placed over the glans of the clitoris in hopes it will increase the blood flow and create more sensitivity.

CLOCKED—when a stranger has identified an MtF transsexual as being a biological or factory-equipped male; aka read.

CLUBBING—a term that is sometimes used in porn-movie making, when the male who is receiving oral sex uses his penis to whack the side of the face of the person who is giving the oral sex. For most couples, this would not be a big deal, but with the size of the average porn star's penis, facial trauma can occur; aka a danza. Also refers to the trendier version of bar hopping.

CLUSTER FUCK—army term for being in a bad situation. Also, three-way sex.

COCK-AND-BALL TOYS—harness-like assemblies that snap around the base of the male genitals to pull the testicles up and apart. Some men hang weights on their CBT toys to stretch or pull down the scrotum.

COCK AND BALL TORTURE (CBT)—for the man who can't get enough abuse from life Involves being punched, slapped or kicked in the genitals as part of a sexual turn on. Can include being zapped in the testicles with electric devices, having the testicles placed in vices, or having the genitals tied up until they swell and look like they are going to pop. Add an extra T (CBTT) and you get Cock and Ball and Tit Torture.

COCK BLOCK—when one male interferes with another male's efforts or intentions to get laid. For the opposite, see wingman.

COCK RING—a ring made of rubber, steel or leather that fits tightly over the base of a penis or over the penis and testicles like a halter. The purpose is to help maintain an erection when the mind and body are otherwise not willing, or to make the male genitals appear larger. Cock rings hold shut the veins near the surface of the penis so the penile blood pressure does not escape. They are of somewhat dubious value, and should not be worn for more than 20 or 30 minutes without being taken off for a few minutes. Otherwise, there is a risk of permanent damage. In BDSM, a cock ring can be used on a submissive to denote ownership. Can also be worn as jewelry when hung from a chain around the neck. (See Cock-Ring Ken in the Chapter 67 on Barbie and Ken.) Regarding rings made of steel, if it gets stuck on a swollen penis, it will require a trip to a hospital to have it removed, where they may actually have to call in a locksmith or welder. This is why it is best if the ring is made of rubber or leather, or if it is metal, it should have a hinge for easy opening.

COCK SOCK—slang for a condom. This is also a gender bending term. If a woman goes out dressed as a guy, or has FtM fever and wants to become a guy, she might wear a cock sock (athletic supporter-like harness) to hold a soft pack (artificial penis and balls) between her legs; see packing.

COITUS—scientific term for sexual intercourse, taken from the root word Coit, which is a carpet- and drapery-cleaning business in Northern California. Coit is also the name of an extremely phallic-looking tower. Roll the tower in the carpets and drapes, and you have coitus.

COJONES—Spanish for testicles. Often misspelled as cajones, which means big boxes rather than testicles.

COKE WHORE—person who is so strongly addicted to cocaine that he or she will do anything (or anyone) to feed the habit; also meth whore.

COME CUP—a device that attaches to the head of a vibrator and fits over the glans of the penis. Be sure to use lots of lube.

COMING TOO SOON—when a male sexual partner consistently ejaculates in a minute or less and both he and his partner are distressed that he doesn't last longer. aka Premature ejaculation, PE or rapid ejaculation. See Chapter 53: *Premature Ejaculation—Dyslexia of the Penis*

COMMANDO—not wearing underwear. When it's a woman, our gyno consultant feels it's good for vulva health, especially while sleeping under hot covers with no air circulation.

CONDOM—another name for a rubber.

CONSENT—please see Chapter 13: *Consent*.

CORNHOLE—means the anus or anal sex. The term probably originated from the use of dried corn cobs in the place of toilet paper.

COTTONTAIL—term that nude sunbathers sometimes use for a person who wears a bathing suit; see textile.

COWGIRL—intercourse position where the woman is on top in a face-to-face orientation with the guy. If she is on top but facing his feet, the position is called reverse cowgirl.

COWPER'S GLANDS—tiny structures near the urethra inside the base of the penis which produce the clear, silky drops of fluid known as precum.

CRABS—what people often see on Card 10 of the Rorschach (ink blot) test. Also, sexually transmitted lice that live on pubic hair and sometimes make a person itch to the point of near insanity. Crabs have six legs, with two of them looking like the claws of a crab. They live on human blood and will often die within a day or two of leaving a body, as they can't live without the body's warmth or blood.

CRACK A FAT—Australian term for have an erection.

CRANK—speed (methamphetamine). The nasal decongestant propylhexedrine is often used to get a quick crank-like rush.

CREAMPIE—a vagina with male ejaculate dripping out of it; aka a wet deck. Porn-speak for when a man comes inside a woman's vagina or rectum and viewers see a close-up of ejaculate oozing out of the orifice. Provides reassurance that the actor has truly ejaculated. Different from the standard money shot where he pulls out and shoots semen on her body. See the Chapter *Porndoggie's Dirty Dozen*.

CROSS-DRESSER—when a man gets joy from wearing a woman's clothes and make-up; transvestite,

CROSSDRESSING—when a person of one sex makes a serious attempt to dress like a member of the other sex—and not a woman simply wearing her boyfriend's shirt or boxer shorts.

CRUISING—primarily a gay term for when men are on the prowl for a quick sexual encounter; aka jonesing for bone. Cruising spots can include parks, parties, bars, baths, or any established area where men are looking for sex. In traditional cruising, there is no need for conversation or small talk; business is business. The cruising of the '70s, '80s and '90s has increasingly been replaced by making contact on the Internet or with an app like Grindr, and then meeting in person twenty minutes later for sex.

CRUMPET—British term for sexual activity. Also a bakery product.

CRUSH—intense romantic feelings unencumbered by the burden of good judgment.

CRYPTORCHIDISM—Greek for a hidden gonad. See undescended testicle.

CRYSTAL DICK—impotence caused by crystal meth. Men who use crystal as a party drug sometimes take Viagra to counter crystal dick, which can create its own health hazard.

CUM (COME)—male ejaculate, the majority of which is produced by the seminal vesicles and prostate gland. Most males produce one-half to one teaspoon per ejaculation. Varies in consistency and taste. Contains sperm, hormones, polyamines, prostaglandins, PSA and other substances. Slang terms include: Splooge, Man Chowder, Spunk, Population Paste, Manthrax, Gizzum, Jizz, Love Juice, Baby Gravy, Pearl Necklace, Wad, Baby Batter, Pimp Juice, Dong Water, Man Jam and Number 3. See Chapter 6: *Semen Confidential*.

CUM SHOT—see money shot.

CUNNILINGUS—cunnus is Latin for vulva (the part of a woman's genitals that is on the outside) and lingere means to lick—put them together and see what you get. Has any living human being ever used the term cunnilingus outside of an academic setting? aka muff diver, go down on her, carpet munching, or eating her out.

CUNT—from the Latin cunnus (meaning vulva).

CUNT TORTURE—cock'n'ball torture for the BDSM-woman who has everything but a cock and balls. Intense stimulation that may or may not include pain.

CUP—see Shock Doc.

CUPID'S HOTEL—a vagina.

CURVED DICK—a penis that curves as it gets hard, most likely due to a tight ligament. This is perfectly normal unless it causes physical pain, or becomes increasingly worse with time, in which case you should consult with a physician. Since some men with curves feel self-conscious, consider the following:

one highly experienced woman explained to us that the best sex she ever had was with an Italian guy who had a curved penis. If you have a curve, experiment with different intercourse positions that might provide an advantage over men who don't have a curve. If your curve is a new occurrence, see Peyronie's Disease.

CUT—refers to a male who has been circumcised. Also a weightlifting term for muscles with great definition.

CYBERSEX—a sexual communication between at least two people that is focused on sexual relations and occurs via synchronous Internet modes (according to Shaughnessy, Byers and Thornton).

CYSTITIS—see bladder infection.

DAIRY QUEEN—a gay man who likes to suck on guy's nipples.

DARKROOM—designated place in clubs, bars, baths, parties where men who enjoy sex with men can have orgy sex.

DAISY CHAIN—sex involving multiple participants where the genitals are being pleased in a multitude of ways.

DATE—without this event, men might never cut their toenails.

DATE RAPE—when a woman is raped by someone she knows or someone who won't stop after she indicates that she wants the sex to stop.

D/D—in sex-related ads, this means drug and disease free.

DELIVERING THE WOOD—to have intercourse with.

DEPILATORY—cream for removing body hair.

DEPTH PLAY—refers to liking a dildo placed deep inside of your favorite orifice. Requires an extra-long dildo, sometimes a foot or longer and perhaps with a special shape.

DHAT SYNDROME—an excessive preoccupation with semen loss. This is a fairly common obsession in India and Pakistan where the belief exists that semen is a perfect and powerful body fluid; loss of it robs the body of its vitality.

DIAMOND CUTTER—the mother of all erections. It is so hard it feels like you could cut diamonds with it. Thank goodness not all erections are diamond cutters, because the pressure inside the penis gets so intense it can actually hurt.

DIAL-A-PORN—phone sex at the rate of $2 or more a minute. Masturbation enhancement for those who like their stimulation over the phone. The women who give phone sex usually work with the caller to create his favorite role-playing fantasy, often something he is too embarrassed to act out with a real-life partner. A massive source of income for phone companies; aka dial-a-fuck.

DIAPHRAGM—a contraceptive barrier device that holds contraceptive jelly against the cervix. A cross between a condom and a frisbee.

DICK FLICKS—movies with lots of guns and violence, as opposed to chick flicks.

DICKNOTIZED—when a girl has such a serious crush on a man that her life becomes defined by wanting to hold him, touch him, talk to him and be with him. Brain researchers are able to see the brain structures being lit up when a lover looks at a picture of his or her idealized lover. They can see how the parts of the brain that help us to have good judgment are being shut down, while the reward parts that are involved with things like drug addiction are having a fireworks display.

DIESEL DYKE—a manly lesbian; butch or bull dyke. Opposing terms are lipstick lesbian, diamond dyke and femme.

DILDO—sex toy that brings much happiness. Can be used freestyle, or when mounted in a harness. Also slang for a person who is being a jerk or an ass.

DILDO HARNESS—a rig that holds a dildo in place at the same angle as a penis. Looks somewhat like a man's athletic supporter. Gives the dildo penis-like properties of suspension and thrustability, but without the maneuverability of the real thing; strap-on.

DOCKING—when an uncircumcised male pulls his foreskin over the head of another man's penis. A straight version might be when the foreskin is pulled over a woman's nipple. Also cyberslang for having sex; to dock.

DOGGIE STYLE—intercourse from behind, not to be confused with intercourse in the behind. More popular than the missionary position in some parts of the world. Can also refer to anal intercourse, but not usually.

DOGGING—formalized voyeurism, where couples who like to be seen having sex log onto special dogging forums and announce the time and place where they will be having sex in their car. Spectators who show up get to watch. Takes most of the risk and long hours of waiting out of being a voyeur. Started in the UK. The term originally referred to peeping Tom action, which was not necessarily done with the consent of the couple. Then came the Internet.

DOG'S BOLLOCKS—an expression in the UK which means "The best!" such as "Marty's new car is the dog's bullocks!" Also, "The mutt's nuts."

DOM—a dominatrix.

DO-ME QUEEN—in BDSM, a bottom whose entire existence revolves around getting the attention of others while giving little in return. In the entertainment industry, an actress or actor.

DORK—a whale's penis.

DORMCEST OR HALLCEST—having sex with someone who lives on the same hall or in the same dorm. Does not always turn out well.

DORMGASM—trying to stay very quiet when having sex or masturbating while your roommate is present, or if the contractor was over-budget and didn't put insulation in the dorm walls. For roommate wanking protocol, see Chapter 25: *Playing with Yourself.*

DOUBLE ANAL—simultaneous penetration of the anus by two penises.

DOUBLE BAGGED—wearing two condoms at once. Not a good idea.

DOUBLE DILDO—dildo that seats two. See Feeldoe dildo.

DOUBLE PENETRATION—penises in the vagina and rear end at the same time; sandwich. Can also be two penises in one vagina at the same time.

DOUCHE BAG—less-than-complimentary term for a woman or prissy man. A gravity-driven device for feminine hygiene. Does not win a nod of approval from the average gynecologist.

DOWNLOW—slang term in the black community for a gay or bisexual black man who is not out but who has sex with men. He can often be married or have a girlfriend but the man-to-man sex is kept quiet so he isn't banished from the straight part of the community.

DRAG—when a man wears women's clothing.

DRAG KING—a factory-equipped female who is dressed like a man. Judith Halberstam divides the drag kings into two groups: the *butch drag king* who's such a natural at it that not even the manly guys mess with her, and the *femme drag king* who has to work really hard at it. Can include anyone of any gender who makes hyper-manliness an act, performance, or parody.

DRAG QUEEN—men who love to dress up and become female characters. A drag queen often refers to her female character as if she were another person: "Cynthia had a bad day and is feeling like a total bitch" or "Crystal was dressed to the nines tonight!" Drag queens tend to be a bit more boisterous about their gender identities than either transsexuals or transvestites; when you are in a room with a drag queen you often know she's there because she so loves giving life to the female character she is playing.

DRAINING THE WEASEL—taking a leak.

DRESSED TO THE RIGHT OR LEFT—guys who wear boxer shorts have to make a decision in life: on which side of the fly to rest their genitals. This is no big deal (sorry) unless you get your pants tailor-made, in which case the tailor will inquire, "Sir, do you dress to the right or to the left?" He will then leave extra material on whichever side you indicate. Deciding which side your package should rest on is usually a no-brainer, since it naturally feels better on one side or the other.

DRUNK DIAL (NOUN) OR DRUNK DIALING (VERB)—a phone call that would be better made while sober, or not at all. Often results in the receiver of the call finding the caller to be a pathetic ass, especially when an ex- is involved. Can refer to texting as well, but "drunk text" doesn't roll off the lips nearly as well as "drunk dial." Good friends do not let friends dial (or text) while drunk.

DRY HUMP—traditional sport of young couples, where pubic regions are feverishly rubbed together while both participants are fully clothed or in their underwear. Can result in chafing, irritation, orgasm or all three; frottage.

DRY SEX—intercourse where the woman tries not to lubricate, as practiced in parts of Africa. If the woman lubricates as much as Western women, she risks having bad things thought about her character.

DTF—down to fuck, means ready, willing and wanting to have sex. Can refer to a person, place or condition, eg. "I'm getting some tonight, she's DTF" or "That's the most DTF dorm on campus."

DVDA—porn-speak for double vagina, double anus. Refers to the penises of four men simultaneously penetrating a woman's vagina and rectum. It is not humanly possible, but was alluded to in the B-movie satire *Orgazmo*.

DYKES ON BIKES—an all-girls motorcycle club.

DYSPAREUNIA—a persistent or recurrent genital pain associated with sexual intercourse. May have multiple causes and can be a bear to treat. Associated terms are vulvarvestibulitis and vaginismus.

ECTOPIC PREGNANCY—a pregnancy in which the embryo implants into the wall of the Fallopian tube instead of the uterus. A very dangerous condition which can result in maternal death.

EDGEPLAY—in the world of BDSM, there's your mainstream whip, chain and collar play, and then there's the edge, which refers to the edge of what is safe. People into edgeplay are willing to take the extra risk of serious harm and sometimes even death for the added rush or thrill.

ELBOW GREASE—a brand of lubricant often used for masturbation or anal play, well known in the gay community.

ELECTROPLAY—using different types of electrical current on the genitals and other body parts. Requires special equipment. Some kinds of electroplay use the current in an attempt to enhance pleasure. Other forms of electroplay are used to administer pain, which people who are into BDSM can perceive as pleasurable. See e-play.

ELLA—pill approved for emergency contraception. Effective closer to the time of ovulation than Plan B.

EMERGENCY CONTRACEPTION—1. let's say you didn't use birth control, or your method failed (the condom broke, you forgot to take the pill for a few days or you were raped). If you don't want to become pregnant, you've got three choices: roll the dice and do nothing, have a copper IUD installed within 5 days—which would take care of your birth control needs for the next 7 to 10 years safely and hassle free, or take Plan B or Ella ASAP. 2. Both Plan B and Ella work by preventing the egg from leaving the ovary. So if you take them after the egg has entered the Fallopian tubes, they do not work. Contrary to what some abstinence-only groups have claimed, neither Plan B nor Ella cause an abortion. In fact, this is why you need to take them as soon after unprotected intercourse as possible, because once you ovulate, they don't work. 3. Plan B is one pill, while the generic version of Plan B is two pills. You can take both of the generic pills at once, and you've got the same dose as if you took one Plan B. Plan B does not require a prescription and males can buy it as well as women. However, Plan P may not work for women who weigh more than 176 pounds. 4. Ella is more effective than Plan B, but you need a prescription for it. 5. Plan B has been shown to be extremely safe, even if taken multiple times. 6. People often confuse Plan B with Mifepristone which causes an abortion. (Mifepristone was known as RU-486 and in the US it is called Mifeprex.)

EMERGENT SEX—when cybersex occurs in games that were not designed for players or avatars to have sex in. Can range from simple avatar-avatar flirting in an MMORPG like *World of Warcraft* to entire sexual economies in an MMO such as *Second Life*. While it might feel safer because it is not real life, emergent sex can take on some of the emotions that accompany real-life sex.

ENDOCRINE DISRUPTERS—see phthalates.

ENDORPHINS—hormones secreted during exercise, laughter and orgasm. These hormones are pain-relieving and share similarities with morphine. Endorphins are also secreted when the body is being stressed or when pain is applied, such as in BDSM, which is said to result in pain reduction and euphoria.

ENGLISH CULTURE—refers to being turned on by spanking or caning.

ENURESIS—peeing in your sleep. Happens to almost as many girls as guys and can last until adulthood. It can be a really lousy thing to have and is sometimes very difficult to shake. Modern pee-absorbing underwear makes it less embarrassing.

EPHEBOPHILIA—where an older man has a sexual obsession for teens who are approximately 15 to 18 and who look young for their age. The term Lolita used to be associated with straight men who have this desire, and "twinks" are the object of desire for gay men with ephebophilia (the boy's genitals are fully adult, but his beard hasn't come in and he looks young for his age).

EPIDIDYMIS—tightly coiled tube that sits on the top and back of the testicles; a storage space where the sperm can mature. The scrotal version of oak barrels where wine or whiskey mellows and ages.

EPIDIDYMITIS—when a man's epididymis gets an infection.

EPISIOTOMY—an incision made in the bottom of a woman's vaginal opening to increase its size so she can deliver a baby without tearing herself.

EPISPADIAS—a developmental problem where the urethra comes out the top of the penis. Related to hypospadias but different and much less common.

E-PLAY—using electricity in a way that is sexually exciting. Can be mild (e-stim or e-jo, electrical jerk off), or painful for BDSM. See electric play.

EROTICISM—state of tension fueled by sexual desire.

EROTOPHILIC—refers to people who have positive feelings about sex.

ESCORT—sex worker or prostitute, can provide social as well as sex services.

EUNUCH—man without testicles; sometimes without a penis as well. This can be a self-administered fetish or is done at the man's request. In past centuries, it was done to slaves and choir boys. Eunuchs could rise to positions of influence or power, given how they were not seen as the kind of threat that a man with sexual urges might be. In the later Roman Empire, the real power was thought to be in the hands of the Emperor's Chief Eunuch. In the Byzantine era, it was not unusual for parents to have one of their sons castrated, with the hope that he would rise to a trusted position, and would then be able to offer help and aid to his other family members. In the modern era, parents don't have this done to their sons, but it doesn't mean they haven't thought about it.

FACEBOOK WHORE—a person who does not seem to experience his or her life unless it's posted on FB. Someone who regards FB wall posts as the building blocks of life. See Myspace whore for historical reference.

FACE SITTING—when a woman straddles the face of the person who is giving her oral sex; queening.

FACIAL—when a male ejaculates on his partner's face. A staple of mainstream male porn. It is difficult to not view this as being degrading toward women, but men who watch a lot of porn (and some women) will argue otherwise.

FAG HAG—a woman who hangs out with gay men, claims to want sex with straight men, yet seems to fear intimacy with straight men or doesn't particularly like them.

FAP—term for male masturbation derived from the "fapping" sound a guy makes when he's masturbating. Also can be used in reference to someone or something that looks hot, because they make you want to fap or masturbate.

FARANG—Thai term for whites or Westerners. Farang prostitution refers to the flesh trade that revolves around the pocketbooks and penises of Westerners. It wouldn't be unusual for the Thai to say "These are Farang sex tourists on a two-week shagging spree." Related term: sexpat.

FAYGELEH—Yiddish term for gay male.

FANNY—in Britain and Australia, the vulva or vagina; in America, the arse.

FANNY MAGNET—British for something that attracts swarms of women, "You should see his brother's Aston Martin, a right fanny magnet!"

FAUXMOSEXUAL—man who appears gay by his mannerisms but who sleeps with women; aka metrosexual.

FEELDOE DILDO—a two-headed dildo that stimulates both the doer and receiver. If a woman is physically robust, she might get away wearing this kind of dildo without a harness. It has a bulb-like end that goes in the vagina of the wearer that helps it stay put. The company makes a model with a smaller dildo end, which is often preferred by male-female couples in pegging or 'bend over boyfriend' situations. The model with the bigger dildo end is more often preferred when the receiver has a vagina.

FEEL UP—to touch or stimulate a partner's genitals with your hand; grope.

FELCHING—when a man ejaculates into a partner's mouth, vagina or anus, and then sucks or licks his ejaculate out of whichever orifice he shot it into.

FELLATIO—from the Latin fellare meaning "that which stops after marriage."

FEMBOT—a droid commissioned by Dr. Evil to do in Austin Powers.

FEMDOM—a term born from the fusion of female and domination, where a woman has control or dominance in a relationship because it fits the emotional chemistry of both partners, and they want it that way. Femdom can be as extreme as a full-time mistress/slave arrangement including serious cock'n'ball torture, or it might include only occasional role-playing and perhaps foot worship, bondage or queening.

FEMALE EJACULATION—some women squirt extra fluid as part of having an orgasm; varies in volume and frequency. See further discussion in Chapter 7: *What's Inside a Girl*.

FEMALE MASTURBATION—when a woman stimulates her own genitals for sexual pleasure, aka she bop, diddle, frig, jill off, muffin'buffin', slam the clam.

FEMORAL INTERCOURSE—when a lubricated penis slides between the labia like a hot dog would if it slid up and down the length of a hot-dog bun.

FEMME—feminine-looking lesbian as opposed to butch. The majority of lesbians would be considered femme, assuming you have an overwhelming need to use labels. Femme covers a much broader spectrum than a lipstick lesbian, as lipstick lesbians are almost always assumed to be straight and have a tendency to be high maintenance. Very high maintenance.

FENCE PAINTING—term for when a male porn actor performs oral sex on a woman The camera's view of a woman's genitals is far more important in porn than her pleasure, so the male actor sticks his tongue way out and wags it at her genitals like he's painting a fence with it.

FETISH—a particular prop (leather, rubber, underwear, shoes, etc.), body part (feet, hair, breasts, etc.), or a scenario that a person relies on to get off sexually; a paraphilia. The prop can be fantasized or exist in actuality. One philosopher has described a fetish as when a hungry person sits down at a dinner table and feels full from simply fondling the napkin. Also a lucky charm or object that is believed to have special or magical powers.

FIFTY-FOOTER—someone who looks hot from across the room, but starts looking less inviting with each approaching step.

FIFTY SHADES OF GREY—a book that made reading about being spanked while having ben wa balls in your vagina a popular literary pastime. Rarely does a blockbuster national best seller receive so many bad reviews from people who really wanted to like it. That's because it's not very well written. The selling points are when the leading male character is perfect (young, great looking, brilliant, with a big dick and billions of dollars in the bank) and never has to work, but instead spends all of his time worshipping and being fixated on the protagonist who he enjoys having kinky sex with. It's what you'd expect from a nation that has spent 2 billion dollars on abstinence-only sex education.

FIGGING—when a peeled piece of ginger is inserted into the anus as you would a suppository to create a burning feeling. It is said to increase sexual enjoyment. Why figging and not gingering? The term probably comes from the 19th century expression feague or feaguing which meant to put a piece of peeled ginger up a horse's arse which caused the horse to march with its tail held high. This was a popular practice among mounted military regimens.

FIGMO—military term meaning "fuck it, got my orders;" used when someone wants you to do something but you are already occupied.

FIST FUCKING (FISTING OR HANDBALLING)—placing a fist into the rectum or vagina, hopefully with lots of lube. It can be a male fist or a female fist, but if you hold the average male hand against the average female hand, some people might prefer the woman's hand while those with a skosh more room in their orifices might prefer the male hand. The term is a misnomer, since the hand goes in with the fingers extended and fingertips bunched together rather than in a fist. However, once it's inside, all bets are off.

FLAMING—term for an effeminate male; nellie, a nancy boy, fem, queen, the opposite of being butch. In the cybersphere, flaming is an extreme and perhaps pointless argument in a chat room or forum; aka flaming out.

FLAPPER—term used to describe a sexually liberated woman during the 1920s who flaunted her unconventional approach to life. Also refers to a style of fashion during the 1920s.

FLIP & FUCK—a cheap fold-out chair made of large foam cushions that easily turn into an imitation futon. Comes in handy for couples as a quick place for sex in college dorm rooms and student apartments.

FLOG THE LOG—to masturbate or fap.

FLUFFER—a person who keeps male porn stars erect when they are not on camera. Fluffers aren't used as much these days, as today's male porn stars are supposed to have trained wood (erect on cue), often aided by lots of Viagra.

FORCED MILKING—A term borrowed from the BDSM community, where a male is made to ejaculate repeatedly.

FORDYCE SPOTS—tiny yellowish or white bumps on the scrotum, shaft of the penis, labia, nipple and lips that occur when sebaceous or oil-producing glands in the skin get clogged up. Fordyce spots aren't filled with pus like a zit might be, but they do start to form during puberty when testosterone kicks the sebaceous glands into high gear. Often smaller than the head of a pin, these little bumps can make the skin look like that of a plucked chicken. Fordyce spots are not contagious and they aren't caused by a sexually-transmitted infection.

FORESKIN—male equivalent of the clitoral hood. A sensitive flap of skin with thousands of nerve endings that extends from the shaft of the penis over the glans to keep the latter moist and safe. Also allows the penis to more easily glide during intercourse, and makes lube less necessary for masturbation and hand jobs. The part of the penis that gets chopped off during circumcision.

FORNICATION—intercourse between people who are not married.

FOUCAULT—a French philosopher who philosophized about sex. What's more fun, reading Foucault or Lacan?—get back to you on that one. One of the things Foucault believed: Once the church decided we needed to confess our sins to a priest in order to save our souls, we needed to find ways to put our sins into words. And so we started describing sex, which was sinful, with words, and this gave governments and religions ways to regulate it, and sex became a way of having power over someone, even in intimate relationships. (Unless you've got Red Bull or Rockstar handy, be very wary of paragraphs containing the names of both Foucault and Nietzsche.)

FRAZIER—manliest lion to ever live in captivity; once had intercourse more than 160 times in three days. Died shortly thereafter.

FREEBALLING—when a guy isn't wearing any underwear, aka commando.

FRENCH—term for oral-genital contact, not to be confused with French kiss, although one often leads to the other.

FRENCH EMBASSY—term for a place where there's lots of gay sex going on.

FRENCH KISSING—kissing with mouths open as opposed to closed. Usually involves transfer of tongues (in the nonbiblical sense); suck face.

FRENCH TICKLER—any form of condom that has bumps, projections or ridges that are marketed to increase a woman's sexual pleasure. Some women will like these, while others find them to be uncomfortable or obnoxious. Ask first!

FRENULUM—sensitive part of the penis just below the head on the side of the shaft that faces away from the belly when the penis is erect.

FRESHMAN 15—urban myth that college freshmen put on 15 pounds their first year. Research shows it's actually two to five pounds. How much of it is from beer and how much from dorm food has not been determined.

FRIENDS WITH BENEFITS (FWB)—see fuck buddy.

FRIG—British for jerk off; wank, five-against-one.

FROG KISSER—person who believes that she can turn a loser into a winner.

FROT—gay term for when aroused males rub their erect penises together; C2C, bone-on-bone.

FROTTAGE—see dry hump.

FSD—stands for Female Sexual Dysfunction. Beyond that, all bets are off as to the specific meaning, or as we say, "The definition and correlates of female sexual response and female sexual dysfunction continue to evolve."

FUCK BUDDY—friend or acquaintance you occasionally (or often) have sex with. While the sex might be serious, the relationship isn't, or not in an engagement-ring way; buddy sex, hooking up, friends with privileges.

FUN AND GAMES—in the swinging lifestyle, a term that refers to having sex.

FURRY—someone who is fascinated by the idea of animals having human qualities, like being able to talk or having a body that is a blend of human and animal qualities. The correct terminology for animals with human-like qualities is anthropomorophic animals. For those who want to take their intrigue with animals a step further, there is an entire furry community with websites like furcadia.com and conventions where people dress up like their favorite animals. There is special furry art and furry fiction. Do not assume that people who are furries are into furry sex. That is only a subset of furries. See yiff.

GANG BANG—when a woman enjoys having intercourse with several men in rapid succession, at her invitation; pulling a train. This is something that some women who are in the swinging lifestyle can do without much fuss.

GANG BANGER—member of a street gang.

GAPE OR GAPE SHOT—the flower of Gonzo Porn, where the camera does a close-up interior shot of a woman's anus right after anal intercourse. The hallmark of the gape shot is that the woman's anus is still open and male ejaculate is dripping out. Can be of a vagina as well. See Gonzo Porn.

GENDER-BENDER—person of one sex who has become, is becoming, or fantasizes about being the other sex. Requires a fluid sexual identity; see transgendered.

GENDER DYSPHORIA—when the genitals you have and the genitals you wish you had are not the same. This is when a guy seriously wishes he were a woman or a woman seriously wishes she were a guy. May lead to taking feminizing or masculinizing hormones of the desired gender, and sometimes sex-reassignment surgery (SRS).

GENDER FUCK—mixing and matching gender attributes, such as wearing a lacy bra with an athletic supporter, having a beard and wearing a dress, or wearing a hard hat with high heels. A watered-down version is when a woman wears a frilly dress with Carhartt boots or Doc Martens. While the latter was originally a gender fuck, it is now an acceptable part of fashion and no longer has the defining elements of being a gender fuck (in most cases).

GENDERQUEER—when the normal definitions of male and female don't quite do it for you. Has become a blanket term for all things having to do with gender and transgender.

GENITAL ACNE—a condition caused by the eruption of small glands on the labia and scrotum called apocrine glands. Looks like zits, but isn't really.

GENITAL BEADING—a form of body modification where beads are implanted under the skin that's on the shaft of the penis.

GENITALS—the part of yourself that you play with under the covers; in the UK, the term bits is often used, especially for female genitals.

GETTING OFF—coming or having an orgasm; getting your rocks off.

GFE—stands for *The Girlfriend Experience,* which is when an escort or prostitute goes that little extra and acts like a girlfriend for the night, including kissing, hugging and holding hands. BFE is *The Boyfriend Experience.*

GIVE HEAD—to perform oral sex; a blow job. The term give head usually refers to performing oral sex on a male, as opposed to going down which can involve either sex, or munching carpet or eating out, which are specific to doing oral sex on a female.

GLANS—head of the penis.

GLORY HOLE—a crotch-high hole in a partition between two enclosed areas that a penis can be stuck through. Located in places where gay men cruise: the baths, video booths, tea rooms, etc. The penis can be sucked or played with by whoever is on the other side of the glory hole, or the other person can look through the glory hole to watch what you are doing with yours. Can also be used for anal sex if the giver is long enough. It is not wise to ask a guy on the other side of a glory hole to go outside and have sex in your car, as sex in cars that are parked anywhere but your garage is illegal in most municipalities and why would you want to invite someone you've never said two words to into your car? (Some people would ask why you would want to have sex with someone who you've never said two words to, but that's a different discussion for a different time.) Also, don't assume the glory hole is legal–it depends on the location. Origin of the term might be from British ships, where a glory hole was a small storage space between decks where treasure or unwanted items were hidden or stored. See cruising.

GLORY-HOLE PROTOCOL—one shouldn't just stick his penis through a glory hole and hope for the best. He might try looking through it first. If the person on the other side is hard and stroking, he might then poke a finger through. If a finger from the other side returns the gesture, it's time to play ball. Or he might stroke his own penis as a sign of availability until a guy on the other side bites. All is nonverbal. There is no room for small talk in the world of cruising and glory holes. And whatever you do, next time you are at the Minneapolis-St. Paul Airport, don't tap your shoes under the stall.

GOATSE.CX—for a bit of cyber-history: an Internet shock site that housed the infamous Hello.jpg which shows the rear end, dangling penis and testicles of a skinny man who is reaching back and spreading his rectum wide. Uh, **very** wide. Put a flashlight beam up that man's gaping anus and you could see the roof of his mouth.

GO DOWN ON—to perform oral sex on.

GOING COMMANDO—no underwear.

GOLDEN ENEMA—a kinky enema where "the nozzle" is another man's urinating penis.

GOLDEN DOUCHE—kinky douche where "the nozzle" is a man's urinating penis.

GOLDEN SHOWERS—peeing on or being peed on as a sexual turn-on; water sports. Silviculturally speaking, a tree of the legume family that's native to India whose Latin name is *cassia fistula*.

GONAD—sex gland, nads, wank tanks, testicles or ovaries.

GONZO PORN—a style of adult movie making that intentionally appears to be low budget and over the top. It is filled with close-up shots and has even more sex and fewer attempts at cheesy plot lines than mainstream porn. The actors are often brash, highly enthusiastic and playing to the camera. The camera angle is frequently from the male point of view (aka POV). The term Gonzo is associated with Hunter S. Thompson's tendency to be over the top and in your face, not that Mr. Thompson ever directed porn. One of the more unfortunate twists of Gonzo porn is that it has become particularly disrespectful and increasingly violent toward the female actors. Names often associated with Gonzo porn are directors Seymore Butts and John Buttman Stagliano.

GRAMP STAMP—tramp stamp on someone who is forty or older.

GREEK—usually refers to anal intercourse or to the author of *The Guide.*

GRINDR—GPS-based social networking app to locate the nearest gay or bisexual penis.

GROMMET—a rookie surfer who often substitutes gumption for intelligence, and hyperactivity for poise; grom, surf rat. Sex is a matter of great concern and mystery for the young grom: What does one do? For how long? Is it all right if I don't get completely naked?

GROT SITE—a term used in the UK for a porn site. In the UK, grot is a similar term to filth, but not quite as strong, e.g. in the same way you could say that something is filthy, you could also say it's grotty.

GROUP SEX—sexual activity by more than two people at once, see swinging, Roman culture or terms that begin with poly.

G-SHOT—the latest sex scam where a so-called healthcare professional gives a woman a shot of collagen in what they claim is her G-spot to somehow make it bigger and miraculously increase her sexual pleasure. Do not be naive or dumb enough to fall for this inane and potentially dangerous scheme. What if it causes long-term damage inside of your vagina?

G-SPOT—area of sensation enhancement for some women on the roof of the vagina. For others, not so. See more in Chapter 7: *What's Inside a Girl.*

G-STRING—about a quarter of a bikini bottom.

GUICHE—a piercing on the male perineum.

GUSHER—term for when a man has an orgasm at the same time that his prostate is being stimulated. For some men, it feels spectacular; others find it annoying. Can also refer to female ejaculation when large amounts of fluid are expelled.

GYNECOMASTIA—when boys appear to be developing breasts; happens to about 20% of boys during puberty and usually goes away in two years. Also, a frequent side effect in men who are using performance enhancing drugs.

HANDBALLING—see fist fucking.

HAND JOB—bringing either yourself or a partner to orgasm with your hand.

HAND WARMERS—Australian term for breasts.

HAPPY ENDING—if you are in Thailand receiving a massage and your masseuse asks if want a happy ending or han-mei, smile, and say, "Yes, please!" And be sure to remember the *Guide To Getting It On* in your prayers.

HARD-ON—when the penis becomes erect; wood, trouser tent. For a rap variation, Dr. Dre might say, "Ya dick's on hard." In the UK: stiffy or pitch a tent. In Australia: crack a fat.

HAVING IT OFF—British slang for having sex, "My roommate and his girlfriend were having it off while they thought I was asleep;" aka, "Have a naughty."

HEART—that which contains all love, caring, passion, tenderness, happiness, courage, loyalty, gentleness, awe, hope, beauty, feeling, play, laughter, trust, charity and joy. An important thing to have.

HEBEPHILIA—when an adult man is sexually attracted to pubescent children and teens, roughly between the ages of 11 to 14, which is different from pedophiles who are attracted to younger children. While some men are both pedophiles and hebephiles, they usually are in one camp or the other, with the majority of incarcerated offenders being hebephiles. A hebephile who cherishes 11-year old boys might find little arousing about the same boys at age sixteen, and nothing arousing about young children.

HELLO.JPG—see goatse.cx.

HENTAI—animated Japanese pornography. Includes Japanese cartoon porn, or graphic novels in the anime, manga, or doujinshi forms. Can be described as amine with all female orifices occupied by large penises. Massive breasts that are unaffected by the forces of gravity are obligatory. In Japanese, hentai means pervert or abnormal. See anime tentacle sex.

HERMAPHRODITE—A misleading term that is hopefully going out of usage. See Intersex.

HERPES—a virus that is transmitted through sexual contact including intercourse, oral-genital contact, and rubbing naked genitals together. Seventy percent (70%) of new herpes cases are transmitted by someone who shows no obvious symptoms. Most genital herpes symptoms are mild. They are easy to miss. See Chapter 52: *Gnarly Sex Germs* for a discussion on herpes that is different than most.

HERSHEY HIGHWAY—refers to anal sex or specifically to the anus or rectum.

HETEROFLEXIBLE—a person who identifies as straight but is not beyond occasional same-sex hook-ups after having enough beers.

HICKEY—love bite resulting in a bruise. A source of embarrassment for some, a badge of honor for others. For how to cover a hickey, see Chapter 3: *Kissing*.

HIPSTERS—low-rise briefs that offer full coverage without looking like granny panties. Close cousin to boy shorts. Hipsters stop higher on the thigh while boy shorts have the start of a leg. Materials range from cotton to lace.

HIRSUTISM—male-pattern hair growth in women.

HIT A HOME RUN—to have intercourse.

HOBBYIST—slang term for a man who likes to visit prostitutes and makes it a lifestyle. Prostitution is referred to as the hobby and the Johns prefer to be known as hobbyists. One of the more famous websites for hobbyists that rates the providers in different cities is www.TheEroticReview.com.

HOLMES—wanna-be gangster talk for "dude."

HO CAKE—rap term for vagina.

HOOCH—illegal liquor. A hut or shack, often where a prostitute or sex worker lives. Also slang for vagina.

HOOCHIE MAMA—term used to describe a woman, can refer to a woman who is hot and generally unreserved with her sexual favors. 2 Live Crew demonstrated a the versatility of hoochie derivatives in their song *Hoochie Mama*, which is a whimsical evaluation of a woman's sexual charms as well as sexual excesses. Historically, the hoochie coochie was a type of belly dance that became a cultural phenomenon during the late 1800s. It was associated with sexual allure.

HOODED CLITORIS—when the hood of the clitoris is either bonded to the surface of the clitoris or does not retract easily. This is not uncommon, and it frequently causes no problems. If it makes sexual enjoyment difficult, speak to a gynecologist. Surgery should be avoided if at all possible, as the results are not always good. If surgery is recommended, get a second or third opinion.

HOOKING-UP SEX—refers to casual sex or to a one-night stand. The sex is usually without expectations (or with low expectations), where neither party has immediate plans to become emotionally involved with the other. Alcohol is generally the foreplay. The term "hooking up" itself has become more generic or ambiguous. It can refer to anything from making out or having casual sex to meeting a friend for coffee.

HOOKING UP (prison)—prison slang for when a jocker, daddy or pitcher enters a relationship with a punk. The daddy controls the relationship and provides protection for the punk who provides anal and oral sex at the whim of the dominant daddy or jocker. Even if the punk is 100% straight and masculine, the jocker may want him to act more feminine so he can better imagine the punk as a woman. The jocker sometimes shares the punk with others or can keep him to himself. Hooking up in prison can sometimes evolve into a loving, protective and caring experience, given the unusual world of prison culture, or it can be an extension of life in hell; see punk.

HORNY—having the sexual urge. The term in Australia is randy.

HOSE MONKEY—fireman, although this term can be used in a less charitable way when referring to someone who isn't a fire fighter, as in a male who plays with his penis more than most.

HO STRO—rap term which means whore stroll, which refers to a street or neighborhood where hookers work.

HOT COFFEE MOD—a fascinating sex-related reference in the history of video games. The Hot-Coffee Mod was an interactive mini-game that allowed players of *Grand Theft Auto: San Andreas* to go inside with CJ when a woman invited him to have coffee. Without the mod, players could only hear love-making sound effects. This mod created a huge scandal and public moral outrage in 2005, which is amazing considering how technologically crude the portrayal of sex in the mod was. Games that were focused on killing and blowing people up never got congressional panties in a wad, but a single crude portrayal of sex in a game and US senators began lashing out at the entire gaming industry.

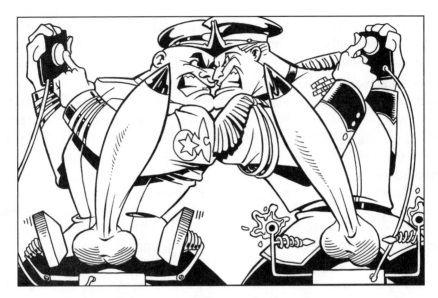

The Cold War. Hopefully gone but not forgotten.

HOT-PILLOW TRADE—slang used in the hotel business for guests who rent rooms just for sex, usually by the hour; aka hot sheet hotel. It's best when the parking lot is not visible from the street;

HOTWIFING—when a man and his wife get off by her having sex with other men. The husband either watches, listens, or has sex with her afterward while she tells him the details. Can include him orally tidying her up while the other man's trail is still fresh.

HPV—human papilloma virus; a virus that lives in the flat cells on the surface of the skin and on the moist mucosal membranes in the body. These include the urethra (peehole), vagina, cervix, penis, anus and throat. There are at least 120 types or strains of human papilloma virus. While many of the HPV strains cause no symptoms, others can cause warts, like the warts people get on their hands and feet, or on their genitals, anus and thighs. Some of the HPV strains can cause cancer. Please see Chapter 52: *Gnarly Sex Germs*.

HUMAN VITAE—the pope's master plan for semen. Every act of intercourse must be open to conception. Sex that can't result in conception is wrong, including oral sex, intercourse with birth control, and masturbation. There appears to have been an exemption for priests who have sex with boys.

HUNG—refers to a male whose sex organs displace more area than most. "Eli is hung" would be correct usage, where "Eli is hung like an elephant" would be redundant. Also, an HBO series from 2009 to 2011 about a financially-strapped teacher with a large penis who rented his sexual services to women.

HUSTLER—male prostitute, usually gay; rent boy, joy boy or escort with a client known as a John.

HYMEN—a small collar or ring of tissue located just inside the opening of the vagina where the vulva and vagina meet. Not visible unless the labia are pulled apart. The hymen is made from two different kinds of embryonic tissue, with one side being sensitive to testosterone and the other being sensitive to estrogen. As for the hymen or cherry getting popped or torn after the first intercourse, that would be a myth. As a girl approaches puberty and her body produces more estrogen, her hymen starts to change. The ring of tissue becomes more elastic. After puberty, the hymen often becomes more like an o-ring or a collar of tissue rather than a barrier, in anticipation of intercourse. Researchers often have trouble distinguishing between the hymens of teenage girls who are sexually active and hymens of teenage girls who are still virgins. The hymen can bleed during a first intercourse if it isn't fully estrogenized (elastic enough) or if the lovemaking is clumsy. While the hymen may become less prominent with age, it never goes away, and it does not become worn down due to athletic activity. See Chapter 8: *The Hymen.*

HYPOSPADIAS—a developmental anomaly where the urethra does not go all the way to the end of the penis, but exits on the lower shaft. See Chapter 57: *Hypospadias.*

IMPOTENCE—when a guy can't get it up on a regular basis, or can get it up most of the way but it isn't rigid or hard enough for intercourse; erectile dysfunction or ED.

IM SEX—sexual banter while messaging; can include cams or not.

INCEST—sex among immediate family members or blood relatives.

INCOMPETENT CERVIX—when a cervix is weakened and can't hold the fetus in the uterus to term. No doubt, named by a male.

INDOOR SPORTS—swinging or group sex.

INFIBULATION—the process of piercing the male foreskin or female labia and installing jewelry to prevent sexual intercourse.

IRIE—rasta or reggae term meaning cool, relaxing, calm, and collected; how you hopefully feel after making love.

INTERSEX—term for a variety of conditions in which a person is born with a reproductive or sexual anatomy that doesn't fit the typical definitions of female or male. Please see the Chapter 77: *Intersex.*

INTERSTITIAL CYSTITIS—pain or discomfort in the pelvis that is related to the bladder. Symptoms often include a persistent urge to pee or the need to pee frequently. Called painful bladder syndrome, as the urge to urinate can feel extreme and be accompanied by spasms and pressure. People with interstitial cystitis can have pain while urinating, pain while driving, and pain while having sex. In men, there can be painful ejaculation. The cause or causes are not known. There are different treatments, with one of the goals being to decrease the pain. People with this disorder are often very depressed as a result, in part due to the pain and discomfort, and in part because it causes incredible interference in their lives.

JACKING OFF—when males stoke their genitals in ways that cause pleasing sensations. Other terms include jerking off, choking your chicken, beating your meat, wanking, fapping, masturbating, cranking the shank, blowing your load, dishonorable discharge, flogging your log, massaging your muscle, pud whacking, rubbing one out, playing with yourself, sending out the troops, spanking your monkey, stroking it, five-on-one, and Code 20 (prison slang–Texas Dept. of Corrections).

JACK'N'JILL PARTIES—gatherings of sexually uninhibited men and women who attend in their underwear and masturbate in front of each other. A by-product of concern about AIDS.

JADE STALK—Chinese Taoist term for penis.

JANEY—lesbian slang for vagina.

JELLY ROLL—jazz term for female genitals.

J-LUBE—a powdered lube that veterinarians mix with water to help them slide their hands up the vaginas and rectums of livestock. Is said to work great for fisting, anal sex and for jerking off, except for how a 1,100 lb horse will drop dead within a few hours if very small amounts of J-Lube get into their peritoneal cavity. Beware.

JOCKSTRAP—jog bra with only one cup.

JOHN—someone who pays a sex worker or prostitute for sex, trick.

JOHNSON—old-fashioned term for penis.

JOHN THOMAS—British term for penis; old fella.

JUNKIE—a drug addict, as well as anyone who is infatuated with someone or something; not necessarily a negative term.

KEGEL EXERCISES—genital aerobics. When a person squeezes or contracts the muscles surrounding his or her genitals in a way that would stop the flow of urine, and then they totally release the muscles. Some people claim these exercises will fix everything pelvic-related. Research results do not always support these claims. The exercises can be useful in becoming more aware of genital sensations, and some people find they result in stronger orgasms as well as being helpful for certain types of incontinence and for improving vaginal and male genital tone. Kegels have never been proven to help nonorgasmic women, although there is much mythology that they do. You should not do Kegels if you are experiencing vaginal or pelvic pain without an evaluation by a pelvic pain specialist.

KILLER PUSSY—group who sang the classic *Teenage Enema Nurses in Bondage* and *Pepperoni Ice Cream, Pocket Pool* and *Bikini Wax*. Also a term men occasionally use for a vagina that feels particularly pleasing or to women they perceive as being attractive, e.g. "There's some killer pussy in that dorm."

KINK—beyond vanilla.

KINSEY AVERAGE—about two-and-a-half minutes. The amount of time sex researcher Alfred Kinsey estimated it took the average American male during the 1950s to ejaculate during intercourse.

KNICKERS—British for panties.

KNOCKED UP—pregnant.

KNOCKING BOOTS—rap term for having intercourse; with boots meaning booty, and knocking referring to the slapping sound a man's hips make when hitting a woman's thighs while having intercourse doggie style. Can also mean anal sex. See lay pipe.

KY JELLY—a brand name of a water-soluble lube that people have historically used to help increase the slip'n'slide coefficient during intercourse. There are newer *KY Personal Lubes* for sex as opposed to the traditional tube of lube that's still used for medical procedures. .

LABIA MINORA—the inner lips of the vulva which attach to the underside of the glans of the clitoris and run inside of the outer lips to the bottom of the vulva. The labia minora are made of the same tissue as the head of the penis. They contain nerve endings, swell when a woman is sexually aroused, and are sexually reactive.

LABIAPLASTY—cosmetic surgery of the inner labia. Usually unnecessary, except to increase the cashflow of the physicians who perform it.

LAD MAGS—a dying genre of men's magazines, somewhere on the Cro-Magnon spectrum between porn and Car & Driver. Best read with beer in hand.

LADYBOYS—term for transsexuals in Cambodia.

LANDING STRIP—medium to severe form of bikini waxing where the pubic hair that remains is in a small rectangle on the mons pubis.

LAPAROSCOPY—visual examination of the ovaries, Fallopian tubes and uterus with an instrument that's inserted just below the navel.

LAWRENCE V. TEXAS—2003 Supreme Court decision declaring it constitutional for two men from Texas to have oral sex in the privacy of their own home; ditto for anal penetration. If you have ever been anywhere in Texas besides Austin, you will appreciate the magnitude of this decision. Since the court's majority decision focused on the right of liberty rather than on the right of privacy, we must assume that the court was speaking directly to the liberties that Mr. Lawrence was taking with Mr. Garner's bum. How this decision is being interpreted by lower courts and applied to other decisions is interesting, eg. while it is no longer a crime for a woman to use a vibrator in Alabama, it may still be a crime to sell one.

LAY PIPE—rap term for having sex, e.g. "I lay pipe with all the lonely bitches while da husbanz hard at work." How thoughtful. Also: to freak, bag up with, bag up bitches, get busy.

LEFT HAND—what a right-handed person sometimes uses to masturbate with so it feels like another person is doing it.

LEG SPREADER—a bar with ankle cuffs on each end that keeps a woman's legs spread open; spreader bar. Also can be a type of mixed drink, although no two recipes for it are even remotely the same; often includes some or all of the following: Bacardi 151, Wild Turkey, Jack Daniels, tequila, vodka, sweet vermouth, and a cherry.

LESBIAN—woman who prefers sex with women.

LESBIAN BED DEATH—the lesbian equivalent of when straight couples are married, have kids and are both working full time.

LIBIDO—what Freud said is the fuel for our desire to make an emotional connection with others; he did not limit the term to erotic feelings or sexual desire as is often done in the present day.

LICHEN SCLEROSUS—a chronic inflammatory disorder of the skin that affects women far more often than men, usually impacting the vulva and greater crotch area but also the breasts and upper arms. The exact cause is unknown.

LIFESTYLES ORGANIZATION—a large organization for couples who like to have sex with other couples (thousands of couples belong), located near Anaheim, California—home of God, Country and the Housewives of Orange County. If you went to one of the dinners or dances sponsored by this organization, you might be surprised at how many police, military and teachers belong.

LINGAM—Sanskrit term for penis.

LIPSTICK LESBIAN—feminine-appearing woman (in a traditional or stereotypical sense) whose choice in sexual partners is other women.

LONG FLANNEL NIGHTGOWN—very effective birth-control device.

LOSING YOUR V-CARD—losing your virginity. Please see Chapter 40: *Bye Bye V-Card—Losing Your Virginity.*

LOVE—a very special way that we have of relating to one another.

LUCKY PIERRE—a gay or bisexual term, referring to three-way sex, with Lucky Pierre being the man in the middle.

LUG—Lesbian Until Graduation.

M2M—means man-to-man, and is used to signify same-sex attraction or sex between men. Replace the humans with computers, and M2M stands for machine-to-machine, which in telemetry systems means data-sharing or sex between two machines.

MAGIC WAND—Hitachi's contribution to women's sexual pleasure; has two speeds, a big round head and vibrates like a Federation freighter at warp 9.

MAINTAIN—cream or spray for the penis to numb it out and supposedly help it last longer during intercourse. Also what you try to do when parents or authority figures are around.

MAKE A MILK RUN—gay term for cruising.

MAN'S SHIRT—object of male clothing which girlfriends often lay claim to and love wearing, especially to bed. The feel and smell of it can give a woman comfort. A man who had a similar attachment to a piece of woman's clothing would be called strange or a paraphiliac, but who's complaining?

MAP OF TASMANIA (TAZZY)—dated slang in Australia for vulva.

MASOCHIST—a person who invites pain and passively controls others in the process; bottom or submissive. The term masochism was coined by Havelock Ellis and named after Leopold Von Sacher-Masoch, a nineteenth-century author who begged his wives to whip and humiliate him. An ideal day for Leopold began with a good whipping; otherwise, he struggled to get into a productive groove.

MASTURBATION—a date with your own genitals.

MATANUSKA THUNDERFUCK—an herbal with a distinctive, burning-rope smell that is sometimes used to enhance the enjoyment of sexual relations. Grown in Alaska's Matanuska Valley, an area known world wide for its legendary herb production as well as being home to the town of Wasilla.

MDMA—ecstasy.

MEAN QUEEN—a drag queen who is into BDSM.

MEATOTOMY—a form of body modification where the penis is sliced in half.

MEATSEX—real-live sex as opposed to cybersex.

MENAGE A TROIS—(sounds like may-naj-ah-twa) when three people are sharing sexual intimacy. Includes either two men and a lucky woman or two women and a lucky man; threesome. See Chapter 44: *Threesomes*.

MENSTRUAL CUP—a soft, flexible container made of soft silicone rubber or latex that is inserted into the vagina to collect menstrual fluids. It looks a bit like a small, upside down funnel, although the stem is not hollow and the body of the cup is more rounded than a funnel. There are from six to eight different kinds of menstrual cups, such as the Lunette, Diva, Moon Cup, Lady Cup, Femmecup, Miacup Keeper and Pink Cup. Most are made of medical grade silicone, with each having a slightly different length, softness, rim, stem and color. Once it's in place, a menstrual cup forms a seal against the wall of the vagina which allows it to collect the flow. Unlike a tampon which also absorbs a vagina's natural secretions in addition to period flow, a menstrual cup holds only period flow until it's removed and washed out. So it won't dry out a vagina like tampons can.

MERCY FUCK—intercourse done from a sense of duty or pity rather than burning desire.

MERKIN—wig for the pubic area; supposedly originated in past centuries to hide syphilis lesions. Was held in place by toupee glue or a small G-string.

METEROSEXUAL—men who live at the intersection of heterosexuality and narcissism; straight guys who shop, wax, accessorize, and use enough body products to fill a landfill. aka mirror men

MILE-HIGH CLUB—to have had sex in a plane while it is airborne.

MILF—acronym for a Mother I'd Like to Fuck, which is when you have lust in your heart for a PTA mom, a soccer mom, or any mom; yummy mummy. Used in the movie *American Pie* where the term refers to having lust for a friend's mom, but its origin may have been the movie *Milk Money*.

MISSIONARY POSITION—an intercourse position where the man and woman are horizontal and face to face, usually with the man on top. The term was possibly coined by savages who were saved by missionaries.

MISTRESS—the other woman. Also, BDSM-speak for dominatrix.

MONEY SHOT—a cornerstone of traditional porn, where the male unloads a wad of white splooge somewhere on his partner's body; cum shot.

MONILIA—type of vaginal yeast infection that can cause a woman to have thicker discharge than is normal, extreme itching, and painful intercourse.

MONS PUBIS—fleshy mound at the top of the vulva where pubic hair grows.

MONTGOMERY NODES—small bumps that often form on the nipples after puberty, especially prominent when you feel a chill or are sexually aroused.

MORNING-AFTER PILL (PLAN B)(ELLA)—see emergency contraception.

MOTHER FIST AND HER FIVE DAUGHTERS—British masturbation term; the equivalent American term is Rosie Palm and her five sisters. In Australia, one would say, Mrs. Palmer and her five daughters; aka "five on one."

MOUSE POTATO—person whose whole social life occurs online.

MTF—transgender term, means male to female, or changing physical appearance from male to female. The order designates which way the sex is changing, as FTM is a bio-woman changing sex to become a male.

MUFF DIVING— going down on a woman; lip service; cunnilingus.

MUMMIFICATION—a BDSM practice where the individual is wrapped tightly like a mummy with plastic wrap or other materials for immobilization.

MUNCH—social events in the swinging and kink communities which are held in neutral locations where no sex occurs. These meetings allow people who are interested but not active to meet with experienced members of their respective lifestyles. They also allow regular members to meet in an environment that does not include overt sex play.

MYSPACE WHORE—myspace? Who dat? A historical term demonstrating the fickle nature of social media. The current term is Facebook whore.

NAPPY DUGOUT—slang for female genitals. Nappy refers to the pubic hair, and the dugout is the recessed part of a baseball stadium where the players sit. In rap, this term refers to what a woman will do sexually, e.g. "Those hos give up the nappy dugout."

NASCA—the North American Swing Club Association. One r short of going to the races. See also lifestyles organization.

NATURAL FAMILY PLANNING (NFP)—has taken the place of the rhythm method for birth control. Uses various means including examining the cervical mucus to determine when it is safe to have intercourse with a lower risk of pregnancy. NFP is a fertility-awareness method that is used by people who abstain from intercourse during a woman's fertile period. This differs from other forms of fertility awareness where couples use barrier methods of birth control during their fertile period. When used correctly, can be fairly effective.

NATURIST VS. NUDIST— in the US, a naturist would be the average birdwatcher. But in the UK, naturist means nudist, and it would be a different type of pecker that's being observed.

NELLY—an effeminate male.

NIPPLE CLIPS—variation of a roach clip that is placed on each nipple as part of sex play aka, nipple clamps. Used by people who like to "have their titties tweaked" although some like them on their labia or scrotum. Can apply varying degrees of pressure, depending on the type of clip used. There are many styles, including vibrating and electrified nipple clips.

NOCTURNAL EMISSION—sexual dream of the male that includes ejaculation; aka wet dream. A lot of men don't have wet dreams, and they can be scarce for those who do. Most will occur in the mid- or late teens. There is also no reason why a sex dream has to include an ejaculation, as plenty are dry.

NONOXYNOL-9—active ingredient in most contraceptive foams and jellies that renders the male ejaculate infertile by changing its pH (acid-base balance). Can increase the chance of getting an STI, as it can irritate tender tissues. If you swallow some during oral sex, you're not going to die. *Note: spermicides are not as effective for birth control as was once thought.*

NPVA—acronym for No Practical Vertical Application, which refers to a person who is good for sex but not much else.

NSU (NONSPECIFIC URETHRITIS)—common infection of the urinary tube.

OFF PREMISE—in the swinging lifestyle, a place where swingers meet socially but don't have sex; a social.

ONANISM—means masturbation, named after the Bible's Onan who spilled his seed (pulled out and came on the side). However, Onan was doing coitus interruptus rather than masturbating.

ONE-EYED—slang terms for the penis in the UK and Australia often begin with one-eyed, such as one-eyed wonder worm, one-eyed trouser snake, one-eyed pant python, one-eyed willie, etc.

ON THE OTHER BUS—UK slang term for gay.

ON THE RAG—to be having your period. Before tampons and sanitary napkins were invented, rags were used to catch menstrual flow.

OPEN MARRIAGE—when people who are legally married agree to have sex with others outside of the marriage. A consensually nonexclusive relationship.

OPEN SWINGING—having sex with others in the same room as opposed to "closed door" which is one couple per room.

ORIENTATION PLAY—a BDSM term for when individuals are made to perform sexual acts not customary for their sexual orientation, eg. two straight women or two straight men being ordered to have sex with each other.

OTPHJ—stands for Over-The-Pants-Handjob. Done when it's private enough to fool around but public enough that pulling it out would be unwise, or just because it's what a partner wants to do. Talk about a gross feeling afterward, unless you manage to pop tissue or a napkin over the head in time.

OUTING—a process where gays publicly expose gays who aren't out of the closet. Sometimes done in a petty and nasty way to slap down a gay person who remains in the closet, sometimes done to show the straight world that some of its biggest heroes and stars are really gay, and sometimes done to expose anti-gay public figures who are gay and who deserve to be exposed. Used more benignly when referring to your own person, as in "I outed myself to my family and friends, and couldn't believe they weren't surprised."

PACKING—when a woman who is cross-dressing wears a penis-shaped object in her pants to make it look like she is well hung. More realistic when made of a soft material rather than silicone (a good packing device does not make a good dildo). Done by some male rock'n'roll singers to help maintain a certain image.

PANDERING—pimping.

PAPERVINE— drug injected into the penis that causes it to get hard; for ED.

PARAPHILIA—kinky stuff. See fetish.

PASS—if you are transgender, means being able to walk through the market or go to work without being clocked, which means people don't recognize you are a TS. You'll know you pass if they hold the rest-room door open for you without giving it a second thought.

PDE5 INHIBITOR—short for phosphodiesterase type 5 inhibitor, aka Viagra, Cialis, Levitra or Stendra. Works by inhibiting cGMP specific phosphodiesterase type 5, which is an enzyme that regulates blood flow in the penis. Was originally to be a drug for hypertension. It's most interesting use to date, other than the obvious and by porn stars, is among track and field athletes, and not just the pole vaulters. Athletes are using it to increase blood flow to the lungs and muscles. They call it Vitamin V, and the World Anti-Doping Agency (WADA) has considered adding PDE5 inhibitors to its list of illegal substances.

PEARL NECKLACE—coming on a woman's chest.

PECKER CHECKER—prison slang for a guy who looks at others guys' genitals in the shower; shower shark or peter gazer.

PEDERAST—man who has sex with boys or young men; chicken fox.

PEEING WITH A HARD-ON—a misery inflicted on the human male in the morning, though much worse when he's a teen. Peeing with a hard-on is a difficult act to achieve, since the passageway to the bladder is closed off when a male gets an erection. A phenomenon that originally caused Hindus to invent meditation, with the earliest mantra being "Lord, let this hard-on subside before my bladder bursts." Even if you can pee when your penis is erect, what do you do—a toilet plank? Stand back three feet and hope the stream ends up in the toilet?

PEGGING—when a woman who is wearing a dildo in a harness does a man in the rear. The winning term for the act selected by Dan Savage's readers; aka bend over boyfriend.

PELVIC INFLAMMATORY DISEASE (PID)—inflammation of the female reproductive organs, often the Fallopian tubes, usually caused by a bacterial infection.

PENIS STUFFER—see sounds.

PERINEUM—demilitarized zone of the human crotch. The area between the anus and genitals in men and women. The perineum is twice as long in males as in females; aka taint.

PERIOD PANTIES—underwear that women reserve for when they are having their periods. Often underwear that is no longer a woman's favorite, or can be budget wear. Some women just wear dark panties during their periods, so they don't have to worry about stains.

PERSISTENT GENITAL AROUSAL DISORDER (PGAD)—when a woman's genitals are physically aroused or engorged for hours or days, but she is distressed by the situation and doesn't feel any desire to have sex. Having sex and orgasms provides little or no relief. This would be like if a man had an unwanted erection that wouldn't go down, and the most earth-shaking orgasm and ejaculation would not bring satisfaction or a dent in the erection. PGAD is poorly understood. In some women it has been related to Tarlov cysts on the spine, in others to restless leg syndrome, and in others to discontinuing SSRI antidepressants.

PURINE'S DISEASE (PD)—a condition that results in a curving or bending deformity of the penis that can range from mild to so severe that intercourse is not possible and there can be pain with erection. PD results from plaques forming on the tunica albuginea of the penis. This results in scar tissue that prevents that side of the penis from expanding during erection. This causes curvature during erection and sometimes pain. (Think of putting a piece of tape on one side of a long balloon, then blowing it up.) Most PD patients are between 45 and 65 years of age, with the average onset occurring at 53 years. The causes of PD are not fully understood and there is no approved treatment. Treatment options and success often depend on the stage and severity of the PD. While there is spontaneous repair in some cases, these would be in the minority. Men with serious cases are often clinically depressed, "feeling like a freak." Pyronie's-related depression can take its toll on a relationship.

PHTHALATES—esters of phthalic acid that are added to plastics to make them more flexible. Used in a massive range of products, from baby bottles and detergents to shower curtains, certain glues, and jelly rubber sex toys. Phthalates are endocrine disruptors which cause genital abnormalities in the fetus. The distance between the scrotum and anus in baby boys who are born to mothers with higher levels of endocrine disruptors are often shorter than normal, which is significant because this makes the male's anogential distance more like that of a female. This shorter distance would indicate the male's genitals may not have been as fully masculinized as nature intended. Infertility is more common in men with a shorter anogenital distance. Phthalates and endocrine disruptors pose a huge environmental hazard, including concern that they are contributing to a lower birth rate of males and an increase in undescended testicles.

PIERCING—placing jewelry, a safety pin or facsimile through a person's nose, lip, nipples, navel, genitals, etc. A form of body mod. See Chapter 43: *Piercings & Tattoos.*

PINK PEARL—pink, bullet-shaped vibrator; can be inserted into the vagina.

PILLOW BITER—refers to anal sex, or when receiving anal sex is painful.

PISTON SHOT—in porn, when the camera is doing such an extreme close-up you can see the woman's inner labia slide in and out with each stroke of the penis; related terms: gyno shot and P&P (pimples & penetration).

PITCHER—partner who is doing the insertion in anal sex; top.

PIT JOB—intercourse using the armpit as a vagina.

PLAN B—see emergency contraception.

POCKET POOL—rubbing the testicles or penis when a male has his hands in his front pockets. It often looks like a guy is doing this when he's got his hands in his pockets and is rubbing coins or his fingers together.

POLYAMORY—in this form of lifestyle, people have sex in more than one committed relationships that are ongoing. It is different from swinging, where you have sex with other swingers but aren't in a committed relation-ships with them. Can include everything from open marriage to polygamy.

POLYCYSTIC OVARY SYNDROME (PCOS)—a hormone imbalance that can result in irregular periods, unwanted hair growth, acne, extra weight gain, baldness, and patches of dark skin on the back of a woman's neck and inner thighs.

Nearly 1 of every 10 to 20 women have it, and it tends to be especially common in young women. Cases can be mild or severe. Researchers still don't know what causes PCOS, but they suspect insulin resistance may play a role. The symptoms of PCOS start when a woman's pituitary makes too much leutinizing hormone (LH) and/or her pancreas makes too much insulin. This causes her ovaries to make more testosterone than her body needs, which helps explain the extra acne and body hair. Too much testosterone can also cause cysts in ovaries. These aren't so much cysts as they are immature follicles which started to develop but stopped before they could release an egg. The most common treatment for PCOS is the birth control pill, which lowers testosterone in a woman's body, as well as diet and exercise. PCOS is also associated with diabetes and obesity, and can result in making it difficult to conceive. Consultation with an endocrinologist who specializes in PCOS is highly advisable.

POLYMORPHOUS PERVERSE—kinky

PON FARR—the Vulcan mating cycle, which causes logic to crumble and the normally stoic Vulcan to become an emotional mess. See Star-Trek sex.

POONTANG—word of dubious origin that refers to a woman's genitals, or of having had sex with her.

PONY BOY—BDSM-speak for a man who pretends to be a horse while his master or mistress rides him, sometimes with crop in hand. There are specially made halter gags, pony tail butt plugs and leather pony-feet trainers for pony boys and pony girls. Pony training is BDSM-speak for schooling a submissive.

POOFTER—British term for a gay male; anal amigo, bum chum, starfish trooper, sausage jockey or on the other bus.

POP A COD—to seriously injure a testicle.

POP A SQUAT—to sit down, or when a woman has to pee outside.

POPPERS—sold over the counter as a liquid air deodorizer, poppers were originally made of amyl nitrate (which is for heart patients). Then the formula was switched to butyl nitrate because the amyl formulation could no longer be legally sold over the counter. When butyl nitrate was outlawed, popper makers switched the formula to a type of isopropyl alcohol which is fairly dangerous, but legal nonetheless. Poppers are very popular in the gay community. Popper vapors are inhaled immediately before orgasm with the resulting sensation described by some as amazing and indescribable. One problem with poppers is that the current formulation can kill you if you have hidden heart problems. It is especially dangerous to combine poppers and Viagra, as both lower blood pressure. Some people feel that popper usage might weaken the immune system, but there's no research on the matter.

POSER PORN—generic term that refers to 3-D adult erotic animation. Some of the first and best software for creating 3-D erotic animation was Poser from Curious Labs, and this is how the entire genre came to be called Poser Porn; renderotica; see adult graphics community or www.Renderotica.com.

POV PORN—a type of porn that is filmed from the male actor's perspective or point of view. The camera is either placed behind the male actor or he holds the camera while performing. Allows the viewer to imagine he's *the man*.

PRECUM—slick, clear fluid that drips out of the penis when it is excited. It is made by the Cowper's glands. Most people assume it is nature's own sex lube. Precum also helps to neutralize or deacidify the urethra to make conception more likely. Precum makes the walls of the urethra more slick so ejaculate has less resistance. It also helps the foreskin slide more easily over the head of the penis. Approximately 40% of men have live sperm in their precum, which casts doubt on the alleged high effectiveness of the withdrawal method of birth control.

PREPUCE—the foreskin.

PRIAPISM—an erection that won't quit. Having an erection for more than four hours straight without its going down can result in permanent penile paralysis. Not a common occurrence, but emergency room visits should be planned accordingly. Priapism is named after Priapus, son of Aphrodite and Dionysus, god of male reproductive power. It can occur in boys between the ages of 5 and 10 (causes include leukemia, sickle-cell disease, and physical injury), as well as in older males, where causes can range from drugs or black-widow spider bites to bicycle injuries, disease, or a kick in the crotch while martial-arts sparing. In many cases, the cause is not determined. There are two types of priapism, low-flow and high-flow. It is important to diagnose which type it is, as this can help determine proper treatment and follow-up. Low-flow priapism is often more dangerous than high-flow priapism. In some types of priapism, the glans or head of the penis is not erect, though the shaft is. Priapism usually has little to do with sexual arousal.

PRIMARY ORGASMIC DYSFUNCTION—when a woman is able to feel sexually aroused or sexually excited, but has never been able to have a satisfying orgasm, either from masturbation or with a partner. See secondary orgasmic dysfunction.

PRINCE ALBERT—male genital piercing where the ring goes in through the urethra and comes out on the underside of the penis. Named after the husband of Queen Victoria, who allegedly had it done so he could strap his well-endowed penis to his leg to keep it from showing through the tight-fitting trousers that were in fashion. But this is probably more rumor than truth. Queen Victoria never mentioned it in her state papers. See showerhead effect and Chapter 43: *Piercings and Tattoos.*

PROMISCUOUS—term used to describe a person who is having more sex than you, often said with a tone of moral superiority.

PROSTATE—walnut-shaped gland located on the floor of a man's rectum nearly a finger's length up his bum. It generates about 30% of the fluid in each ejaculation. The prostate contracts seconds before orgasm, resulting in fine sensations. It enlarges with age, sometimes making it difficult to pee. Some men (straight, gay—it doesn't matter) enjoy the feeling that results from having the prostate rubbed; others would sooner die. See Chapter 18: *The Prostate and Male Pelvic Underground* and Chapter 6: *Semen Confidential.*

PROSTATITIS—according to the excellent Prostatitis foundation, Prostatitis is an inflammation of the prostate gland, often resulting in swelling or pain. Prostatitis can result in four significant symptoms: pain, urination problems, sexual dysfunction, and general health problems, such as feeling tired and depressed. Less than 5% of cases of prostate pain are from infection. The problem often isn't in the prostate itself, but from the tissues and muscles that surround the prostate. For more information, go to www.prostatitis.org.

PSA—abbreviation for prostate specific antigen, which is made by the prostate and helps liquefy semen after it's been ejaculated. The liquefying action of PSA is what makes male ejaculate more easily drip down a partner's legs after intercourse, as well as contributing to the wet spot on the mattress. PSA tends to be elevated in men who have prostate cancer. Can be checked via a routine blood test, but is never definitive by itself. PSA is present in very small amounts in breast milk and amniotic fluid. PSA is also what Southwest Airlines used to be called. See the Chapter 18: *The Prostate and Male Pelvic Underground* and Chapter 6: *Semen Confidential.*

PUDENDA—anatomical term for women's external genitals (vulva); from the Latin word pudere, which means to be ashamed.

PULLING A TRAIN—see gang bang.

PUNANNY—rasta or reggae term for sex; "I wan' punanny!"

PUNK—a prison term for a submissive and often younger male who is on the receiving end of anal sex. The punk is seldom in the relationship because he is gay or because it is his choice; see hooking up (prison). The term punk was adopted in the late 1970s to describe a movement within rock'n'roll. Punk bands had a rougher and more immediate edge than mainstream bands.

PUSSY POSSE—the vice squad. Or, this describes a group of women who are obsessed with the same man.

PUSSY WHIPPED (PW)—where the male grovels and begs in excess of what is normally required to have sex.

PUSSY WHIPPER—a sexual partner who is controlling and rarely satisfied. She often wishes aloud that her man would be more aggressive, yet would annihilate him the second he dared.

QAF—*Queer As Folk*, the ground-breaking television series about the lives of six gay men and a lesbian couple. A wildy-successful American-Canadian production that ran from 2000 to 2005.

QUEEF—a vagina fart.

QUEENING—when a woman straddles a man and rubs or grinds her vulva into his face; face sitting.

QUEER EYE FOR THE STRAIGHT GUY—A successful TV show that ran from 2003 to 2007 where five gay men transformed a style-deficient and culturally-challenged straight man from drab to fab.

QUIM—very dated British term for a vulva,vagina or fanny.

RANDY—Australian term for horny.

RAPE—sexual bodily assault. Because the developmental issues are so profound and the capacity for empathy is so diminished, rapists rarely seek psychotherapy. There are men who commit rape and an hour later go home to have what appears to be normal sex with their wives. Most rapists don't view their acts as being criminal or brutal and are apt to justify themselves by saying the woman wanted it, needed it or deserved it. Fortunately, juvenile sexual offenders can often be helped. This is one of many reasons why they should never be placed with hardened adult offenders. See Chapter 13: *Consent.*

RAPE FANTASY—a common fantasy where a person is aroused by the thought of being raped, but would rarely want it to happen in real life. The rapist in rape fantasies is often (but not always) someone the victim would like to have sex with. A person having a rape fantasy is in control of her or his fantasy, while a real rape victim has no control at all.

RAW DOG IT—to have intercourse without protection.

REACH AROUND—when a woman with a strap-on or a man is providing anal or vaginal intercourse from behind and reaches around to simultaneously masturbate their partner.

REAM JOB—licking the anus; rimming, reaming, tossing salad. Also what a conscientious plumber does to the inner lip of pipe that's just been cut.

RED WINGS—what a man earns when he's performed oral sex on a woman who is having her period. Also the name of Detroit's team in the National Hockey League.

RENDEROTICA—see adult graphics community, poser porn or go to the website renderotica.com.

RENT BOY—male prostitute, usually a gay male, but sometimes straight.

REPARATIVE THERAPY—during the early 1900s, the testicles of straight men were transplanted into the scrotums of gay men to help the latter become heterosexual. Today, conservative Christian therapists aim for a similar outcome but without the surgery.

RETARDED EJACULATION—when a guy's sexual hang time is so long his partner has mentally completed the plot line for her new novel before he comes; delayed ejaculation. See Chapter 54: *Delayed Ejaculation*.

RETROGRADE EMISSION—when an ejaculating penis backfires. Can be caused by prostate problems, diabetes, MS, spinal-cord injury, neurological wiring issues, and because a man clamps the end of his penis shut when he's masturbating—to name a few. Men who don't have the luxury of ejaculating into toilet paper, Kleenex, or a sock when masturbating will sometimes clamp the penis shut when they come so nothing shoots out. Intentionally doing this can cause severe plumbing problems and should only be done in the most dire of circumstances unless a man wants to end up at the doctor's office doubled over with pain having to answer some really embarrassing questions.

REVERSE COWGIRL—intercourse position where the female is on top, facing the man's feet. Since the woman is on top and facing south, she can watch her partner's toes curl with delight each time she squeezes the muscles around her vagina. She might also get to see her partner's testicles rise up and hug the shaft of his penis when he begins to ejaculate or she can reach down with her hand and feel them do this (it's more pronounced in some men than in others). This is also a good position for a woman to massage her clitoris or for using a vibrator during intercourse.

RIMMING (RIM JOB)—kissing ass, literally, ass-blowing, tossing salad or E-coli pie.

RING TOSSING—when a NuvaRing comes out during sex or while a woman is having a bowel movement. No problem. It can be out for three hours with no decrease in effectiveness. Longer than that, and she should put it back in but check with her healthcare provider as soon as possible.

ROAD ERECTION—spontaneous erections can happen any time to a guy who is sitting in a vehicle that vibrates (bus, car, tractor, etc.). It is caused by a combination of the vibration, which sends extra blood into the penis, and sitting, which tends to shut the veins that carry blood out of the penis.

ROAD HEAD—blow job while driving.

ROMAN CULTURE—refers to swinging and group sex.

ROOFIES—date-rape drugs such as rohypnol, sometimes GBH, and perhaps ketamine. While very real and a reason for concern, way more women who experience date rape had been drinking or smoking with the moron than were actually drugged. So if harm reduction dollars are in short supply, they should be focused on sexual coercion and alcohol use. Ambien may be replacing roofies as the date rape drug. See ambien sex.

ROID RAGE—unpleasant mood which occurs in some people who take steroids and performance enhancing drugs.

RU-486—the name given to mifepristone when it was in its testing phase, which is a drug that causes an abortion if taken within 49 days of conception.

RUBBERS—a somewhat dated name for condoms. Before the invention of latex, condoms were made of vulcanized rubber, and so the name "rubbers." In the UK, a rubber is an eraser.

SADOMASOCHISM—where people find it erotic when there's an imbalance in power in a relationship and one person submits while the other dominates. Aside from psychiatric situations where there truly is sadism or masochism, the idea that one person is totally dominant and the other does whatever the dominant person wants is giving way to more equality and mutual agreement in the BDSM scenarios that couples enjoy.

SAFE—prison slang for vagina or place to hide drugs or contraband.

SAME-ROOM SEX—when two couples (or more) have sex in the same room.

SANGER, MARGARET—(1883-1966) famous birth-control advocate at a time when dispensing information about birth control was illegal in America.

SAPPHO—poetess on the island of Lesbos. Sappho's name has been synonymous with lesbian love. There is debate about whether she was really gay.

SAFE WORD—BDSM-speak for a prearranged word or gesture that means to stop or to ease up.

SAUSAGE FEST—an event or gathering where the men greatly out number the women;aka brodeo.

SAVAGE, DAN—highly intelligent American author and journalist, creator of the world's most popular sex advice column "Savage Love," co-creator of the "It Get's Better" project for LGBT youth, and former editor-in-chief and now editorial director of one of the nation's best and few remaining alternative weekly newspapers.

SCABIES—small mites that burrow under the skin, causing a rash approximately a month after infestation. Since it takes a month for symptoms to form, it is likely that other family or living-group members are infected and require treatment. Should be treated by a physician; be sure to follow instructions carefully. Soften your skin by taking a bath before applying pesticide treatment. Since scabies can't live away from human skin for more than 24-hours, you don't need to nuke your carpets and surroundings. However, do wash your clothes and sheets at the time of treatment. Scabies look a little like beach crabs when magnified. See chigger, which is a mite of a different kind.

SCAT—when brown is a turn-on and the phrase "Look at that sexy shit!" means just that; coprophilia.

SCHLONG—Jewish term for penis.

SCISSORING—a sexual act where two women rub their vulvas together. Can be used in a more general way like the words tribadism or tribbing are used. Or it can refer to when the women's bodies are pointing in opposite directions with one woman's head and shoulders being at the head of the bed and the other's at the foot, with their vulvas rubbing together in the middle—as if the women's open legs are two open pairs of scissors that you push together at a slight angle.

SCUMBAG—referring to a person as a used condom. After being in use for nearly 200 years (long before condoms were invented), the term eventually started referring to a condom, but not in a nice way. It was usually used as a term for someone you don't like.

SECONDARY ORGASMIC DYSFUNCTION—when a woman has been able to have orgasms in the past, but is unable to currently have orgasms although she is able to feel sexually aroused and excited. There can be numerous reasons, from illness to a change in partner.

SEMEN ALLERGY—an immune response against allergens contained in male ejaculate. Symptoms include vaginal burning, swelling and itching occurring approximately ten minutes after intercourse. While not rare, not overly common. Can develop right away, or suddenly after a few years with the same partner. To differentiate from chronic vaginitis, see if using a condom stops the problem. (You might try a polyurethane condom, as a latex allergy could mimic semen allergy symptoms.) Aside from a complete gynecologic exam, diagnosis should include intradermal testing, where a tiny bit of the semen is injected under the skin. Treatment under the supervision of an allergist or immunologist can include a graded challenge where dilute solutions of semen are placed in the vagina every 20 minutes until the patient can tolerate undiluted semen. The couple has to have intercourse at least once every 48 hours to maintain the desensitization. As is the case with food allergies, the semen allergy might go away as fast as it came.

SERIAL MONOGAMY—sounds like a dangerous criminal activity when it really means getting married, then divorced, then married again.

SEX BEFORE THE GAME—refers to masturbating or having sex fewer than twenty-four hours before taking part in a sporting event. It is unlikely there is any correlation between sex before the game and decreased athletic performance as long as the athlete has gotten a full night's sleep. As Casey Stengel said: "It isn't sex that wrecks these guys, it's staying up all night looking for it."

SEX DREAMS—nature's way of making sleep more interesting.

SEXILED—to be kicked out of your room while your roommate is having sex.

SEX-ON-THE-BEACH—a mixed drink with as many different formulations as there are intercourse positions.

SEXTASY—refers to when people combine ecstasy and Viagra; aka trail mix. The ecstasy is not good on erections, so Viagra is used to help. No one knows the long-term effects of this combination or what's really in the ecstasy or Viagra that you get on the street.

SEXTING—using mobile devices for foreplay or taking pictures of yourself and forwarding them to a lover or potential partner.

SEXUALITY—an altered state of mind that's often quite enjoyable. Includes various degrees of erotic or sensual feelings and sensations.

SEX WORKER—can be a prostitute, but now includes anyone who helps other people get off: phone-sex and cam-sex providers, erotic dancers, sex surrogates, etc.

SEXUAL ORIENTATION—refers to your gender in relation to the gender you are turned on by, often with the term gay, straight or bisexual being attached. Men tend to be more category specific in their sexual orientation, meaning they are mostly interested in either women or men but not both. Many women, on the other hand, can find both men and women to be sexually interesting—but this doesn't mean the woman is bisexual or gay. See Chapter 74: *Orientation in Flux*.

SHAGADELIC—someone who looks good enough to shag; a person you'd like to have sex with; vintage Austin Powers: "She shags like a minx, baby!"

SHAKE 'N' BAKE—to make love; do the wild thing.

SHE-HE, SHE-MALE, or HE-SHE—see transgendered.

SHOCK DOC—a popular brand of a cup, which is a device that men wear to protect their genitals from dick-high line drives, bad hops, elbows, lacrosse implements, kicks, etc. Which cup you wear depends on the sport and your position in that sport, for instance a goalie or catcher is looking for protection over mobility, where a shortstop or attackman is going to value mobility, as will someone in the martial arts. Along with new designs in cups, improvements have also come in the design of compression shorts, which hold the cup in place and are like a cross between bicycle short and an athletic supporter. Unfortunately, the sporting goods stores and other chain stores don't always carry the better cups, so you might visit shockdoctor.com and sawsports.com.

SHORT-ARM INSPECTION—military term for examining an enlisted man's penis. Supposedly for the detection of sexually transmitted infections.

SHORT HAIRS—pubic hair.

SHOT MY WAD—ejaculated, came, popped, splooged or blew a load.

SHOWERHEAD EFFECT—when a piercing like a Prince Albert or an apadravya goes through a man's urethra, it tends to make urine spray like a showerhead instead of a stream. This can make peeing while standing quite a mess. Often the only solution is to pee while sitting down. A man with this type of piercing will tend to ooze rather than shoot when he ejaculates.

SISTERS OF PERPETUAL INDULGENCE—a spirited, benevolent organization of drag queens who delight in taking the convent out of conventional. Their mission statement: *The Sisters devote ourselves to community service, ministry and outreach to those on the edges, and to promoting human rights, respect for diversity and spiritual enlightenment.* Visit the sisters at thesisters.org.

SIXTY-NINE (69)—when two people perform oral sex on each other at the same time. When French people do 69 they call it soixante-neuf.

SIZE QUEEN—a woman who likes guys who are seriously well-hung; best for men who are not well hung to avoid. Also a guy who likes guys who are well-hung.

SKANK—a person who is short on physical and social graces; hard or harsh. Also refers to the person's sexual choices in a less-than-kind way.

SKIN FLICK—porn film.

SKYPE SEX—when geography gets in the way of having sex in person, couples can use services like Skype (or Facetime, Snapchat, Vine or whatever) to not only say sexy things to each other, but to see each other doing sexy things.

According to an article about Skype sex in the Stony Brook Statesman, make sure your door is locked and the blinds are drawn to prevent unexpected visitors, remove the clutter around your desk which the person on the other end will have to see, check your equipment (do they mean the webcam or whether you have shaved or trimmed?), be sure the lighting and sound are good, and enjoy!

SLASH—type of fan fiction where famous male characters end up having sex with each other, eg. Spock & Kirk, Starsky & Hutch, Harry & Snape. Fem Slash is a sub genre focusing on female characters, as in Janeway & Seven-of-Nine.

SLICK—refers to male or female genitals that have been shaven. Some people enjoy the look or feel of being slick as a sexual turn-on. Women often shave to accommodate thongs, bikini bottoms, or because it's the current fashion; men might shave to make their units look bigger, neater or more porn like, or if a partner prefers it that way for oral sex.

SLOPPY SECONDS—having intercourse when you are not first in line.

SLOW DANCING—an event that sometimes causes males to get erections, especially during the teenage years. When girls congregate in the women's restroom during dances, they might say, "Justin got a raging boner while we were slow dancing."

SLUT HUT—a dorm-room version of a bed canopy. Created when you have bunk beds and drape a sheet down from the top bunk so it encases the bottom bunk. Keeps your roommate from seeing you having sex if he or she walks in.

SLUT SHAMING—criticizing a woman for enjoying sex or for being sexual.

SMEGMA—cheesy stuff that forms beneath the foreskin and under the hood of the clitoris; knob cheese. Calling someone smeg is an insult.

SNAP-ON TOOL—slang term for a dildo that some women wear in a harness and use as if it were an erect penis.

SNAP QUEEN—a gay male where the snap refers to the snap of fingers that's done with an exaggerated spin-and-prance attitude. Can also refer to a woman who ranks high on entitlement and is demanding of others.

SNOWBALLING—when a man swallows his own ejaculate after it's been somewhere else; for instance, his partner gives him oral sex, he ejaculates in his partner's mouth, and then he kisses his partner and his partner transfers the ejaculate back into his mouth.

SNOW QUEEN—slang term for a gay black man who only dates white men.

SOAPY MASSAGE—a Thai sex experience where the woman undresses and bathes you, massaging your body with her wet soapy body.

SOAPY TIT WANK—masturbating between a woman's well-lubricated breasts.

SOCIAL SWING CLUB—a private membership organization for couples who swing.

SODOMY—any kind of sex that is declared illegal by local statute. In some areas, it can be oral sex or regular intercourse, in others, specifically anal sex.

SOFT SWINGERS—a couple who is in a long term relationship and who enjoys having most kinds of sex with others except for intercourse, which they only do with each other.

SOUNDS—medical instruments used to help dilate the urethra. Used in urethra play or penis stuffing. There are different types of sounds with different shapes and thicknesses, including the Pratt, Van Buren, Hegar, Hank and Dittel.

SOUTHERN COMFORT—sex with someone from the south.

SPANISH FLY—alleged aphrodisiac made from powdered blister beetles; causes severe irritation of the bladder and urethra. Can be very toxic. Women have died from it. The effect is not dissimilar to drinking Draino. Giving her roses and a foot rub will get you much further and won't endanger anyone's health.

SPASM CHASM—a vagina; gristle gripper.

SPECTATORING—sex therapist-speak: describes when a person is worried or obsessing about his or her sexual performance instead of being able to enjoy having sex. Can result in performance anxiety.

SPIT ROASTING—in a threesome, when the person in the middle is on all fours and is being penetrated from behind while sucking on the penis of the person in front. When viewed from the side, it gives the appearance of a chicken on a two-penis rotisserie.

SPLASH CONCEPTION—getting pregnant from anal sex, after semen oozes out of the woman's anus and drips into her vagina. People conceived this way do not necessarily become anal retentive.

SPLIT BEAVER—slang for when a woman spreads her labia wide open.

SPLOSHING—smearing yourself or a partner with wet and gooey things such as raw eggs, paint, or mud as part of a fetish or sexual turn-on. Became a bit popular in the late 1980s in the UK, growing out of the fetish wank mag *Splosh!* A related term is: WAM or wet and messy. Does not include excrement, which is a fetish of a different smell and color.

SPREADER BAR—see leg spreader.

SRPE—SLEEP-RELATED PAINFUL ERECTIONS—results in waking with painful erections. This understudied problem may occur more often than is reported, and can result in serious pain and loss of sleep. Daytime erections are not painful for these men, only those that occur during sleep. Sleep erections and waking erections are governed by different parts of the brain, and it appears that SRPEs may be the result of spasms or ischemia. Oral baclofen currently appears to be the experimental treatment of choice, but that may change when more is learned about SRPEs.

SSRIs—a class of overly prescribed antidepressants which include Prozac, Zoloft, Paxil, Luvox, Celexa, Lexapro, Effexor, Serzone and Remeron. According to the *Journal of Sexual Medicine*, any person who has been given a prescription for an SSRIs should be given a warning such as the following: *There is a high probability of sexual side effects while on SSRI medications. There are indications that in an unknown number of cases, the side effects may not resolve with cessation of the medication and could be potentially irreversible.* Not to be taken lightly.

STAR-TREK SEX—*Denobulans:* Denobulans practiced polygamy. Each Denobulan had three partners, and each of these had two other partners. Denobulans were liberal about sex, with sex occurring during Denobulan mating cycles. *Deltans:* Deltans were so highly sexed they were forbidden from having sex while in Starfleet. Deltan sex was such an intense activity that a member of another species who had sex with a Deltan could go insane as a result. *Vulcans:* Vulcans were ruled by strict logic except every seven years during pon farr, which was the Vulcan mating cycle when a Vulcan lost all emotional control. *Klingons:* There is not a single thing about Klingon sex that could ever be described as gentle.

STONE BUTCH—A lesbian with stereotypical male gender role behavior; as described in Leslie Fineberg's book *Stone Butch Blues*.

STONEWALL—refers to the 1969 Stonewall Riots, when New York City police raided a gay bar in Greenwich Village and large numbers of gay people resisted arrest. A landmark event in the gay-rights movement. In gay-rights, epochs of time are often divided into pre-Stonewall and after Stonewall.

STRAP-ON—abbreviation for strap-on dildo, usually worn and used by women on women or on men, but can also be worn by men for double penetration or if their own penis can't get hard.

STUNT BABE—a woman who poses as a gay soldier's girlfriend at military events and whose picture he keeps on his desk.

SURFER—person who has sex with waves.

SWEET DEATH—refers to orgasm or the release that comes with orgasm, from the French term *la petite mort*. The term has become so dated it isn't used very often.

SWINGER—partner swapper, enjoys having sex with lots of people.

SWING LOW—rap term for oral sex.

SWINGERS—couples in committed relationships who enjoy having sex with a variety of sexual partners.

SWITCHES—people into BDSM who enjoy alternating between the top and the bottom roles.

TAINT—perineum, the area between the genitals and anus, slang for "isn't" or "it ain't" as in "*'taint his balls or ass*," or "*'taint her vagina or ass;*" see perineum.

TAR BEACH—rooftop of a tall building in large urban setting where people do things like sunbathe, grow plants, make out, or shoot up drugs.

TEA-BAGGING—when a man lowers his testicles into his partner's mouth. Not to be confused with "tea party."

TEA ROOM—public rest-room where gay men go to have sex; in Britain they are called cottages. In Australia they are known as beats.

TEDDY—women's lingerie that is a combination of tank top and panties, sometimes snaps at the crotch, usually made of silk, lace, acetate, or leather.

TENTACLE SEX—the full name is Tentacle-Hentai Sex, where monsters and octopuses wrap their penis-like tentacles around the bodies of shocked and surprised female Hentai characters, who then experience the kind of intense sexual sensations that any woman might if an octopus slid its slimy tentacle inside of her vagina. See Hentai.

TEXAS TWO-STRAP—highly regarded brand of dildo harness.

TEXTILE—term that nude sunbathers sometimes used for a person who wears a bathing suit; see cottontail.

THE EXCLUSIVITY TALK—when you've spent the past month texting your new lover more than everyone else combined, it's time to consider taking your relationship to the next level, going from casual to committed. The conversation or vehicle by which that happens is known as the exclusivity talk. No matter how many loving and wonderful things a partner might say to you, don't assume exclusivity until you've had the talk.

THE GAY SEAT—the empty seat that homophobic teenage boys and college bros leave between them when they are in a theater, given the social and emotional dangers of sharing an arm rest.

THIGHBROW—pubic hair that's sticking out from the sides of a bikini or thong.

THONG—a narrow piece of material that passes between the legs and up through the butt cheeks where it attaches to a waistband. Thongs have traditionally been the underwear of strippers. Different types of thong include the G-string or T-back, which are the underwear equivalent of dental floss, the Tanga, which has more material in the seat, and the Rio which has straps on the sides. Thongs are even popular for some guys to wear. Our gyno-consultant warns about thongs causing vulvar irritation. Thongs are also a zipline for bacteria from the anus to easily hop into the vagina.

THREESOME—sex with two women and a man or two men and a woman. See menage a trois. Hopefully, having a menage a trois is not as complicated as spelling it. See Chapter 44: *Threesomes*.

THRUSH—vaginal infection caused by candida or monilia fungus. Men can also get it, but not in the vagina.

TICKET—for a guy in the swinger's lifestyle to show up without a woman is like arriving at a church potluck without a casserole. Single men usually aren't allowed. To get around this dilemma, single males will occasionally invite females who aren't necessarily into swinging—just to get through the door. Such a woman is known as a ticket. This is seriously frowned upon.

TIJUANA BIBLES—pornographic pulp parodies that were popular in America from the 1920s until after World War II. These 8-page booklets were printed on cheap paper and often found themselves in the knapsacks of soldiers and schoolboys. The crudely illustrated booklets (approximately 4" by 6") often poked fun at actors, politicians, and public figures, although their main focus was another kind of poking. They were irreverent, usually humorous, and always dirty—featuring sex-starved characters from Popeye and Donald Duck to baseball heroes, with their pants down and penises proud. They were eventually relegated to paper graves by the then-new glossy magazines such as *Playboy*. The pin-up powerhouse *Esquire* probably served a death notice or two as well.

TIPPED UTERUS—a woman's uterus is usually parallel to her spine; a uterus that is tipped points in various angles toward the back. Can make rear entry or doggie-style intercourse uncomfortable. See Chapter 7: *What's Inside a Girl*.

TIT-FUCKING—when a well-lubricated penis is thrust back and forth between a woman's breasts; aka Russian or soapy tit wank.

TOOTHING—a media hoax that claimed people were using their Bluetooth devices for proposing sex or hooking up with strangers in their immediate vicinity, such as at a cafe or on the train. It sounded so convincing that it got wide airplay and became part of modern urban legend.

TOP AND BOTTOM—a top is someone who prefers doing, and a bottom is someone who prefers having it done to them. In anal sex, the bottom is the one who is catching or receiving.

TOSS or TOSSING SALAD—licking a lover's anus, aka rimming. Can also be a UK term for masturbating, to toss off or toss oneself off.

TOXIC SHOCK SYNDROME—very rare and sometimes lethal infection. Was associated with use of the ultra absorbent Rely tampon.

TRAINED WOOD—necessary requirement of a male porn star, meaning he can pretty much get an erection on cue. Failure to do so means he has untrained wood, which puts he and his bulge in the same unemployment line as many of the legit actors in town. Viagra is often used as an aid.

TRAINING BRA—training wheels for the growing chest.

TRAMP STAMP—a lower back tattoo that rides on the pants line. It peeks out when the owner—usually a woman—wears low-rise jeans and/or a cropped T-shirt, or she bends over and her pants go low or her shirt goes high. Tramp stamps are often v-shaped and point down toward the sexual anatomy below. Designs range from flowers, butterflies, dolphins and tribal art to unusual symbols and geometric art.

TRANNY—slang for someone who is transsexual, transgendered, or a cross-dresser. Also, that which helps give automobiles their go.

TRANSGENDERED—when the sex you were born with is different from the sex you want to be. People who are transgendered challenge notions of what it is to be male and female.

TRANSSEXUAL—person who uses surgery, makeup, electrolysis, and hormones to correct mother nature's assignment of sex or gender.

TRANSVESTITE—see crossdresser.

TRAUMA QUEEN—person who is highly skilled at finding or creating chaotic scenes, then feeds on it and fans it, complaining the whole time about it.

TRIBADISM—two women rubbing their vulvas together, resulting in sexual pleasure; aka tribbing. The way they shake hands on the island of Lesbos.

TRICK—customer of an escort or prostitute; aka John. Can also be a sexual act as done by a sex worker, as in turning a trick.

TRIPLE PENETRATION—porn-film term for where there's a wealth of penii and only one taker; triple play.

TROLL—when someone gets on the Internet and posts messages that are designed to enrage people, such as posting cat-meat recipes on a pet-lover